Tumors of the Lung

Volume 24 in the Series
MAJOR PROBLEMS IN PATHOLOGY

OTHER MONOGRAPHS IN THE SERIES MAJOR PROBLEMS IN PATHOLOGY

Published

Whitehead: *Mucosal Biopsy of the Gastrointestinal Tract, 3rd ed.*
Azzopardi: *Problems in Breast Pathology*
Frable: *Thin-Needle Aspiration Biopsy*
Wigglesworth: *Perinatal Pathology*
Jaffe: *Surgical Pathology of Lymph Nodes and Related Organs*
Wittels: *Surgical Pathology of Bone Marrow*
Finegold: *Pathology of Neoplasia in Children and Adolescents*
Taylor: *Immunomicroscopy*
Fu & Regan: *Pathology of the Uterine Cervix, Vagina and Vulva*
Wolf & Neiman: *Disorders of the Spleen*
LiVolsi: *Pathology of the Thyroid*
Striker, Olsen & Striker: *The Renal Biopsy, 2nd ed.*
Whitehead: *Mucosal Biopsy of the Gastrointestinal Tract, 4th ed.*
Virmani, Atkinson, & Fenoglio: *Cardiovascular Pathology*

Forthcoming

Hendrickson & Kempson: *Surgical Pathology of the Uterine Corpus, 2nd ed.*
Nash & Said: *Pathology of Acquired Immune Deficiency*
Frable: *Fine Needle Aspiration Biopsy, 2nd ed.*
Ordóñez & Mackay: *Soft Tissue Tumors*
Crissman & Zarbo: *Surgical Pathology of the Upper Aerodigestive Tract Mucosa*
Variokojis & Vardiman: *Pathology of Myeloproliferative Disorders*
Henson & Albores-Saavedra: *Pathology of Incipient Neoplasia, 2nd ed.*
Azzopardi: *Pathology of the Breast, 2nd ed.*
Fox, Young & Buckley: *Pathology of the Ovary and Fallopian Tube*
Ellis, Auclair & Gnepp: *Pathology of the Salivary Glands*
Fox: *Pathology of the Placenta, 2nd ed.*
Jaffe: *Surgical Pathology of the Lymph Nodes, 2nd ed.*
Lack: *Surgical Pathology of the Adrenal Glands*
Lloyd: *Surgical Pathology of the Pituitary Gland*
Kornstein: *Pathology of the Anterior Mediastinum*

Contents

BRUCE MACKAY, M.D., Ph.D.
Professor of Pathology
The University of Texas
MD Anderson Cancer Center
Houston, Texas

JOHN M. LUKEMAN, M.D.
Professor of Pathology
The University of Texas
MD Anderson Cancer Center
Houston, Texas

NELSON G. ORDÓÑEZ, M.D.
Professor of Pathology
The University of Texas
MD Anderson Cancer Center
Houston, Texas

Tumors of the Lung

Volume 24 in the Series
MAJOR PROBLEMS IN PATHOLOGY

1991
W.B. SAUNDERS COMPANY
Harcourt Brace Jovanovich, Inc.
PHILADELPHIA LONDON TORONTO MONTREAL SYDNEY TOKYO

W. B. SAUNDERS COMPANY
Harcourt Brace Jovanovich, Inc.

The Curtis Center
Independence Square West
Philadelphia, PA 19106

Library of Congress Cataloging-in-Publication Data

Mackay, Bruce
Tumors of the lung / Bruce Mackay, John M. Lukeman, Nelson G. Ordóñez.
p. cm.

ISBN 0–7216–5807–5

1. Lungs—Cancer—Histopathology. I. Lukeman, John M. II. Ordóñez, Nelson G. III. Title.
[DNLM: 1. Lung Neoplasms—pathology. WF 658 M153t]

RC280.L8M24 1990

616.99'224—dc20

DNLM/DLC 90-8526

Editor: Jennifer Mitchell
Designer: Ellen Bodner
Production Manager: Ken Neimeister
Manuscript Editor: Jeanne M. Carper
Illustration Coordinator: Cecelia Kunkle
Indexer: Victoria Boyle

TUMORS OF THE LUNG ISBN 0–7216–5807–5

Printed in the United States of America

Last digit is the print number: 9 8 7 6 5 4 3 2 1

Editor's Foreword

For years, pathologists have attempted to find in the morphology of lung cancers features that can be used to sort them into groups with predictable behavior patterns. In spite of our having made considerable progress in understanding the histogenesis and the direction of cellular differentiation of the various types of lung cancer, no subsets have emerged as having uniquely favorable natural histories, and only small cell cancers of the lung have proved to be susceptible to adjuvant cytotoxic chemotherapy.

As we attempt to further delineate the contribution of cytogenetic abnormalities and the effect of environmental carcinogens on the genesis of lung cancers, and as we continue our search for effective chemotherapeutic agents, the need for accuracy and precision in classification assumes increasing importance. *Tumors of the Lung* provides an answer to this need. It covers in detail the characteristic light microscopic features of all known types and variants of primary lung cancers along with detailed discussion of electron microscopic and immunocytochemical features helpful in their diagnosis and classification.

Drs. Mackay and Lukeman are well known for their work in pathology and cytology of neoplastic diseases of the lung, and both have made many important original contributions to this field. Their great wealth of knowledge and diagnostic expertise is reflected in this well written, comprehensive, and scholarly update on the pathology of lung cancer. The practical experience of Dr. Ordonez in the field of immunocytochemistry is reflected in the sections on this aspect of the study and diagnosis of lung tumors. All physicians who deal with cancer of the lung, particularly surgical pathologists, thoracic surgeons, oncologists, and radiation therapists, will find *Tumors of the Lung* invaluable.

JAMES L. BENNINGTON, MD
Consulting Editor

Preface

If the current trend in the incidence of lung cancer in the United States persists, it is estimated that approximately 200,000 new cases will be diagnosed annually by the year 2000. The frequency of mesothelioma may be diminishing by then, but it is likely to continue at its present rate through the 1990s. Responsiveness to warnings concerning the effects of tobacco and asbestos is producing some improvements in the situation in the United States, but in less developed countries the number of smokers is not decreasing. In North America, the earlier male predominance in lung cancer is being eroded as the incidence curve in females rises.

These trends are continuing in spite of intensive clinical and laboratory studies. Our understanding of the different types of lung carcinoma has improved from two decades ago, methods for early detection are better, and the techniques available to the pathologist are considerably more sophisticated, but the outlook for a patient with lung cancer is still dismal. Significant improvements in the management of small cell carcinoma were achieved with combination chemotherapy, but there has been little further advance in the past decade. Early diagnosis and therapy are the best hope for the patient, and the pathologist plays an important role. To the clinician, the significant subdivision of lung carcinoma is into small cell and non–small cell types; subtyping of the non–small cell tumors is less important in management. However, the pathologist must strive for as much precision as is possible in the diagnosis of lung carcinomas, regardless of their type, since we cannot predict how pertinent this information will be in the future.

Given our inability to cure most patients with lung carcinoma today, it is clearly necessary to intensify therapeutic efforts in the hope of achieving at least gradual improvements in survival. The pathologist plays a pivotal role in this regard, but in order to provide the most information, good biopsy material is essential. The specimens that the pathologist obtains from patients with lung cancer are often less than optimal, and this can lead to an incorrect interpretation or to inability to provide a diagnosis. There is a greater degree of inaccuracy in the diagnosis of primary lung tumors than many pathologists are willing to admit.

In this book, our main objective has been to review the basic histopathology of primary lung tumors. Since the interpretation of lung tumors by conventional light microscopy can be greatly enhanced when the light microscopic findings are correlated with those from immunocytochemistry and electron microscopy, we place emphasis on relating the information these techniques can provide with the basic features seen in histologic and cytologic preparations.

The first World Health Organization classification of lung tumors brought organization where earlier there had been essentially chaos, and the revised version improved on the original in a number of areas. Further modifications were introduced by study groups including the Veterans Administration Oncology Group, the Working Party for the Therapy of Lung Cancer, and the current Lung Cancer Study Group. It can be anticipated that more changes will be instituted as data from pathologic and biologic studies accrue and are shown to be clinically relevant.

Acknowledgments

We wish to extend our sincere appreciation to Karen Gray, Carol Cherry, Lydia Shanks, Elsa Ramos, Mannie Steglich, Hazel Dalton, Sharon Thompson, Fatima Natar, and Thomas E. Brooks for their valuable technical assistance, and to Madonna Yancey for her secretarial expertise. We are grateful to Dr. Clifton F. Mountain and the editors of *Chest* for their permission to reproduce his paper on the staging of lung cancer. The preparation of this book was encouraged from the outset by Dr. James L. Bennington, at that time editor of the *Major Problems in Pathology* series, and we are deeply indebted to him and to the editorial staff of W.B. Saunders for their support and patience.

Chapter

1

STRUCTURE AND FUNCTION OF THE RESPIRATORY TISSUES

Some familiarity with the structure and function of the cells that form the respiratory passages is helpful when it comes to interpreting the histopathology of the various tumors that arise in the lung. Most pathologists see the tumor cells in routine cytologic and histologic preparations, but information about their structure and function has been greatly expanded in recent years by ultrastructural studies and immunocytochemistry. Throughout this book, therefore, descriptions and illustrations of tumors of the lung as shown by light microscopy and cytology are correlated with the contributions of special staining procedures and electron microscopy.

DEVELOPMENT OF THE RESPIRATORY TISSUES

The development of the respiratory system[8, 36] is briefly summarized in the following section.

Intrauterine Development

The earliest indication of the impending formation of the larynx and trachea occurs during the fourth week of intrauterine life when a laryngotracheal groove appears in the ventral wall of the primitive pharynx. As the groove deepens, its lips move together to create a tube with the lumen separated from the esophagus but opening into the pharynx at its upper end. Even at this early stage, the lung buds are visible as two outgrowths from the caudal end of the lengthening tube. They expand laterally, and lobules appear, three on the right and two on the left.

Formation of new branches continues through the 16th week of gestation under the inducing influence of the surrounding mesenchyme. The thick epithelium during this period gives the developing lung a glandular appearance. Through the 24th week, branches to the level of the terminal bronchioles are formed and the surrounding mesenchyme differentiates to form the tissues of the bronchial and bronchiolar walls and the accompanying blood vessels. Primitive respiratory bronchioles then begin to form, and alveolar sacs grow out from them. Initially, the alveoli are pouches in the walls of the alveolar sacs and respiratory bronchioles, but they subsequently proliferate by budding.

Postnatal Development

The lungs continue to develop after birth.[45, 82] New bronchi and alveoli are formed, and the alveoli increase in size.[11] The lung weighs only about 60 g at birth, but its volume enlarges some 28 times by the age of 8 years. It has been estimated that an adult lung contains at least 300 million alveoli.

ANATOMY OF THE RESPIRATORY PASSAGES

Trachea

The adult trachea is approximately 10 cm long, and its bifurcation lies slightly to the right of the midline. Because it is constructed from incomplete rings of elastic cartilage and smooth muscle, the trachea can lengthen and shorten quite rapidly. At rest the carina is opposite the sternal angle, but during deep inspiration it descends as far as the level of the sixth thoracic vertebra. The isthmus of the thyroid gland crosses the second, third, and fourth tracheal rings. The esophagus separates the trachea from the vertebral column, and the recurrent laryngeal nerves ascend in the grooves between the sides of the trachea and esophagus. The lower trachea is intimately related to the great vessels, and the remnant of the thymus lies in front of it. The lumen is about 12 mm in the anteroposterior direction and under 2 cm in transverse diameter. In cross section, the trachea is flattened posteriorly where its wall is formed by bundles of transversely oriented smooth muscle fibers.

Bronchi

The right main bronchus is more vertical, wider, and about half the length of the left main bronchus. It gives off the upper lobe bronchus before entering the hilum, where it divides into branches to the middle and lower lobes. The left main bronchus is roughly 5 cm in length, and it divides into its two lobar branches within the hilum.

The primary branches of the lobar bronchi are termed *tertiary bronchi* or *segmental bronchi* because each is associated with a bronchopulmonary segment. The layer of connective tissue that envelops a bronchopulmonary segment will sometimes limit the spread of nonneoplastic processes such as infections, but tumors do not respect such flimsy boundaries.

Plates of cartilage in the wall of the bronchus are more complete than those of the trachea, but their arrangement is not as regular, and distally they gradually become thinner, smaller, and more widely spaced, disappearing completely as the bronchi become bronchioles.

Bronchioles

The first bronchioles are about 1 mm in diameter. With continued branching, they become progressively smaller until they enter the lobules, where each gives rise to about six terminal bronchioles. From a terminal bronchiole, up to three respiratory bronchioles are formed, and at this point the columnar epithelial lining of the respiratory passages terminates and the respiratory tissue itself begins. From the respiratory bronchioles, thin ducts lead into the alveolar sacs.

Alveoli

Alveoli are rather like square rooms with one wall missing. They open directly into respiratory bronchioles and alveolar ducts and sacs, and neighboring alveoli communicate through small pores.[67] An alveolus is roughly 200 μm across.

CELLS OF THE RESPIRATORY EPITHELIUM

The epithelial lining is similar throughout the trachea and bronchi, but changes in the distribution of the various cell types occur toward the periphery. The respiratory epithelium is pseudostratified, and most of the cells bear cilia (Fig. 1–1). The physical properties of respiratory tract secretions play an important role in the nonspecific defense mechanisms of the lung.[53] As many as ten different cell types have been described in animal lungs, but they have not all been identified in the human lung.[9, 10, 38, 39, 69]

It is rare to see mitoses in the differentiated cells of the trachea and bronchi. Surface cells that die or are lost by desquamation are replaced by proliferation of the basal cells. It is not certain whether the endocrine cells are replaced in this manner, although there is evidence that such a mechanism occurs in the gut.[14, 15, 78]

Ciliated Cells

Most of the epithelial cells in the trachea and bronchi are ciliated (Fig. 1–2). Each cell is columnar, but it tapers toward its base (Fig. 1–3), which is a necessary modification to

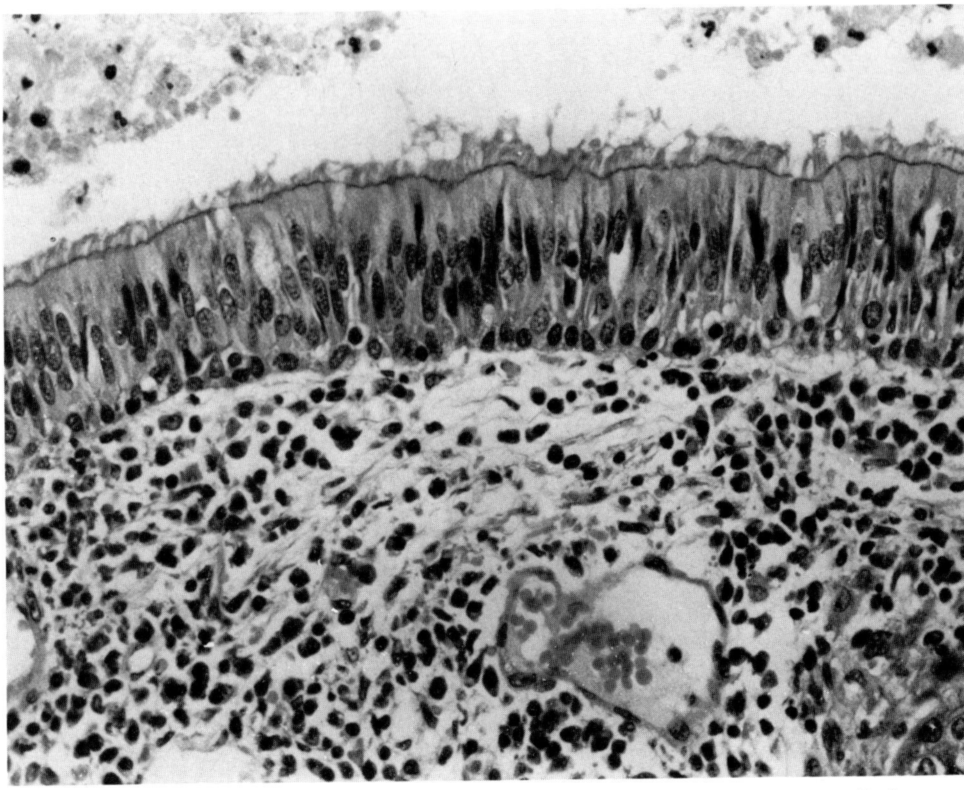

Figure 1–1. Normal respiratory epithelium. Most of the cells are ciliated. The reserve cells form an almost continuous row.

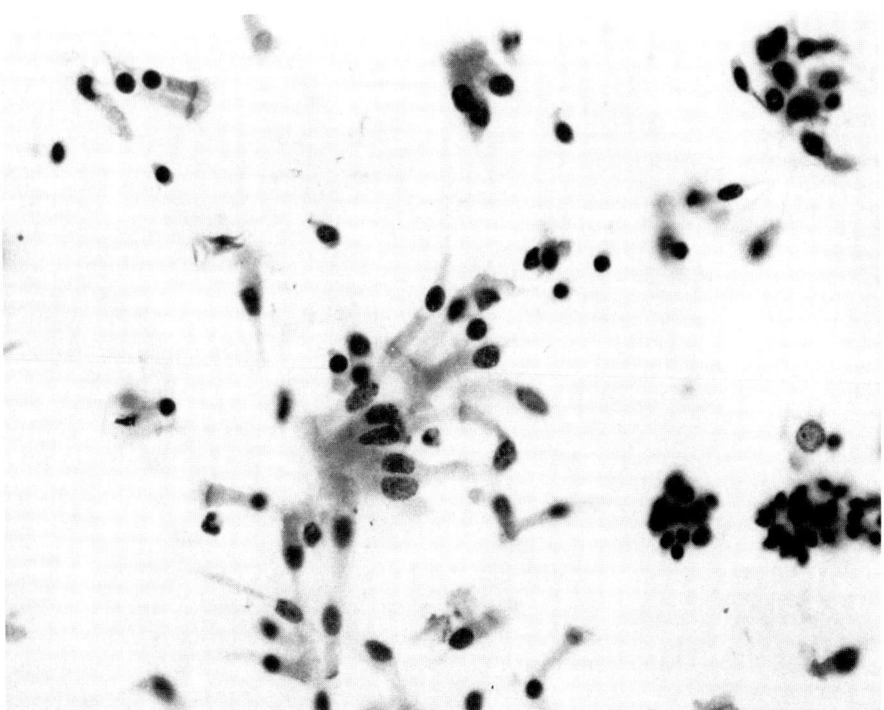

Figure 1–2. Cells from a bronchial brushing. Ciliated columnar cells and small groups of basal cells are present.

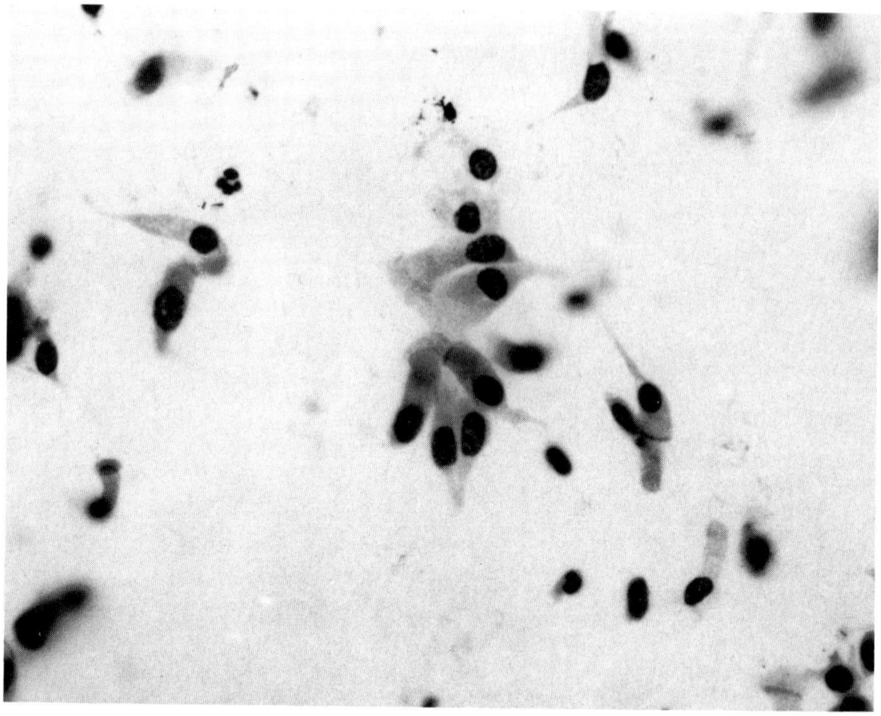

Figure 1–3. Ciliated epithelial cells from a bronchial brushing: the cytoplasm tapers below the level of the nucleus.

make room for the basal and endocrine cells located at this level. The ciliated cell contains lakes of glycogen in its basal cytoplasm, and a well-developed Golgi complex is positioned above the nucleus. Some 250 cilia protrude from the apical surface together with a small number of microvilli.

A cilium is longer and thicker and has a more elaborate internal construction than a microvillus (Fig. 1–4).[2] Each cilium is about 6 μm long, and it contains a system of microtubules (its axoneme) that are arranged in nine peripheral pairs with one central doublet. The microtubules continue below the level of the apical cell membrane into the basal body of the cilium, a cylindrical structure that closely resembles the centriole from which it is derived. The row of basal bodies in the apical cytoplasm produces a linear density that cytologists refer to as the terminal bar (Fig. 1–5). A tapering, striated rootlet of contractile filaments extends down from the basal body into the cytoplasm. The cilia are surrounded by watery periciliary fluid that bathes their surface. The actual mucus layer lies above this fluid, and only the tips of the cilia penetrate it.

In a variety of nonneoplastic conditions and many tumors, occasional cells possess a rudimentary cilium, either confined within the cytoplasm where it invaginates the endoplasmic reticulum or protruding from the surface covered by cell membrane. These aberrant cilia are common and merely represent disordered centriolar activity. They do not provide an indication of the cell type and are of no value in differential diagnosis.

Abnormal cilia have been described in many conditions, including the immotile cilia syndrome.[1, 3, 21, 22, 58] The anomalies include cilia with aberrant numbers of microtubules and compound cilia that are larger than normal with increased numbers of microtubules (Fig. 1–6). The practice of obtaining a biopsy specimen of respiratory mucosa from the nasal cavity or nasopharynx in order to examine the cilia with the electron microscope is controversial since similar abnormalities to those seen in the immotile cilia syndrome can be found in infectious and other nonneoplastic disorders. In a study of 22 specimens of hyperplastic, metaplastic, and dysplastic human bronchial mucosa, Gonzales and associates[23] found a variety of atypical ciliary structures, including abnormal configurations of the plasma membrane, varying amounts of matrix, disorganization of basal bodies, and alterations in the pattern of the microtubules. More than one deviation was present in a single case, and there was no

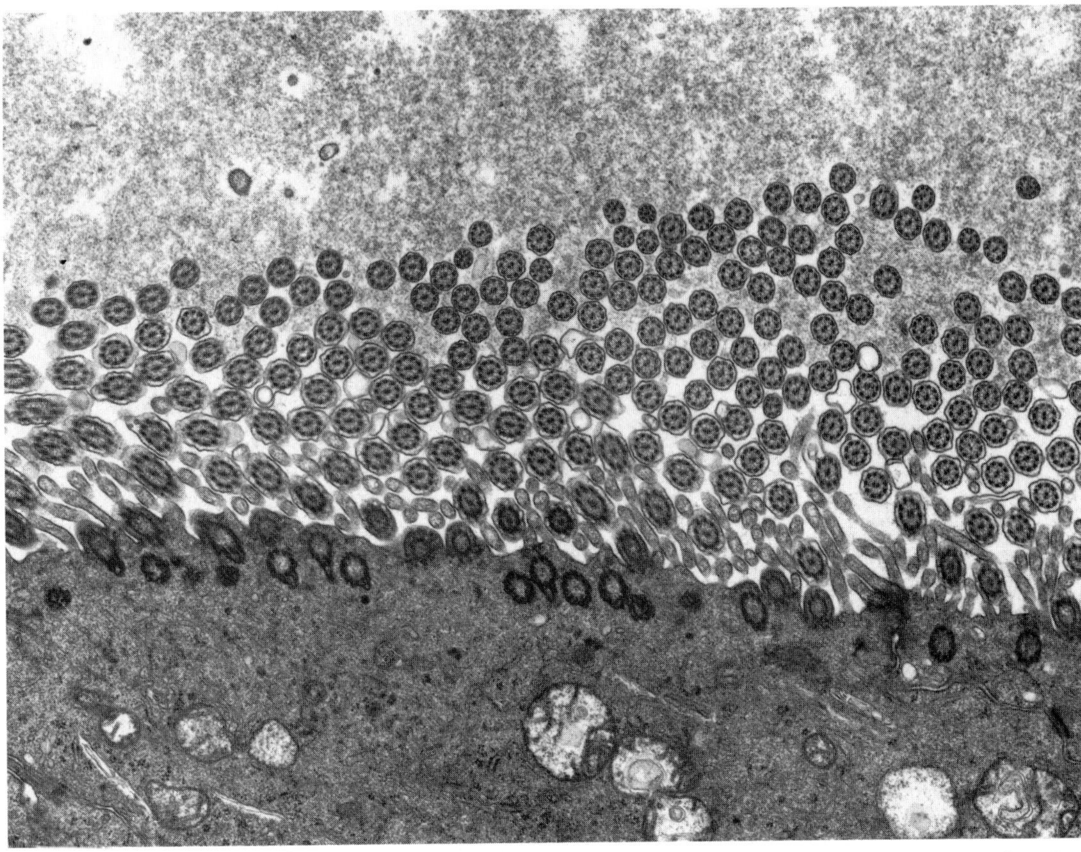

Figure 1–4. The surfaces of two adjacent ciliated cells are shown. Most of the cilia are cut in cross section. Some microvilli and a number of basal bodies can be seen. (× 5,500).

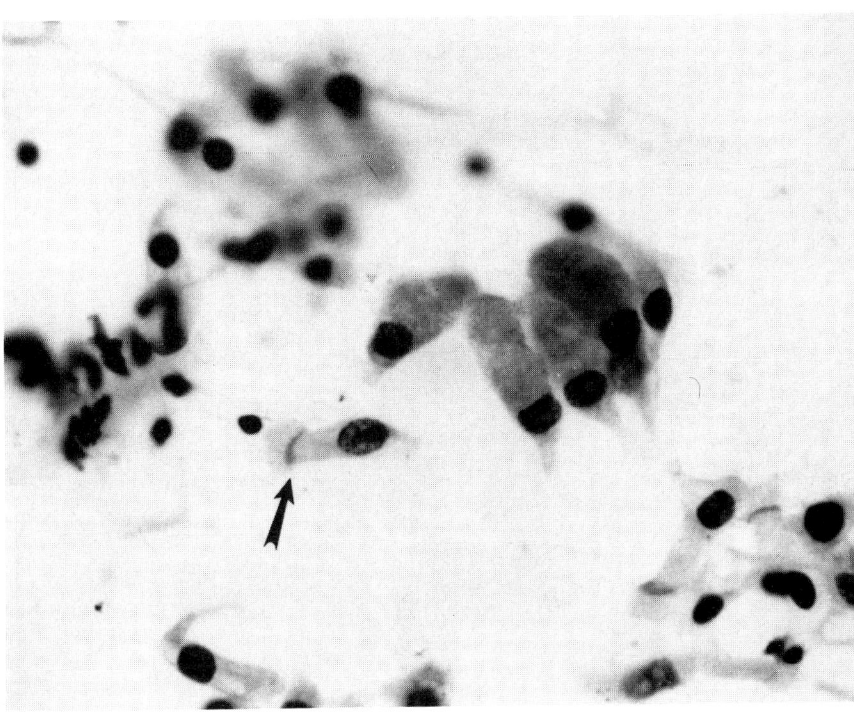

Figure 1–5. Cells from a bronchial brushing. A small group of goblet cells is present. In the ciliated cell indicated by the arrow, the dense line in the apical cytoplasm *(terminal bar)* is produced by the basal bodies of the cilia.

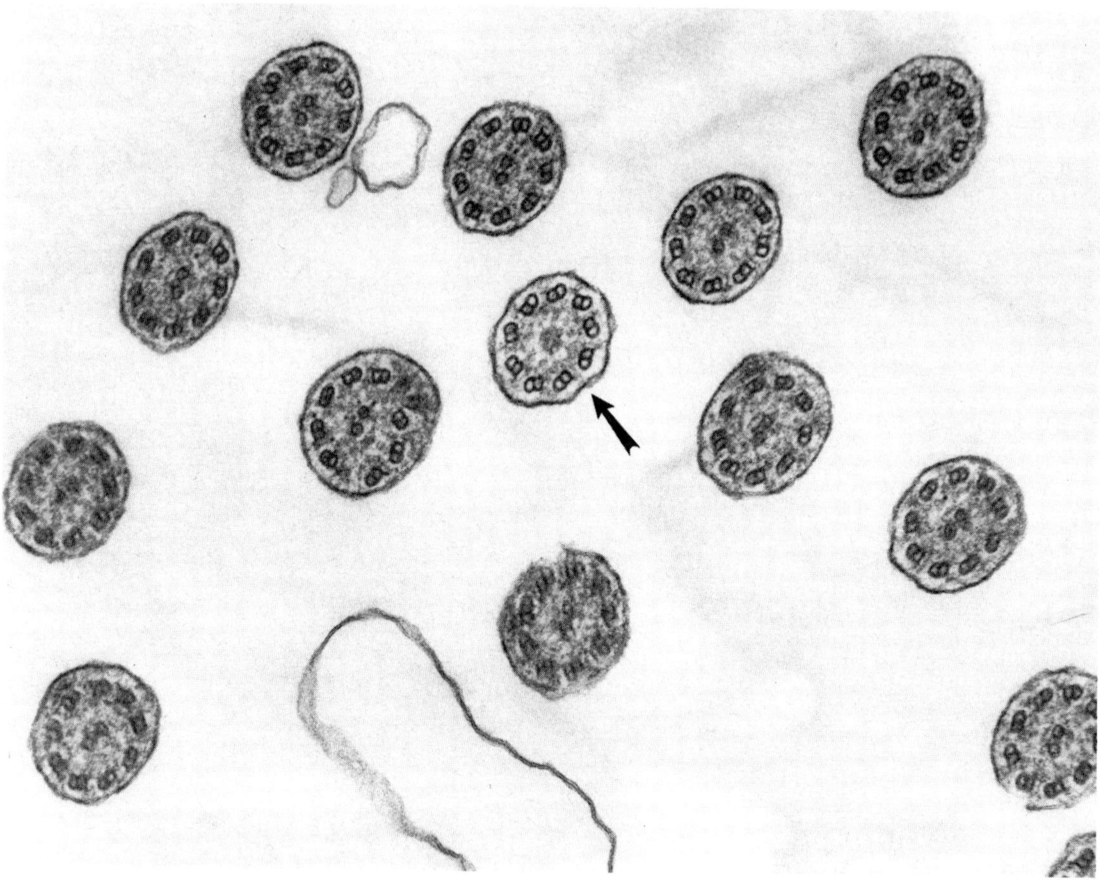

A

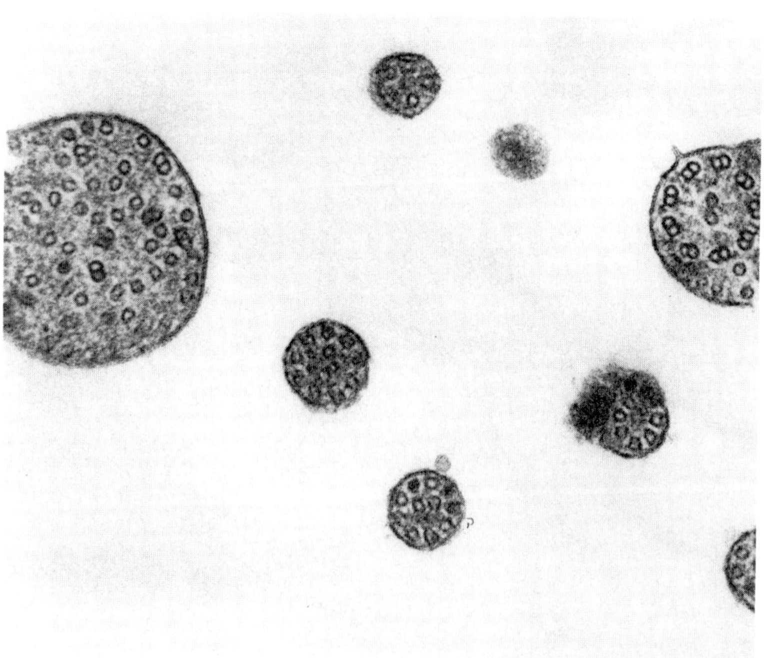

B

Figure 1–6. *A*. The pattern of the microtubules that form the axoneme of a cilium is only seen to good advantage in a true transverse section. In the cilium indicated by the arrow, the central doublet is missing. *B*. Markedly abnormal cilia from a patient who had clinical symptoms of the immotile cilia syndrome. (× 62,000).

evidence of a correlation between the type of ciliary deformation and the extent of the dysplastic process. These abnormal cilia evidently are the result of disordered regeneration of damaged cells, and diagnostic significance should not be attributed to them unless the clinical context is that of the immotile cilia syndrome.

Goblet Cells

The number of goblet cells has been estimated as roughly 7,000/mm^2 of respiratory surface, but the frequency varies at different levels of the respiratory tract and it is increased in some pathologic conditions.[12, 37] In chronic bronchitis, the number of goblet cells may be much greater than normal. Goblet cells are abundant in the trachea, particularly its lower portion, and in contrast are relatively sparse in the bronchioles.

Like the ciliated cells of the respiratory epithelium, goblet cells taper as they approach the basal lamina (Fig. 1–7). Goblet cells accumulate mucin in droplets, which coalesce to become over 1 μm in diameter. The droplets are electron lucent, but they have a fine granularity and may contain a dense core that, at low magnification, can simulate an endocrine granule. When the goblet cell is full of mucin, its luminal end protrudes above the surrounding ciliated cells, and the mucin is discharged into the lumen through breaches in the apical cytoplasm.[66] Some cytoplasm is lost in this apocrine type of secretion, and shreds of cell membrane left adhering to the surface of the cell are quickly detached. In this way, the cell membrane adjusts to the changes in cell volume. While the cell is accumulating mucus, a few microvilli project from the apical surface.

Surface Serous Cells

Serous cells contain large electron-dense granules. They have been described in animals, but identical cells have not been documented in human respiratory epithelium.

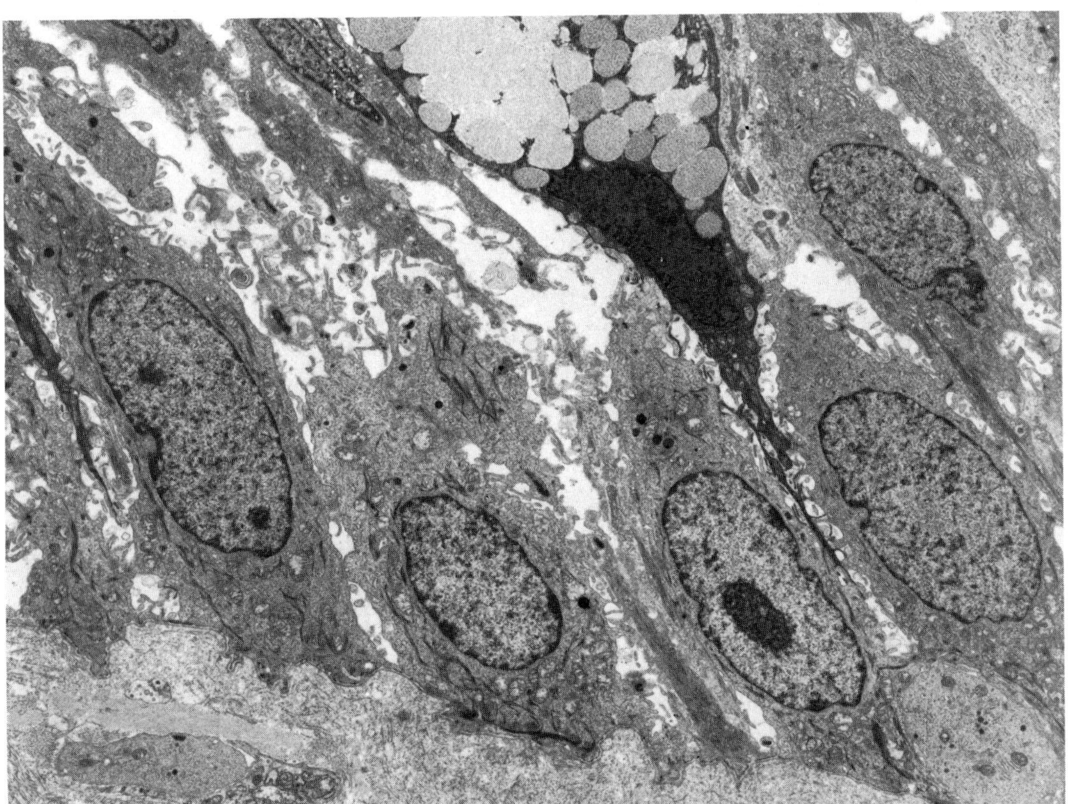

Figure 1–7. Several basal cells are shown. They rest on the basal lamina, and slender bundles of cytokeratin filaments are present in the cytoplasm. The lower part of a goblet cell can be seen: the cytoplasm tapers below the level of the nucleus, and the distended cytoplasm above the nucleus is filled with droplets of mucin. (× 4,000).

Brush Cells

It is also not certain that brush cells, which have been described in animals,[10] occur in the human respiratory mucosa. The animal cell is suspected to have an absorptive function. Brush cells are columnar, and they contain cytoplasmic glycogen and filaments and have many long slender microvilli with microfilament cores that extend down into the apical cytoplasm, an appearance similar to that seen in cells lining the gastrointestinal tract. Since occasional lung adenocarcinomas have microvilli of this type, it is conceivable that brush cells do exist in the human bronchi, but if so they must be present only in small numbers. An alveolar brush cell has been described in the rat lung.[60]

Endocrine Cells

The endocrine cells of the respiratory mucosa are currently of particular interest because of histogenetic implications with regard to bronchial carcinoid and small cell lung carcinoma.[5, 28] Paradoxically, some non–small cell lung carcinomas also contain cells with cytoplasmic granules of endocrine caliber.

Pulmonary endocrine cells have been studied extensively in animals and humans,[6, 24, 54, 55, 57, 63, 68, 81] and they have been given many synonyms, including Feyrter cells, argyrophil cells, and Kulchitsky cells. Endocrine cells are present throughout the trachea and bronchi, and they extend into the bronchioles and the ducts of peribronchial glands. They are present in greater numbers in the fetal lung,

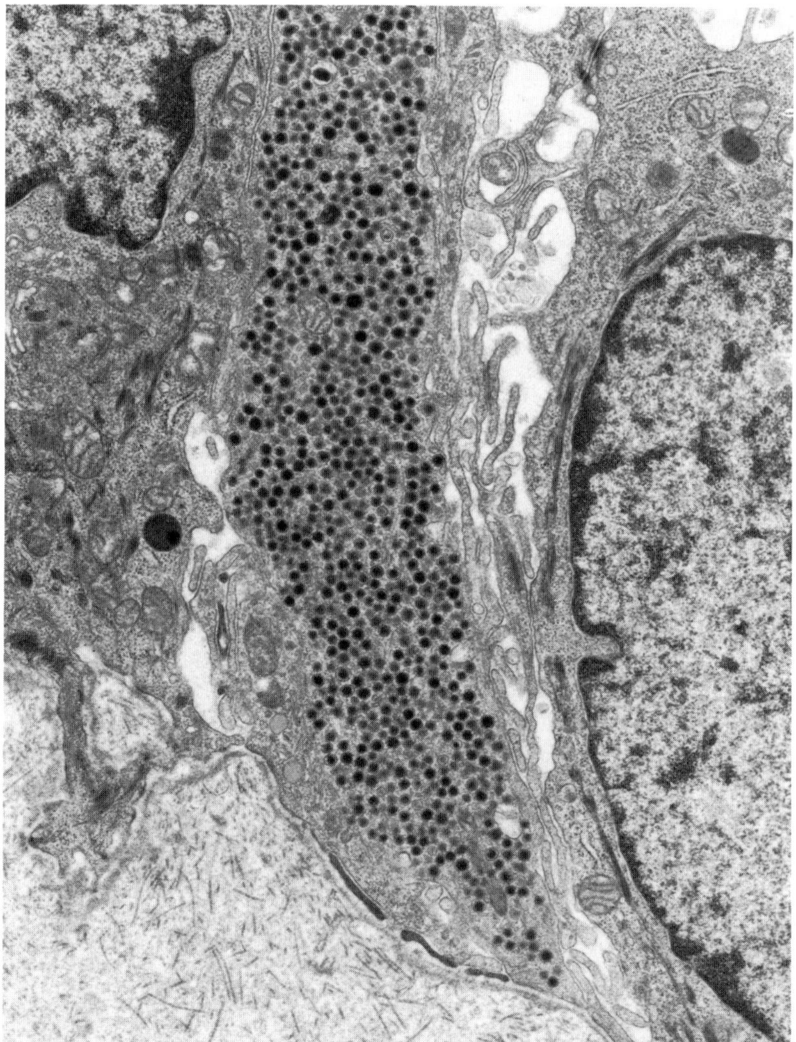

Figure 1–8. An endocrine cell from bronchial epithelium rests on the basal lamina and contains many small dense-core granules. (× 12,000).

where more than one structural type of granule has been described.[19] Most of the endocrine cells are solitary, but they also form small clusters called neuroepithelial bodies,[26, 27] and these cell groups have been studied in animal lungs and in the human fetal lung.[13, 46–49, 79, 80]

The endocrine cells are broadest at their base where they attach to the basal lamina (Fig. 1–8), and they are intimately sandwiched between neighboring columnar cells so that each is triangular in profile, tapering apically and rarely reaching the lumen. The cytoplasm contains many small dense-core granules, which vary in size between 120 and 250 nm but fall within a narrow range of calibers in a particular cell.

The cells can be identified by light microscopy using argyrophil stains such as Grimelius' silver nitrate method[29, 30] or the Sevier-Munger stain.[76] Argentaffin cells (containing reducing agents capable of reducing silver solutions) apparently do not occur in normal tracheobronchial epithelium.

Attempts have been made to classify the endocrine cells of the lung on the basis of the caliber of their dense-core granules[31–33] and by their functional properties as revealed by immunostaining. It appears that more than one type does occur, but it is difficult to relate the normal cells to those seen in tumors because the neoplastic cells display a variety of immunocytochemical and ultrastructural features.

The immunocytochemical demonstration of cytokeratin and desmoplakin in both the solitary neuroendocrine cells and the neuroepithelial bodies confirms their epithelial nature.[52] Immunocytochemical studies have shown reactivity in both the solitary neuroendocrine cells and in neuroepithelial bodies to general neuroendocrine markers such as neuron-specific enolase,[25] chromogranin,[51] and synaptophysin,[52] as well as some regulatory peptides and specific endocrine products, including bombesin, calcitonin, serotonin,[17, 20, 25] somatostatin,[20] and calcitonin gene-related peptide.[50] Leu-enkephalin has been demonstrated only in solitary endocrine cells.[52]

The function of the solitary pulmonary endocrine cells has not been clearly defined, although they presumably elaborate secretions that affect tissues in their immediate vicinity, such as smooth muscle cells in the walls of the respiratory passages and vessels. Stahlman and Gray[81] examined the lungs of 34 human fetuses and 22 newborns using electron microscopy and identified axons, cholinergic terminals, and nonadrenergic-noncholinergic terminals, including some in contact with endocrine cells and deep within neuroepithelial bodies. They suggest that the function of these cells may include reflex mechanisms integrated with the autonomic nervous system and postulate that the cells may have a tropic role in lung development and regeneration. Lauweryns and Van-Lommel[49] report that the cells in neuroepithelial bodies synapse with both afferent and efferent nerves and conclude that the bodies function as neuroreceptors that are locally modulated by axon reflexes.

Oncocytes

The eosinophilic cytoplasm of oncocytic cells results from the presence of large numbers of mitochondria.[10] Similar mitochondrion-rich cells are found in other tissues, notably endocrine organs such as the thyroid (Hürthle cells) and parathyroid (oxyphil cells), and in salivary tissues (oncocytes). They occur in some tumors of these tissues, and similar cells are seen in low-grade renal neoplasms. In the normal respiratory tract, oncocytes have been observed in the trachea, and varying degrees of oncocytic change can be seen in the duct cells of the bronchial glands (Fig. 1–9).

Basal Cells

Basal or reserve cells are found in the respiratory epithelium as far distal as the bronchioles, but they are more numerous proximally. They may be sufficiently plentiful to form a continuous row along the basal lamina, and some stratification can occur (Fig. 1–10), but usually the layer of basal cells is incomplete. Their presence at the base of the epithelium creates an impression of two distinct rows of nuclei (see Fig. 1–1).

In Figure 1–11, the small, round to polygonal basal cells can be seen sitting on the basal lamina. They are in contact with their neighbors or adjacent columnar epithelial cells at various points along their surface, and small desmosomes connect the apposed cell membranes. The basal cells have very few organelles, but slender bundles of cytokeratin filaments are often evident, and a thin strand of smooth muscle myofilaments can sometimes be found in the cytoplasm close to the attachment of the cell to the basal

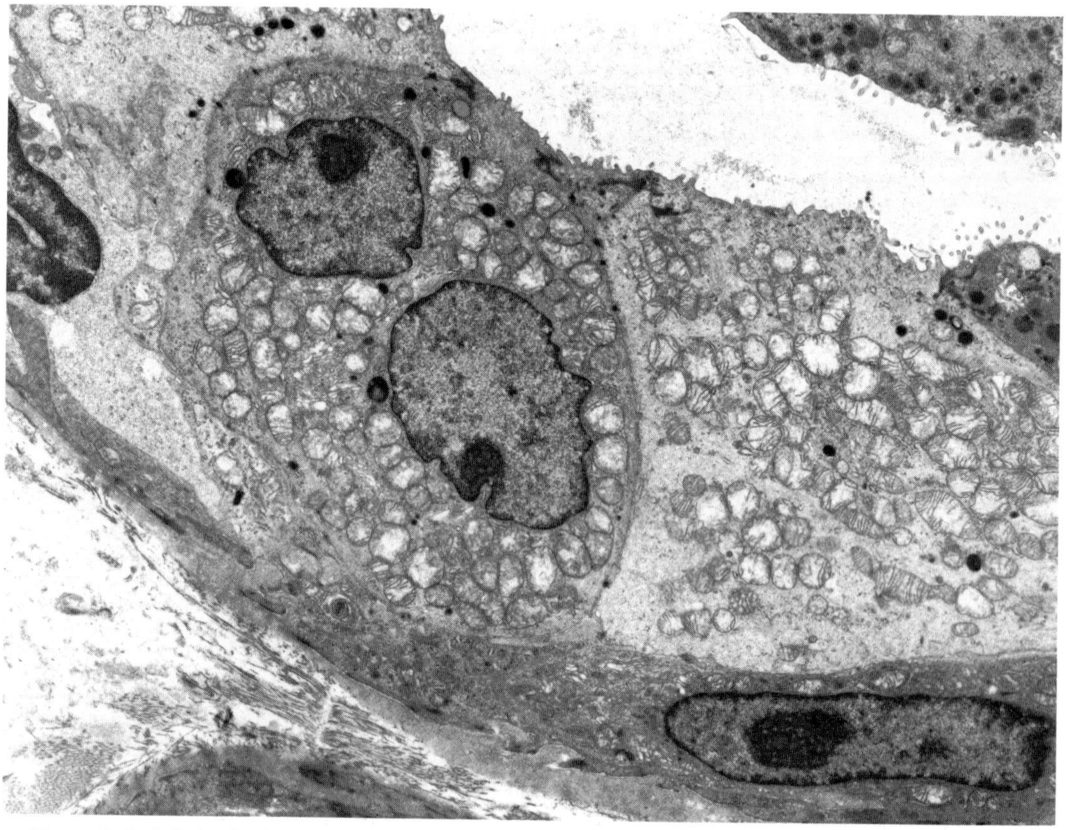

Figure 1–9. Cells in the duct of a bronchial gland contain moderate numbers of mitochondria. (× 5,500).

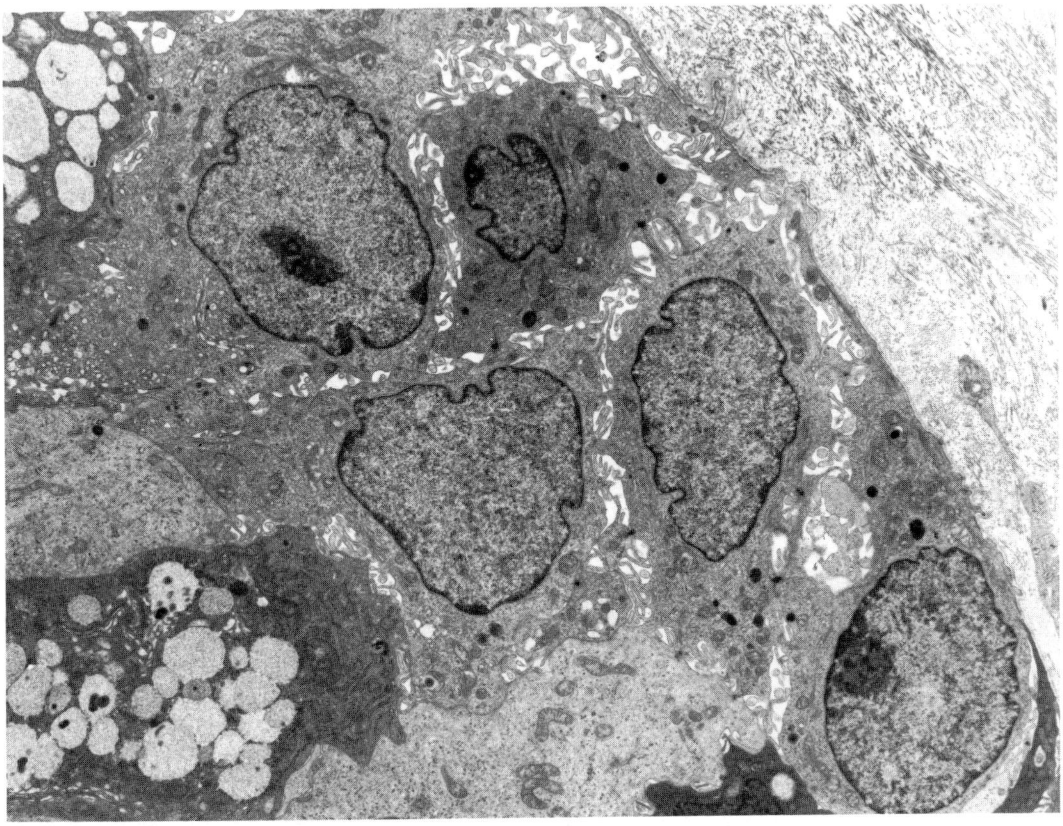

Figure 1–10. Basal cells showing some stratification. Filopodia project into clefts between the cells. The sparse dense bodies in the cytoplasm are probably lysosomes. (× 4,900).

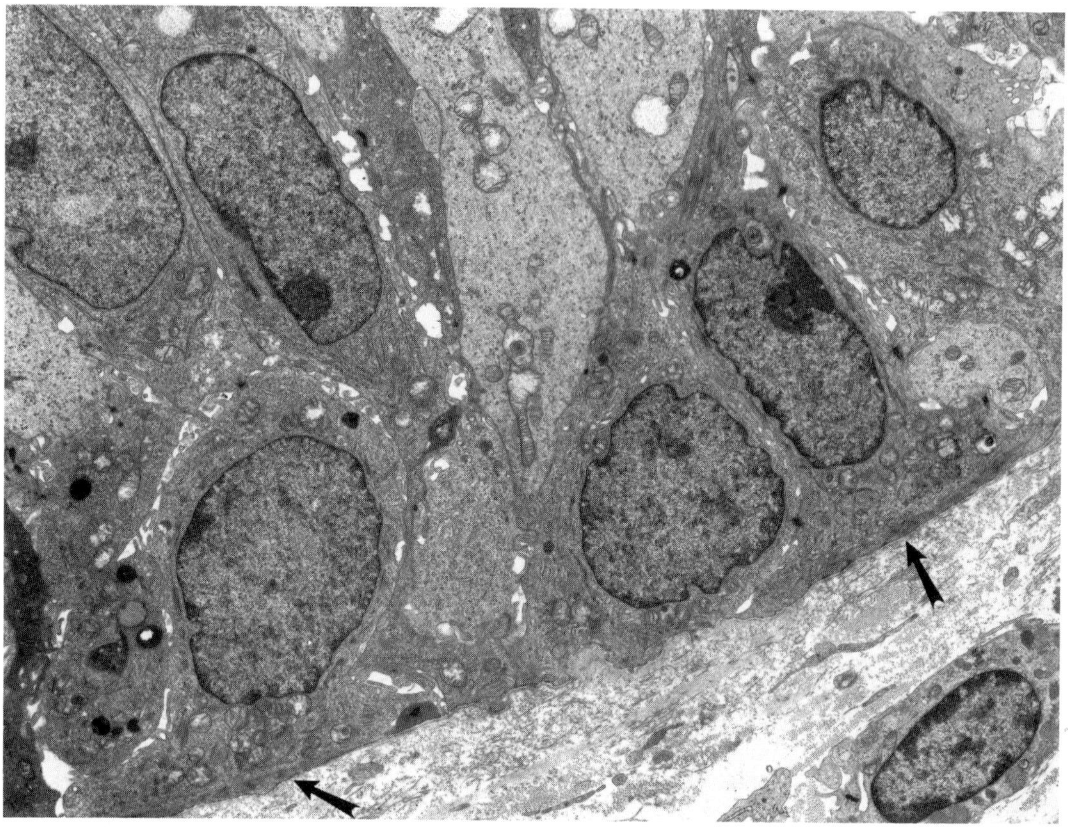

Figure 1–11. Slender bundles of smooth muscle myofilaments may be present in the basal cytoplasm of the basal cells *(arrows)*. (× 4,900).

lamina. Sparse dense granules in the cells are probably primary lysosomes: basal cells are not richly granulated like the true endocrine cells of the mucosa, although an occasional small membrane-bound granule can be found.

It may be that the basal cells have the ability to proliferate and mature in order to replace defects in the epithelium, passing through transitional or intermediate forms before producing the tall columnar cells. More probably, their potential for differentiation into specialized cells like the ciliated columnar cells is limited and they may be able to form only squamous or relatively undifferentiated cells.

BRONCHIAL GLANDS

Three regions have been described in a bronchial gland.[39] A ciliated duct leads via a connecting duct into several secretory tubules, which are blind pouches lined by mucous and serous cells (Fig. 1–12).[61, 62] The mucous cells are similar in appearance to the surface goblet cells, but their mucin is more evenly distributed through the cytoplasm. Large, dense, zymogen-type cytoplasmic granules confer a distinctive ultrastructural appearance on the serous cells.

Secretion empties from the secretory tubules into the collecting duct, which is lined by tall columnar cells containing many mitochondria but no mucin. From the collecting ducts, the secretion passes into the ciliated duct, which has a wider lumen lined by tall columnar cells with cilia on their apical surfaces.

The secretion of the bronchial glands is influenced by the action of sympathetic and parasympathetic efferent fibers. Myoepithelial cells surround the tubules and ducts (Fig. 1–13), and fine branches of the efferent fibers approach the basal lamina and release transmitter substances that diffuse across the lamina.

BRONCHIOLES

The terminal bronchioles in the adult human lung are approximately the 16th divisions formed by the dichotomous branching of the bronchial tree. Nonciliated bronchiolar cells (Clara cells) intermingle with ciliated cells in the terminal bronchioles. They were first reported by Kolliker[42] in 1881, but Clara[16] described them in detail in 1937. Some bulge into the lumen,[73] and the apical caps of the cells in the rat lung are traversed by filaments[74]; we have not observed the filaments in human Clara cells, but apparently the apical cap is not an apocrine droplet. The ultrastructural hallmark of the Clara cell is large dense-core granules that accumulate in the apical cytoplasm. The granules contain protein that is secreted from the apical surface to form a component of the surfactant.[18, 56]

ALVEOLI

Most of the alveolar surface is lined by type 1 pneumocytes (Fig. 1–14), which are flattened cells with attenuated cytoplasm that bulges at its center where the nucleus is located so that the cell has the shape of a fried egg.[71] The type 1 pneumocytes may be called squamous or squamoid because of their flattened, platelike architecture. Scattered cells with a more cuboidal profile are the type 2 pneumocytes. The type 1 cells have very few organelles in their thin cytoplasm, but the type 2 cells contain concentrically laminated "lamellar" bodies (Fig. 1–15), which are extruded from the cell to furnish the phospholipid portion of the surfactant.[4, 40, 43, 77, 83, 86, 87] Synthesis of the lamellar bodies requires an intact microtubular system, and their secretion is mediated by actin filaments. Type 2 cells proliferate in response to noxious agents, progressively replacing the type 1 cells, and in so doing they reduce the effective area for gas exchange.

The interalveolar septa are normally very thin. On each side they are bounded by the pneumocytes of the adjacent alveoli. The basal lamina of the many capillaries within the septa are intimately related to the basal lamina of the alveolus.[35, 72, 73] Pulmonary endothelium is a metabolically active tissue that regulates the composition of the arterial blood, affects target organ functions, and contributes to thrombosis, hemostasis, and immune functions.[73] The area for gas exchange in the lungs is more than 100 m^2. Each septum contains a small amount of

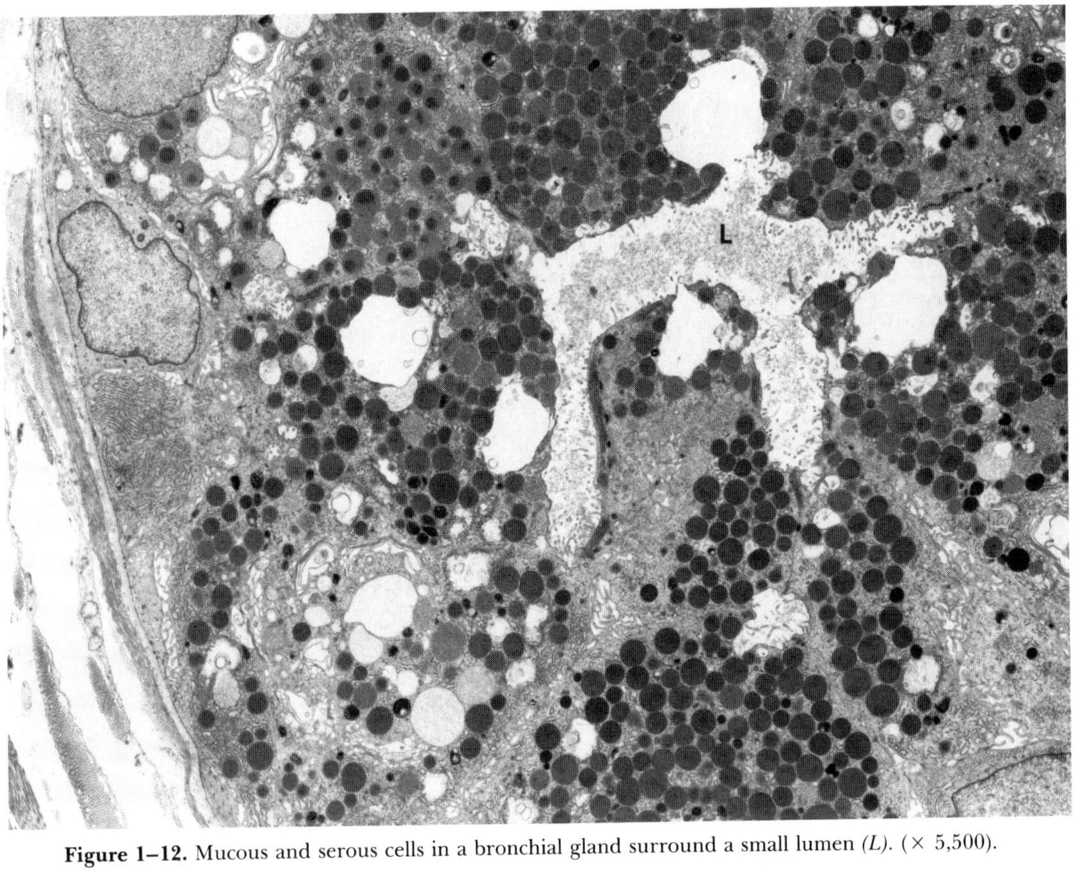

Figure 1–12. Mucous and serous cells in a bronchial gland surround a small lumen *(L)*. (× 5,500).

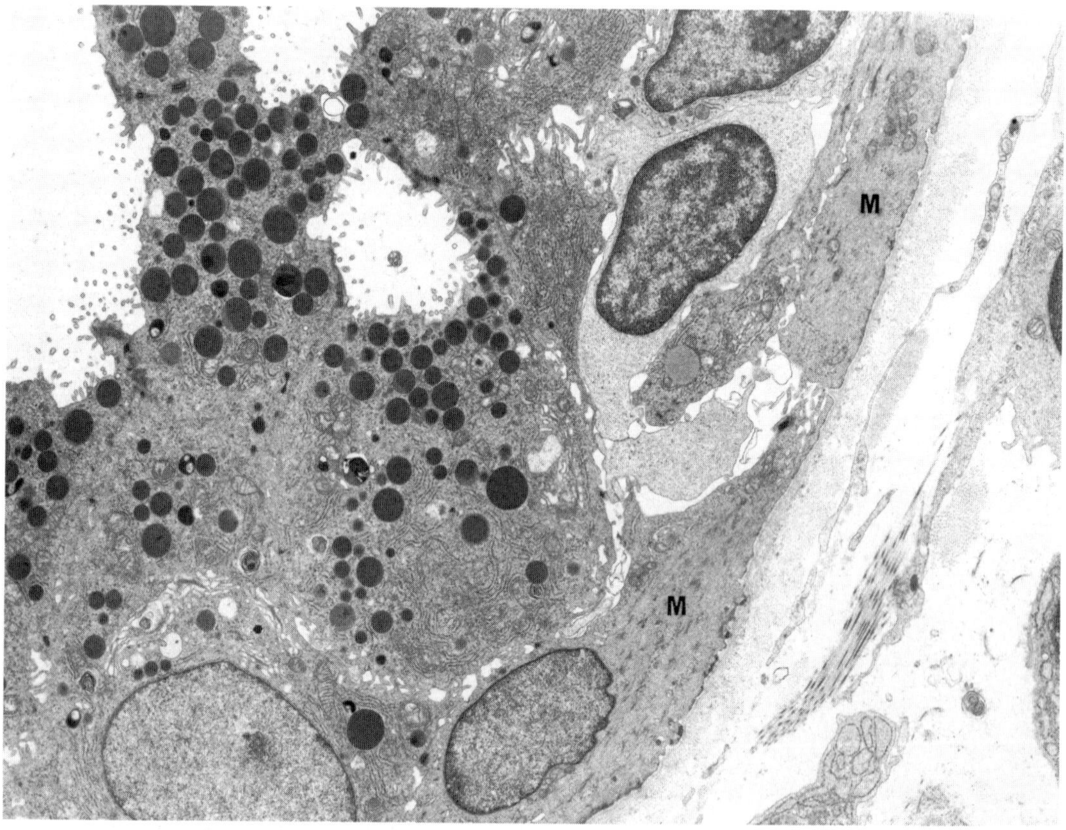

Figure 1–13. Myoepithelial cells *(M)* are present at the periphery of a bronchial gland. They lie within the basal lamina and contain smooth muscle myofilaments. (× 5,500).

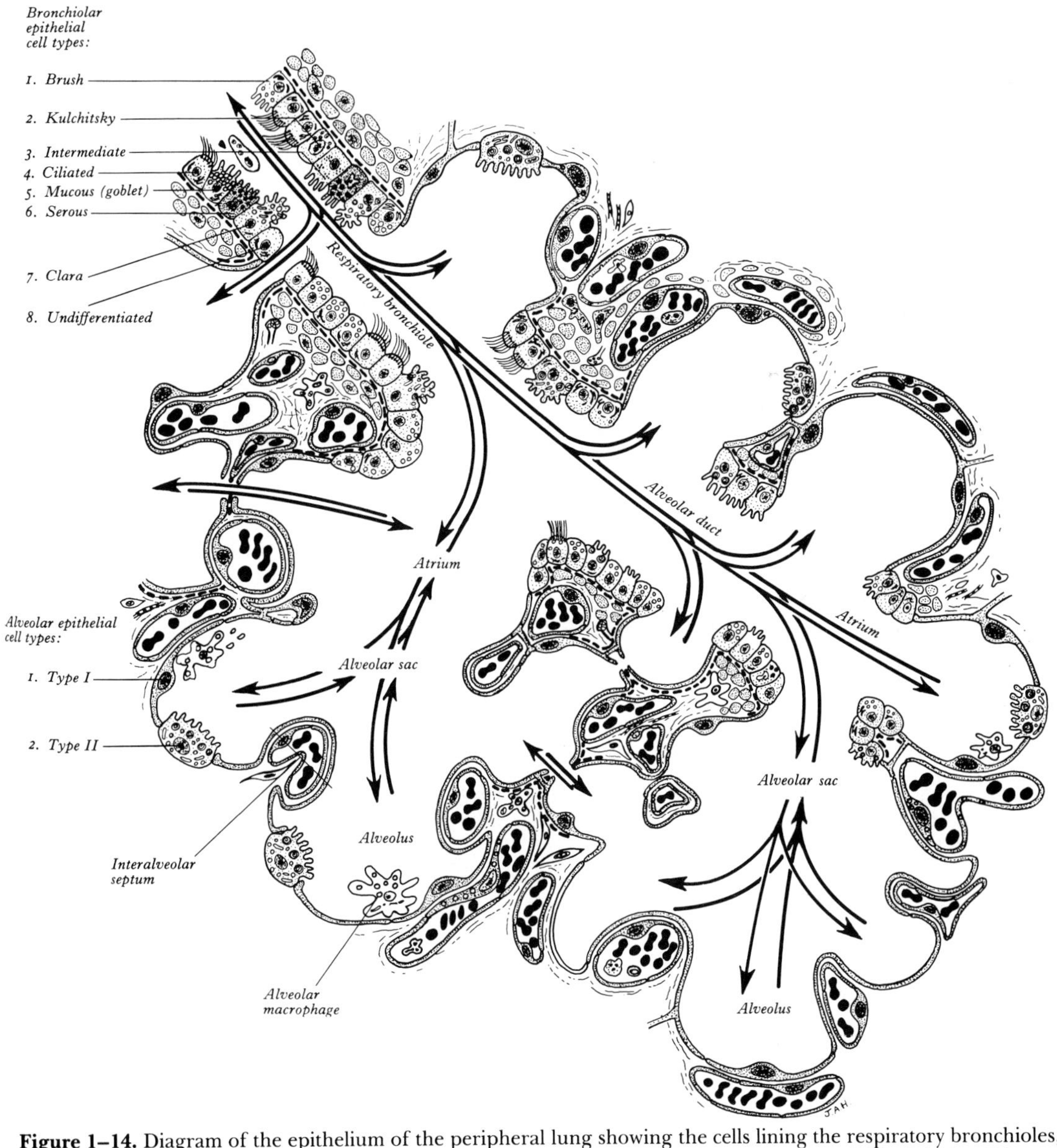

Figure 1–14. Diagram of the epithelium of the peripheral lung showing the cells lining the respiratory bronchioles, alveolar ducts and sacs, and alveoli. (Williams PL, and Warwick R [eds]: Gray's Anatomy, 36th British edition, p 1261. London, Churchill Livingstone, 1980.)

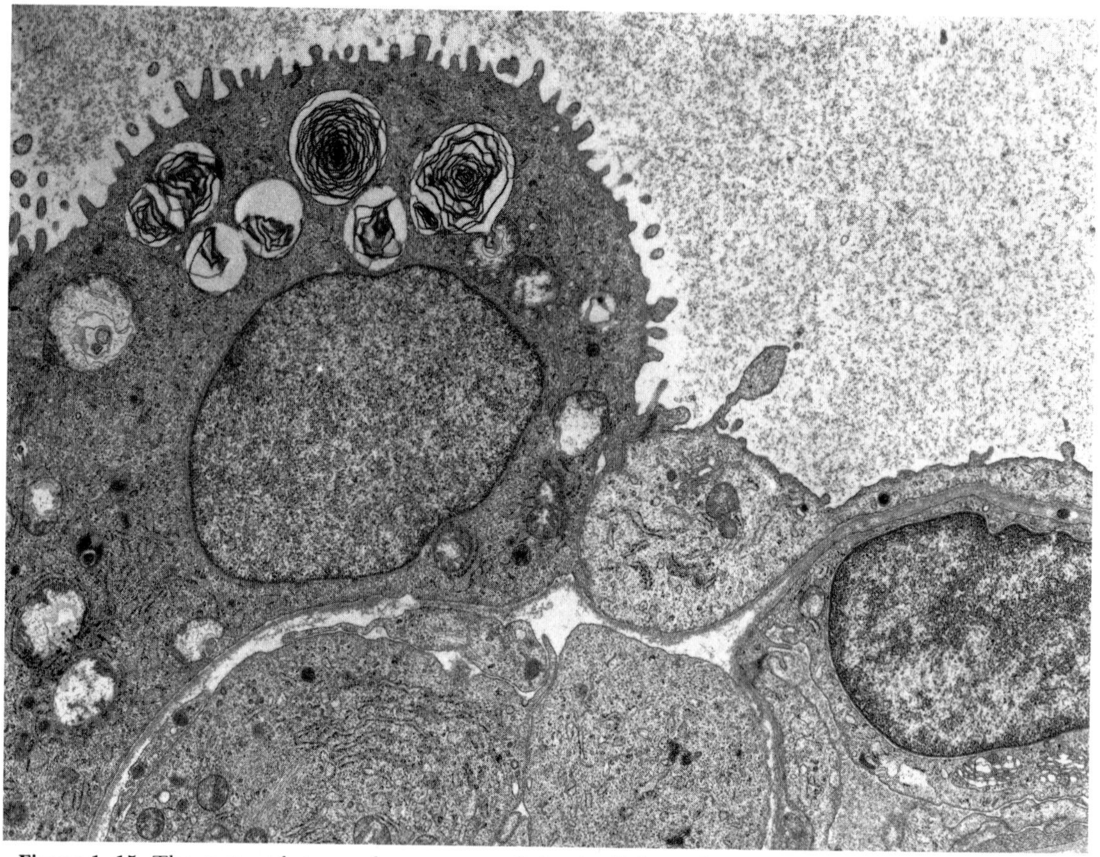

Figure 1–15. The contrast between the two types of alveolar lining cells is evident in this electron micrograph. The type 2 cell is almost spherical, and it contains lamellar bodies in its cytoplasm. The adjacent type 1 cell has very thin cytoplasm. Both cells rest on the alveolar basal lamina. A capillary lies close to the base of the type 1 cell. (× 9,000).

collagen and a few fibroblasts and migratory cells, including macrophages[7, 34, 59, 64, 65] and mast cells.[75, 84]

VESSELS OF THE LUNG

Branches of the pulmonary arteries accompany the bronchi, usually on their posterolateral aspect. Rich plexuses of capillaries permeate the interalveolar septa and surround the alveolar sacs and respiratory bronchioles. The pattern of the venous return is quite variable compared with the arterial distribution, and each bronchopulmonary segment is drained by more than one segmental vein. A plexus of veins also ramifies beneath the visceral pleura. The bronchial arteries conveying arterial blood from the descending aorta or intercostal arteries form a plexus in the bronchial wall and extend peripherally to the level of the respiratory bronchioles. They also supply the interstitial connective tissue of the lung and the visceral pleura.

PULMONARY LYMPHATICS

Lymphatic capillaries ramify on the lung surface deep to the pleural epithelium and within the walls of the respiratory passages as far distal as the respiratory bronchioles. In the larger bronchi, lymphatic plexuses are present in the submucosal connective tissue and in the loose connective tissue that surrounds the bronchi and bronchioles. The lymph drains into subsegmental and segmental nodes and the peribronchial and hilar nodes and from them to the mediastinum (Fig. 1–16). At the base of the oblique fissure, connections exist between the lymphatics of the upper and lower lobes.

NERVES OF THE LUNG

Branches of the vagi and sympathetic chains form the anterior and posterior pulmonary plexuses around the hilum of each lung, and efferents accompany the bronchial

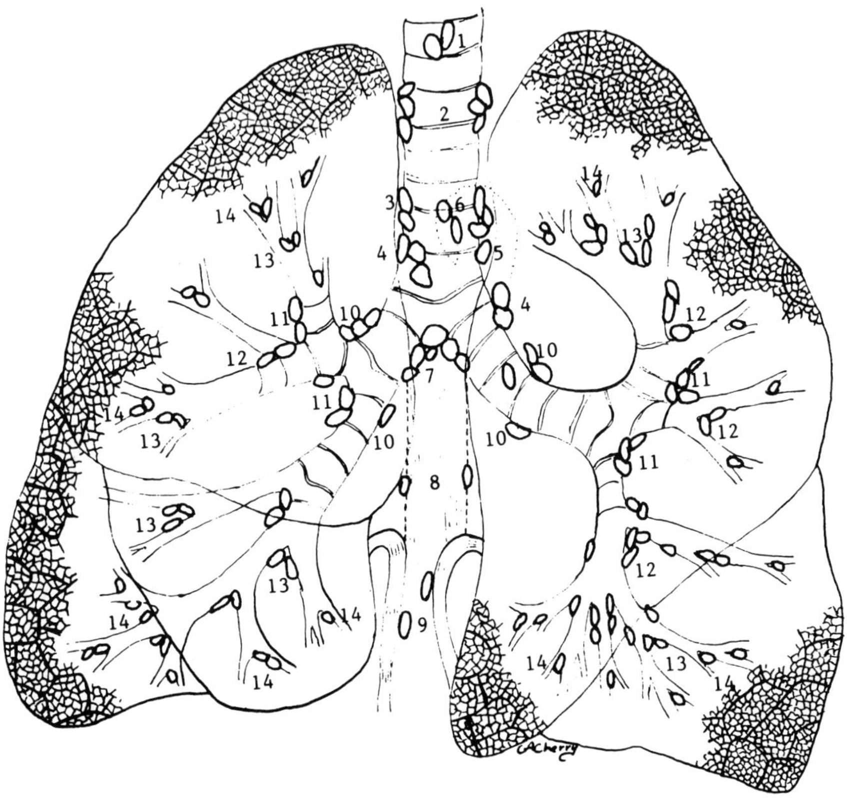

Figure 1–16. Location of intrathoracic lymph nodes. (1) Superior or highest mediastinal; (2) upper paratracheal; (3) pretracheal and retrotracheal (anterior and posterior mediastinal); (4) tracheobronchial (lower paratracheal); (5) subaortic (aortic window, Botallo's); (6) para-aortic (ascending aorta, phrenic); (7) subcarinal; (8) paraesophageal (below carina); (9) pulmonary ligament; (10) hilar; (11) interlobar; (12) lobar; (13) segmental; (14) subsegmental.

N2 Nodes

Superior Mediastinal Nodes

1. Highest mediastinal
2. Upper paratracheal
3. Pretracheal and retrotracheal
4. Lower paratracheal (including azygos nodes)

Aortic Nodes

5. Subaortic (aortic window)
6. Para-aortic (ascending aorta or phrenic)

Inferior Mediastinal Nodes

7. Subcarinal
8. Paraesophageal (below carina)
9. Pulmonary ligament

N1 Nodes

10. Hilar
11. Intralobar
12. Lobar
13. Segmental
14. Subsegmental

tree supplying smooth muscle in the bronchial wall and myoepithelial cells in the bronchial glands.[41, 42, 44, 70, 85] Afferent fibers arborize in the bronchial mucosa and extend distally as far as the interalveolar septa.

PLEURA

The structure of the normal pleura is described in Chapter 13.

REFERENCES

1. Afzelius BA: A human syndrome caused by immotile cilia. Science 193:317, 1976.
2. Afzelius BA: Ultrastructural basis for ciliary motility. Eur J Respir Dis 128(suppl):280, 1983.
3. Ailsby RL, Ghadially FN: Atypical cilia in human bronchial mucosa. J Pathol 109:75, 1973.
4. Balis JU, Paterson JF, Paciga JE et al: Distribution and subcellular localization of surfactant-associated glycoproteins in human lung. Lab Invest 52:657, 1985.
5. Becker KL, Gazdar A: The pulmonary endocrine cell and the tumors to which it gives rise. In Reznick-Schuller HM (ed): Comparative Respiratory Tract Carcinogenesis, vol 2, p 161. Boca Raton, FL, CRC Press, 1983.
6. Bonikos DS, Bensch KG: Endocrine cells of bronchial and bronchiolar epithelium. Am J Med 63:765, 1977.
7. Bowden DH, Adamson IYR: Role of monocytes and interstitial cells in the generation of alveolar macrophages: I. Kinetic studies on normal mice. Lab Invest 42:511, 1980.
8. Boyden EA: Development and growth of the airways. In Hodson WA (ed): Development of the Lung, p 3. New York, Marcel Dekker, 1977.
9. Breeze R, Turk M: Cellular structure, function and organization in the lower respiratory tract. Environ Health Perspect 55:3, 1984.
10. Breeze RG, Wheeldon EB: The cells of the pulmonary airways. Am Rev Respir Dis 116:705, 1977.
11. Brody JS, Vaccaro C: Postnatal formation of alveoli: Interstitial events and physiological consequences. Fed Proc 38:215, 1979.
12. Cerkez V, Tos M, Mygind N: Goblet-cell density in the human lung: Whole mount study of the normal left lower lobe. Anat Anz 162:205, 1986.
13. Chen MF, Wang NS, Kimizuka G: Increase of neuroepithelial bodies in human fetal lungs of smoking mothers. Lab Invest 52:13A, 1985.
14. Cheng H, Leblond CP: Origin, differentiation and renewal of the four main epithelial cell types in the mouse small intestine: III. Enteroendocrine cells. Am J Anat 141:503, 1974.
15. Cheng H, Leblond CP: Origin, differentiation and renewal of the four main epithelial cell types in the mouse small intestine: V. Unitarian theory of the origin of the four epithelial cell types. Am J Anat 141:537, 1974.
16. Clara M: Zur Histobiologie des Bronchial-epithels. Z Mikrosk Anat Forsch 41:321, 1937.
17. Cutz E, Chan W, Track NS: Bombesin, calcitonin and leu-enkephalin immunoreactivity in endocrine cells of human lung. Experientia 37:765, 1981.
18. Cutz E, Conen PE: Ultrastructure and cytochemistry of Clara cells. Am J Pathol 62:127, 1971.
19. Cutz E, Gillan JE, Bryan AC: Neuroendocrine cells in the developing human lung: Morphologic and functional considerations. Pediatr Pulmonol 1(suppl):S21, 1985.
20. Dayer AM, DeMey J, Will JA: Localization of somatostatin-, bombesin-, and serotonin-like immunoreactivity in the lung of the fetal rhesus monkey. Cell Tissue Res 239:621, 1985.
21. Eliasson R, Mossberg B, Camner P et al: The immotile cilia syndrome. N Engl J Med 297:1, 1977.
22. Gonzales S, von Bassewitz DB, Grundmann E et al: Atypical cilia in hyperplastic, metaplastic and dysplastic human bronchial mucosa. Ultrastruct Pathol 8:345, 1985.
23. Gonzales S, von Bassewitz DB, Grundmann E et al: Rudimentary cilia in hyperplastic, metaplastic and neoplastic cells of the lung and pleura. Pathol Res Pract 180:511, 1985.
24. Gould VE: Editorial: The endocrine lung. Lab Invest 48:507, 1983.
25. Gould VE, Lee I, Warren WH: Immunohistochemical evaluation of neuroendocrine cells and neoplasms of the lung. Pathol Res Pract 183:200, 1988.
26. Gould VE, Linnoila RI: Pulmonary neuroepithelial bodies, neuroendocrine cells, and pulmonary tumors. Hum Pathol 13:1064, 1982.
27. Gould VE, Linnoila RI, Memoli VA et al: Neuroendocrine components of the bronchopulmonary tract: Hyperplasias, dysplasias, and neoplasms. Lab Invest 49:519, 1983.
28. Gould VE, Linnoila RI, Memoli VA et al: Neuroendocrine cells and neuroendocrine neoplasms of the lung. Pathol Annu 18(Part 2):287, 1983.
29. Grimelius L: A silver nitrate stain for alpha-2 cells in human pancreatic islets. Acta Soc Med Uppsala 273:243, 1968.
30. Grimelius L, Wilander E: Silver stains in the study of endocrine cells of the gut and pancreas. Invest Cell Pathol 3:3, 1980.
31. Hage E: Endocrine-like cells of the pulmonary epithelium, thesis. University of Odense, 1976.
32. Hage E: Light and electron microscopic characteristics of the various lung endocrine cell types. Invest Cell Pathol 3:345, 1980.
33. Hage E, Hage J, Juel G: Endocrine-like cells of the pulmonary epithelium of the adult lung. Cell Tissue Res 178:39, 1977.
34. Hoogsteden HC, van-Dongen JJ, van-Hal PT et al: Phenotype of blood monocytes and alveolar macrophages in interstitial lung disease. Chest 95:574, 1989.
35. Huang TW: Composite epithelial and endothelial basal laminas in human lungs: A structural basis for their separation and apposition in reaction to injury. Am J Pathol 93:681, 1978.
36. Inselman LS, Mellins RB: Growth and development of the lung. J Pediatr 98:1, 1981.
37. Jeffery PK, Ayers M, Rogers DF: The mechanisms and control of bronchial mucous cell hyperplasia. Chest 81:27S, 1982.
38. Jeffery PK, Reid LM: Ultrastructural features of airway lining epithelium in the developing rat and human lung. J Anat 120:295, 1977.

39. Jeffery PK, Reid LM: Ultrastructure of airway epithelium and submucosal gland during development. In Hodson WA (ed): Lung Biology in Health and Disease, Vol 6, Development of the Lung, p 87. New York, Marcel Dekker, 1977.
40. King RJ: Utilization of alveolar epithelial type II cells for the study of pulmonary surfactant. Fed Proc 38:2637, 1979.
41. Kneussl M: Regulation of the tracheobronchial and lung vascular system: Innervation and receptors. Wien Klin Wochenschr 98:7013, 1986.
42. Kolliker A: Zur Kentniss des Baues der Lunge des Menschen. Verh Physik Med Ges Wurtzburg 16:1, 1881.
43. Kumar RK, Lykke AW, Truscott SY et al: Immunohistochemical identification of type 2 pneumocytes by an antibody to a lamellar body enriched fraction of lung homogenate. Lung 163:243, 1985.
44. Laitinen A: Ultrastructural organisation of intraepithelial nerves in the human airway tract. Thorax 40:488, 1985.
45. Langston C, Kida K, Thurlbeck WM: Lung growth up to 1 month of postnatal age. Lab Invest 40:307, 1979.
46. Lauweryns JM, de Bock V, Verhofstad AAJ et al: Immunohistochemical localization of serotonin in intrapulmonary neuroepithelial bodies. Cell Tissue Res 226:215, 1982.
47. Lauweryns JM, Goddeeris P: Neuroepithelial bodies in the human child and adult lung. Am Rev Respir Dis 111:469, 1975.
48. Lauweryns JM, Van-Lommel A: The intrapulmonary neuroepithelial bodies after vagotomy: Demonstration of their sensory neuroreceptor-like innervation. Experientia 39:1123, 1983.
49. Lauweryns JM, Van-Lommel A: Ultrastructure of nerve endings and synaptic junctions in rabbit intrapulmonary neuroepithelial bodies: A single and serial section analysis. J Anat 151:65, 1987.
50. Lauweryns JM, Van Ranst L: Calcitonin gene related peptide immunoreactivity in rat lung: Light and electron microscopic study. Thorax 42:183, 1987.
51. Lauweryns JM, Van Ranst L, Lloyd RV et al: Chromogranin in bronchopulmonary neuroendocrine cells: Immunocytochemical detection in human, monkey, and pig respiratory mucosa. J Histochem Cytochem 35:133, 1987.
52. Lee I, Gould VE, Moll R et al: Synaptophysin expression in the bronchopulmonary tract neuroendocrine cells, neuroepithelial bodies and neuroendocrine neoplasms. Differentiation 34:115, 1987.
53. Lopez-Vidriero MT: Biochemical basis of physical properties of respiratory tract secretions. Eur J Respir Dis 153(Suppl):130, 1987.
54. Marchevsky AM, Kleinerman J: Immunocytochemical studies of APUD cells in airways: Effects of nitrosodiethylamine and nitrogen dioxide. Arch Pathol Lab Med 106:400, 1982.
55. Marchevsky AM, Kleinerman J: Quantitative and immunocytochemical studies of APUD cells in airways and gut. Lung 161:67, 1983.
56. Massaro GD, Fischman CM, Chiang M-J et al: Regulation of secretion in Clara cells. J Clin Invest 67:345, 1981.
57. McDougall J: Endocrine-like cells in the terminal bronchioles and saccules of human fetal lung: ultrastructural study. Thorax 33:43, 1978.
58. McDowell EM, Barrett LA, Harris CC et al: Abnormal cilia in human bronchial epithelium. Arch Pathol Lab Med 100:429, 1976.
59. McGowan SE, Thompson RJ: Extracellular matrix proteoglycan degradation by human alveolar macrophages and neutrophils. J Appl Physiol 66:400, 1989.
60. Meyrick B, Reid L: The alveolar brush cell in rat lung: The third pneumocyte. J Ultrastruct Res 23:71, 1981.
61. Meyrick B, Reid L: Ultrastructure of cells in the human bronchial submucosal glands. J Anat 107:281, 1970.
62. Meyrick B, Sturgess JM, Reid L: A reconstruction of the duct system and secretory tubules of the human bronchial submucosal gland. Thorax 24:729, 1969.
63. Mosca L, Ceresoli A, Anzanello E et al: Neuroendocrine structures in normal and diseased human lung. Appl Pathol 4:147, 1986.
64. Nakahashi H, Yasumoto K, Nagashima A et al: Antitumor activity of macrophages in lung cancer patients with special reference to location of macrophages. Cancer Res 44:5906, 1984.
65. Nakstad B, Lyberg T, Skjorten F et al: Subpopulations of human lung alveolar macrophages: Ultrastructural features. Ultrastruct Pathol 13:1, 1989.
66. Neutra MR: The functional ultrastructure of mucous cells. Chest 81(suppl):14, 1982.
67. Parra SC, Gaddy LR, Takaro T: Ultrastructural studies of canine interalveolar pores (of Kohn). Lab Invest 38:8, 1978.
68. Polak JM, Bloom SR: Regulatory peptides and neuron-specific enolase in the respiratory tract of man and other mammals. Exp Lung Res 3:313, 1982.
69. Reid L, Jones R: Bronchial mucosal cells. Fed Proc 38:191, 1979.
70. Richardson JB: Nerve supply to the lung. Am Rev Respir Dis 119:785, 1979.
71. Rosenbaum RM, Picciano P: The type I alveolar lining cells of the mammalian lung: II. *In vitro* identification via the cell surface and ultrastructure of isolated cells from adult rabbit lung. Am J Pathol 90:123, 1978.
72. Ryan US: Metabolic activity of pulmonary endothelium: Modulations of structure and function. Annu Rev Physiol 48:263, 1986.
73. Ryan US, Ryan JW: Cell biology of pulmonary endothelium. Circulation 70:46, 1984.
74. Sasaki J, Takehara Y, Fujii Y et al: Presence of abundant filaments in apical caps of the nonciliated bronchiolar epithelial (Clara) cells. Am J Anat 179:1, 1987.
75. Schulman ES, MacGlashan DW, Peters SP et al: Purification and characterization of human lung mast cells. Fed Proc 41:377, 1982.
76. Sevier AC, Munger BL: A silver method for paraffin sections of neural tissue. J Neuropathol Exp Neurol 24:130, 1965.
77. Shimura S, Aoki T, Takishima T: Morphological aspects of the surfactant system in human lungs: A freeze-fracture study. Respiration 50:139, 1986.
78. Sidhu GS: The endodermal origin of digestive and respiratory tract APUD cells: Histopathologic evidence and a review of the literature. Am J Pathol 96:5, 1979.
79. Sonstegard K, Wong V, Cutz E: Neuroepithelial bodies in organ cultures of fetal rabbit lungs. Cell Tissue Res 199:159, 1979.

80. Sorokin SP, Holt RF, Grant MM: Development of neuroepithelial bodies in fetal rabbit lungs: I. Appearance and functional maturation as demonstrated by high-resolution light microscopy and formaldehyde-induced fluorescence. Exp Lung Res 3:237, 1982.
81. Stahlman MT, Gray ME: Ontogeny of neuroendocrine cells in the human fetal lung: I. An electron microscopic study. Lab Invest 51:449, 1984.
82. Thurlbeck WM: Postnatal growth of the lung and its significance in disease. Hum Pathol 9:492, 1978.
83. Van Golde LMG: Synthesis of surfactant lipids in the adult and fetal lung: Pathways and regulatory aspects. Eur J Respir Dis 67:19, 1985.
84. Warton A, Papadimitriou JM, Goldie RG et al: An ultrastructural study of mast cells in the alveolar wall of normal and asthmatic lung. Aust J Exp Biol Med Sci 64:435, 1986.
85. Widdicombe JG: Nervous receptors in the respiratory tract and lungs. In Hornbein TF (ed): Regulation of Breathing, part I, p 429. New York, Marcel Dekker, 1981.
86. Wright JR, Clements JA: Metabolism and turnover of lung surfactant. Am Rev Respir Dis 136:426, 1987.
87. Zimmermann B: Secretion of lamellar bodies in type II pneumocytes in organoid culture: Effects of colchicine and cytochalasin B. Exp Lung Res 15:31, 1989.

Chapter

2

STAGING OF LUNG CANCER

Advances in the diagnosis and treatment of lung cancer have been related, primarily, to the application of a multimodality therapeutic concept and to refinements in the treatment selection process. Accurate, reproducible classification of the anatomic extent of disease and of histologic cell type in a given patient is fundamental to the rational application of these elements of management. The new international staging system for lung cancer meets this need for disease extent classification because it has consistent meaning among physicians and scientists throughout the world. The system is based on TNM (T—primary tumor, N—regional lymph nodes, M—distant metastasis) classification principles. Some useful and valid definitions of the earlier staging recommendations of the American Joint Committee on Cancer (AJCC) and the International Union Against Cancer (UICC) are included; however, the international system contains new elements that resolve staging problems not met by prior staging systems. Newly defined categories for specific levels of extrapulmonary extension and regional lymph node involvement, along with new stage grouping rules, provide for classification of 21 TNM levels of disease progression that are combined in five stage groups. Each stage has generally similar expectations for survival and options for therapy. As we apply the new system, the limitations of a workable classification must be kept in mind. In practice, we can use only a classification that discriminates the majority of patients within a definable subgroup; otherwise, we will become involved in a hopelessly complex and unmanageable number of subcategories.

The following article, reproduced with permission from *Chest,* volume 89, pp. 225S–233S, April 1986 (supplement), describes and illustrates the new international staging system. A selection of pertinent publications that have appeared since this paper was written can be found following the article.

A NEW INTERNATIONAL STAGING SYSTEM FOR LUNG CANCER*

Clifton F. Mountain, M.D., F.C.C.P.

Staging of lung cancer according to the TNM system is an accepted principle used by oncologists as a guide to estimating prognosis and selecting treatment in a given patient and for reporting end results. The two most widely used recommendations for TNM classification are those of the American Joint Committee on Cancer (AJCC)[1–3] and the Union Internationale Contre Cancer (UICC).[4] As investigators throughout the world have put these staging systems to work, the need for refinements to meet their individual practices has resulted in variations in the use of the classifications. A proposal now is made for a new and universal staging system for lung cancer that is acceptable to the international community charged with the responsibility for unifying staging systems (see Appendix).

THE TNM SYSTEM

The TNM system, as originally proposed by Denoix,[5] provides a consistent, reproducible description for the anatomic extent of disease in cancer patients at a specific time in the life history of the cancer. Clinical staging is the best estimate of disease extent made prior to the institution of any therapy; surgical-pathologic staging is the classification of disease extent as determined from pathologic examination of resected specimens. The letter "T" represents the primary tumor and numerical suffixes describe increasing size and involvement or both. The "N" category represents regional lymph nodes with appropriate suffixes to describe levels of metastatic disease. The letter "M" represents distant metastasis with appropriate suffixes to describe the absence or presence of metastasis to distant sites. The various TNM subsets thus classified are then grouped into a small number of stages of disease so that patients in each stage group have a similar life expectancy.

Focus of Problem Areas

To present the new international staging proposal in a meaningful context, I would like to discuss the problems with present systems and some of the data used to propose solutions. I collected and studied variations in the use of the TNM system that have been reported in the literature and expressed in letters and recommendations of various groups of treatment specialists. A new data base of contemporary case records of lung cancer patients was assembled to examine some of the questions raised by the variations study.

Methods. The data base for the classification research project consisted of 3,753 patient records and is described in Table 1. All patients were at risk at least 24 months, and follow-up was complete through December 1984. Survival curves were generated according to the method of Gehan.[6–8] Zero time was the date of first treatment. Operative deaths are excluded. The terminal event is death from cancer or unknown cause.

Table 1—***New Stage Data Base for Classification Research 1975–82***

University of Texas M.D. Anderson Hospital*	2,749
Reference Center for Anatomic and Pathologic Classification of Lung Cancer†	1,004
Total cases	3,753

*Consecutive patients treated for primary lung canc[er] 1975–80; surgical patients only 1981–82.

†Patients treated for primary lung cancer b[y] National Cancer Institute cooperative Lung [Cancer] Study Group—representative slide material a[nd] documentation submitted to the Reference Ce[nter for] Anatomic and Pathologic Classification of Lung [Cancer] for confirmation of staging and histology 1977-

*From the Department of Thoracic Surgery, The University of Texas System Cancer Center, M. D. Anderson Hospital and Tumor Institute, Houston.

This project was supported by the following organization, foundations, private donors, and government agencies: American Joint Committee on Cancer, Hawn Foundation of Texas, Herman Neel Hipp Fund for Research in Thoracic Surgery, Kelsey-Seybold Foundation grant 996, National Cancer Institute Division of Cancer Treatment (contract CA 34503 Reference Center for Anatomic and Pathologic Classification of Lung Cancer of the Lung Cancer Study Group), Private Donors Fund for Research in Thoracic Surgery (Department of Thoracic Surgery, University of Texas System Cancer Center M. D. Anderson Hospital).

Stage Grouping. A number of end-results reports suggest that the present stage grouping of TNM subsets includes wide variation in survival characteristics.[9-11] The end results for patients with T1 N0 M0 tumors—70-85% expected to survive 5 years—have prompted many to question whether such tumors should be assigned to a separate stage group. One of the major differences in the two most widely used staging systems is the assignment of T1 N1 tumors. The experience of the Japanese Cancer Committee,[12] which represents a carefully classified data base, suggests that the outcome for patients with T1 N1 tumors more closely resembles the survival pattern of patients with stage II lung cancer than that of the other stage I subsets. The surgical oncologists have identified specific groups of patients with stage III-M0 disease who have a superior prognosis compared with those with stage III-M0 tumors that are not operable.[13-15]

It is common among treatment specialists to subdivide stage III disease into "limited" or "extensive" categories, but there are notable inconsistencies in the use of these terms. The need for greater specificity for these groups of patients has been emphasized, particularly by medical oncologists treating patients with undifferentiated small cell lung cancer.[16]

The present UICC staging recommendations designated all distant metastasis as stage IV, whereas in the AJCC recommendations, patients with M1 disease are classified as stage III. There is no problem with modifying the AJCC rules to include a stage IV classification for all distant metastatic disease; however, the question of whether to assign patients with supraclavicular or scalene lymph mode metastasis to a stage III or stage IV group remains to be answered.

Our starting point for examining the questions regarding stage grouping was to examine the survival characteristics of each TNM subset classified according to present recommendations of the AJCC for clinical and surgical staging and to review the differences overall and for each cell type. The cumulative proportion of patients expected to survive 5 years and the median survival time for each of the clinical and surgical TNM subsets are shown in Table 2. The ordering of the end results and similarities and statistically significant differences in outcome between the subsets indicate that a number of stage groupings are rational for combining patients with similar prognoses. The present recommendations still work very well for identifying 3 or 4 stage groups, each with a unique survival pattern. There are several other ways[17] that the TNM subsets can be combined that will provide 3, 4, or even 5 stages of disease with significantly different survival rates; however, these proposals make no attempt to meet the needs of treatment specialists for staging that is consistent with contemporary treatment planning as well as for estimating prognosis.

TNM Descriptors

We found that classification problems with the TNM categories were related to the T3 descriptor for extrapulmonary, but intrathoracic, primary tumors; to the N2 descriptor for mediastinal lymph node metastasis, and to the M1 descriptor for distant metastasis.

T3 Descriptor. The current definition for T3 is "a tumor of any size with direct extension into an adjacent structure such as the parietal pleura or chest wall, the diaphragm, or the mediastinum and its contents; or a tumor demonstrable bronchoscopically to involve a main bronchus less than 2.0 cm distal to the carina; or any tumor associated with atelectasis or obstructive pneumonitis of an entire lung or pleural effusion." This definition encompasses a broad spectrum of primary tumors with varying degrees of extrapulmonary extension.

The clinical staging system for lung cancer proposed by the Radiation Therapy Oncology Group (RTOG) in the United States (personal communication, G. Seydel, April 1985) provides for sep-

Table 2–***Cumulative Percentage Surviving Five Years and Median Survival by Clinical and Surgical TNM Subsets (1979 AJCC Definitions)***

TNM Subset			Clinical No.	Clinical % Surviving	Clinical Median Survival, mo.	Surgical No.	Surgical % Surviving	Surgical Median Survival, mo.
T1	N0	M0	591	61.9	60+	429	68.5	60+
T2	N0	M0	1,012	35.8	26	436	59.0	60+
T1	N1	M0	19	33.6	20	67	54.1	60+
T2	N1	M0	176	22.7	17	260	40.0	29
T3	N0	M0	221	7.6	8	57	44.2	26
T3	N1	M0	71	7.7	8	29	17.6	16
Any	N2	M0	497	4.9	11	168	28.8	22
Any	M1		1,166	1.7	6	—	—	—
Total			3,753			1,436		

aration of lung tumors with extrapulmonary extension into two categories—one for whom local control by radiation therapy is feasible and another with extensive intrathoracic spread in whom palliation is the only treatment objective. These categories are further subdivided by the RTOG into specific subsets of patients according to technical factors of treatment planning.

The surgical oncologists have identified patients with T3 tumors who are candidates for complete resection and thus have the potential for an improved survival compared with inoperable patients in this category. These tumors are (1) peripheral tumors invading the chest wall, (2) tumors with direct extension to involve the mediastinum or pericardium, (3) superior sulcus tumors in patients with no true Pancoast's syndrome, and (4) tumors involving the proximal main bronchus and carina that are amenable to tracheobronchial or sleeve resection.[18]

N2 Descriptor. Mediastinal lymph node metastasis, whether ipsilateral or contralateral, is classified N2 in present systems. Within this N2 group, selected patients with metastasis limited to the ipsilateral mediastinal lymph nodes may undergo complete resection. A far better outcome is anticipated for such patients than for those with more extensive mediastinal metastasis, which obviates consideration for surgical treatment.

M1 Descriptor. The supraclavicular and contralateral hilar lymph nodes are classified as M1 disease in current recommendations. These lymph nodes are usually included in the field of irradiation treatment. They are considered regional by the radiation oncologist and are not approached by them in the same manner as disseminated disease.[19] The prognoses for patients with contralateral mediastinal lymph node involvement fall with this group. The contralateral mediastinal lymph nodes are included in the regional treatment field of radiotherapy with the contralateral hilum and supraclavicular nodes, so there is sound logic for assigning all of these groups to an N3 designation.

Table 3–*TNM Definitions*

	Primary Tumor (T)
TX	Tumor proven by the presence of malignant cells in bronchopulmonary secretions but not visualized roentgenographically or bronchoscopically, or any tumor that cannot be assessed as in a retreatment staging.
T0	No evidence of primary tumor.
TIS	Carcinoma *in situ*
T1	A tumor that is 3.0 cm or less in greatest dimension, surrounded by lung or visceral pleura, and without evidence of invasion proximal to a lobar bronchus at bronchoscopy.*
T2	A tumor more than 3.0 cm in greatest dimension, or a tumor of any size that either invades the visceral pleura or has associated atelectasis or obstructive pneumonitis extending to the hilar region. At bronchoscopy, the proximal extent of demonstrable tumor must be within a lobar bronchus or at least 2.0 cm distal to the carina. Any associated atelectasis or obstructive pneumonitis must involved less than an entire lung.
T3	A tumor of any size with direct extension into the chest wall (including superior sulcus tumors), diaphragm, or the mediastinal pleura or pericardium without involving the heart, great vessels, trachea, esophagus or vertebral body, or a tumor in the main bronchus within 2 cm of the carina without involving the carina.
T4	A tumor of any size with invasion of the mediastinum or involving heart, great vessels, trachea, esophagus, vertebral body or carcina or presence of malignant pleural effusion.*

*See Table 6

THE NEW INTERNATIONAL STAGING SYSTEM FOR LUNG CANCER

We have derived a new nomenclature for staging lung cancer that retains the valid and useful components of current systems and has new elements to meet the needs of treatment specialists for classification relating to therapeutic options—as well as for estimating prognosis.

International Agreement

Members of the Task Force on the Lung of the AJCC made their evaluation of my data and recommendations, along with their own end results and the end results of others,[20–22] and the proposals made by the international TNM study committees of the UICC with specific recommendations from Japan and Germany. This group then made recommendations for modifications of the AJCC staging system for lung cancer to be consistent with international objectives (see appendix). The UICC groups made their recommendations for modification of that nomenclature, and the proposal shown in Tables 3 to 7 was agreed on by all of the international representatives (see appendix).

Table 4–*TNM Definitions*

	Nodal Involvement (N)
N0	No demonstrable metastasis to regional lymph nodes.
N1	Metastasis to lymph nodes in the peribronchial or the ipsilateral hilar region, or both, including direct extension.
N2	Metastasis to ipsilateral mediastinal lymph nodes and subcarinal lymph nodes.
N3	Metastasis to contralateral mediastinal lymph nodes, contralateral hilar lymph nodes, ipsilateral or contralateral scalene or supraclavicular lymph nodes.

Table 5–*TNM Definitions*

Distant Metastasis (M)	
M0	No (known) distant metastasis
M1	Distant metastasis present—Specify Site(s)

TNM Definitions

The new definitions for the TNM categories are shown in Tables 3 to 6, and selected new elements are illustrated in Figures 1 to 6.

T—Primary Tumor. The descriptors for the primary tumor provide for classification of 4 distinct levels of tumor progression that have different implications for treatment selection and prognosis, depending on the status of the regional lymph nodes and the presence or absence of distant metastasis. The *T1* designation is assigned to those small tumors with no invasion proximal to a lobar bronchus and no involvement of the pleura. To aid in the classification of the uncommon superficial tumor with the invasive component limited to the bronchial wall, which may spread along the main bronchus, the footnote shown in Table 6 has been added to the definitions. The *T2* classification is assigned to tumors larger than 3 cm or those involving the visceral pleura or main bronchus, regardless of size, and those with atelectasis or obstructive pneumonitis extending to the hilar region. Tumors with limited, circumscribed, extrapulmonary extension involving the chest wall, the proximal main bronchus, mediastinal pleura or pericardium are assigned to the *T3* category (Fig 1). Included are tumors originating in the superior sulcus that have no accompanying Pancoast's syndrome or invasion of the vertebral body (Fig 2). *T4* defines those tumors with extensive extrapulmonary extension involving the mediastinum, major vessels, nerves, or, in the case of Pancoast's tumors, the vertebral body (Figs. 3 and 4). To aid in the classification of pleural effusion a footnote has been added to the definitions regarding the implications of pleural fluid as a

Table 6–*TNM Definitions*

Footnote to TNM Definitions	
T1*	The uncommon superficial tumor of any size with its invasive component limited to the bronchial wall which may extend proximal to the main bronchus is classified as T1.
T4*	Most pleural effusions associated with lung cancer are due to tumor. There are, however, some few patients in whom cytopathological examination of pleural fluid (on more than one specimen) is negative for tumor, the fluid is nonbloody and is not an exudate. In such cases where these elements and clinical judgment dictate that the effusion is not related to the tumor, the patients should be staged T1, T2 or T3, excluding effusion as a staging element.

Table 7–*Stage Grouping of TNM Subsets*

	Stage Grouping		
Occult Carcinoma	TX	N0	M0
Stage 0	TIS	Carcinoma in situ	
Stage I	T1	N0	M0
	T2	N0	M0
Stage II	T1	N1	M0
	T2	N1	M0
Stage IIIa	T3	N0	M0
	T3	N1	M0
	T1-3	N2	M0
Stage IIIb	Any T	N3	M0
	T4	Any N	M0
Stage IV	Any T	Any N	M1

staging element. Pleural effusion in patients with lung cancer is usually related to the malignancy and is a poor prognostic sign; however, in a few patients cytopathologic examination of pleural fluid—on more than one specimen—is negative for tumor, is nonbloody, and is not an exudate. If these elements and clinical judgment dictate that the effusion is not related to the tumor, the patient should be staged T1, T2, or T3, excluding effusion as a staging element. Patients with malignant pleural effusion, as determined clinically or from cytologic examination of the fluid, are classified as *T4*.

N—Regional Lymph Nodes. Involvement of the intrapulmonary lymph nodes by direct extension or metastasis is classified as *N1*. Metastasis to the ipsilateral mediastinal lymph nodes and subcarinal nodes is designated *N2* in the new definitions (Fig. 5). Metastasis to the contralateral mediastinal nodes, contralateral hilum, or ipsilateral and contralateral supraclavicular or scalene lymph nodes is classified as *N3* (Fig. 6). Although the prognosis for patients with supraclavicular lymph node metastasis was not found to be markedly superior to those with other M1 disease, particularly that of single sites, the *N3* designation is rational for treatment planning. Also, this designation provides for separate stage groupings for patients with "limited" and "extensive" disease.

M—Distant Metastasis. The designation for dissemination of tumor to distant metastatic sites is *M1*.

Stage Grouping

Stage grouping of the TNM subsets is shown in Table 7. The new international proposal for staging excludes tumors with lymph node metastasis from *stage I disease* (Fig. 7). The deleterious effect on prognosis of lymph node metastasis has been shown in many studies, such as those of the Japanese Cancer Committee[13] and the Sloan-Ket-

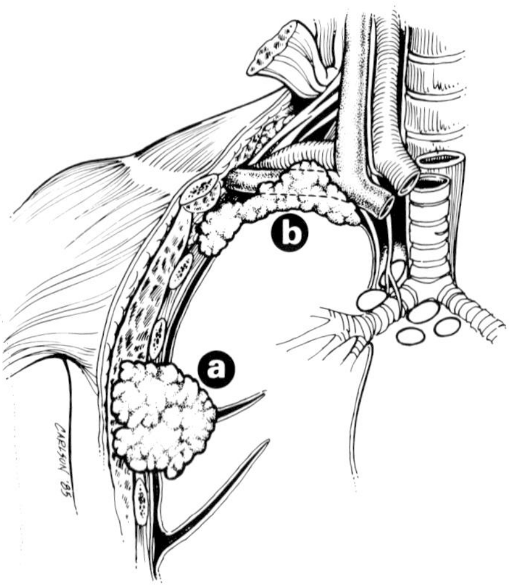

T3

A tumor of any size with direct extension into the (a) chest wall (b) (including superior sulcus tumors), diaphragm or the mediastinal pleura or pericardium, without involving the heart, great vessels, trachea, esophagus or vertebral body, or a tumor in the main bronchus within 2 cm. of the carina without involving the carina.

Figure 1. T3: A tumor of any size with direct extension into the *(a)* chest wall *(b)* including superior sulcus tumors.

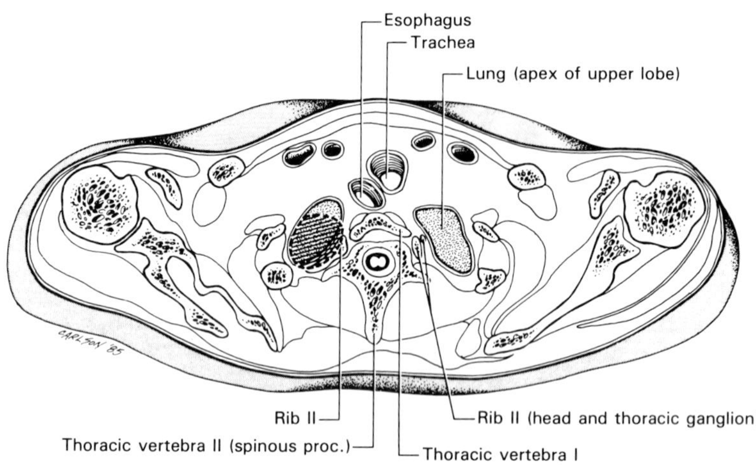

Figure 2. T3: Superior sulcus tumor with no involvement of the vertebral body.

T3 A tumor of any size with direct extension into the chest wall (including superior sulcus tumors)....without involving the vertebral body.

Superior Vena Cava Syndrome

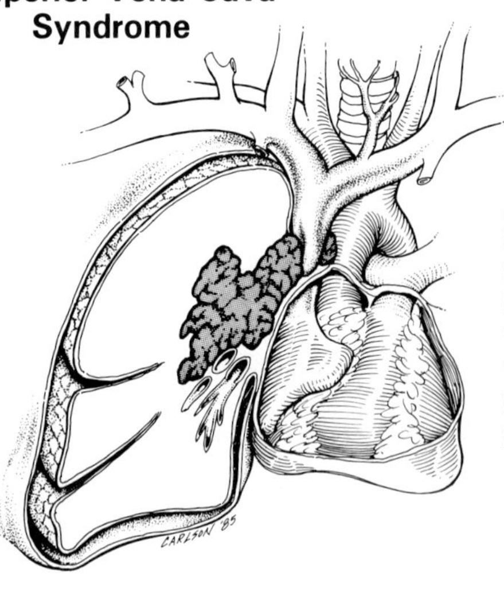

T4

A tumor of any size with invasion of the mediastinum, or involving heart, great vessels, trachea, esophagus, vertebral body or carina or presence of malignant pleural effusion.

Figure 3. T4: Superior vena cava syndrome—tumor involving great vessels.

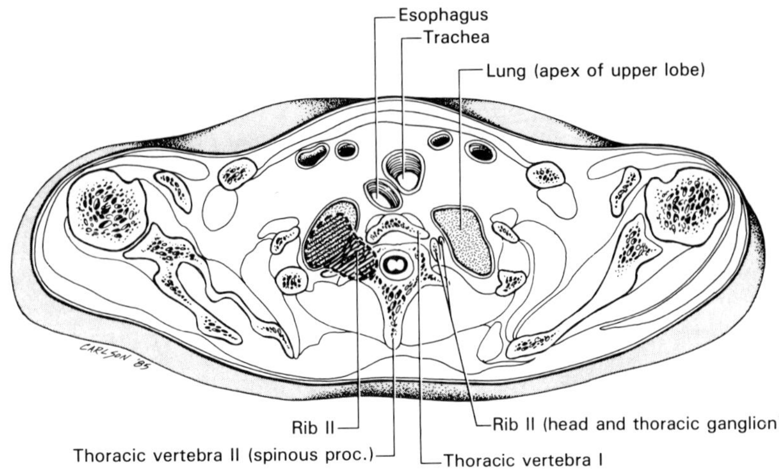

Figure 4. T4: Tumor invading the vertebral body—unresectable, produces Pancoast's syndrome.

T4 A tumor of any size with invasion of the vertebral body (unresectable - true Pancoast's Syndrome).

N2 -

Involvement of ipsilateral mediastinal and/or subcarinal lymph nodes

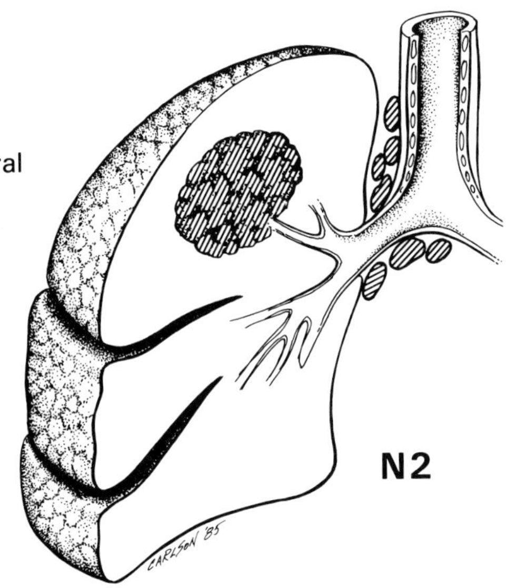

Figure 5. N2: Involvement of ipsilateral mediastinal and/or subcarinal lymph nodes.

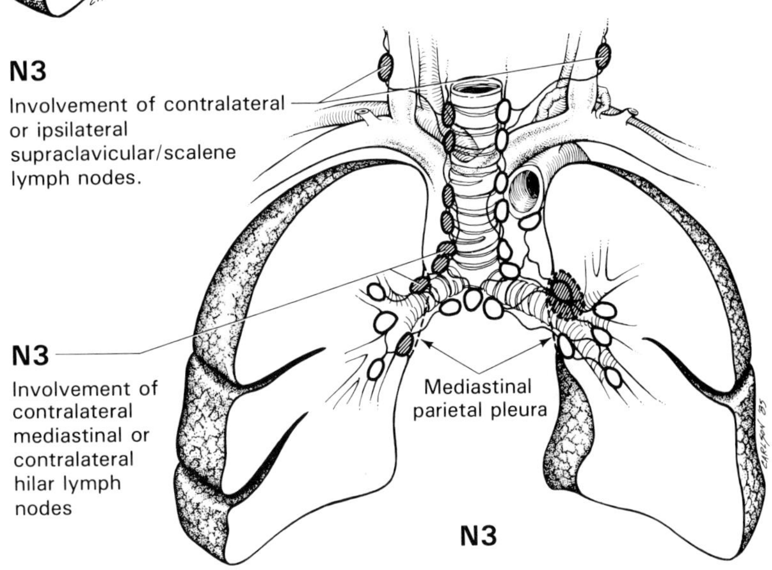

Figure 6. N3: Involvement of contralateral or ipsilateral scalene or supraclavicular lymph nodes; contralateral mediastinal or contralateral hilar lymph nodes.

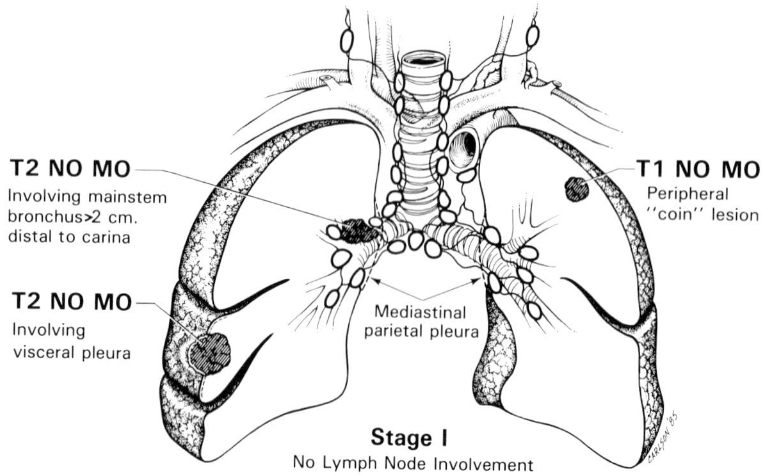

Figure 7. Stage I disease.

tering Cancer Center.[22] In our own studies, intrapulmonary metastasis was particularly unfavorable in patients with adenocarcinoma.

Stage II lung cancer includes all patients with T1 and T2 tumors with metastasis to the peribronchial, lobar, and hilar lymph nodes, including those involved by direct extension. The new stage grouping rules specify the T1 N1 and T2 N1 subsets as *stage II* disease (Fig. 8).

Stage III disease is subdivided into *stage IIIa* and *IIIb* categories. Patients with T2 N0 or N1 disease and those with T1-3 primary tumors with metastasis limited to the ipsilateral mediastinal and subcarinal lymph nodes are classified as having *stage IIIa* disease (Fig. 9). The new staging nomenclature specifies that *stage IIIb* disease include patients with extensive extrapulmonary tumors, T4, that have no distant metastasis. Patients with metastasis to the contralateral mediastinal and hilar nodes or the supraclavicular or scalene lymph nodes, whether ipsilateral or contralateral, or both are classified as having *stage IIIb* disease. This stage group includes patients with the T4 component and any N value or with an N3 component and any T value (Fig. 10). Patients classified as having *stage IIIa* or *stage IIIb* disease have no distant metastasis. Only patients with distant metastasis are classified *stage IV*.

End Results According to the New Staging Proposal

When the TNM definitions and stage grouping rules are applied to a large contemporary data base, the end results shown in Fig. 11 are obtained. These survival patterns are derived from clinical estimates of disease extent. Each stage has a unique survival experience and relationship to treatment planning. Patients with clinical stage I, II, or IIIa non-small cell lung cancer usually are candidates for definitive surgical treatment, and those with stage IIIB and stage IV disease are generally assigned to radiotherapy, chemother-

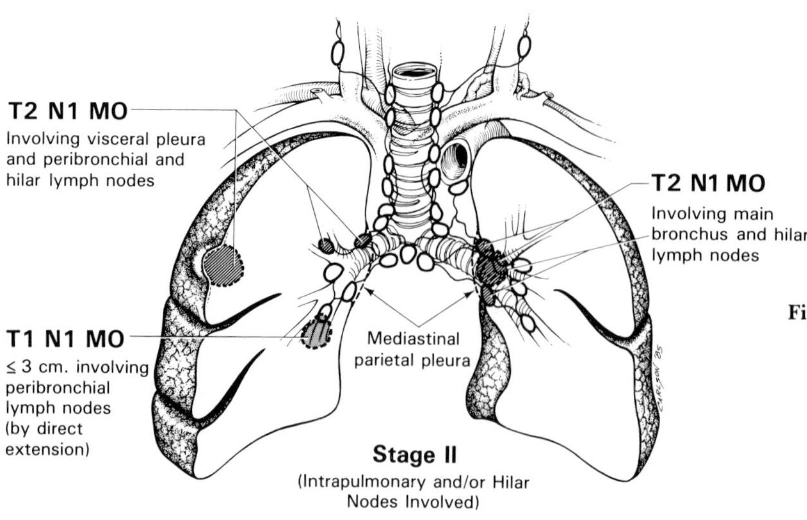

Figure 8. Stage II disease.

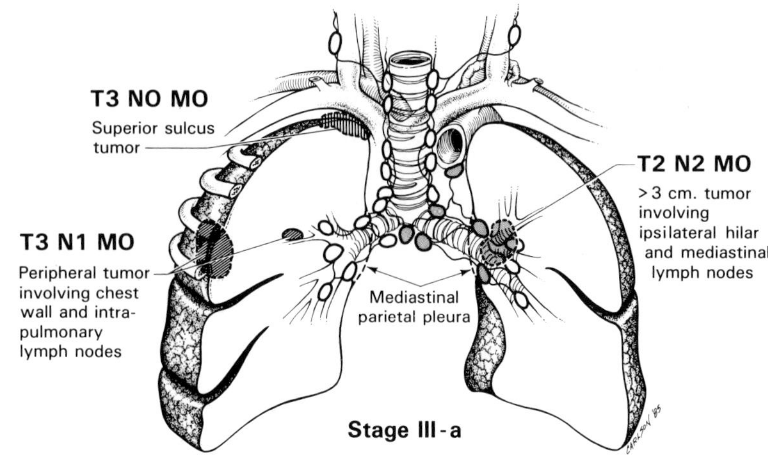

Figure 9. Stage IIIa disease.

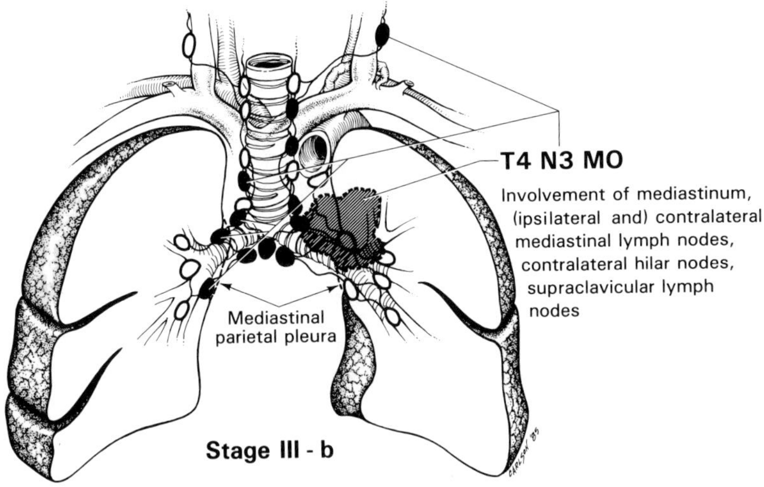

Figure 10. Stage IIIb disease.

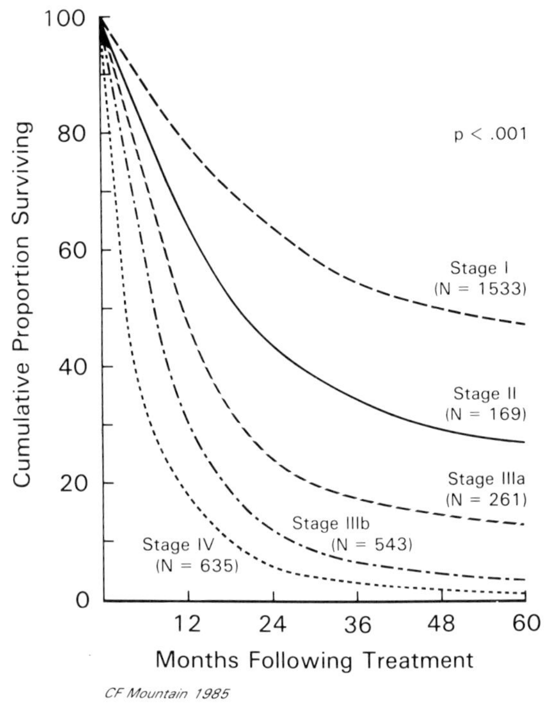

Figure 11. Cumulative proportion of patients surviving 5 years by clinical stage of disease.

apy, or combined modalities. Chemotherapy or combined programs are usually the treatment of choice for patients with undifferentiated small cell carcinoma, regardless of stage; however, the proportion of patients expected to achieve the complete response necessary for long-term survival varies with the stage of disease. The treatment regimen is related to the stage classification of small cell tumors just as it is for stage IIIb or IV non-small cell lung cancer.

CONCLUSION

The new international proposal for stating lung cancer has five stages of disease, including a *Stage 0,* that provide for the classification of six groups of patients who have similar prognostic expectations and therapeutic options. *Stage I* includes only patients with the best prognostic expectations—those with T1 or T2 tumors and no evidence of metastasis. *Stage II* disease includes those patients with a primary tumor classification of T1 or T2 metastasis to the intrapulmonary (including hilar) lymph nodes. *Stage IIIa* disease designates those patients, usually within the realm of the surgical oncologist, with extrapulmonary extension of the primary tumor and/or ipsilateral mediastinal lymph node metastasis. *Stage IIIb* includes patients with more extensive extrapulmonary involvement than in the potentially operable group, those having malignant pleural effusion and those with metastasis to the contralateral mediastinum, hilum, or supraclavicular and scalene lymph nodes. *Stage IV* disease is reserved for patients with metastasis to distant sites.

These new recommendations for staging fill the need for specific definitions for "limited" and "extensive" disease that can be reproduced and compared. Further, they meet the goal of modifying present classifications to provide a universal, single staging system for lung cancer that is responsive to the needs of all those involved in the treatment and study of lung cancer.

Appendix

Meeting for Unification of Staging Definitions
Hawaii, December 6–7, 1985

AJCC Representatives:
Harvey Baker, M.D., Chairman AJCC
David Bragg, M.D.
Robert V. P. Hutter, M.D.
B. J. Kennedy, M.D.
Clifton F. Mountain, M.D.
Elliot Strong, M.D.
Madelyn A. Murray, staff

UICC Representatives:
Leslie Sobin, M.D., Chairman, TNM Committee
Arnold Levine, M.D.
Japanese Cancer Committee
Heizaburo Ichikawa, M.D., Head of delegation
Toshifumi Iizuka, M.D.
Takeshi Iwanga, M.D.
Keiichi Maruyama, M.D.
Kasakazu Maruyama, M.D.
Kiyoshi Miwa, M.D.
Tsuguo Naruke, M.D.
Mitsumasa Nishi, M.D.
Yukio Ohmori, M.D.
Isamu Ono, M.D.
Sunichi Sakai, M.D.

American Joint Committee Task Force on Lung Staging Revision Meeting—Houston, Texas, March 30, 1985

Clifton F. Mountain, M.D., Chairman
David T. Carr, M.D.
Nael Martini, M.D.
Frederick P. Stitik, M.D.

Reviewed Recommendations:
Herbert Derman, M.D.
Willis J. Taylor, M.D.

UICC Annual Meeting–Geneva, April 20, 1986

Robert V. P. Hutter, M.D., transmitted recommendations of the American Joint Committee for consideration of the UICC.

Final Liaison Meeting–Stockholm, June 19, 1986

AJCC Representatives:
Harvey Baker, M.D.
Robert V. P. Hutter, M.D.
Clifton F. Mountain, M.D.
Donald E. Henson, M.D.

UICC Representatives:
Leslie Sobin, M.D.
Arnold Levine, M.D.
German TNM Committee:
Walter C. Reiner, M.D.
Paul Hermanek, M. D.
Japanese TNM Committee:
Heizaburo Ichikawa, M.D.

ACKNOWLEDGMENT: The author wishes to acknowledge the substantial contributions of Kay E. Hermes, Senior Research Assistant, Department of Thoracic Surgery, to the research and writing of this report, and of Anne Murphy, Assistant Epidemiologist, Department of Thoracic Surgery, for data management and programming.

REFERENCES

1. American Joint Committee on Cancer, Task Force on Lung. Staging of Lung Cancer 1979. Chicago: American Joint Committee on Cancer, 1979
2. Mountain CF, Carr DT, Anderson WAD. A system for the clinical staging of lung cancer. AJR 1974; 120:130-38
3. Carr DT, Mountain CF. The staging of lung cancer. Semin Oncol 1974; 1:229-34
4. Harmer EM. TNM Classification of malignant tumors. Geneva: Union Internationale Contre le Cancer, 1978:41-45
5. Denoix PF. Enquete permanent dans les centres anticancereux. Bull Inst Nat Hyg 1946; 1:70-75
6. Gehan EA. Statistical methods for survival time studies. In: Staquet MJ, ed. Cancer therapy, prognostic factors and criteria of response. New York: Raven Press, 1975:7:35

7. Smith T, Putnam JE, Gehan E. A computer program for estimating survival functions for the life table. Comput Prog Biomed 1970; 1:58-64
8. Lee E, Desu M. A computer program for comparing K samples with right-censored data. Comput Prog Biomed 1972; 2:315-21
9. Melamed MR, Flehinger BJ, Zaman MB, Heelan RT, Hallerman ET, Martini N. Detection of true pathologic stage I lung in a screening program and the effect on survival. Cancer 1981; 47:1182-87
10. Williams DE, Pairolero PC, Davis CS, et al. Survival of patients surgically treated for stage I lung cancer. J Thorac Cardiovasc Surg 1981; 82:70-76
11. Mountain CF, Gail MH. Surgical adjuvant intrapleural BCG treatment for stage I non-small cell lung cancer: preliminary report of the National Cancer Institute Lung Cancer Study Group. J Thorac Cardiovasc Surg 1981; 82:649-57
12. Ishikawa S. Staging system on TNM classification for lung cancer. Jpn J Clin Oncol 1973; 6:19-30
13. Gilbert A, Deslauriers J, McLish A, Piraux M. Tracheal sleeve pneumonectomy for carcinoma of the proximal left main bronchus. Can J Surg 1984; 27:583-85
14. Naruke T, Suemasu K, Ishikawa S. Lymph node mapping and curability at various levels of metastasis in resected lung cancer. J Thorac Cardiovasc Surg 1978; 76:832-39
15. Patterson GA, Ilves R, Ginsberg RJ, Cooper JD, Todd TRJ, Pearson FG. The value of adjuvant radiotherapy in pulmonary and chest wall resection for bronchogenic carcinoma. Ann Thorac Surg 1982; 34:692-97
16. Bunn PA Jr, Cohen MH, Ihde DC, Fossieck BE, Matthews MJ, Minna JD. Advances in small cell bronchogenic carcinoma. Commentary. Cancer Treat Rep 1977; 61:333-42
17. Yoshimura K. A clinical statistical study of lung cancer patients in Japan with special reference to the staging system of TNM classification: a report from the Japan Joint Committee of Lung Cancer associated with the TNM system of clinical classification (UICC). Radiat Med 1983; 1:186-95
18. Mountain CF. The biologic operability of stage III non-small cell lung cancer. Ann Thorac Surg 1985; 40:60-64
19. Cox JD. Radiotherapeutic management of complications of carcinoma of the lung. Clin Chest Med 1982; 3:415-20
20. Piehler JM, Pairolero PC, Weiland LH, Offord KP, Payne WP, Bernatz PE. Bronchogenic carcinoma with chest wall invasion: factors affecting survival following en bloc resection. Ann Thorac Surg 1985; 40:60-64
21. Martini N, Flehinger BJ, Zaman MB, Beattie EJ Jr. Results of resection in non-oat cell carcinoma of the lung with mediastinal lymph node metastases. Ann Surg 1983; 198:386-97
22. McCaughan BC, Martini N, Bains MS, McCormack PM. Chest wall invasion in carcinoma of the lung: therapeutic and prognostic implications. J Thorac Cardiovasc Surg 1985; 89:836-41
23. Martini N, Flehinger BJ, Nagasaki F, Hart B. Prognostic significance of N1 disease in carcinoma of the lung. J Thorac Cardiovasc Surg 1983; 86:646-53

ADDITIONAL REFERENCES ON LUNG CANCER STAGING

Aisner J, Whitley NO: Current staging of lung cancer: An overview of current and newer approaches. In Hansen HH (ed): Basic and Clinical Concepts of Lung Cancer, p 183. Boston, Kluwer Academic Publishers, 1989.

This update of some of the current approaches to the pretreatment assessment of patients with lung cancer puts emphasis on both standard staging and newer techniques. Small cell and non–small cell carcinomas are discussed separately. The authors provide 97 references.

Byhardt RW, Hartz A, Libnoch JA et al: Prognostic influence of TNM staging and LDH levels in small cell carcinoma of the lung. Int J Radiat Oncol Biol Phys 12:771, 1986.

An expanded TNM type staging system was investigated in a series of 73 patients with small cell lung cancer. A clear statistical advantage for predicting chemotherapy response or survival could not be shown, but trends suggested that the TNM system could divide patients into three prognostic subgroups. Higher serum lactic acid dehydrogenase levels were seen with more extensive tumor, and they predicted poorer responses to chemotherapy and lower survival within similar stage subgroups compared with patients with normal lactic acid dehydrogenase levels.

Kayser K, Bulzebruck H, Probst G et al.: Retrospective and prospective tumor staging evaluating prognostic factors in operated bronchus carcinoma patients. Cancer 59:355, 1987.

A retrospective study was conducted on a series of 1,332 patients with potentially curative resections of lung carcinoma; 282 patients were included in a prospective study. Cell type and relative frequency of T1 stage were similar in the two groups. Major differences were obtained in relative frequencies of T3, N0, N1, and N2, and the authors suggest that T1 N1 and T2 N1 tumors should be stage II.

Little AG, DeMeester TR, Ferguson MK et al: Modified stage I (T1 N0 M0, T2 N0 M0) non–small cell lung cancer: Treatment results, recurrence patterns, and adjuvant immunotherapy. Surgery 100:621, 1986.

Among 96 surgical patients with T1 or T2 (N0 M0) non–small cell carcinomas, the overall 5-year survival was 70%. Disease recurred in 9.1% of T1 N0 patients versus 23.4% of T2 N0 patients. Survival of T1 N0 and T2 N0 patients was 72.1% and 68.3%, respectively, and survival was not affected by type of surgery, cell type, sex, age, or race.

Mountain CF: The New International Staging System for Lung Cancer. Surg Clin North Am 67:925, 1987.

The stage I and stage II definitions provide for classification of two levels of disease extent completely contained within the lung that have different prognostic and therapeutic implications. Definitive resection is the first therapeutic choice for patients with non–small cell lung carcinoma in these two groups. The stage II category takes into account the erosion of survival expectations in the optimum group of T1 and T2 patients as a consequence of intrapulmonary lymph node involvement. Small cell carcinoma is infrequently encountered in stage I and stage II disease, but the classification may be useful in the structure of investigational programs involving adjuvant surgery. The exclusion of distant metastases and the division of stage III into two levels of extrapulmonary disease allow for selection of patients for specific treatment plans. Patients with stage IIIA non–small cell carcinoma are usually candidates for definitive surgical treatment. The specificity of the T and N definitions in the stage IIIA and IIIB categories identifies patients for whom particular radiation therapy treatment plans are structured and protocol assignments are made.

Mountain CF: Prognostic implications of the International Staging System for Lung Cancer. Semin Oncol 15:236, 1988.

The new nomenclature is sufficiently uncomplicated to be applicable in environments at all levels of sophistication yet is sufficiently specific for use by the research community. The prognostic implications of each category are a reflection of the relationship between extent of disease and the potential for cure of available therapies.

Mountain CF, Lukeman JM, Hammar SP et al: Lung cancer classification: The relationship of disease extent and cell type to survival in a clinical trials population. J Surg Oncol 35:147, 1987.

Survival characteristics were generated for 1,121 patients who underwent complete resection of non–small cell lung cancer and subsequently were entered into protocols to receive either adjuvant treatment or no further therapy. Patients with squamous cell carcinoma had an outcome superior to that of patients with adenocarcinoma in every TNM subset. The differences in survival according to these major cell types were significant overall and in the T1 NO, T1 N1, and T2 N1 subsets, but not in the TNM subsets in stage III disease.

Naruke T, Goya T, Tsuchiya R et al: Prognosis and survival in resected lung carcinoma based on the new international staging system. J Thorac Cardiovasc Surg 96:440, 1988.

The review includes 1,737 Japanese patients who underwent pulmonary resection for lung cancer: 3 patients had occult carcinoma; 821 had stage I; 248, stage II; 465, stage IIIA; 82, stage IIIB; and 118, stage IV. Five-year survival figures were stage I, 50.1%; stage II, 31.2%; stage IIIA, 20.2%; stage IIIB, 5.1%; and stage IV, 7.9%. Based on postoperative staging, the numbers of patients in each group and their 5-year survival figures were stage 0,4; stage I, 536, 65.0%; stage II, 221, 42.9%; stage IIIA, 559, 22.2%; stage IIIB, 159, 5.6%; and stage IV, 258, 7.5%. In both clinical and postoperative stages, prognostic differences were significant between stages I and II, II and IIIA, and IIIA and IIIB, but not between IIIB and IV.

Plaja S, Puccia V, Russo A et al: Carcinoma of the lung, stage III: Experience with the new TNM-AJCC classification. Scand J Thorac Cardiovasc Surg 22:139, 1988.

One hundred fifteen patients (94 men, 21 women) with stage III disease among 228 resections were retrospectively analyzed. Stage IIIA disease was present at operation in 87 cases, and stage IIIB was evident in 28 cases. Actuarial analysis of survival rates showed that the subclassification of stage III disease permits identification of those patients who may benefit from surgical therapy.

Roeslin N, Chalkiadakis G, Dumont P et al: A better prognostic value from a modification of lung cancer staging. J Thorac Cardiovasc Surg 94:504, 1987.

Among 538 post-resection patients, 279 had stage I disease; 113, stage II; and 146, stage III. Overall survival rates were 72% at 1 year, 54% at 2 years, 47% at 3 years, 43% at 4 years, and 39% at 5 years. The survival curves of the three stages were significantly different. The 5-year survival of 71% for stage I, T1 N0 tumors differed significantly from those of all other groups. Survival curves for stage II tumors differed according to a hilar or lobar location of N1. The survival rate of T2 N1 hilar tumors was similar to that of T2 N2 tumors. In stage 3, survival of T3 N2 tumors was the worst of all classifications. Recommended changes in the staging system include the following. Stage II can comprise T2 N0, T1 N1 lobar, and T2 N1 lobar. Stage III or IIIA would comprise T2 N1 hilar, T1 N2, T2 N2, and perhaps T3 N0 and T3 N1. T3 N2 should probably be isolated in a IIIB or IV stage.

Sobin LH, Hermanek P, Hutter RV: TNM classification of malignant tumors: A comparison between the new (1987) and the old editions. Cancer 61:2310, 1988.

The major revision of the TNM classification eliminates previous differences between the versions of the International Union Against Cancer (UICC) and American Joint Committee on Cancer (AJCC). It also updates existing site classifications and includes previously unclassified tumors.

Vincent MD, Ashley SE, Smith IE: Prognostic factors in small cell lung cancer: A simple prognostic index is better than conventional staging. Eur J Cancer Clin Oncol 23:1589, 1987.

In a study of 333 consecutive patients, possible prognostic factors for small cell carcinoma were analyzed. The combination of clinical performance status and serum albumin and serum alanine transaminase levels defined three groups (good, medium, poor) of better prognostic significance (survival at 1 year 50%, 27%, 3%) than conventional limited/extensive disease staging (survival at 1 year 48%/18%).

Chapter

3

FINE-NEEDLE ASPIRATION BIOPSY

The first recorded needle aspiration biopsy of the lung was performed by Leyden, a Berlin physician, in 1863.[9] He was interested in inflammation as a cause of lung disease and was seeking to confirm the presence of pneumonia in one of his patients. In 1866, Ménétrier used a needle aspiration of the lung to identify cancer cells.[12] Aspiration was initially regarded as a curiosity and was only occasionally attempted prior to the turn of the century with 16- and 18-gauge and cutting-edge needles. Horder reported in 1909 that it was a useful procedure for culture and tumor diagnosis,[7] but enthusiasm was not great because of the high incidence of hemorrhage, pneumothorax, air embolism, and fear of infection or the spread of cancer cells in the needle tract.

In the 1930s, Martin and Ellis[10, 11] and Stewart[20] reported excellent results, but others had difficulty duplicating their success, and fear of complications persisted. Rosemond and colleagues,[15] in 1949, and Godwin,[6] in 1956, advocated the method as being useful and feasible, but it still did not gain widespread acceptance and most surgeons continued to prefer thoracotomy as a diagnostic procedure.

As it became appreciated that the high incidence of complications could be reduced if the needles then in use were replaced by smaller-caliber 20- to 23-gauge needles without a cutting edge, the technique found more favor. With the technical advances in image amplification fluoroscopy, computed tomography, ultrasonography, and efficient methods for treating pneumothorax, radiologists, pathologists, and surgeons progressively developed increased confidence in the use of fine-needle aspiration as a diagnostic tool.[8, 18] The escalating costs of inpatient care added further impetus to its widespread use since it contributed significantly to the rapidity with which a diagnosis could be obtained, thus appreciably shortening the length of hospitalization. Use of the procedure has continued to increase, and lung, pleura, and the mediastinum are now routinely aspirated with assurance.[4, 19] While there may occasionally be difficulty determining the correct diagnosis, particularly with some metastatic cancers, fine-needle aspiration is considered to be a simple, safe, rapid, and cost-effective procedure. A critical factor that contributes to the accuracy of the procedure is the quality of the preparations. Unless they are technically excellent, the results may not be diagnostic. A persistent problem is the shortage of experienced cytopathologists.

INDICATIONS

There are many indications for the use of fine-needle aspiration biopsy of the lung.[2, 3] They include the following:

1. To identify a pulmonary tumor when the noninvasive procedures and sputum sampling, washings and brushings, and bronchoscopic biopsy are not diagnostic
2. To differentiate between a possible recurrent carcinoma and a second primary lesion
3. To distinguish between an inflammatory process and lymphoma or lymphangitic spread from a metastatic breast carcinoma or other carcinoma

4. To establish a diagnosis in high-risk cardiac patients when radiation therapy will be the only treatment[5]
5. To identify by culture the causative microbial agent responsible for an inflammatory coin lesion
6. To distinguish between a cavitary carcinoma and cavitary pulmonary tuberculosis when sputum and other cultures have not identified the organism
7. To establish a diagnosis in patients who refuse thoracotomy
8. To establish a diagnosis in bulky unresectable or bilateral carcinomas so that chemotherapy or radiation therapy can be begun
9. To obtain cells for flow cytometry, tissue culture, chemosensitivity, and genetic studies

CONTRAINDICATIONS

Fine-needle aspiration biopsy is contraindicated in the following:

1. Patients with chronic hepatitis, cirrhosis, idiopathic thrombotic thrombocytopenic purpura, or any other disease associated with a tendency for hemorrhage
2. Patients with pulmonary hypertension secondary to portal obstruction
3. Patients with extensive bullous emphysema in close proximity to a lung mass
4. Patients with severe chronic obstructive pulmonary disease with borderline pulmonary function
5. Patients with radiologic evidence of pneumonia, especially if it lies adjacent to a mass in an immunosuppressed patient
6. Patients who are uncooperative or refuse needle biopsy
7. Patients subject to severe uncontrollable coughing attacks
8. Patients suspected of having an echinococcus cyst, since puncture of the cyst may disseminate the infection
9. Patients with vascular abnormalities or vascular tumors
10. Patients with diffuse chronic interstitial disease. Aspiration biopsy is not adequate to establish the diagnosis, and the incidence of pneumothorax is greater in these patients than in those with discrete lesions.

Thoracic oncology patients who require a diagnosis of a new or recurrent neoplasm will, as a rule, be evaluated with sputum samples, bronchial washings and brushings, and bronchial biopsy. If these are not informative, transtracheal biopsy or percutaneous fine-needle aspiration biopsy will be performed, depending on the location of the lesion.[8] If it lies in close proximity to a large bronchus, a transbronchial endoscopic biopsy may procure representative material, but when the lesion lies in the mid or peripheral lung fields, percutaneous fine-needle aspiration biopsy is the procedure of choice. In most instances, the fine-needle aspiration biopsy is effective, and it has the great advantage of expediting the diagnosis so that therapy may be quickly begun.

Fine-needle aspiration of the lung carries a low morbidity and mortality, but complications, and especially pneumothorax, occur in as many as one third of patients in some reported series. Sinner has shown that patients without emphysema have a lower (16.9%) incidence of pneumothorax, while in those with moderate or severe emphysema, it is substantially higher (47% and 66.6%, respectively).[17] Patients with severe emphysema or chronic obstructive pulmonary disease with borderline pulmonary function should be thoroughly evaluated and aspirated only if emergency procedures such as chest intubation can be rapidly instituted. In these patients, even a small pneumothorax can prove fatal. In Zornoza and colleagues' series of 425 fine-needle aspiration biopsies performed with a 21- to 22-gauge non-cutting-edge needle, 115 (27%) of the patients developed pneumothorax and required chest tube intubation.[22] None of the patients developed pulmonary hemorrhage, hemoptysis, subcutaneous emphysema, infection, or mediastinal shift, and there were no fatalities. The diagnostic accuracy was 85%.

In Zornoza and colleagues' series,[22] the size of the lesion did not appear to be related to the incidence of pneumothorax, but small lesions may nevertheless require multiple aspirations (Fig. 3–1). Sinner[17] noted that tumor masses smaller than 2 cm in diameter required more than one aspirate in order to obtain an adequate sample, whereas a single aspiration sufficed for lesions between 2 and 3.5 cm. Large cavitary lesions require more passes (Fig. 3–2): necrotic debris is generally recovered in the first sample, and it is not always possible to secure a sufficient number of tumor cells from the peripheral (growing) margin. Such tumors frequently require two or more attempts to obtain diagnostic cells, and this increases the possibility of pneumothorax. Feldman and Covell have reviewed the recorded deaths associated with fine-

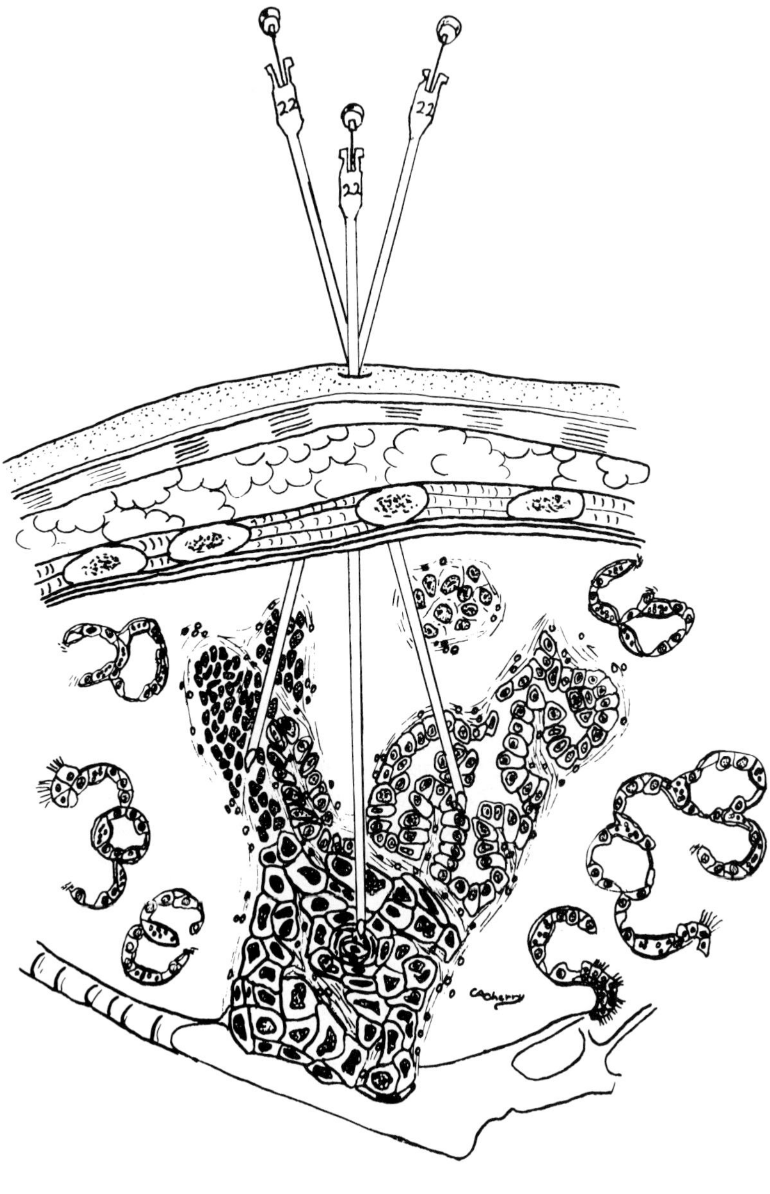

Figure 3–1. It is not always easy to obtain diagnostic material when the lesion is small. Three or four passes may be required. Absence of necrosis will improve the quality of the smears.

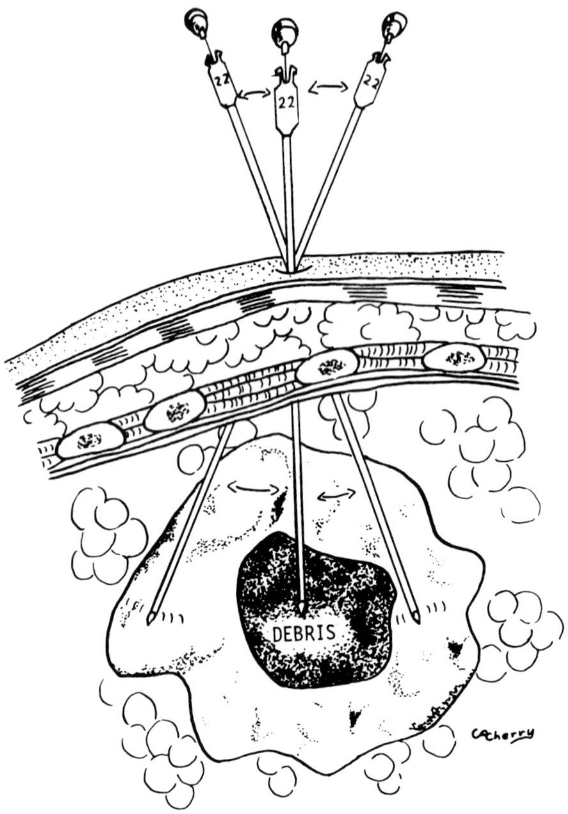

Figure 3–2. Avoid debris at the center of a lesion by aspirating cells at the growing margin. Several passes may be needed to obtain enough material, especially if immunostaining, electron microscopy, microbiologic studies, or cytogenetics is contemplated.

needle biopsy of the lung.[4] In most instances deaths were caused by intrapulmonary hemorrhage or air embolus, and they occurred with the use of large-caliber or cutting-edge needles and because experience of the radiologist or other person performing the aspiration was limited. Patient selection, the experience of the aspirator, and preparedness to perform resuscitation and chest intubation may have been factors. Today, careful selection of patients, improved radiologic techniques for guiding and monitoring the needle, availability of medical teams capable of responding promptly and effectively to chest emergencies, and awareness of the complications that can arise have practically eliminated the problems.

The implantation of malignant cells aspirated from malignant tumors of the lung is mentioned in some reports, most written prior to 1960, before the widespread use of 22- to 23-gauge needles. Berger and colleagues[1] reported two instances, and Sinner[16] and Zajicek[21] reported one each in more than 2,700 aspirations. Failure to release the plunger of the syringe while the needle was still within the tumor in order to equalize the negative pressure may have been a causative factor. The release of pressure is mandatory, and spread of malignant cells into adjacent tissues is extremely unlikely when proper technique is followed.

We have observed one example of tumor implantation, in a patient in whom metastatic melanoma lay adjacent to the visceral pleura and who had an associated pleural effusion. An aspiration biopsy of the mass was performed, and a chest tube was implanted for removal of the recurring effusion. Within a week, melanoma cells were collected from the chest tube and tumor growth was apparent in the soft tissue surrounding it. Not all examples of implantation within a needle tract are detected. When surgery is performed, the resection may remove the needle tract. If radiation therapy is given, malignant cells that have been deposited within the irradiated field may be destroyed.

DIAGNOSTIC ACCURACY

The degree of accuracy varies among different institutions and is influenced by the experience of the radiologist and cytopathologist and the quality of the cytopreparatory techniques. The range of true positive cases is between 70% and 97%. False-positive reports are given in 1% to 4%, and the frequency of false-negative reports ranges from 3% to 28%.[4] Mesenchymal tumors are difficult to aspirate, and the yield is often scanty. If the lesion to be aspirated lies immediately beneath the pleura, a Rotex or cutting-edge needle may be helpful in providing a satisfactory specimen, whereas a lesion in the mid lung may require thoracotomy for procurement of sufficient tissue. Figure 3–3 illustrates three fundamental principles. The aspiration should be attempted from the nearest point on the thorax, and the needle should not pass through emphysematous lung or traverse an interlobar fissure.

As more experienced cytopathologists enter the field, and with progressive improvements in radiologic and cytologic techniques, the accuracy of diagnoses should continue to improve. Studies performed to evaluate the sensitivity and specificity of the technique provide strong support for its overall accuracy and the importance of its contribution in the detection of pulmonary tumors and nonneoplastic processes.[13, 14] The thousands of aspiration biopsies that have been per-

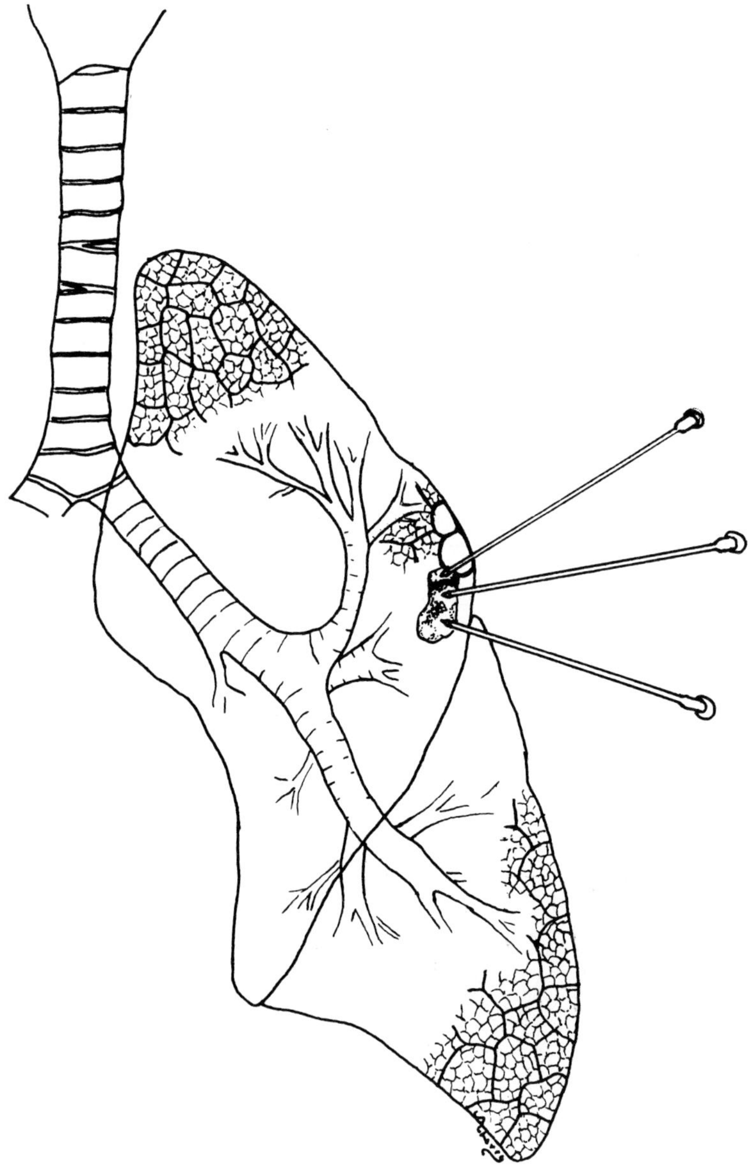

Figure 3–3. Approach the lesion from the shortest feasible route, avoiding emphysematous bullae and interlobar fissures.

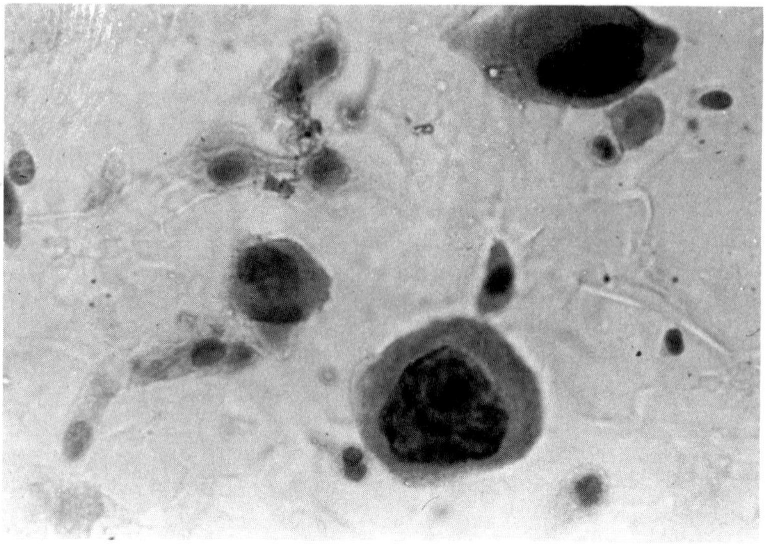

Figure 3–4. Case study 1. The cytologic features are those of a squamous cell carcinoma. The nuclear contour is slightly irregular, and the chromatin is coarsely clumped.

formed in the past decade in the United States and many other countries attest to the success and acceptance of this procedure.

ILLUSTRATIVE CASES

The short selection of cases that follows illustrates some contributions of fine-needle aspiration biopsy of neoplasms in the lung.

Case Study 1. *A 55-year-old man had smoked one to two packs of cigarettes per day for more than 20 years. He noticed that his cough was more persistent and that his sputum was intermittently tinged with blood. Chest radiography revealed a 4.5-cm mass in the right hilum that appeared to involve the main lower lobe bronchus, and lymph nodes in the hilar area were enlarged. The mass was aspirated (Figs. 3–4 and 3–5), yielding cells of squamous cell carcinoma. The right lower lobe was resected, and the diagnosis was confirmed (Fig. 3–6). Postoperative radiation therapy was given, and 5 years later there was no evidence of recurrence or metastases.*

Case Study 2. *A 64-year-old woman who had smoked cigarettes for 30 years developed a chronic cough with blood-tinged sputum. After antibiotics failed to relieve her symptoms, a chest radiograph*

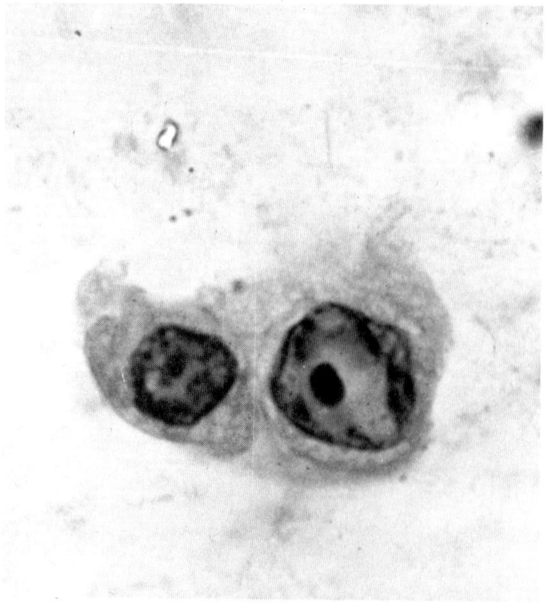

Figure 3–5. Case study 1. Two cohesive cells with nuclei of different sizes, one with a prominent nucleolus.

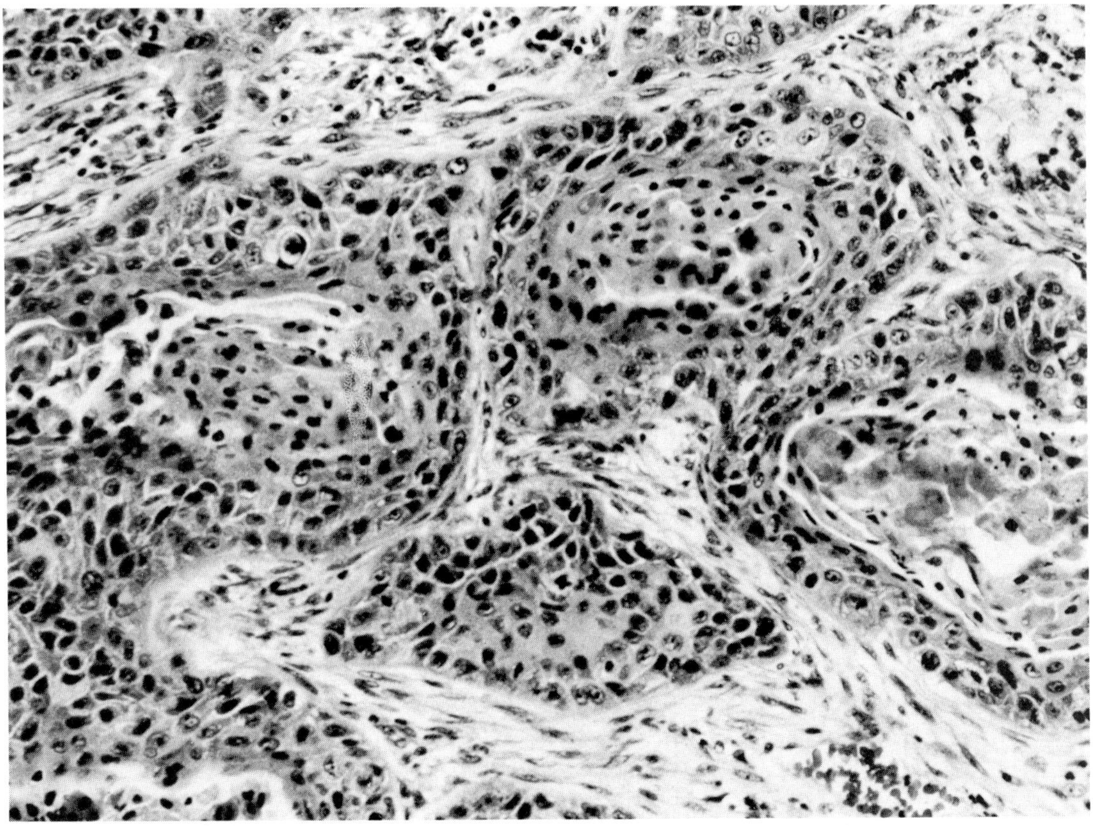

Figure 3–6. Case study 1. Microscopic sections of the resected lobe confirmed the diagnosis of nonkeratinizing squamous cell carcinoma.

was taken and it revealed a 3.5-cm mass in the periphery of the right middle lobe. An aspiration was performed, providing a diagnosis of adenocarcinoma (Fig. 3–7), and the lobe was resected. The adenocarcinoma had a cribriform pattern (Fig. 3–8), which was not detectable in the aspirate smears.

Case Study 3. *A 64-year-old man who had smoked for many years was found to have tuberculosis involving his right upper lobe. He stopped smoking and received treatment with clinical evidence of a good response, but 5 months later he became hoarse and laryngoscopy revealed a squamous cell carcinoma of the right vocal cord. It was treated with surgery and radiation therapy. Six months later, a 3-cm lesion was noted in the periphery of the left upper lobe and a fine-needle aspiration was performed. The cytologic diagnosis was bronchioloalveolar adenocarcinoma (Fig. 3–9), and the lobe was removed. The histology was characteristic of a bronchioloalveolar adenocarcinoma (Fig. 3–10).*

Case Study 4. *A 66-year-old woman was admitted to a local hospital for treatment of pain in the left hip. Radiographs revealed a pathologic fracture of the left upper femur, lytic lesions in the ilium and the right clavicle, and a 3.5-cm left suprahilar mass. Aspiration of the suprahilar mass produced cells with both glandular (Fig. 3–11) and squamous (Fig. 3–12) features, confirmed on resection as a mucoepidermoid carcinoma (Fig. 3–13). A core needle biopsy of the femur showed a similar tumor. Two years later, she died with widespread metastases.*

Case Study 5. *A routine chest radiograph of this 48-year-old man showed an 8-cm left upper lobe mass. Three years earlier an adenocarcinoma of the descending colon had been resected. Aspirated cells from the lung mass were characteristic of a pleomorphic undifferentiated large cell carcinoma (Fig. 3–14). The left upper lobe was removed, and the diagnosis was confirmed (Fig. 3–15). Nodal metastases were not present, and the patient has survived for more than 12 years without further evidence of tumor.*

Case Study 6. *A 48-year-old man had smoked 2 packs of cigarettes a day for 23 years. He developed a persistent cough, which did not improve with*

Text continued on page 44

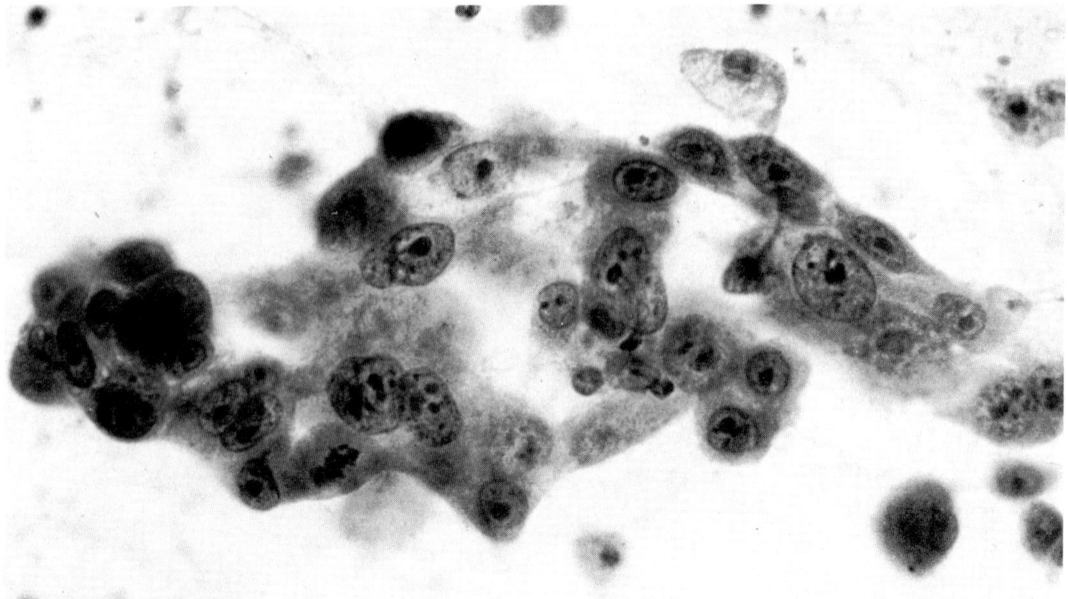

Figure 3–7. Case study 2. Cells from the aspiration biopsy specimen show the characteristics of a moderately differentiated adenocarcinoma. The nuclei are ovoid with smooth profiles, and nucleoli are prominent.

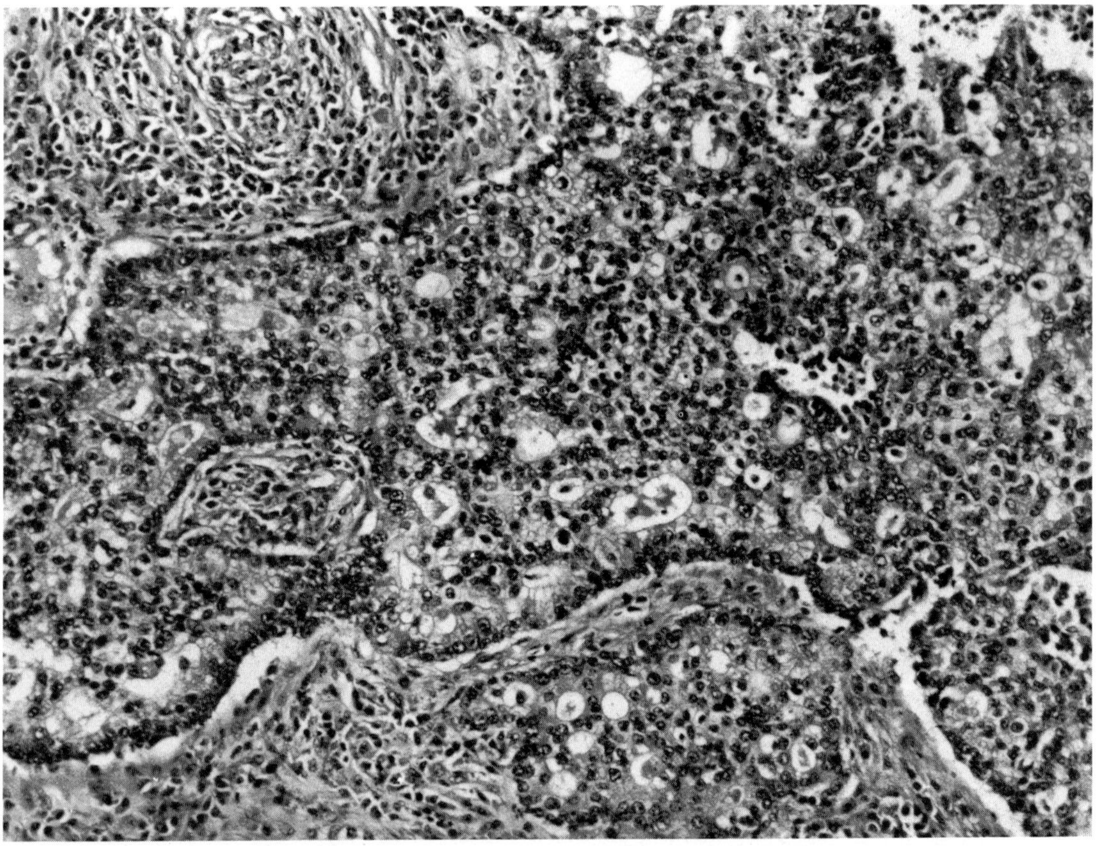

Figure 3–8. Case study 2. Histology of the resected tumor showed a microacinar adenocarcinoma.

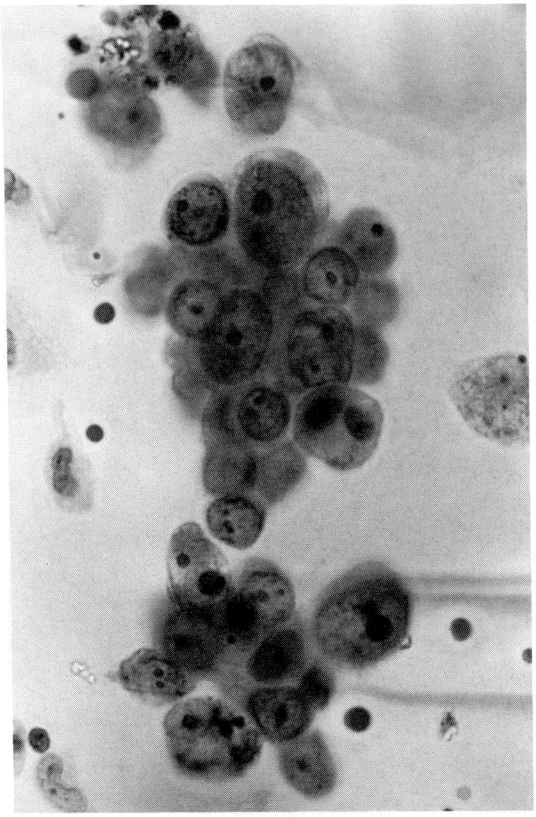

Figure 3–9. Case study 3. Characteristic papillary clusters of cells indicating a bronchioloalveolar adenocarcinoma.

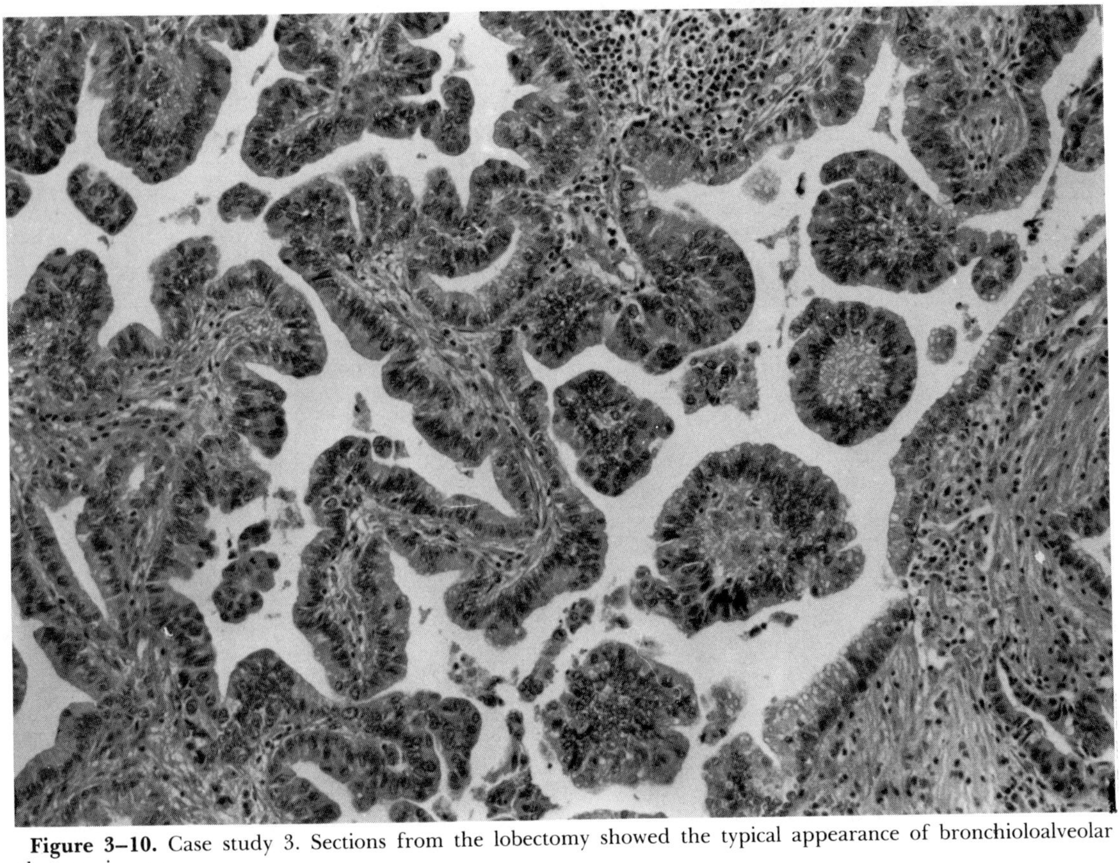

Figure 3–10. Case study 3. Sections from the lobectomy showed the typical appearance of bronchioloalveolar adenocarcinoma.

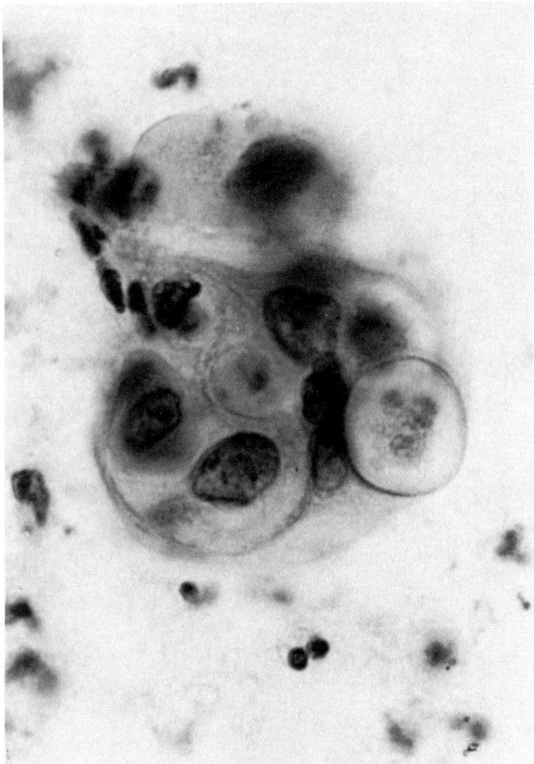

Figure 3–11. Case study 4. A cytologic smear of the fine-needle aspirate of the suprahilar mass shows a cluster of intimately apposed adenocarcinoma cells.

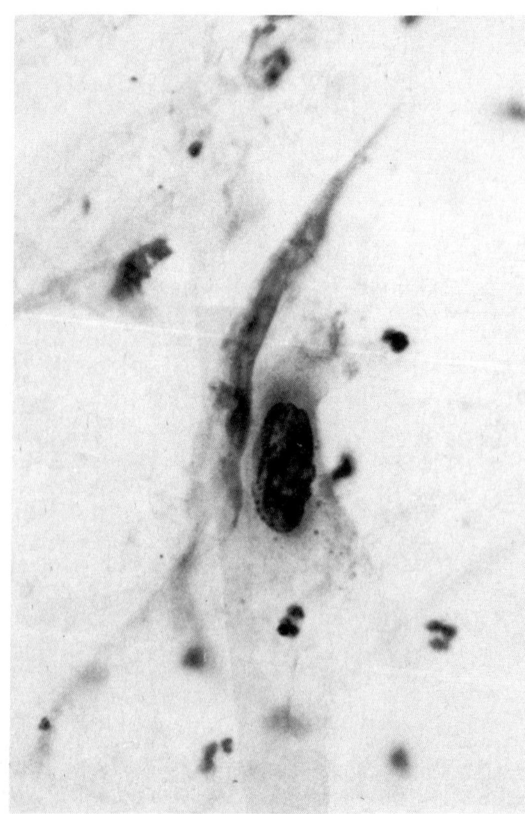

Figure 3–12. Case study 4. Other areas of the same smear as in Figure 3–11 showed epidermoid features.

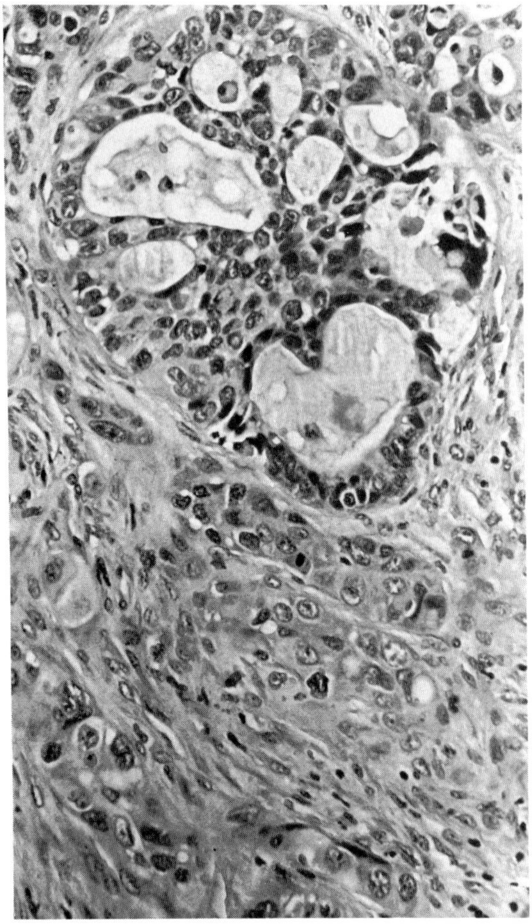

Figure 3–13. Case study 4. Histologic sections of the resected tumor confirmed the diagnosis of mucoepidermoid carcinoma.

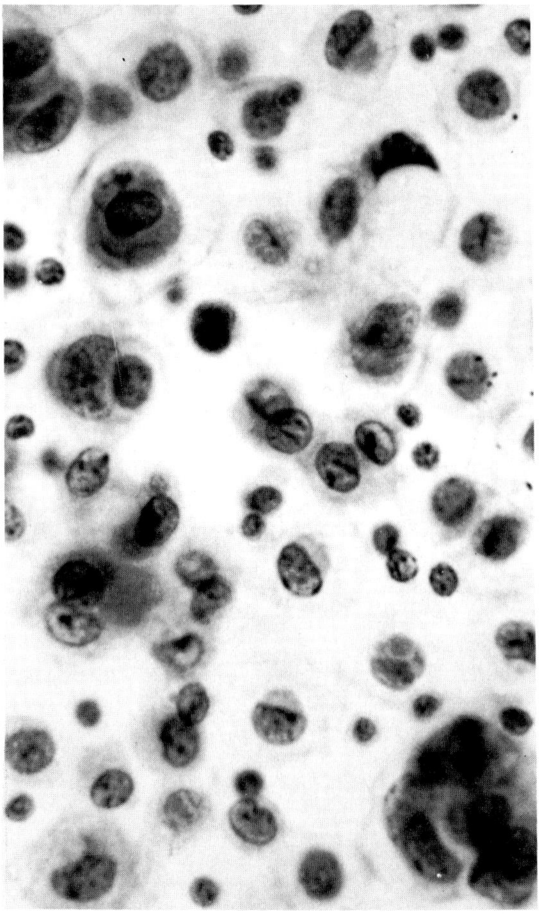

Figure 3–14. Case study 5. Aspirated cells from the lung mass showed pleomorphic tumor cells mixed with lymphocytes.

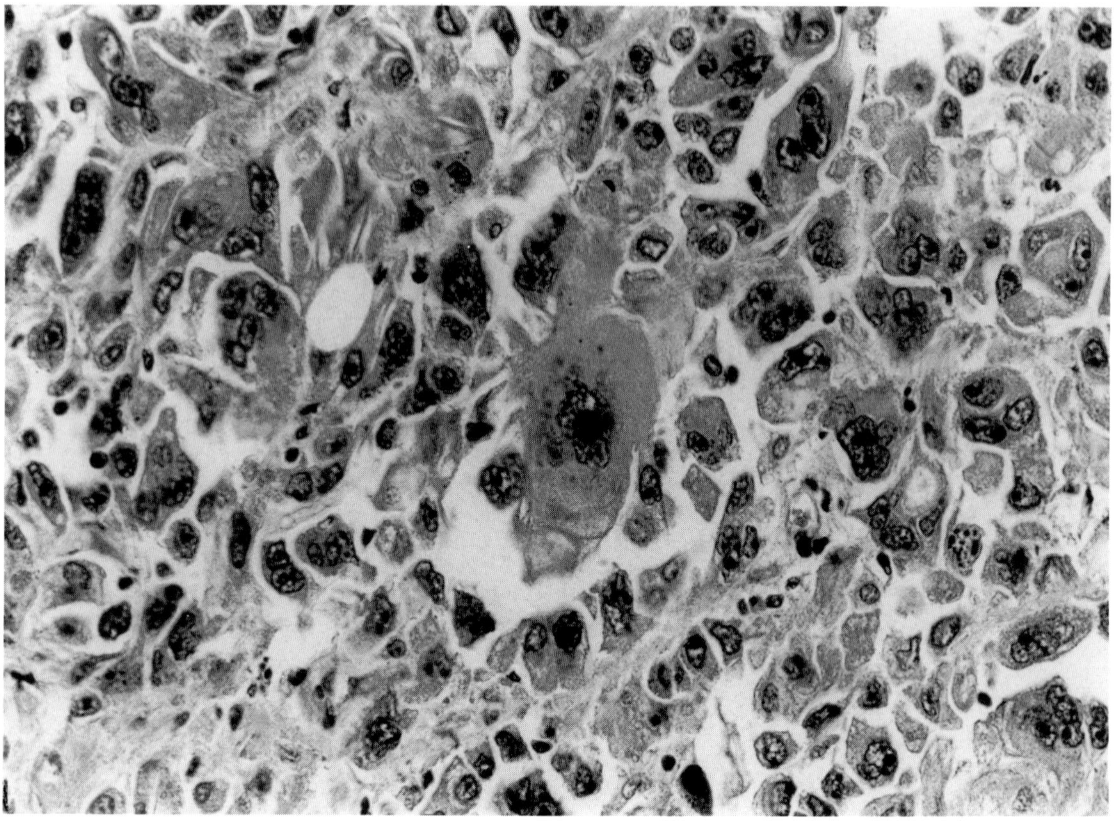

Figure 3–15. Case study 5. Even more variability in cell size and shape was evident within the tumor cells in the resected specimen, characteristic of a pleomorphic undifferentiated large cell carcinoma.

antibiotic therapy, and a chest radiograph showed the presence of a mass surrounding the main right upper lobe bronchus with enlarged hilar and paratracheal lymph nodes. An aspiration biopsy of the lung mass led to the diagnosis of small cell undifferentiated carcinoma (Fig. 3–16). Three months later metastases were documented in liver, vertebrae, and ribs. He died 13 months from the time of diagnosis.

Case Study 7. *A 28-year-old man presented with a complaint of left-sided chest pain. Chest radiography did not reveal a lesion, but it was repeated after 2 months and a pleural effusion was then evident. Aspiration of the fluid produced a bloody specimen, and after the fluid had been removed, multiple nodules could be detected on the parietal pleura and diaphragm. The cytologic diagnosis from smears (Fig. 3–17) and cell block sections (Fig. 3–18) of the pleural fluid was malignant mesothelioma, supported by immunostaining and confirmed by electron microscopy. Despite extensive surgery, the tumor invaded the chest wall (Fig. 3–19) and metastasized to regional lymph nodes.*

Case Study 8. *A 49-year-old woman was seen because of vague lower abdominal discomfort and intermittent constipation. A gastrointestinal radiographic series revealed a mass partially occluding the rectosigmoid colon. It was resected and there were no visible metastases. She was well for 7 years, until a solitary subpleural mass was identified and aspirated with a diagnosis of metastatic adenocarcinoma of colon (Fig. 3–20).*

Case Study 9. *A 60-year-old man had a history of left nephrectomy for renal cell adenocarcinoma 12 years earlier. Chest radiography revealed a subpleural mass with a small pleural effusion. The effusion was tapped, but cells were scanty and a diagnosis could not be reached. Therefore a fine-needle aspiration was performed, leading to a diagnosis of metastatic renal cell carcinoma (Fig. 3–21). Since the nodule was solitary, it was excised (Fig. 3–22).*

Case Study 10. *A level IV melanoma had been removed from the back of a 32-year-old man. Two years later, a chest wall lesion was identified and*

Text continued on page 53

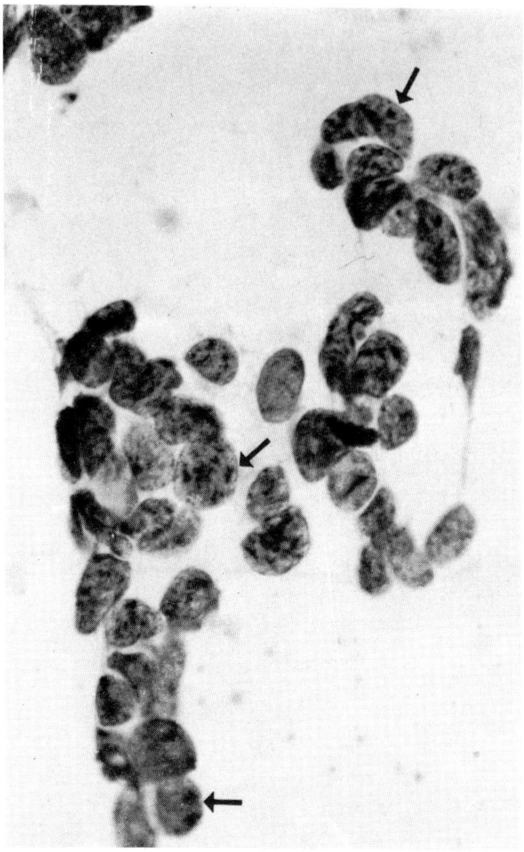

Figure 3–16. Case study 6. An aspiration biopsy specimen of the lung mass showed small, ovoid, naked nuclei with finely granular chromatin and inconspicuous nucleoli.

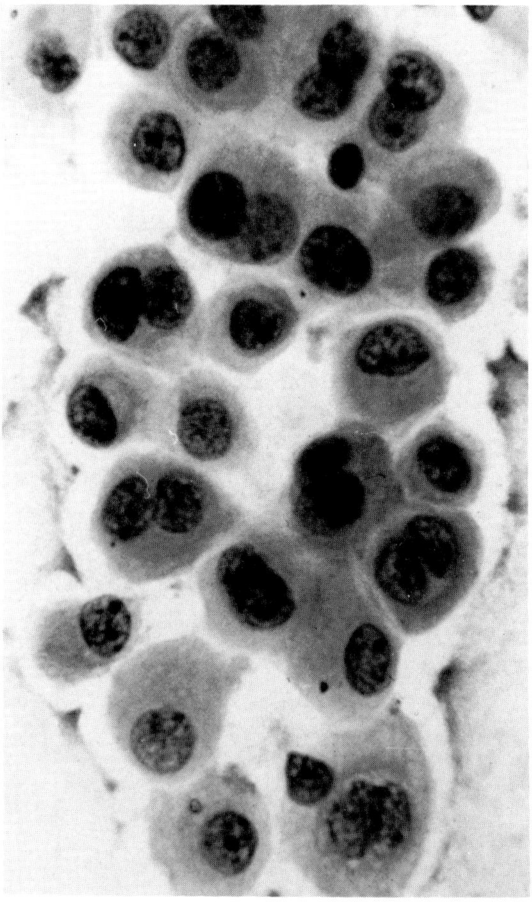

Figure 3–17. Case study 7. Aspirated fluid from the pleural space of this 28-year-old man showed relatively large, uniform cells with one or two nuclei.

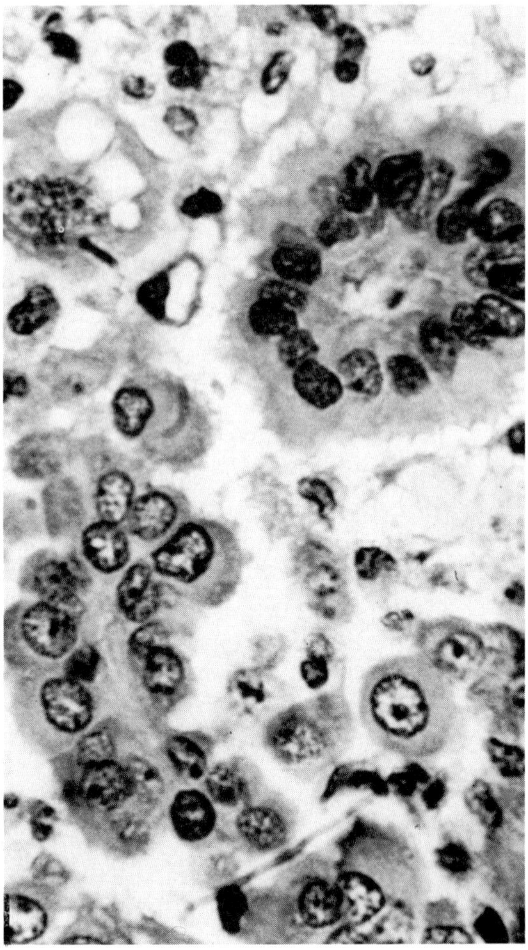

Figure 3–18. Case study 7. A papillary architecture was revealed in sections of the cell block of the aspirated fluid. The diagnosis of mesothelioma was rendered.

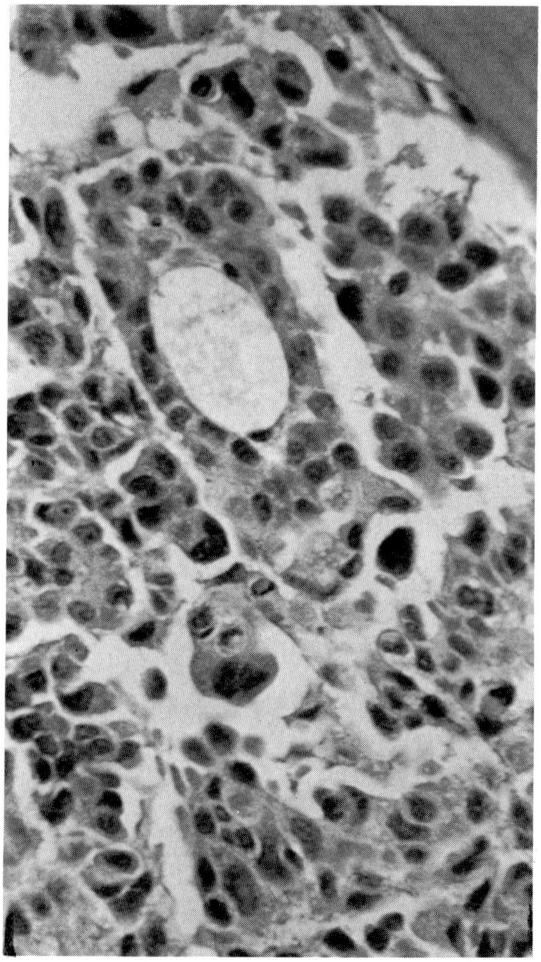

Figure 3–19. Case study 7. Tissue section of a rib metastasis consistent with mesothelioma.

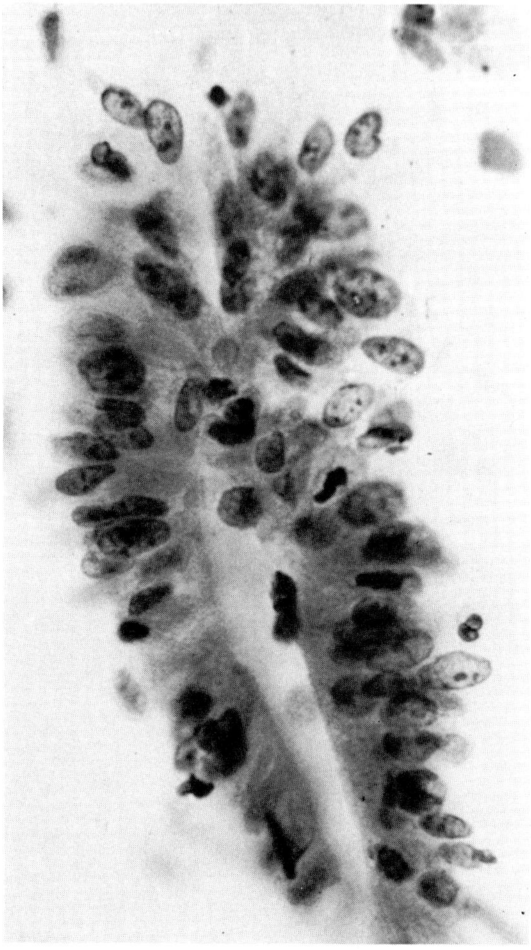

Figure 3–20. Case study 8. Aspiration of the solitary subpleural mass showed a glandular architecture with tall columnar cells consistent with metastatic colonic adenocarcinoma.

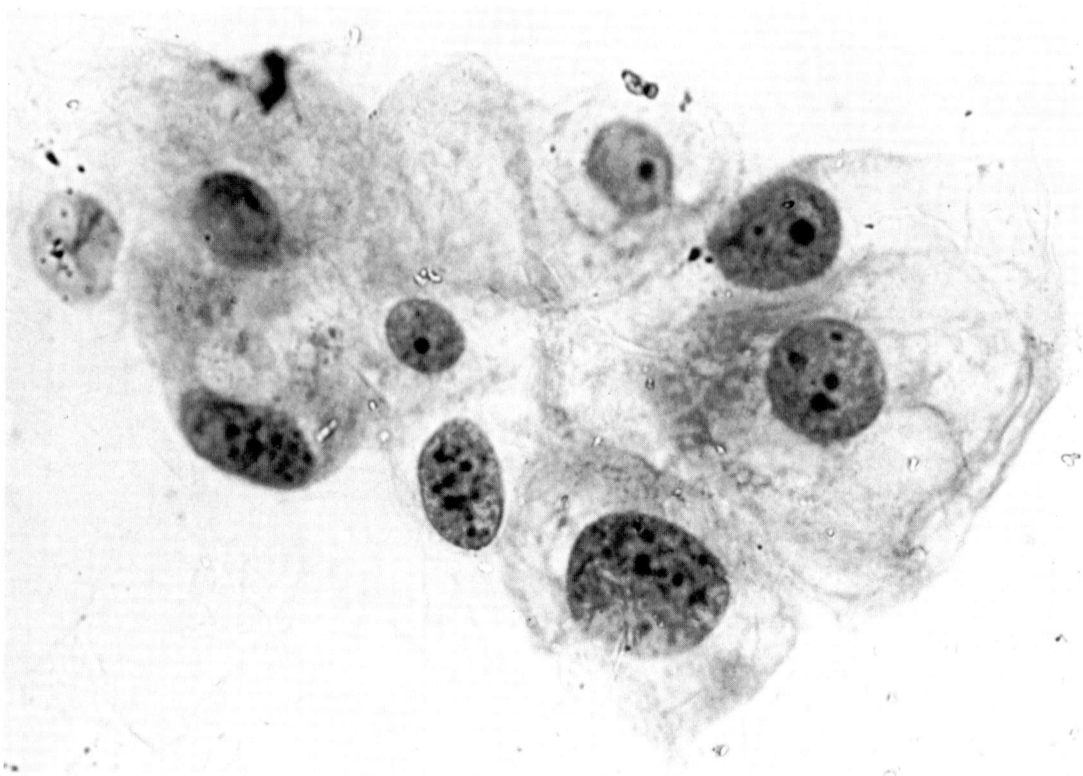

Figure 3–21. Case study 9. Since the pleural fluid from this patient did not yield a diagnosis, a subpleural mass was aspirated. The cells have clear, foamy cytoplasm that contained plentiful glycogen, supporting the diagnosis of metastatic renal cell adenocarcinoma.

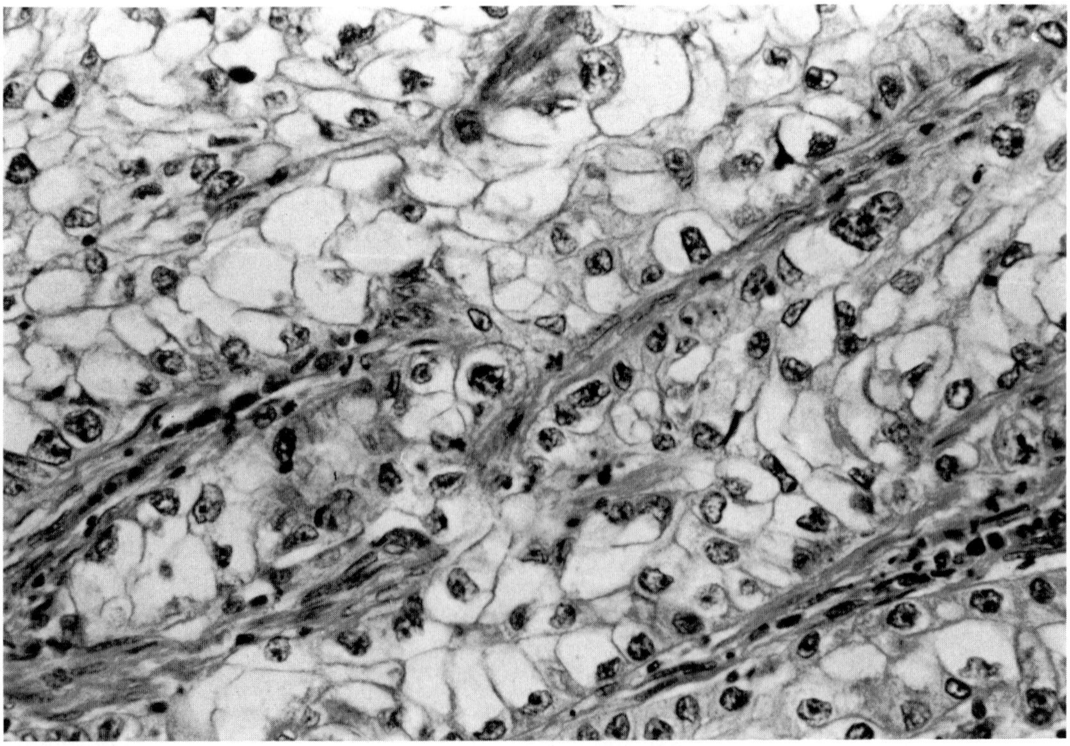

Figure 3–22. Case study 9. Histologic section of the excised subpleural nodule showing the typical appearance of renal cell adenocarcinoma.

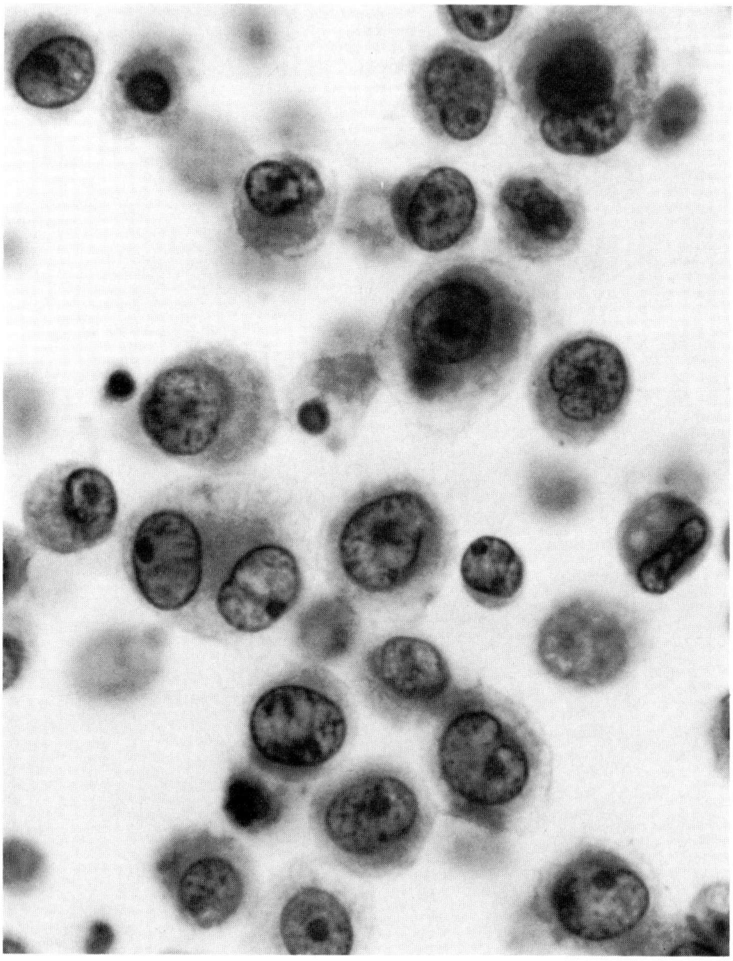

Figure 3–23. Case study 10. Aspirate of a chest wall lesion in a 32-year-old man with a history of cutaneous melanoma. The cytologic features support the diagnosis of metastatic melanoma. Immunostaining for S-100 protein and melanoma-specific antigen was positive.

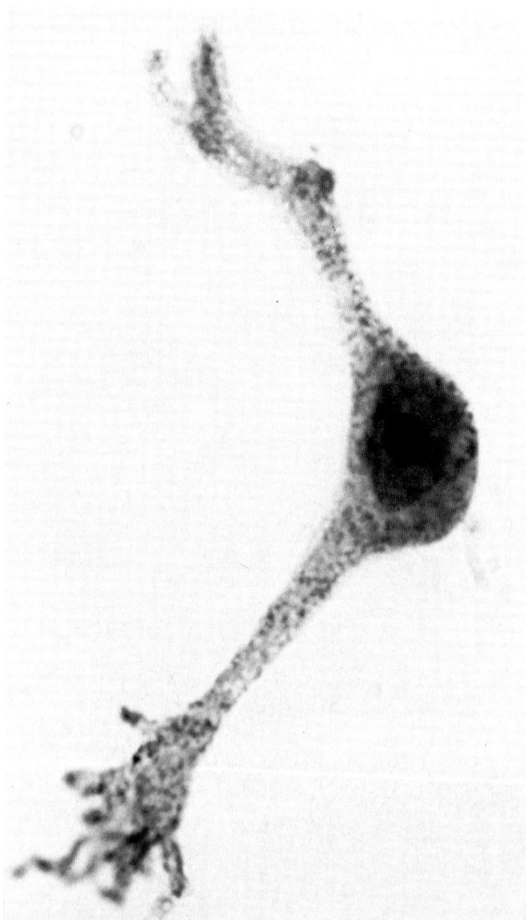

Figure 3–24. Case study 10. Numerous pigmented granules can be seen in the cytoplasm of a cell from the same aspirate as Figure 3–23.

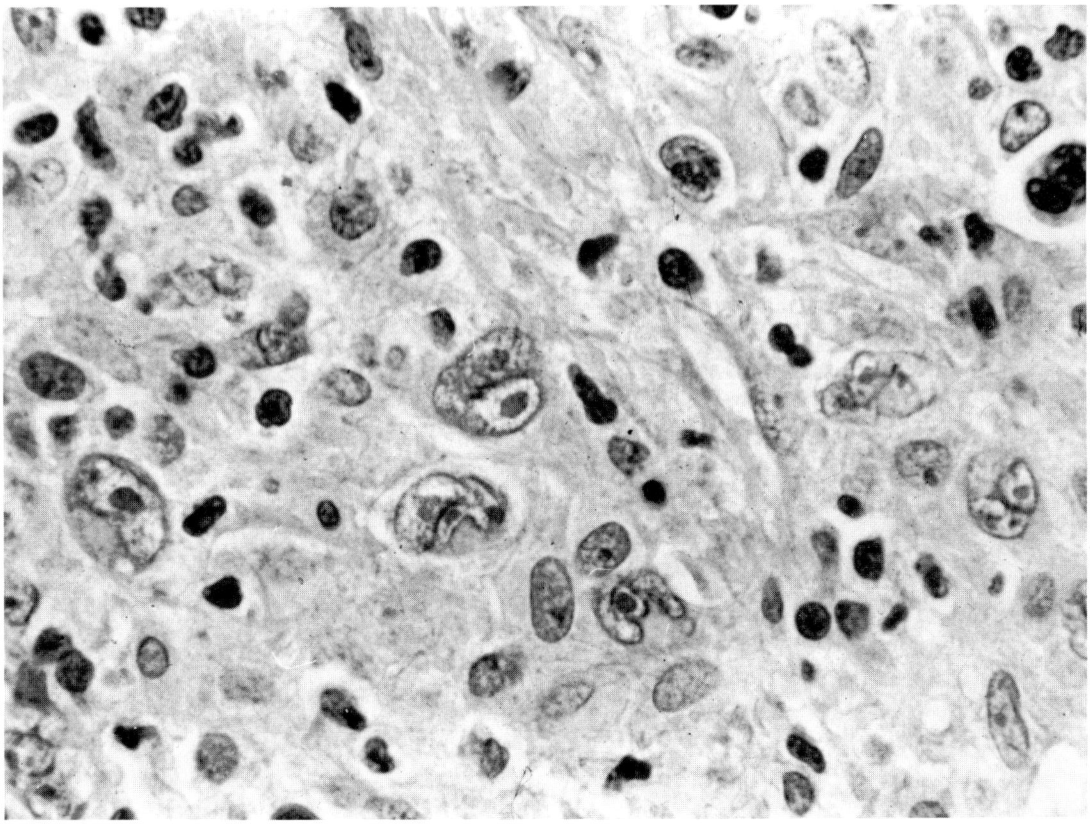

Figure 3–25. Case study 11. Histologic sections of a supraclavicular lymph node showed the features of Hodgkin's disease.

Figure 3–26. Case study 11. A Reed-Sternberg cell from the aspirate of the left upper lobe.

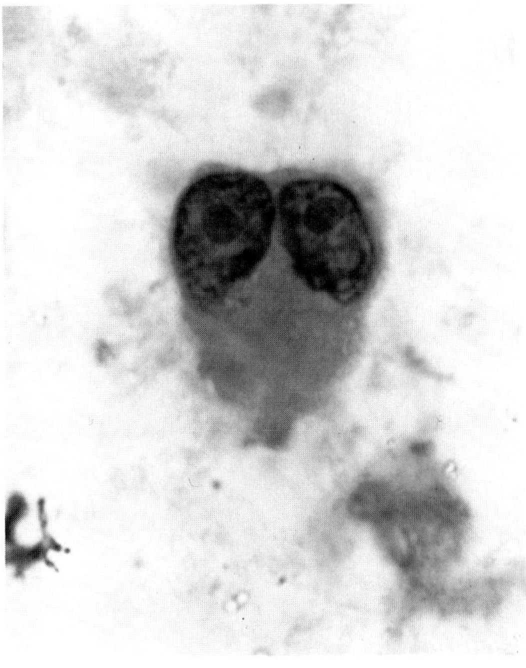

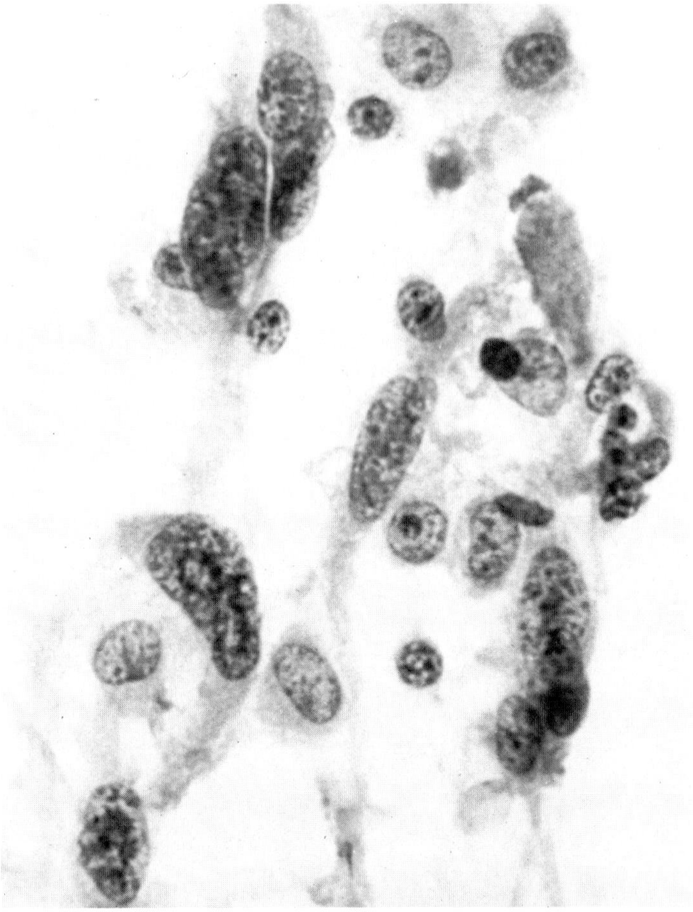

Figure 3–27. Case study 12. Spindle and pleomorphic cells from a left lower lobe aspirate consistent with malignant fibrous histiocytoma.

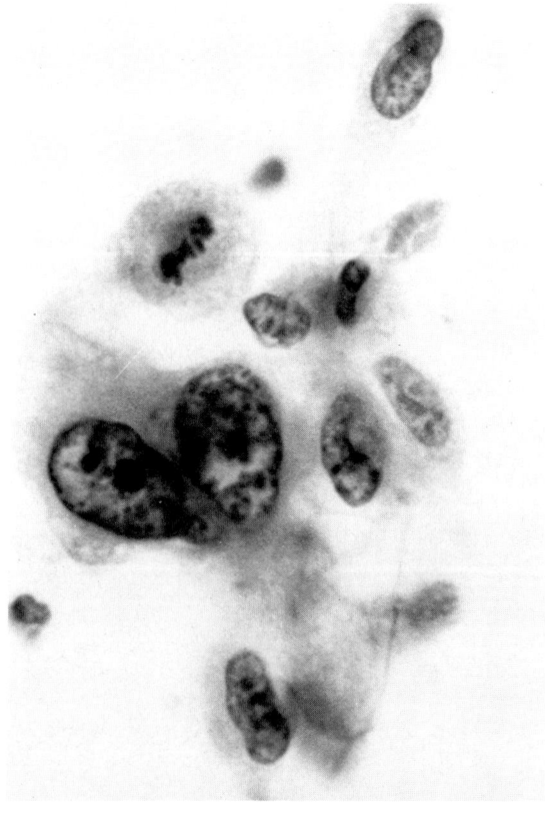

Figure 3–28. Case study 12. A large binucleate cell with prominent nuclei and granular chromatin from the same aspirate as the specimen shown in Figure 3–27. An adjacent cell contains a mitotic figure.

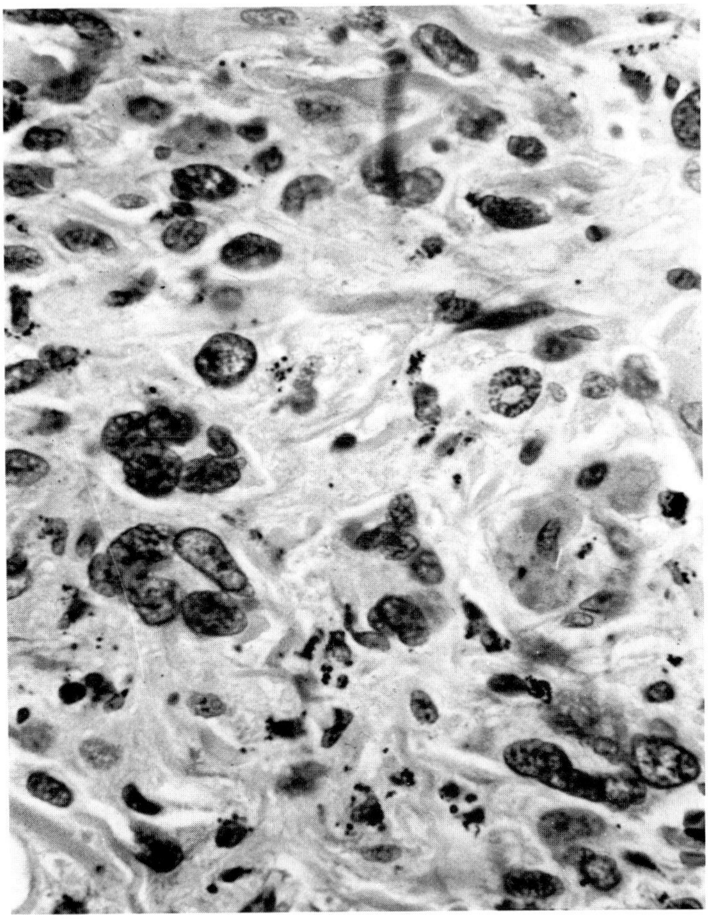

Figure 3–29. Case study 12. Histologic section of the resected lobe confirming the diagnosis of malignant fibrous histiocytoma.

aspirated (Figs. 3–23 and 3–24), establishing the presence of metastatic melanoma.

Case Study 11. *A 21-year-old man felt listless and tired and lost his appetite and 14 pounds in weight. An enlarged left supraclavicular lymph node was biopsied with a diagnosis of nodular sclerosing Hodgkin's disease (Fig. 3–25), and he received chemotherapy and radiation therapy. A local recurrence received similar treatment and responded. Two years later, he was found to have a 5-cm mass in the left upper lobe, and it was aspirated and showed cells of Hodgkin's disease (Fig. 3–26).*

Case Study 12. *For 6 months, a 63-year-old man ignored persistent chest pain, but it became progressively more severe and he saw his physician, who ordered a chest radiograph. A mass that was 10 cm in greatest diameter was found in the left lower lobe, and a fine-needle aspiration was performed. Spindle and pleomorphic cells were considered consistent with a sarcoma (Figs. 3–27 and 3–28), subclassified as malignant fibrous histiocytoma on the resection specimen (Fig. 3–29).*

REFERENCES

1. Berger RL, Dargan EL, Huang BL: Dissemination of cancer cells by needle biopsy of the lung. J Thorac Cardiovasc Surg 63:430, 1972.
2. Bonfiglio TA: Fine needle aspiration biopsy of the lung. Pathol Annu 16(part I):159, 1989.
3. Covell JL, Feldman PS: Fine needle aspiration diagnosis of aspiration pneumonia (phytopneumonitis). Acta Cytol 28:77, 1984.
4. Feldman PS, Covell JL: Fine Needle Aspiration Cytology of Breast and Lung Accuracy, part III, p 137. Chicago, American Society of Clinical Pathologists Press, 1985.
5. Fontana RS, Miller WE, Beabout JW: Transthoracic needle aspiration of discrete pulmonary lesions: Experience in 100 cases. Med Clin North Am 54:961, 1970.
6. Godwin JT: Perspectives in cancer cytology: Aspiration biopsy, technique and application. Ann NY Acad Sci 63:1348, 1956.
7. Horder TJ: Lung puncture: A new application of clinical pathology. Lancet 2:1345, 1909.
8. Jenkens R, Myerowitz RL, Kavic T et al: Diagnostic yield of transbronchoscopic biopsies. Am J Clin Pathol 72:926, 1979.
9. Leyden E: Uber infectiose pneumonie. Dtsch Med Wochenschr 9:52, 1883.
10. Martin HE, Ellis EB: Aspiration biopsy. Surg Gynecol Obstet 59:578, 1934.

11. Martin HE, Ellis EB: Biopsy by needle puncture and aspiration. Ann Surg 92:169, 1930.
12. Ménétrier P: Cancer primitif du poumon. Bull Soc Anat Paris 11:643, 1886.
13. Mitchell ML, King DE, Bonfiglio TA et al: Pulmonary fine-needle aspiration cytopathology. Acta Cytol 28:72, 1984.
14. Poe RH, Tobin RE: Sensitivity and specificity of needle biopsy in lung malignancy. Am Rev Respir Dis 122:725, 1980.
15. Rosemond GP, Burnett WE, Hall HJ: Value and limitations of aspiration biopsy for lung lesions. Radiology 52:506, 1949.
16. Sinner WN, Zajicek J: Implantation metastasis after percutaneous transthoracic needle aspiration biopsy. Acta Radiol Diagn 17:473, 1976.
17. Sinner WN: Complications of percutaneous transthoracic needle aspiration biopsy. Acta Radiol Diagn 17:813, 1976.
18. Sinner WN: Primary neoplasms diagnosed with transthoracic needle biopsy. Cancer 43:1533, 1979.
19. Stevens GM, Weigen JF, Lillington GA: Needle aspiration biopsy of localized pulmonary lesions with amplified fluoroscopic guidance. AJR 103:561, 1968.
20. Stewart FW: The diagnosis of tumors by aspiration. Am J Pathol 9:801, 1933.
21. Zajicek J: Aspiration Biopsy Cytology: I. Cytology of Supradiaphragmatic Organs. Basel, Karger, 1974.
22. Zornoza J, Snow J, Lukeman JM et al: Aspiration biopsy of discrete pulmonary lesions using a thin needle. Radiology 123:519, 1977.

Chapter

4

ATYPICAL AND FALSE-POSITIVE DIAGNOSES IN PULMONARY CYTOLOGY

Abnormal and even malignant-appearing epithelial cells occasionally are found in pulmonary cytology specimens from patients in whom there is no evidence of cancer. The presence of the abnormal cells can often be attributed to exposure of the sensitive respiratory epithelium to vapors, noxious fumes, particulate matter from chemicals or industrial compounds, drugs, antigens, or chemotherapeutic agents. The changes that occur in the epithelial cells reflect their response to the quantity, type, and duration of exposure to the irritant or antigen and the host's ability to react. The changes are conventionally classified as mild, moderate, or severe. Mild alterations are usually reported as atypias: their causes are diverse, and they are of minor consequence. The moderate and severe reactions are, in contrast, worrisome and may cause the unwary pathologist to issue a false-positive diagnosis.

A false-positive diagnosis is a diagnosis of malignancy made by examination of a cytologic or histologic specimen that subsequently proves to be incorrect. When malignant-appearing cells are unexpectedly discovered in a routine specimen, the pathologist should communicate with the clinician and possibly the radiologist. The validity of the diagnosis of malignancy must be thoroughly discussed prior to release of the report.

Changes in epithelial cells simulating those encountered in cancer of the lung occur in sputum and bronchial washings and brushings, and they are sometimes seen in specimens obtained by fine-needle aspiration. Cells in sputa are quite often mildly atypical. They show subtle changes such as cytoplasmic swelling or nuclear hyperchromasia, and one can only surmise that they have been caused by exposure to a noxious agent such as a foreign substance, to a viral or other antigen, to a drug, or perhaps to an industrial compound. It is rarely possible to determine the nature of the inciting factor without clinical information. When an adequate history is given, it may be possible to relate the findings to a causative agent. In association with the rising incidence of lung cancer, there has been a proportionate increase in the use of anticancer chemotherapeutic agents. These chemicals alter the patient's biologic defense mechanisms, and immunosuppression may result. Opportunistic fungi, bacteria, viruses, and protozoan parasites have the ability to invade and proliferate rapidly in immunosuppressed patients.[68, 80, 98, 110] A review of the autopsy files at the M.D. Anderson Cancer Center reveals that more than 30% of patients receiving one or several chemotherapeutic compounds have died of infectious diseases with extensive pulmonary involvement. Recently, patients with the acquired immunodeficiency syndrome (AIDS) have greatly expanded the pool of patients who require courses of broad-spectrum antibiotics and chemotherapy. Some patients suffering from IgE-mediated hypersensitivity reactions such as asthma or occupational disease show alteration of their immunologic defense mechanisms and develop severe symptoms that require treatment.[41, 73] Usually they have been presensitized to bacterial, fungal, viral, or chemical compounds.[128] While minor abnormalities of the epithelial cells lining the pulmonary tree are common in these patients, there are also instances of unexplained marked cellular atypia that simulate adenocarcinoma or squamous cell carcinoma. Fortunately the incidence of false-positive diagnoses is low (less than 1% of positive cases at M.D. Anderson Cancer Center).

In this chapter, many of these cytopathologic changes are illustrated with case histories and photomicrographs. The purpose is to heighten the awareness of the cytopathologist, internist, and surgeon to reactions, processes, or diseases that may produce false-positive cytologic reports.

Before proceeding, it is appropriate to list the changes in cell morphology that occur in cancer cells that can be detected and assessed in cytologic preparations. They include the following:

1. Increase in the nuclear/cytoplasmic ratio
2. Abnormal positioning of the nucleus. An absence of consistency in the location of nuclei in tissue is seen as loss of normal polarity.
3. Increase in nuclear chromatin with variation in the size and shape of chromatin particles
4. Nuclear hyperchromasia
5. Variation in shape, number, and size of nucleoli
6. Abnormal mitoses

It should be remembered that no single criterion or even several in combination are necessarily diagnostic of cancer. Many of these changes may be found in association with acute inflammatory processes and benign disorders. Also, these cytologic changes are often absent in tumor cells, and some biologically malignant cells appear cytologically normal.

PATHOLOGIC PROCESSES ASSOCIATED WITH ATYPICAL OR FALSE-POSITIVE PULMONARY CYTOLOGY

In routine cytologic material where cancer is not suspected, the presence of severely atypical cells usually surprises the cytopathologist. These abnormal cells often appear when specimens are unaccompanied by adequate clinical information that might have yielded a clue toward a specific diagnosis. Fortunately many experienced clinicians recognize the importance of routinely providing pertinent clinical data. Granulomatous inflammation including tuberculosis is the most common nonneoplastic cause for cytologic atypia. Table 4–1 is a list of many of the diseases that can be associated with marked atypia.

Table 4–1. Diseases Associated With Marked Atypia

I. Granulomatous Inflammation
  A. Infectious, acute
    1. Tuberculosis
    2. Fungal infections
    3. Parasitic infestations
  B. Granulomatous, idiopathic
    1. Sarcoidosis
    2. Wegener's necrotizing granulomatosis
II. Lung Abscess
III. Pneumonia
  A. Bacterial pneumonia
    1. Acute
    2. Chronic organizing (nonresolving)
    3. Lipid
  B. Viral pneumonia
    1. Herpes
    2. Cytomegalovirus
    3. Varicella
    4. Rubeola
IV. Bronchial Asthma
V. Pulmonary Infarction
VI. Radiation Therapy
VII. Chemotherapeutic Agents
VIII. Emphysema and Chronic Bronchitis
IX. Bronchiectasis
X. Autoimmune Disease
  A. Rheumatoid lung
  B. Pemphigus
XI. Chemical Pneumonias
  A. Oxygen toxicity
  B. Paraquat poisoning
  C. Industrial compounds

GRANULOMATOUS INFLAMMATION

Acute Infectious Disease

Tuberculosis

Over the centuries and into the first half of the 20th century, tuberculosis was the scourge of humanity.[102] It was prevalent in all areas of the world where poverty, starvation, and debilitation occurred.[46] It still occurs in France, Germany, England, and the United States in spite of pasteurization and the availability of effective antimycobacterial drugs.[46, 61, 102, 125] There are three known pathogenic strains of the bacillus, human, bovine, and avian, but subvarieties (*i.e.*, the chromogenic mycobacteria) also exist, and while they occur less frequently than *Mycobacterium tuberculosis,* they show considerable resistance to therapy.[108] Tuberculosis, the most frequently encountered form of granulomatous inflammation, is responsible for marked cytologic atypia. In tuberculous infections, reactive nodules (tubercles) are present early in the disease. Later, the tubercles become granulomas, with areas of necrotic debris at the center. This caseation necrosis is a hallmark of tuberculosis.[127] In persistent cases, cavitary masses or bronchopleural fistulas develop.[29] Host resistance may produce healing, but in many instances, immunosuppressive antibiotics are required to destroy the bacterium.[46, 120, 121]

Case Study 1. *A 47-year-old black man had a 12-lb weight loss and a persistent productive cough. A chest radiograph revealed a large cavitary mass in the left upper lobe. The radiographic diagnosis was carcinoma versus cavitary tuberculosis.*

The cytologic report read as follows: "Cells suspicious for squamous carcinoma are present. Comment: tuberculosis must be excluded since numerous epithelioid cells and pigment-laden macrophages are present." A second cytologic specimen revealed atypical epithelial cells and macrophages. The patient's tuberculin test was negative, and he had not been in contact with a tuberculous person. The left upper lobe was removed surgically, and the diagnosis of tuberculosis was confirmed (Figs. 4–1 through 4–6).

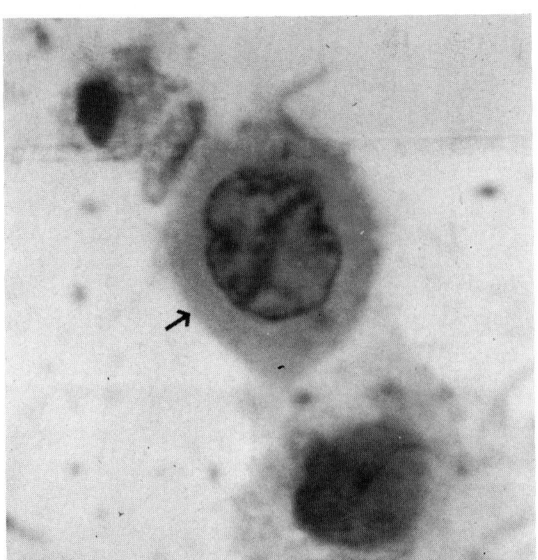

Figure 4–1. Case 1. Pulmonary tuberculosis. Sputum specimen: an epithelioid cell with a nuclear fold and irregular nuclear membrane *(arrow).* The chromatin is clumped beneath the nuclear membrane and adjacent to the nuclear fold. (Papanicolaou, ×425)

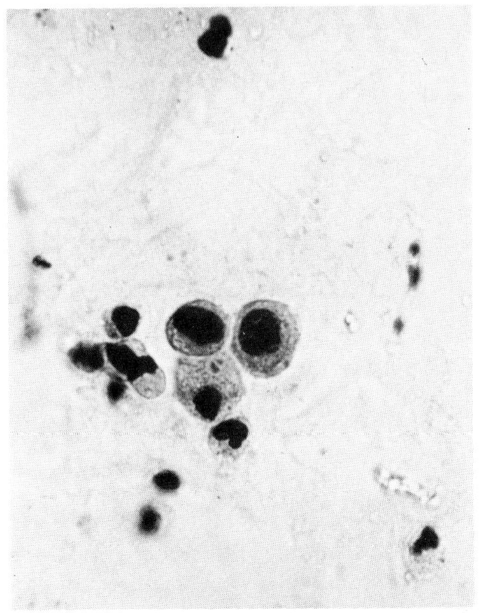

Figure 4–2. Case 1. Sputum specimen: two dyskaryotic squamous cells showing hyperchromasia and high nuclear/cytoplasmic ratio. (Papanicolaou, ×265)

Fungal Infections

Fungi are divided into true pathogens, which invade normal tissues, and saprophytes, which are not normally pathogenic but become so in the immunosuppressed person and are often referred to as "opportunistic" fungi.[6] An area of pneumonia, an abscess, or a bronchiectatic cavity may be secondarily invaded and filled with mycelia.

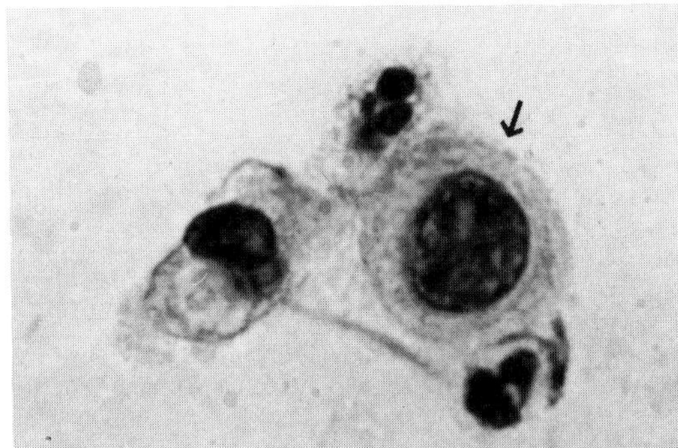

Figure 4–3. Case 1. Sputum specimen: higher magnification of a malignant-appearing cell *(arrow)* strongly suggestive of squamous cell carcinoma. (Papanicolaou, ×425)

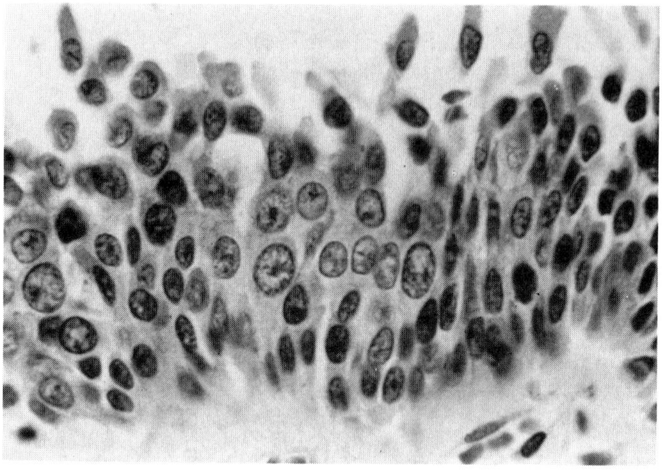

Figure 4–4. Case 1. Tissue section through the wall of the granuloma. Note the tendency toward cohesiveness and, within the aggregates of cells, some variation in size of nuclei. (Hematoxylin-eosin, ×115)

Fungal morphology is not always distinct with the standard hematoxylin-eosin stain, but it is clearly visible with the periodic acid–Schiff or Gomori methenamine silver stains, which have an affinity for the β-linked polysaccharides of fungal walls. Necrosis within a granuloma is an indication for the use of special stains and culture to precisely identify the fungus. Patients treated with corticosteroid therapy for prolonged intervals, diabetic patients, postchemotherapy patients and other immunosuppressed patients (*e.g.*, those with AIDS) require careful surveillance for fungal infection, especially if their neutrophil count is less than 1,000/mm^3. A rapidly spreading infection in any patient with a lowered neutrophil count should alert the clinician to this possibility.[16, 35] The major fungal diseases are listed Table 4–2. Candidiasis and aspergillosis can cause marked cytologic epithelial dysplasia.

CANDIDIASIS

The *Candida* group consists of a number of species of which *Candida albicans* is the most pathogenic.[6, 30, 35] It is common in the oral cavity, gastrointestinal tract, and vagina of healthy persons. When the flora in these areas is altered by drugs, disease, or poor hygiene, the mucosa in which the organisms are dormant becomes vulnerable to invasion.[16, 42] In patients suffering from systemic diseases such as lymphoma, leukemia, cancer, tuberculosis, AIDS, and diabetes, and in young women taking broad-spectrum antibiotics for cervicovaginal or pulmonary infections, rapid multiplication of the organisms can occur.[16, 20, 35, 97] Pulmonary candidiasis is the most common fungal infection complicating chemotherapy.[20, 35, 92, 97]

Table 4–2. Major Fungal Diseases

Disease	Causative Agent
Candidiasis	*Candida albicans*
Aspergillosis	*Aspergillus fumigatus*
Mucormycosis	*Rhizopus, Mucor, Absidia*
Coccidioidomycosis	*Coccidioides immitis*
Sporotrichosis	*Sporotrichium schenkii*
Histoplasmosis	*Histoplasma capsulatum*
Cryptococcosis	*Cryptococcus neoformans*
Blastomycosis	*Blastomyces dermatitidis*
Actinomycosis	*Actinomyces* species

Case Study 2. *A 56-year-old male receiving chemotherapy for lymphoma was found on chest x-ray to have a 3-cm peripheral lung nodule. Sputum specimens showed atypical cells that suggested squamous cell carcinoma. A wedge resection was performed, revealing a granuloma that contained a solid mass of* Candida albicans. *Atypical cells in the resection also simulated cells of squamous cell carcinoma, but tumor was not present (Figs. 4–7 through 4–10).*

ASPERGILLOSIS

Aspergillus is the second most common fungal pathogen seen in debilitated and immunosuppressed patients with cancer.[80, 105] It has a predilection for devitalized tissues[16, 50, 92] and is capable of lying dormant for a period and then invading the regional capillaries and spreading to other organs.[21, 92, 105] Once the organism becomes invasive, it produces a lesion that resembles an abscess (aspergilloma). Within it, the fungus may be indolent, especially if some host resistance is present,

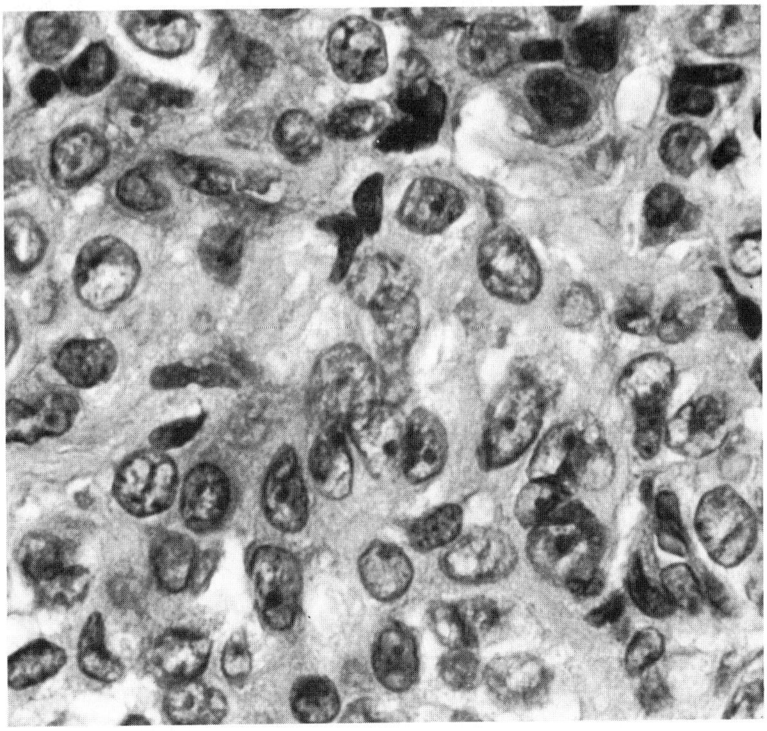

Figure 4–5. Case 1. Tissue section: numerous epithelioid cells are present in the wall of the granuloma. They vary in shape and size, and some resemble histiocytes. (Hematoxylin-eosin, ×665)

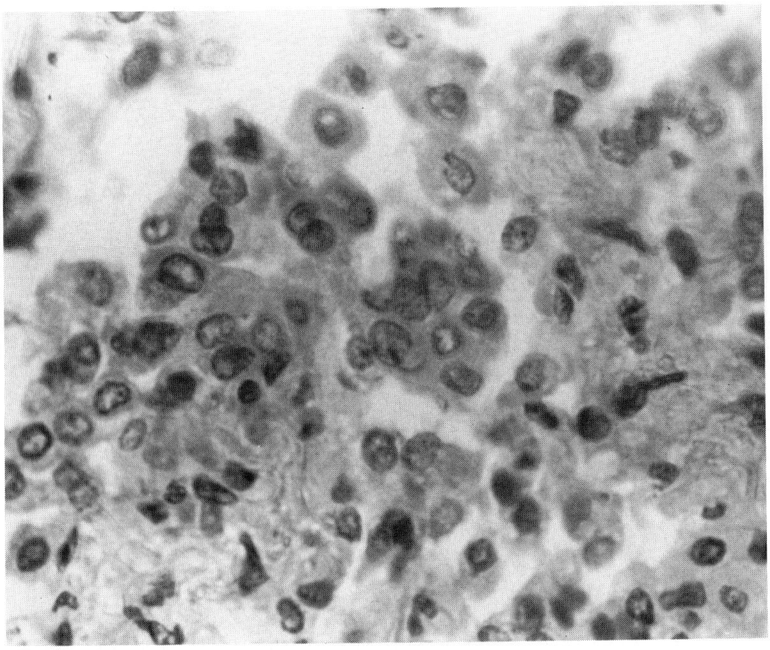

Figure 4–6. Case 1. Tissue section: additional sections through the granuloma revealed a small bronchus with atypical reactive cells in one area of the mucosa. (Hematoxylin-eosin, ×265)

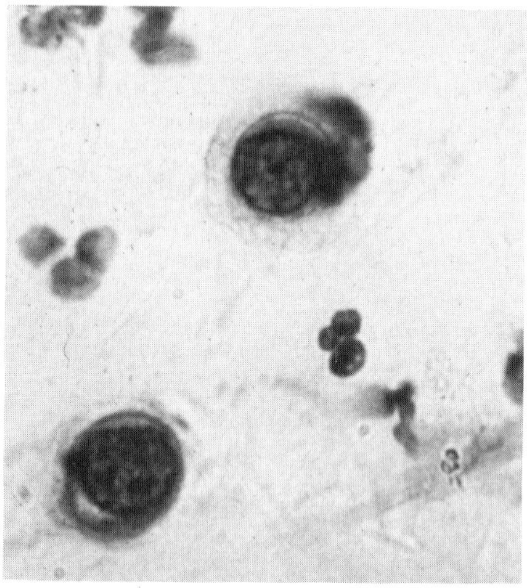

Figure 4–7. Case 2. Pulmonary candidiasis. Sputum specimen: two hyperchromatic malignant appearing cells with high nuclear/cytoplasmic ratio that resemble those often seen in nonkeratinizing squamous cell carcinomas. (Papanicolaou, ×425)

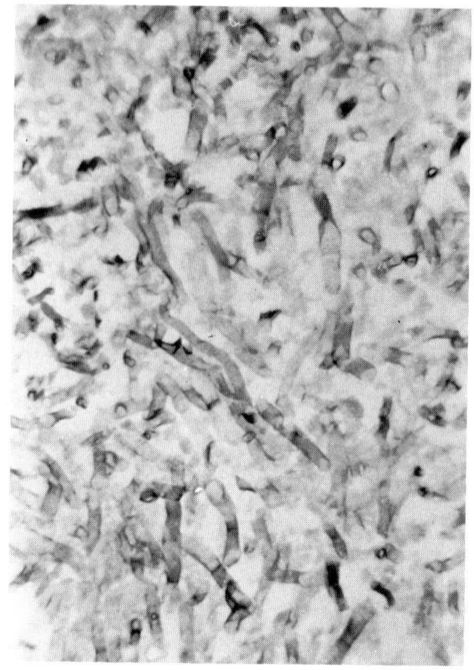

Figure 4–9. Case 2. A histologic section through the lesion stained with periodic acid–Schiff showed the fungal morphology of *Candida albicans.* (×265)

but the infection can progress into a granulomatous lesion and the organism may invade arterial walls, obstruct the flow of blood, and produce mycotic emboli and thrombi.[35, 92] It invades areas of bronchiectasis and is the most common fungus found in abscess cavities, where the hyphae form a mass known as a "fungus ball."[21, 104, 105] Patients being treated with chemotherapy for lung cancer experience a rapid deterioration in their condition when *Aspergillus* invades.[93, 98] It is an extremely aggressive organism, producing

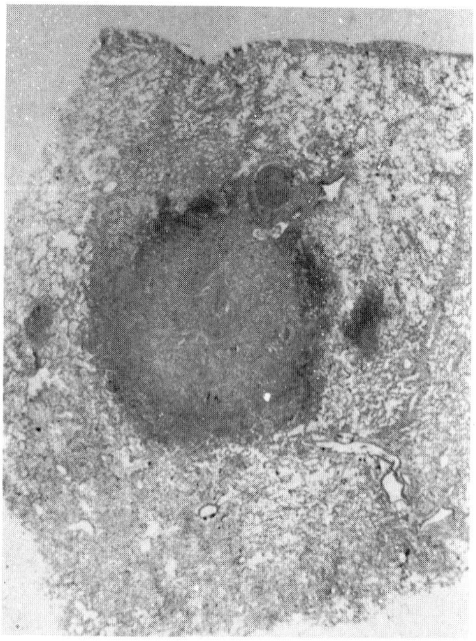

Figure 4–8. Case 2. A 2-×3-cm granuloma found in the wedge resection of the lung. The granuloma contained a solid mass of *Candida albicans.* (Hematoxylin-eosin, ×45)

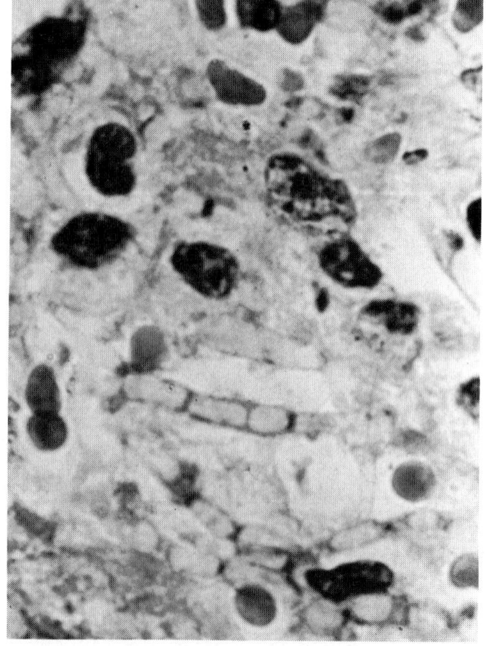

Figure 4–10. Case 2. Histologic section through the granuloma showing hyphae of *Candida*, and abnormal reactive, malignant-appearing cells. (Periodic acid–Schiff, ×265)

necrosis, fistulas, hemorrhage, pulmonary epithelial atypia, and, frequently, death.[29]

Case Study 3. *The appearance of multiple nodules in both lung fields of a male patient who was undergoing chemotherapy for squamous cell carcinoma of the lung led to serial sputum cytology studies that revealed atypical cells suggestive of carcinoma. A wedge resection contained small granulomas with fungal organisms consistent with* Aspergillus, *confirmed by culture. Multinucleated giant cells were present in the reactive zones of the granulomas (Figs. 4–11 through 4–14).*

MUCORMYCOSIS

Mucor ranks third in frequency among the infectious fungi. It is a nonseptate, broad-branching fungus of which there are several species. It shows a predilection for the walls of arteries and veins and causes infarction predominantly in the upper respiratory tract.[33, 40] It may produce a discrete solitary nodule when it initially involves the lung, but it subsequently spreads by the hematogenous route to other viscera. The pulmonary lesions show masses of organisms but little epithelial reaction.

COCCIDIOIDOMYCOSIS

Infection with *Coccidioides immitis*[28] produces epithelial atypia, but it is less pronounced than that found in candidiasis or aspergillosis, possibly because of variation in the biochemical structure of the endosporulating spherules that are so characteristic of the infection. We have observed mild cellular atypia in the sputum of patients with coccidioidomycosis but no dysplasia of significance.

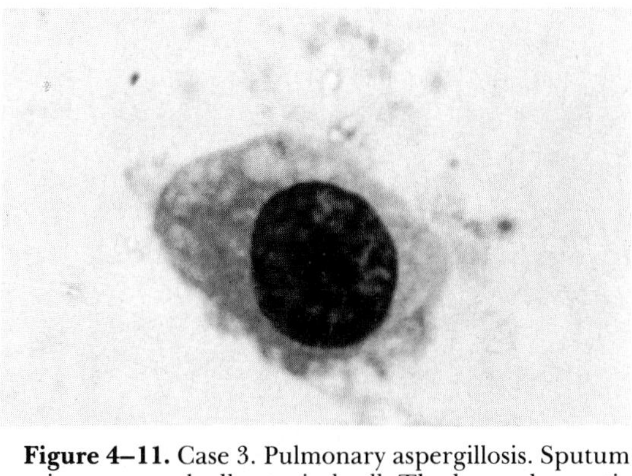

Figure 4–11. Case 3. Pulmonary aspergillosis. Sputum specimen: a markedly atypical cell. The hyperchromatic nucleus shows clumped nuclear chromatin. Although it appears to be undergoing degenerative changes, it is sufficiently atypical to suggest a neoplastic process. (Papanicolaou, ×425)

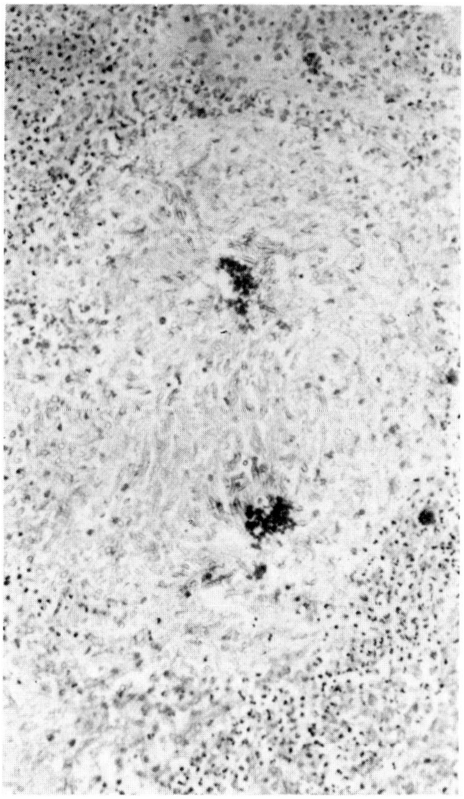

Figure 4–12. Case 3. Tissue biopsy specimen of two confluent, small, fungus-containing granulomas. Atypical single cells were present at the margin. (Hematoxylin-eosin, ×165)

SPOROTRICHOSIS

Rarely one encounters a primary pulmonary infection with *Sporotrichum schenkii.*[52] Foci of granulomatous inflammation with cavitation occur, but epithelial cell atypia within the lung is mild and has not in our experience been associated with a false-positive diagnosis.

HISTOPLASMOSIS

Cavitating granulomas surrounded by a fibrous capsule are formed in histoplasmosis.[6, 7, 54, 65] Within the cavity are necrotic debris and small, budding yeast forms that are easily recognized with the Gomori methenamine silver stain. The organisms are not detected in routine sputum samples. Very little epithelial atypia occurs in sputum with this infection.

CRYPTOCOCCOSIS

Cryptococcosis incites a mild epithelial reaction with little atypia in the acute infection.

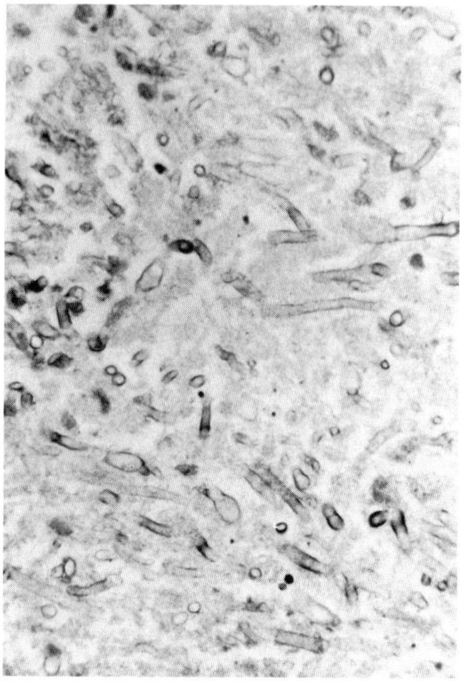

Figure 4–13. Case 3. Same specimen as in Figure 4–12 showing fungi within the granuloma. Culture revealed *Aspergillus.* (Periodic acid–Schiff, ×265)

In chronic cryptococcosis, marked epithelial cell atypia is noted in association with the cryptococcal organisms that are often engulfed in foreign body giant cells.[19, 20] The organisms appear as round intracytoplasmic vacuoles within the giant cells or as free clusters or aggregates within alveoli.[92] In frozen or in formalin-fixed tissues, the periodic acid–Schiff or Mayer's mucicarmine stain demonstrates the mucinous capsule of the fungal organisms, which are found in sputum samples and in sections of the lung.

BLASTOMYCOSIS

Usually blastomycosis is a cutaneous disease, but the organisms may invade the lungs. While it causes pseudoepitheliomatous hyperplasia of the epidermis, the infection in the lung is an acute or chronic granulomatous process,[65, 106] and little epithelial atypia is noted. In our laboratory, the organisms have not been encountered in sputum.

ACTINOMYCOSIS

Actinomyces israelii is a filamentous bacterium frequently encountered in the sputum of cancer patients. Tissue infections commonly occur in the cervicofacial area, thorax, intestine, and female genital tract and may be seen in bone. In the lung it causes abscesses and fibrosis and the formation of secondary sinus tracts to the pleura, chest wall, subcutaneous tissue, and skin. Sulfur granules (large aggregates of organisms) may be observed in sputum or in abscesses. Severe epithelial atypia has not been associated with this infection.

Parasitic Infestation

Pulmonary parasitic lung disease is uncommon in the United States, but amebiasis, echinococcal disease, paragonimiasis, and strongyloidiasis have been reported.[2, 58, 71] Infection with *Paragonimus* species produces multiple necrotizing granulomas.[124] Echinococcal disease is associated with cyst formation, and amebiasis is characterized by abscesses. A case has been reported in which amebas were identified in the sputum of a patient with intestinal amebiasis.[57] We have encountered larvae of *Strongyloides* but not associated epithelial atypia.[58] Infection with the lung fluke *Paragonimus westermani* produces characteristic granulomas, and the golden operculated eggs are readily seen in the necrotic material and surrounding lung

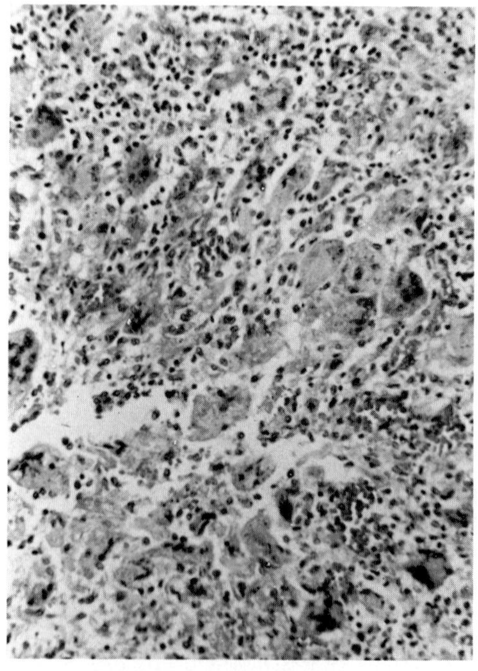

Figure 4–14. Case 3. Tissue section of a reactive area within the *Aspergillus* granuloma showing multinucleated giant cells and inflammation. Fungi were not seen in the area of necrosis (Hematoxylin-eosin, ×165)

tissue. The infection occurs in Americans who have lived for extended periods of time in the Philippines, China, Japan, or Korea. It has also been found in southeast Asia and in some African countries. A case of paragonimiasis has been reported in a cyst of the back of an African boy.[71] A rare species *(Paragonimus kellicotti)* has been recovered from North American mammals that eat shellfish.[71] Persons who eat raw freshwater crayfish or crabs that have ingested the larval form may become infected. The larvae ultimately reach the lungs, mature, and lay their eggs. Acute necrosis, fibrosis, and granulomas occur in response to the adult fluke and the operculated eggs.

Case Study 4. *In a patient with paragonimiasis, the large golden operculated eggs are readily detected. They measure 60 to 100 μ.[124] Figures 4–15 and 4–16 show the appearance in a tissue section of involved lung and illustrate the acute necrosis, fibrosis, and granulomatous inflammation that occurs.*

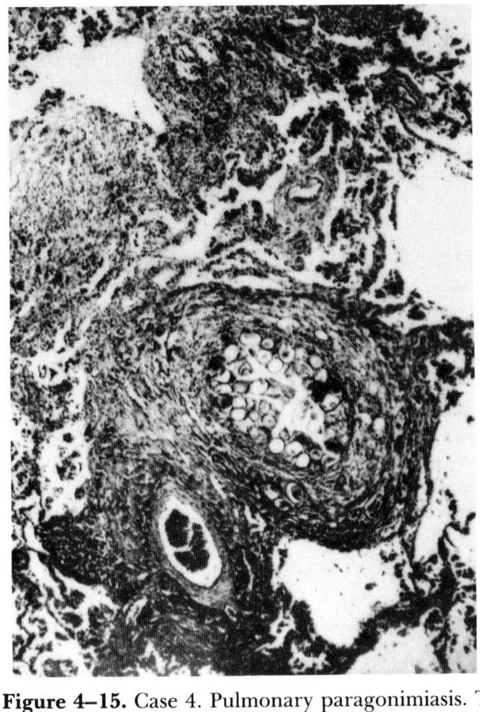

Figure 4–15. Case 4. Pulmonary paragonimiasis. Tissue section: the fibrous wall with granulomatous inflammation surrounds many operculated eggs of *Paragonimus westermani.* Histiocytes filled with hemosiderin and fragments of epithelium sloughed into alveolar spaces can be seen. Many neutrophils and eosinophils are present in the inflammatory exudate. (Hematoxylin-eosin, ×265)

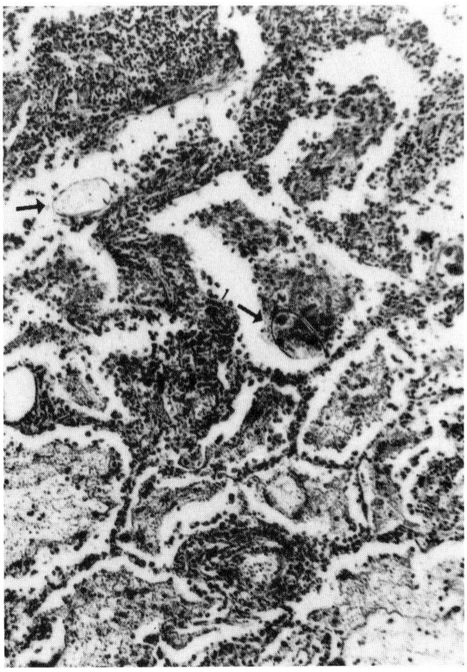

Figure 4–16. Case 4. Tissue section: a section through the inflammatory reaction peripheral to the granuloma showing an egg of *Paragonimus westermani (arrow).* The operculated eggs induce a severe inflammatory response. They appear semitranslucent and may easily be detected in sputum. (Hematoxylin-eosin, ×265)

Idiopathic Granulomatous Disease

Sarcoidosis

Sarcoidosis involves many organs and presents as a variety of clinical symptoms. The eye, conjunctiva, skin, spleen, bone marrow, liver, salivary glands, endocrine glands, and central nervous system may be involved, but the lung is the most common initial site of involvement.[1, 45, 115, 125] Sarcoidosis characteristically is found in persons younger than age 40 and occurs more frequently in blacks than in whites and in female patients more than male patients. In the United States, it occurs more frequently in the southern states. Laboratory studies have revealed that circulating T lymphocytes are reduced in the circulating blood but are present in increased numbers in the granulomas. T lymphocytes and monocytes at the periphery of the pulmonary granulomas are believed to be related to an immunologic process that initiates the granuloma formation. Granulomas are formed by the aggregation of numerous mononuclear cells, which also fuse to form multinucleated giant cells. Numerous single and confluent noncaseating granulomas varying from 1 to 3 cm may be found throughout the pulmonary parenchyma and in mediastinal, hilar, and pulmonary lymph nodes.

In sputum, the cells are single, large, and hyperchromatic with a very high nuclear/cytoplasmic ratio. The nuclei contain dense granular chromatin and are quite similar to single cells of nonkeratinizing squamous cell carcinoma. The cells may also occur in clusters, and multinucleated giant cells may be found.[1]

Case Study 5. *This 38-year-old black woman was asymptomatic, but because of a history of carcinoma of her right breast without lymph node metastases 1 year earlier, she came for her routine follow-up. The physical examination was completely unremarkable, but the chest radiograph revealed bilateral hilar adenopathy and enlargement of the paratracheal lymph nodes. In addition there appeared to be nodularity in the lingula subpleurally. Sputum cytology was reported as positive for squamous cell carcinoma. The cells are illustrated in Figures 4–17 and 4–18. Mediastinal lymph node and pulmonary biopsy specimens were taken and revealed the characteristic noncaseating granulomas of sarcoidosis (Figs. 4–19 and 4–20).*

Wegener's Necrotizing Granulomatosis

Wegener's necrotizing granulomatosis is a rapidly fatal acute necrotizing granulomatous vasculitis that may be found in any organ. The major areas of involvement are the respiratory tract and kidney. The disease affects men predominantly, but fatal cases also occur in women. The vasculitis strikes the smaller arteries and veins, producing thickening and infiltration by neutrophils.[63, 70] In the surrounding tissue, lymphocytes, eosinophils, plasma cells, and multinucleated giant cells occur in large numbers. The pulmonary ar-

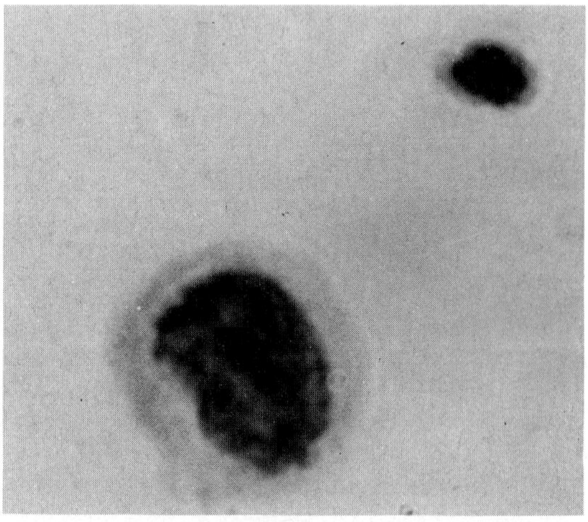

Figure 4–17. Case 5. Sarcoidosis. Sputum specimen: a severely dyskaryotic cell. (Papanicolaou, ×425)

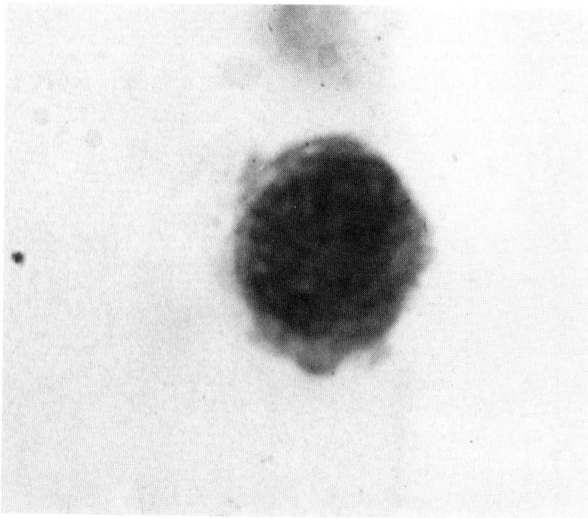

Figure 4–18. Case 5. Sputum specimen: another malignant-appearing cell with high nuclear/cytoplasmic ratio and chromatin clumping resembling a cell of poorly differentiated squamous cell carcinoma. (Papanicolaou, ×425)

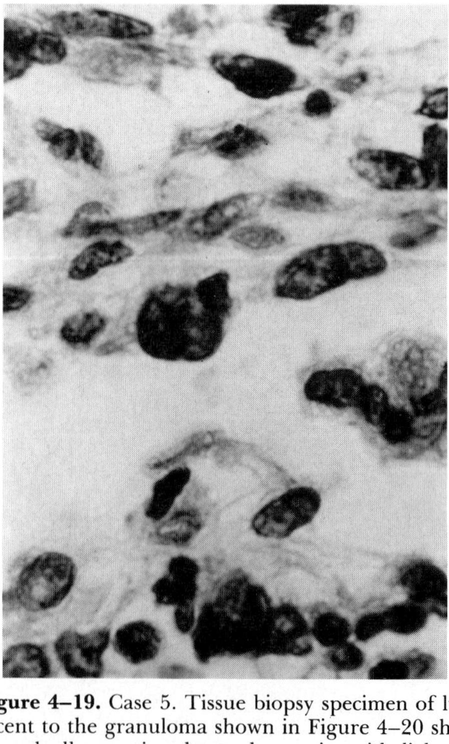

Figure 4–19. Case 5. Tissue biopsy specimen of lung adjacent to the granuloma shown in Figure 4–20 showing markedly reactive, hyperchromatic epithelial cells. (Papanicolaou, ×425)

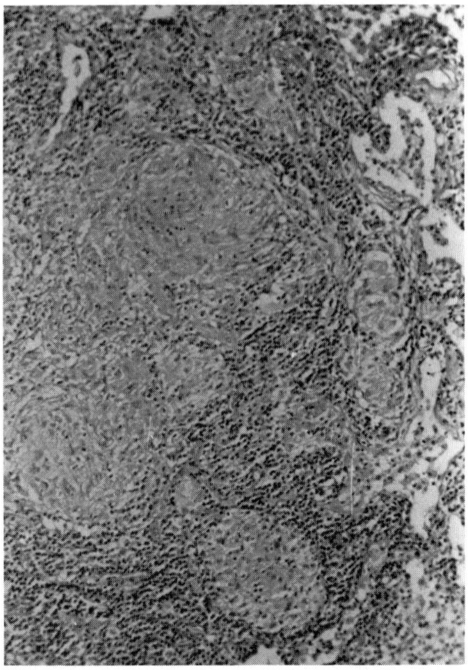

Figure 4–20. Case 5. Tissue biopsy specimen of one of the many granulomas in the lung showing confluent aggregates of reactive histiocytes admixed with numerous lymphocytes. (Hematoxylin-eosin, ×165)

chitecture is destroyed by the necrobiotic process, which is probably a form of hypersensitivity angiitis since immune complex injury has been identified.[45]

The granulomas are usually small; however, larger ones are not uncommon and some become cavitary. The granulomas may show a striking resemblance to those of tuberculosis, but mycobacteria have not been found in the lesions. Hector reported the sputum findings in two cases.[44] The cells occur in small clusters and contain markedly dyskaryotic nuclei with moderate to high nuclear/cytoplasmic ratios, resembling the cells demonstrated in sarcoidosis.

LUNG ABSCESS

A pulmonary abscess is a localized acute suppurative process. Lung abscesses vary in size up to 10 cm, occur in any lobe, and may be single or multiple.[83] The usual causative agents are *Staphylococcus aureus,* pneumococcus, streptococci (aerobic and anerobic), *Bacteroides,* fusobacteria, and other organisms found in the oral cavity.[9, 53]

Usually the causative organisms enter the lung when a primary pulmonary infection already exists; and pathogenic bacteria,

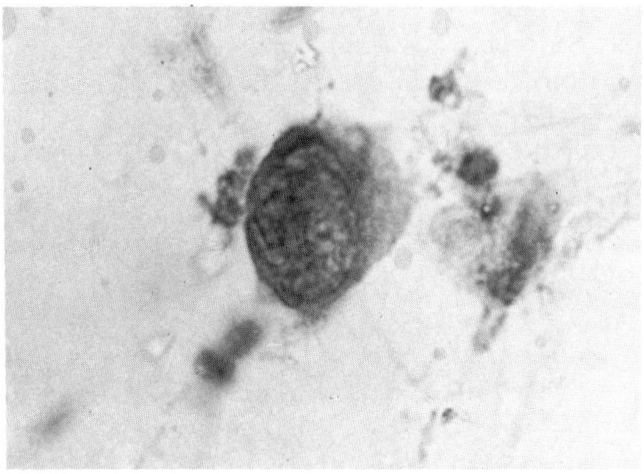

Figure 4–21. Case 6. Lung abscess. Sputum specimen: smudged and enlarged dyskaryotic cells. (Papanicolaou, ×425)

fungi, or viruses invade the devitalized area. Foci of bronchiectasis, septic emboli associated with venous obstruction within the lung, aspiration of regurgitated gastric contents, and tumors that obstruct an airway may be responsible.[9, 53, 83] In many instances an antecedent cause is not apparent. Abscesses of the upper lobes occur following aspiration pneumonitis.[83] They may be associated with empyema, bronchiectasis, or cancer and may be multiple. Necrotic debris, inflammatory cells, saprophytic fungi, and bezoars may be found in the cavity. The parenchyma adjacent to the abscess often shows varying degrees of epithelial atypia, including hyperplasia and dysplasia, which is sometimes severe.

Case Study 6. *A 62-year-old man with a history of heavy smoking presented with intermittent hemoptysis of 1 year's duration, chest pain, and sore throat. A chronic productive cough had increased in severity over the previous 3 months, and weight loss of 40 pounds had occurred over several years. Chest radiography revealed no evidence of pneumonia or a neoplastic lesion. A bronchial biopsy*

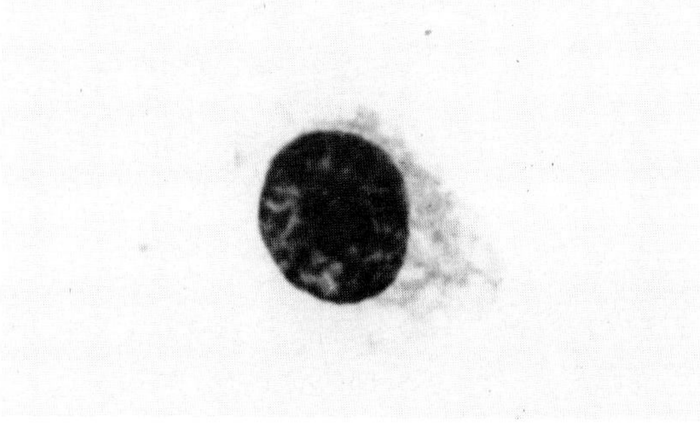

Figure 4–22. Case 6. Sputum specimen: dyskaryotic and hyperchromatic cell with granular chromatin and with most of the cytoplasm lost. (Papanicolaou, ×425)

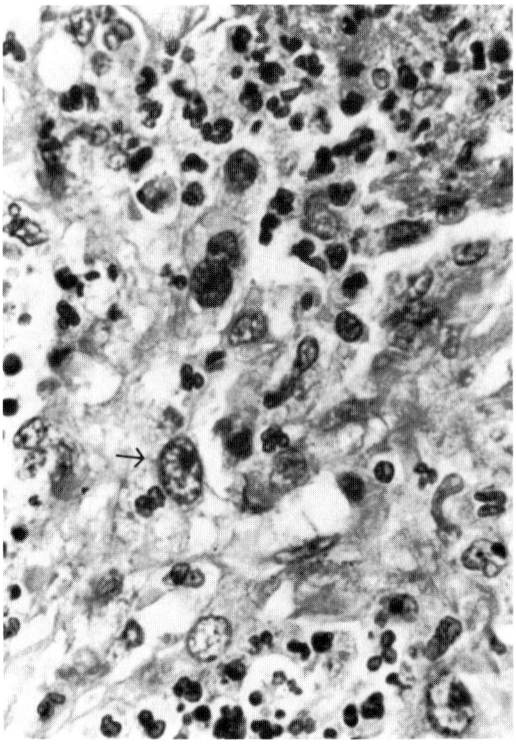

Figure 4–23. Case 6. Tissue section: wall of abscess showing enlarged epithelial cells. One cell *(arrow)* contains a large nucleolus. (Hematoxylin-eosin, ×265)

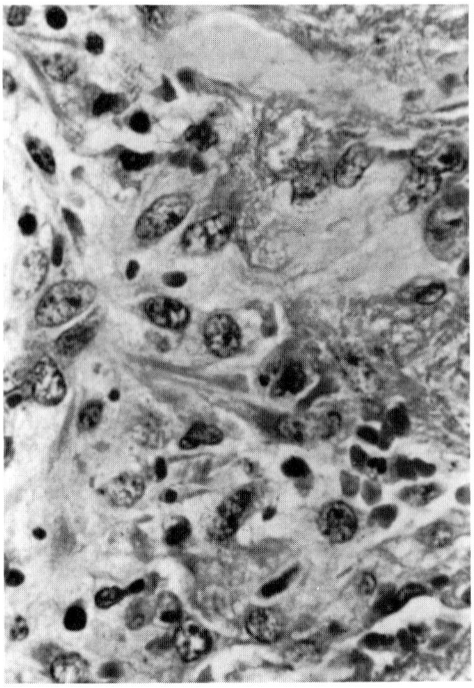

Figure 4–24. Case 6. Tissue section: another section from the wall of the abscess in Figure 4–23. The abscess cavity communicated with a bronchus. (Hematoxylin-eosin, ×265)

specimen showed bronchitis. Radiologic investigation 8 months later revealed pneumonia in the posterior segment of the right upper lobe with an ill-defined margin and lucency that suggested cavitation. Squamous cell carcinoma was diagnosed from sputum cytology. A repeat bronchogram now revealed a lesion in the right upper lobe, and a lobectomy was performed 8 months after the initial admission. The histologic diagnoses were carcinoma in situ, *lung abscess with severe chronic bronchitis, and focal bronchopneumonia. He remains well 11 years later. The atypical cells are illustrated in Figures 4–21 through 4–25.*

PNEUMONIA

Bacterial Pneumonia

Acute Pneumonia

Acute bacterial pneumonia is the earliest and most frequent major complication in the

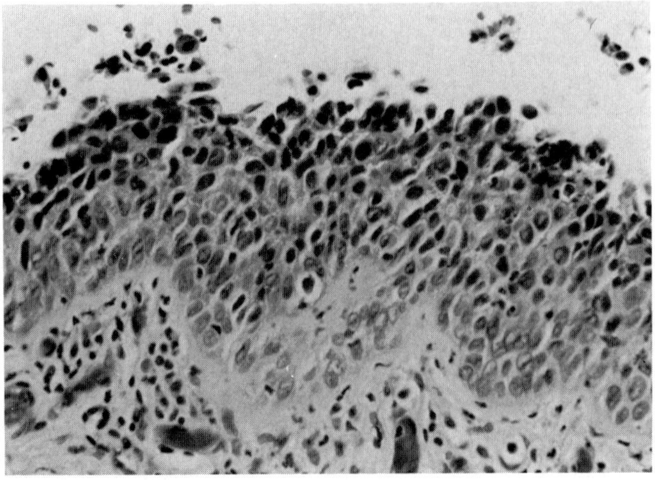

Figure 4–25. Case 6. Tissue section: a section of a bronchus in the resected lobe. While this bronchus was not directly connected with the abscess, its epithelium showed severe dysplasia bordering on carcinoma *in situ.* (Hematoxylin-eosin, ×265)

immunosuppressed patient.[113, 128] It not only follows chemotherapy for cancer but also occurs in diabetics and following a heart, kidney, or other organ transplant.[9, 15, 16, 53] Pathogenic bacteria and fungi (even saprophytes) become invasive and fill the alveoli with a suppurative exudate and cell debris.[15, 113] If treated successfully with antibiotics, the pneumonia resolves. Sputum examinations are rarely requested for a patient with elevated temperature, cough, and focal bronchopneumonia, but with opacification of an entire lobe, especially in elderly patients, lung cancer must be included in the differential diagnosis. The following case reveals a rare instance in which the epithelial cell reaction was severely atypical.

Case Study 7. *A 61-year-old alcoholic patient was admitted obtunded and incoherent to a neighborhood hospital. Results of urine and blood sugar examinations were unremarkable, but the chest radiograph revealed opacification of the lower half of the left chest. His white blood cell count was 10,000/mm^3 with 70% neutrophils, and his respirations were rapid and shallow. At bronchoscopy, red friable mucosa was noted in the lingular bronchus and a biopsy specimen was taken. The biopsy diagnosis was adenocarcinoma. The patient was promptly transferred to a cancer center where several sputa were collected. Because of fluid and opacity in the left lower chest, the pleural cavity was aspirated. Two liters of a yellow-gray purulent exudate were removed. Culture revealed* Staphylococcus aureus, *and antibiotic therapy was begun. Sputa, in the meantime, were reported as positive for adenocarcinoma. The patient responded to antibiotic therapy and was completely well in 12 days. The cleared chest revealed no evidence of residual pneumonia or tumor, and he has remained well for 2 years without evidence of carcinoma. The abnormal cells that occurred with this patient's acute pneumonitis are shown in Figures 4–26 and 4–27.*

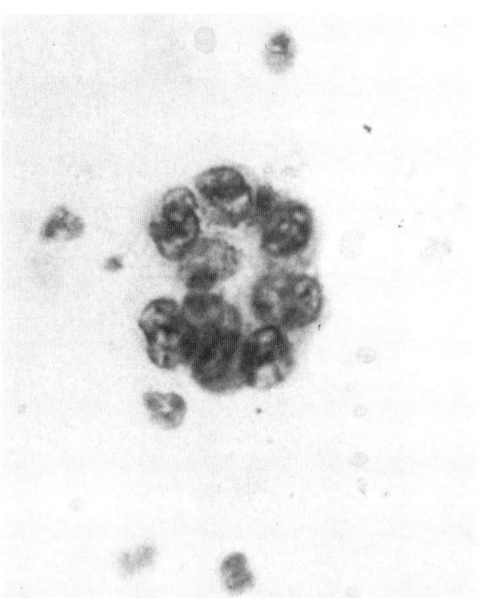

Figure 4–26. Case 7. Acute pneumonia. Sputum specimen: an acinar-like structure. This sputum specimen was diagnosed as adenocarcinoma. (Papanicolaou, ×425)

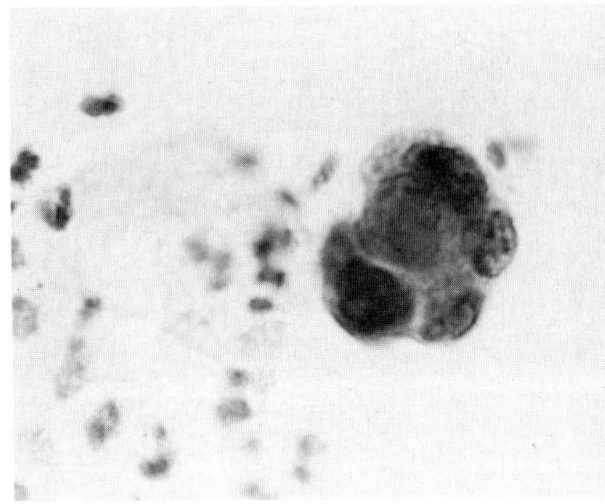

Figure 4–27. Case 7. Sputum specimen: another cluster of cells resembling an acinus of a poorly differentiated adenocarcinoma. (Papanicolaou, ×425)

Chronic Organizing (Nonresolving) Pneumonia

In a small number of patients who have had lobar pneumonia, resolution is not complete and an area of unresolved pneumonia persists.[110] In this area, alveolar walls are thickened and many alveoli contain a fibrinoid material. If the process continues, fibrous tissue obliterates many of the alveolar spaces. Surrounding the persistent pneumonia, alveoli and small bronchioles show squamous metaplasia, epithelial hyperplasia, and even marked atypia.

Case Study 8. *The patient, a 57-year-old man who had smoked two packs of cigarettes per day for more than 25 years, noted a chronic productive cough that was sometimes blood tinged, fatigue, and a 12-lb weight loss in the previous month. Chest radiography revealed a mass in the superior segment of the right lower lobe that did not respond to a course of antibiotics. He was transferred to a cancer center where bronchoscopic examination showed inflammation of the bronchial mucosa but*

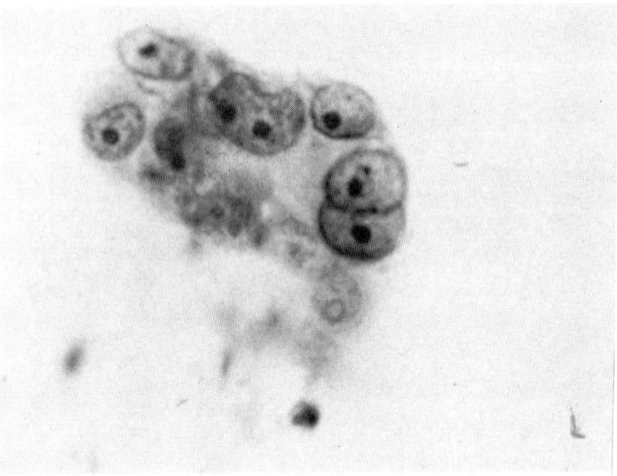

Figure 4–28. Case 8. Chronic organizing pneumonia. Sputum specimen: an acinar-like structure suggestive of adenocarcinoma with prominent nucleoli. (Papanicolaou, ×425)

no intrinsic mass. Tomograms revealed pneumonic consolidation. Three sputum samples were submitted for cytologic examination. Two were diagnosed as positive, and one was suspicious for cells of adenocarcinoma. The lesion did not respond to additional antibiotic therapy, and 17 days later the right lower lobe was resected. The histologic diagnosis was chronic organizing (nonresolving) pneumonia, with fibrosing alveolitis. The process did not spread to other areas and has not recurred in 4 years following surgery (Figs. 4–28 through 4–30).

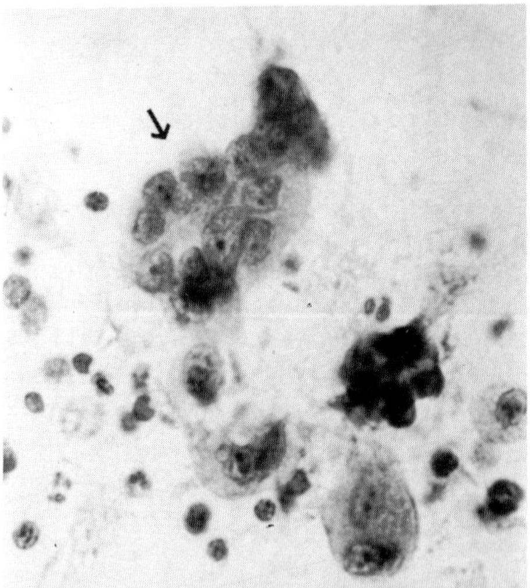

Figure 4–29. Case 8. Sputum specimen: a second acinar-like structure *(arrow)* from the same sputum specimen as Figure 4–28. The lung lesion histologically was chronic nonresolving pneumonia, but the cytologic features were very suggestive of adenocarcinoma. (Papanicolaou, ×265)

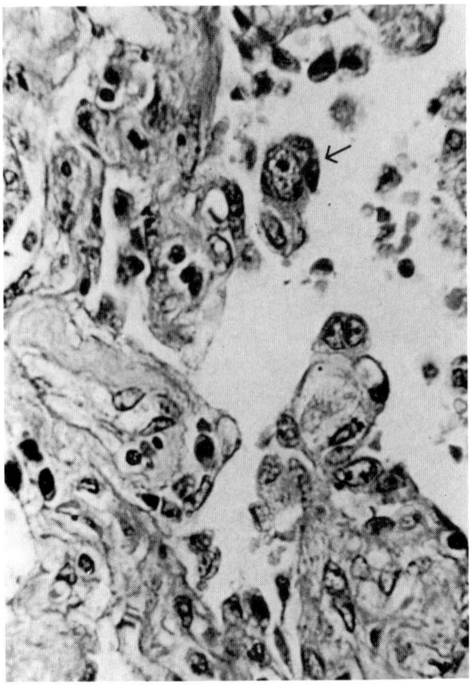

Figure 4–30. Case 8. Tissue section: chronic organizing pneumonia. Interstitial fibrosis was present throughout the area of organization. In the center is an entrapped small bronchiole with a few atypical cells similar to those noted in the sputum *(arrow)*. (Hematoxylin-eosin, ×265)

Lipid Pneumonia

Lipid pneumonia usually occurs in persons taking mineral oil as a laxative or from the use of mineral oil nose drops.[17, 82, 116] Fumes from superheated lipids, fats, or some drugs produce a severe bronchial reaction. Lipid materials that are apparently inert can nevertheless induce a foreign body reaction, empyema, or fistulas and stimulate a marked macrophage response.[17, 82, 117, 119] Grossly the process may be diffuse or form a localized firm yellow granular mass without hemorrhage, necrosis, or calcification. There may be multiple nodules. Lipid droplets are found within alveolar macrophages. In sputum, the aggregates of distended macrophages vaguely resemble cells of adenocarcinoma and may be confused with it. It is not possible to stain for the lipid in sputum smears if it has been removed by processing. An aggregate of fat-laden macrophages from a patient who had used mineral oil nose drops for many years is shown in Figure 4–31.

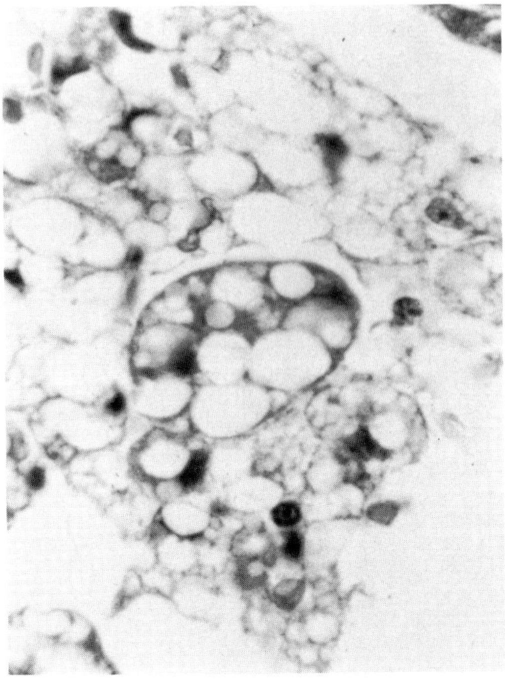

Figure 4–31. Lipid pneumonia. Tissue section: the central ovoid structure lies within a lipogranuloma. It is composed of an aggregate of lipid-filled macrophages that have coalesced to resemble a giant cell. Many single distended macrophages were present in the sputum, and some resembled the cells of a signet-ring adenocarcinoma. The oil-red-O stain was positive for lipids on the touch preparation. (Hematoxylin-eosin, ×265)

Viral Pneumonia

Some viral infections are mild and produce little injury to the host; others are severe, especially in nonimmunized children, following blood transfusion, in organ transplant patients, and in persons with AIDS. Different species and serotypes of virus have affinity for different cell sites. Some strains become attached to specific surface lipid or protein complexes or to other cell membrane receptor sites. The type of attachment site receptor often determines the form of interaction between the host cell and the invading virus. Once attached upon the surface, the virus enters the cell, adheres to cytoplasmic vacuoles (endosomes), and fuses with the endosomal membrane or becomes attached to the nuclear membrane. Affinity for different cell sites is characteristic of different species of virus.

Some viruses produce inclusion bodies that are readily identified in slides, but their absence does not preclude a viral infection. Direct immunofluorescence and tissue culture isolation techniques are commonly used to identify many strains of virus. Characteristic viral inclusions (Cowdry type A) may be formed by adenoviruses, respiratory syncytial virus, cytomegalovirus, herpes, variola, and varicella.[129] Smaller intranuclear virus particles (Cowdry type B) are found in infections such as poliomyelitis. They occur in relatively normal-appearing cells and are not easily detected by light microscopy.

Viral infection results in swelling, vacuolization, nuclear enlargement with hyperchromasia, and cell lysis. Direct invasion of adjacent cells is also promoted by viral gene products, resulting in the formation of multinucleated giant cells like those seen in rubeola and sometimes in varicella. The swelling and cell enlargement, often associated with nuclear hyperchromasia and multinucleation, result occasionally in misinterpretation of the abnormal cells as cancer cells.

Herpes Pneumonitis

In immunosuppressed adults, herpes is the most common viral infection.[81] Next in frequency are cytomegalovirus, in combination with *Pneumocystis carinii,* and varicella.

Case Study 9. *An 81-year-old man was admitted with chest pain, cough of 2 weeks' duration and a low-grade temperature. He had on several occasions noted chills. The chest radiograph revealed small patchy areas of confluent pneumonia in the left lower lobe, and a sputum sample was obtained. The smears were submitted by a medical resident*

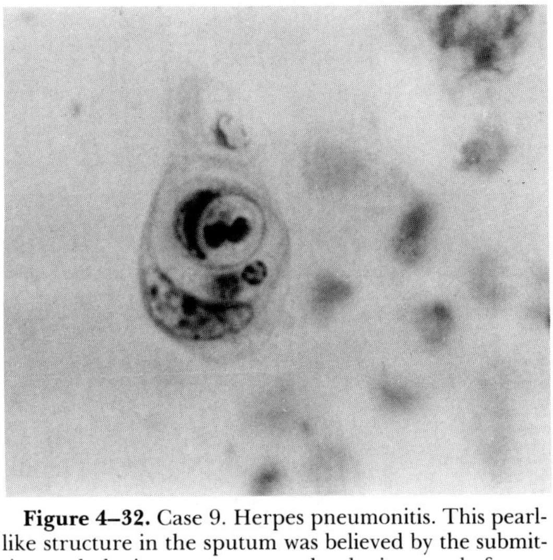

Figure 4–32. Case 9. Herpes pneumonitis. This pearl-like structure in the sputum was believed by the submitting pathologist to represent a developing pearl of squamous cell carcinoma. (Papanicolaou, ×425)

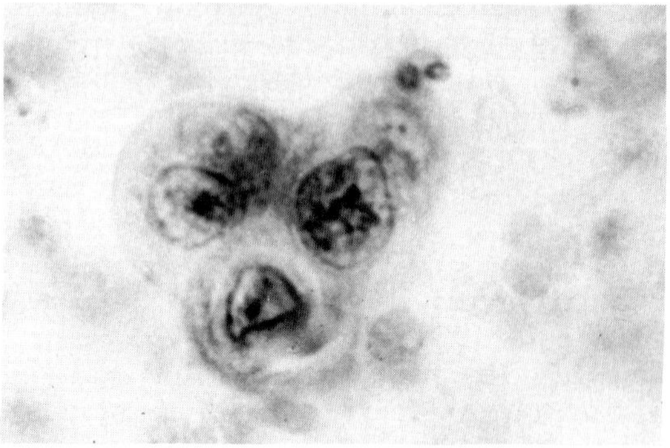

Figure 4–33. Case 9. This cluster of distorted cells with degenerating nuclei was also considered representative of squamous cell carcinoma. (Papanicolaou, ×425)

with the information that the patient had pulmonary "nodules." Abnormal cells were present and were reported as cells of squamous cell carcinoma. A second sputum sample was taken on the following morning, and it contained cells with characteristic herpes inclusions. When the original smears were reviewed, herpes inclusions were also found in sparse numbers. The patient responded to supportive therapy and was discharged in 3 weeks with a normal chest radiograph and no evidence of carcinoma (Figs. 4–32 through 4–36).

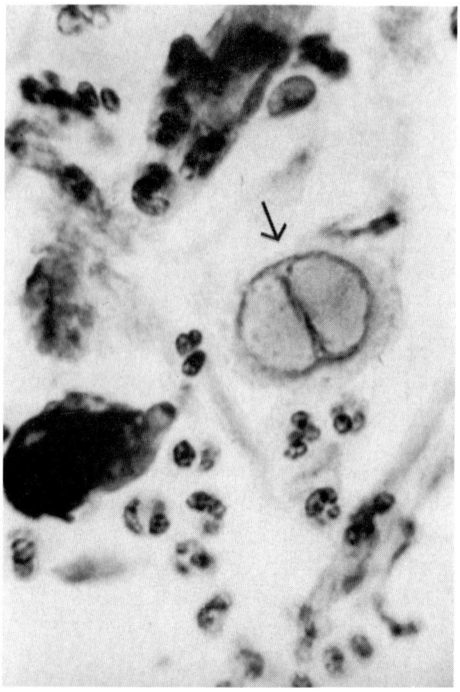

Figure 4–35. Case 9. These herpes inclusion bodies were found in cells of the second sputum specimen, obtained on the following morning. The opaque bodies fill the cytoplasm *(arrow)*. (Papanicolaou, ×425)

Cytomegalovirus

Cytomegalovirus has appeared as a complicating infection of patients receiving renal or other organ transplants. It is a common pulmonary pathogen in patients with AIDS and is frequently found in association with *Pneumocystis carinii* infections in the immunocompromised host. The infection is spread by respiratory droplets, but in about 5% of the fatal cases it is transmitted by blood transfusion. Large intranuclear inclusion

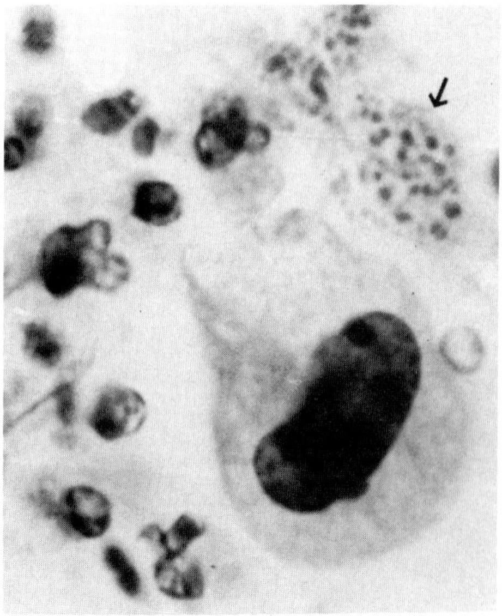

Figure 4–34. Case 9. This large degenerating cell was found in the same sputum. Note the inclusions within an adjacent cell *(arrow)*. (Papanicolaou, ×425)

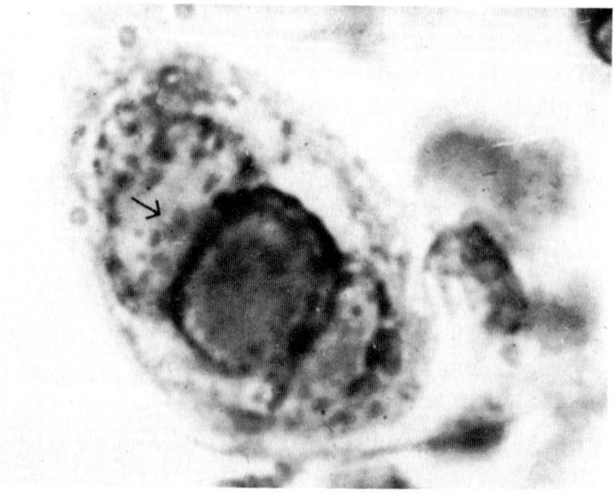

Figure 4–36. Case 9. This epithelial cell contains not only the opaque herpetic inclusion but also the immature reproductive forms that are emerging from the cell *(arrow)*. (Papanicolaou, ×665)

bodies surrounded by a "halo" are characteristic, but cytoplasmic inclusions also occur. Some atypia in uninvolved epithelial cells is often noted.

Varicella

Varicella is an acute infectious communicable disease of childhood that also affects nonimmunized adults and debilitated elderly patients. It involves the skin, mucous membranes, reticuloendothelial tissue, and lungs. The causative agent is a member of the herpes family of DNA viruses that spread by droplet infection and usually involve the trachea and bronchi. Pulmonary involvement is often patchy. Epithelial cells in the lung and buccal mucosa become enlarged, undergo rapid mitotic division, and form multinucleated cells, which are occasionally seen in sputum or in smears of the buccal cavity.

Case Study 10. *An 11-year-old girl being treated for leukemia was in early relapse and she returned to the hospital for a repeat course of chemotherapy. During hospitalization she developed coryza, conjunctivitis, elevated temperature (104.5°F) and a rash. Lymph node enlargement was generalized and especially noticeable in the inguinal, axillary, and supraclavicular areas. On the third day of hospitalization, her respiratory rate increased and a chest radiograph showed patchy peribronchitis and focal bronchopneumonia. Inspection of the oral cavity and buccal surface of the lips revealed a few vesicles. She developed a productive blood-tinged cough, and a sputum specimen was submitted for microscopic examination. The smears showed clusters of cells containing varicella inclusions (Figs. 4–37 and 4–38). With supportive therapy, she recovered slowly and symptoms of infection disappeared. Therapy for the leukemia was continued 1 month later.*

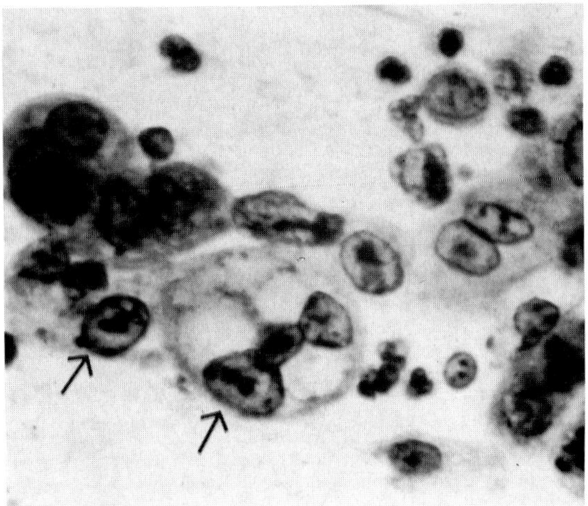

Figure 4–37. Case 10. Varicella. Sputum specimen: marked epithelial enlargement, multinucleation and nucleolar enlargement *(arrows)* in epithelial cells in varicella. (Papanicolaou, ×425)

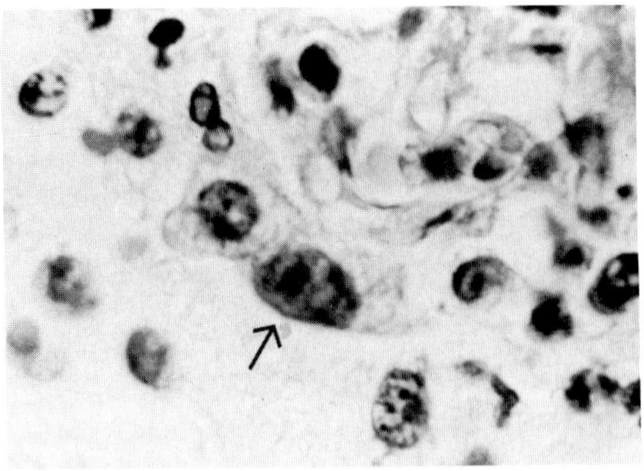

Figure 4–38. Case 10. Lung tissue from a fatal case of varicella showing an enlarged cell with an intranuclear inclusion *(arrow)*. (Hematoxylin-eosin, ×425)

Rubeola and Parainfluenza Viruses

Rubeola and parainfluenza viruses are RNA viruses that are highly contagious but are seldom encountered in vaccinated children. Infections do occur in the young, the aged, and immunosuppressed children being treated for leukemia.[34] They are characterized by marked hyperplasia of alveolar epithelial cells and bronchioles. The epithelial cells enlarge and fuse. Intracytoplasmic and intranuclear inclusions are easily found in many cells. The pneumonic process associated with rubeola (measles) is referred to as "giant cell" pneumonia. The parainfluenza virus produces similar changes.[34]

BRONCHIAL ASTHMA

Asthma is a relatively common immunologic disorder of unknown etiology with an incidence of 4% in the United States.[43, 45, 47] It is characterized by increased irritability of the bronchial tree manifested by coughing, spasm, and wheezing. It has been classified on the basis of elevated IgE serum concentrations and peripheral blood eosinophilia. Type I is the extrinsic form that is associated with allergens and elevated serum IgE.[3, 115] It has been correlated with exposure to foods, animal dander, pollens, dusts, and other allergens.[90] Type II, the intrinsic form, is not associated with elevated serum IgE and appears to be related to pulmonary infections predominantly of viral etiology.[45] Aspirin, chemicals,[48] occupational fumes,[18, 45, 47] exercise,[73] *Aspergillus* spores,[51] stress, and other factors such as the leukotrienes may precipitate asthmatic attacks.[43, 101] The histologic appearance has been well documented. Cytologic specimens contain Curschmann's spirals, epithelial whorls, mucus, Charcot-Leyden crystals, and eosinophils. Eosinophilic granules are not seen in Papanicolaou-stained smears but are seen in smears stained with Wright-Giemsa stain.[90] In cases in which the attack is persistent, aggregates of columnar epithelial cells and goblet cells known as Creola bodies may be present in the sputum. These bodies occasionally resemble clusters of adenocarcinoma cells. A careful search will reveal a terminal bar and cilia and eliminate the possibility that these cell aggregates represent a neoplasm. In a rare instance, severe epithelial dysplasia may simulate squamous cell carcinoma. The following case is unusual.

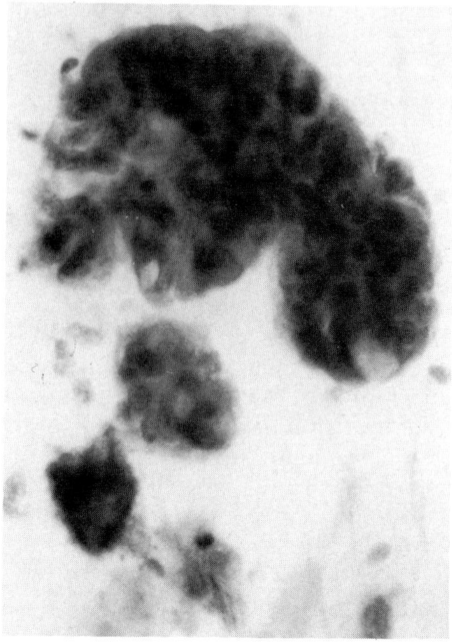

Figure 4–40. Case 11. Sputum specimen: a thick Creola body in a woman with status asthmaticus. Because of a left lower lobe infiltrate, metastatic adenocarcinoma had been considered in the differential diagnosis. (Papanicolaou, ×425)

Case Study 11. *A 20-year-old woman with a long history of recurrent asthmatic attacks developed persistent coughing, wheezing, mucus hypersecretion, and vague chest radiographic changes. Her physician requested a sputum analysis. Atypical epithelial cells were found and were diagnosed as squamous cell carcinoma in a private laboratory where the history was not known. The physician referred the patient to a cancer center where a sputum series was performed and the characteristic findings of epithelial whorls, groups of severely dyskaryotic squamous cells, mucus, and Curschmann's spirals were identified. She was treated with corticosteroids, and a repeat chest radiograph at the time of discharge revealed no abnormality. The dyskaryotic squamous cells and other characteristic findings that occur in some patients with asthmatic bronchitis are shown in Figures 4–39 through 4–42.*

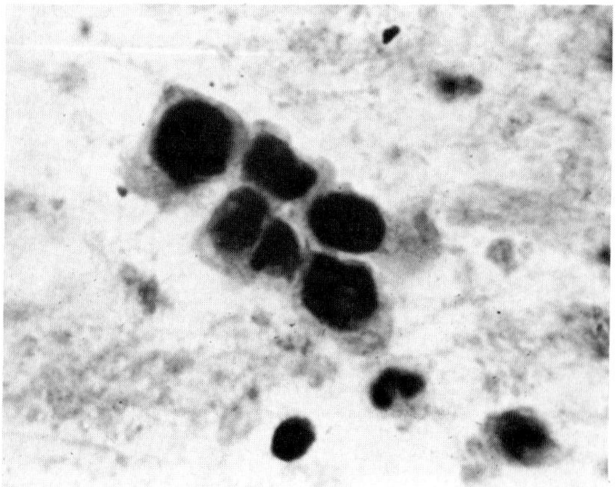

Figure 4–39. Case 11. Bronchial asthma. A cluster of severely dyskeratotic cells in asthma showing features similar to cells of nonkeratinizing squamous cell carcinoma by virtue of their hyperchromasia, pleomorphism, and very high nuclear/cytoplasmic ratio. (Papanicolaou, ×425)

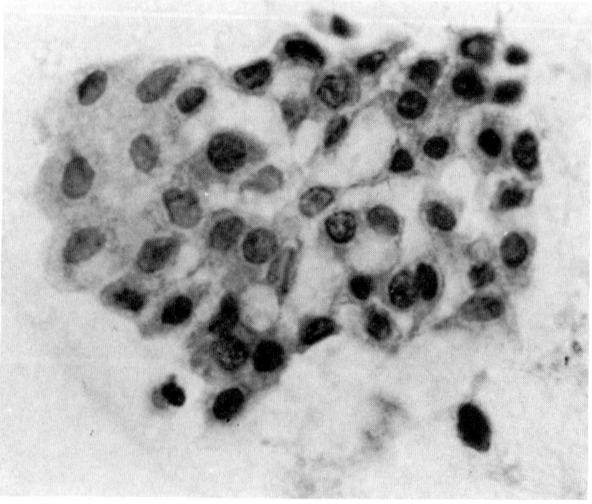

Figure 4–41. Case 11. A cluster of metaplastic and goblet cells in sputum. Such clusters are not uncommon in asthmatic patients. (Papanicolaou, ×425)

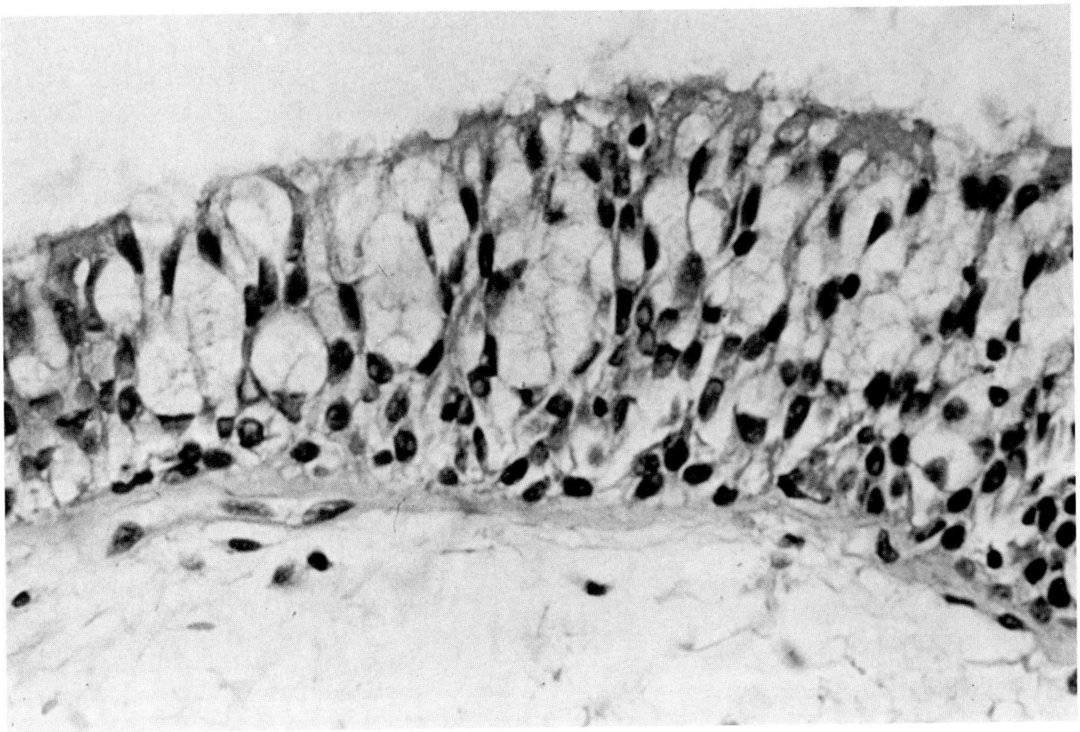

Figure 4–42. Case 11. Tissue section of a bronchus in an asthmatic patient. Hyperplastic goblet cells are present in the mucosa. Squamous metaplasia also may also occur with goblet cell hyperplasia. (Hematoxylin-eosin, ×265)

PULMONARY INFARCTION

Pulmonary embolization, which occurs frequently in hospitalized patients, is the third most common cause of death following cardiovascular disease and cerebral hemorrhage.[23, 24] Annually there are more than 600,000 incidents and 50,000 deaths.[94, 95] It is found in 10% to 15% of hospitalized patients who come to autopsy.[99] Emboli arise in the thrombosed deep veins of the lower extremities and in the iliac or pelvic veins,[12, 13, 77, 78] and from the periprostatic, parovarian, or renal veins or the inferior vena cava.[62] Large emboli are a cause of sudden death, especially if there has been antecedent heart failure or cardiopulmonary disease.[26, 99] Smaller emboli that obstruct the lobar and segmental or subsegmental arteries cause infarction.[11, 14, 100] The infarct grossly is a wedge-shaped, congested peripheral area of the lung usually less than 5 cm in greatest dimension. It becomes apparent on radiography from 12 to 36 hours post embolization. The cardinal clinical signs are a rapid pulse and respiratory rate without elevation of temperature in a relatively asymptomatic patient.[77, 78, 91] Microscopic examination of the infarcted tissue reveals distention of alveolar capillaries and fluid within alveoli. The alveolar lining cells show marked atypia. Small emboli produce peripheral infarcts that often extend to the pleura and are accompanied by a fibrinous exudate on the involved pleural surface; a small amount of hemorrhagic fluid is usually seen within the pleural space on the chest radiograph. The volume of the pleural fluid, which should routinely be recorded on every specimen received in the cytopreparatory laboratory, has not in our experience exceeded 250 ml.

Sputum samples from patients with radiologically recognized infarcts are seldom submitted to the laboratory. The presence of a pleural effusion, however, brings with it requirement for a cytologic examination to eliminate the possibility of a pleural metastasis from an occult carcinoma. Mesothelial cells found in the bloody effusion fluid often aggregate in small clumps. The individual cells are enlarged, and the nuclear/cytoplasmic ratios are sometimes exceedingly high. Nuclei show smudgy hyperchromasia, and nucleoli are prominent.[78] Markedly atypical cells associated with a pulmonary infarct are illustrated in Figure 4–43.

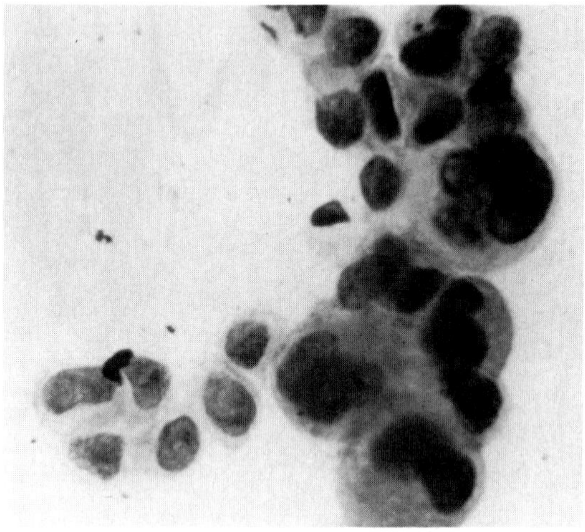

Figure 4–43. Pulmonary infarct. Clusters of hyperplastic reactive mesothelial cells found in pleural fluid associated with a pulmonary infarct. The cells simulate aggregates seen in mesothelioma and metastatic adenocarcinoma. (Papanicolaou, ×425)

RADIATION THERAPY

Normal pulmonary epithelial cells are relatively insensitive to radiation.[5, 49, 85, 96] The nucleus appears to be more vulnerable than the cytoplasm. The initial response to radiant energy is swelling of the entire cell, vacuolization of the cytoplasm, and alteration of the permeability of the plasma membrane.[118] The cytoplasm becomes watery and vacuolated and often appears metachromatic with a lavender-purple hue. The nuclear changes are marked swelling, smudginess, vacuolization, rupture of the nuclear membrane, and, ultimately, karyorrhexis. If the nucleus is partially injured, it may not lose its ability to undergo mitosis. The nuclear DNA develops structural alterations and molecular rearrangements.[25] Uninjured nuclear protein complexes are stimulated to repair those damaged, and they do so in an uncontrolled fashion, with the result that bizarre nuclear forms develop and persist indefinitely. Malignant tumors that show a high mitotic rate are more sensitive to the radiation therapy than those that have a low mitotic rate.[118] Irradiation during the mitotic phase results in chromosome aberrations such as deletions, fragmentation, and translocations.[49] The genetic process often is completely altered, and the cells with modified chromosomes may show haploidy, aneuploidy, or hyperploidy.

At times it is impossible following irradiation to differentiate the cells found in sputum from malignant cells. Consequently, detection of recurrence in sputum samples can be exceedingly difficult. Comparison with smears made prior to therapy may be helpful. Follow-up with additional specimens is man-

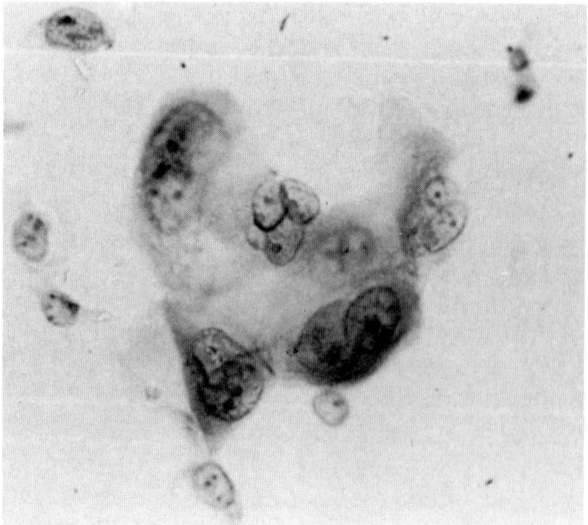

Figure 4–44. Case 12. Radiation therapy changes. Bronchial brushings. Note cytoplasmic swelling and nuclear enlargement with binucleation. (Papanicolaou, ×425)

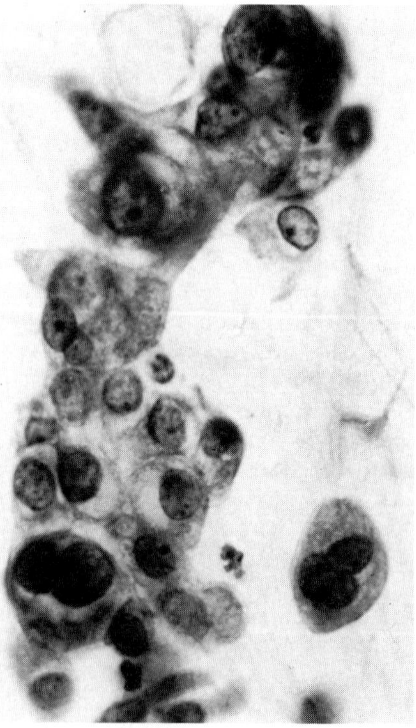

Figure 4–45. Case 12. Bronchial brushing after radiation therapy. The field showed a high nuclear/cytoplasmic ratio and multinucleation with nuclear molding. (Papanicolaou, ×465)

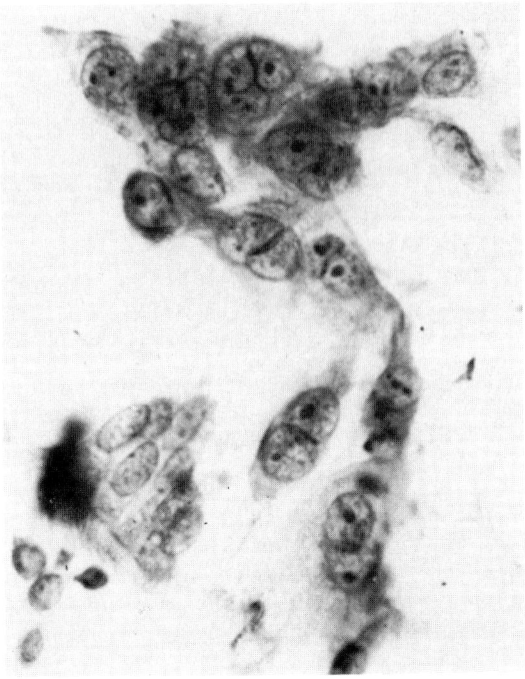

Figure 4–46. Case 12. Same brushing as in Figure 4–45 revealed an area with even more exaggerated changes that by themselves might be considered suggestive of adenocarcinoma. Nucleoli are prominent. The cytoplasm of the cells is fragile and fragmented. (Papanicolaou, ×465)

datory when abnormal cells are found following irradiation.

Case Study 12. *A 27-year-old man received radiation therapy for Hodgkin's disease involving his mediastinum. Several months later, he developed haziness in the right middle and upper lobes, and bronchoscopy was performed. Only an edematous pale mucosa was noted. It was brushed and revealed swelling of the epithelial cells with nuclear enlargement caused by the recent irradiation. Figures 4–44 through 4–46 show the cytology of the bronchial brushings from this patient. Figure 4–47 shows alterations in cells in the sputum specimen from a patient who had been irradiated for small cell carcinoma.*

CHEMOTHERAPEUTIC AGENTS

Chemotherapeutic compounds are derived from a variety of sources. Some exist in nature; others are biochemically synthesized. They fall into the following categories:

1. Alkylating agents
2. Alkaloids
3. Antimetabolites
4. Antibiotics
5. Corticosteroids

Members of each category have been shown to have physiologic effects that include disruption of enzyme systems and cell metabolism. The gastrointestinal tract, liver, kidneys, and hematopoietic organs will frequently mirror these cytopathogenic effects. They occur through the use of both therapeutic drugs, to which there is an unexpected degree of hypersensitivity, and chemotherapeutic agents used in the treatment of cancer.[67] The agents in each of the above categories that have an effect on the lung parenchyma are discussed in the following sections.

Alkylating Agents

The alkylating agents are polycyclic aromatic hydrocarbons that are extracted from fossil fuels or from products that result from incomplete combustion of the fuels. They are true but weak carcinogens. A few compounds in this group that are used as therapeutic

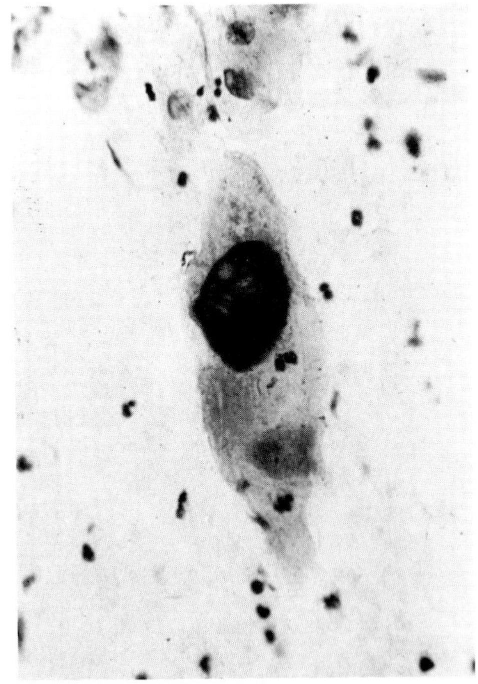

Figure 4–47. Case 12. A patient was treated with radiation therapy for small cell carcinoma. This is a follow-up sputum specimen. The chest radiograph was negative. A markedly enlarged squamous cell has ballooned cytoplasm and a hyperchromatic smudgy nucleus. There was no evidence of recurrent carcinoma. (Papanicolaou, ×425)

agents have also been implicated in the development of certain human cancers.[66, 67, 89] Some compounds in this category are referred to as direct-acting carcinogens. Others have been referred to as procarcinogens since they form intermediate metabolic compounds that are capable of transforming benign epithelial cells into malignant ones by modifying their enzyme systems.

The effects produced by the anticancer chemotherapeutic compounds often are first noted in the gastrointestinal tract where mucosal edema, superficial ulceration, hemorrhage, and eventually necrosis with perforation may occur. The lung is particularly sensitive to a few of these agents, and especially to some of the direct-acting ones, such as busulfan and cyclophosphamide.[38, 59, 60, 66] The changes seen may be summarized as interstitial and intra-alveolar edema, cell edema, and vacuolization, with ultimate dissolution of the cytoplasmic membrane and nuclear degeneration.

Busulfan, chlorambucil, procarbazine, cyclophosphamide, melphalan, and the nitrosoureas are used routinely. Of this group, busulfan and cyclophosphamide are especially cytotoxic to pulmonary epithelial cells and elicit marked interstitial fibrosis.[75]

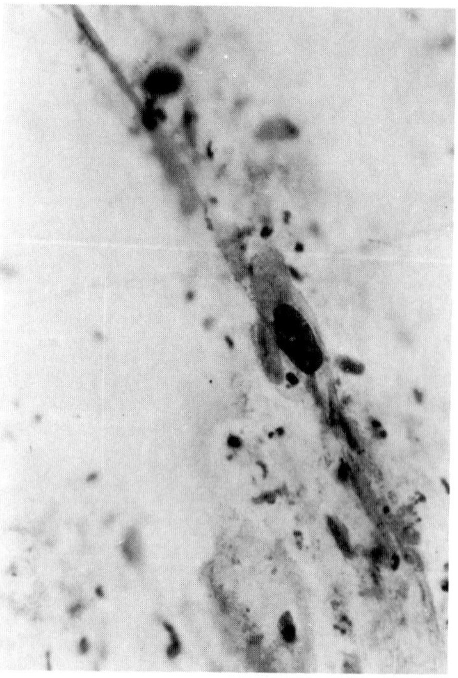

Figure 4–48. Case 13. Busulfan therapy changes. The elongated columnar cell is quite hyperchromatic and resembles a spindle squamous carcinoma cell. (Papanicolaou, ×425)

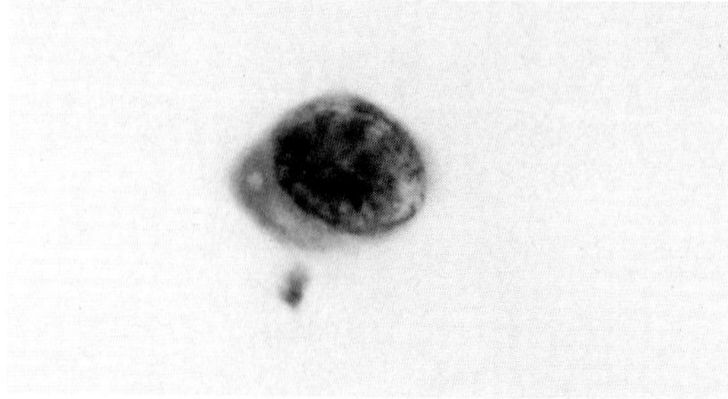

Figure 4–49. Case 13. Busulfan therapy changes. Sputum specimen: a cell from another patient with chronic myelogenous leukemia treated with busulfan showing marked chromatin clumping, hyperchromasia, and a high nuclear/cytoplasmic ratio. Fortunately such cells were few in the sputum specimen. (Papanicolaou, ×425)

Case Study 13. *A patient was undergoing treatment for chronic myelogenous leukemia with busulfan. Because of the presence of a diffuse pulmonary infiltrate, sputum specimens followed by a tissue biopsy were obtained (Fig. 4–48). Cells from a different patient receiving busulfan for leukemia are shown in Figure 4–49.*

Alkaloids

The two alkaloids most often used are vincristine sulfate and vinblastine sulfate. They are employed primarily in the treatment of leukemias, lymphomas, and germ cell tumors and are minimally cytotoxic to pulmonary epithelial cells.

Antimetabolites

Antimetabolites resemble biochemical compounds that are used in normal metabolic processes, and they interfere with the metabolism of malignant cells.

Methotrexate, fluorouracil, mercaptopurine, and cytarabine produce some cytopathogenic effects. Methotrexate is the agent most commonly responsible for cytopathogenic effects in the lung.[10, 109] It has been found to cause hyperemia, with exudation of fluid into alveoli, and interstitial fibrosis. The findings are similar to those of the Hamman-Rich syndrome and other types of hypersensitivity pneumonitis. Peripheral and pulmonary eosinophilia may or may not be present. The extent of the cellular reaction is related to the dose, length of the therapeutic regimen, and degree of hypersensitivity of the individ-

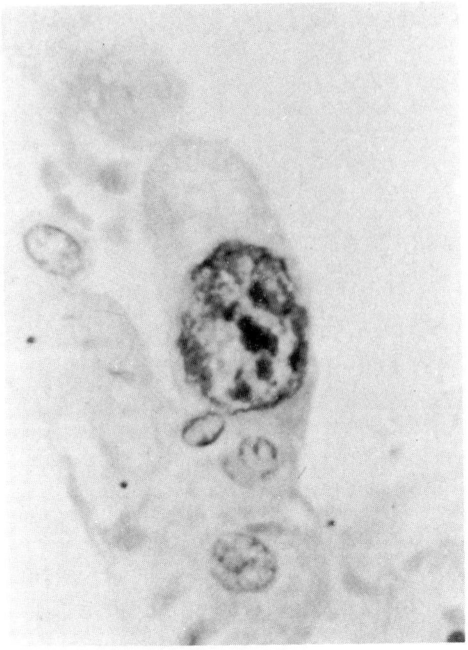

Figure 4–50. Bleomycin therapy changes. The patient received bleomycin in large doses for squamous cell carcinoma. There was marked pulmonary edema and some interstitial fibrosis. The cytologic specimen and the tissue from the lung revealed only a few abnormal cells. The large epithelial cell sloughed into an alveolus shows irregularity of the nuclear membrane and prominence of nuclear chromatin. These cell changes were considered to be induced by therapy. (Papanicolaou, ×425)

ual patient. The reaction simulates that seen with busulfan and bleomycin. It is also similar to the changes found in oxygen toxicity and in some patients with scleroderma.

Antibiotics

Antibiotics are destructive to microorganisms, and some are also cytotoxic to cancer cells. Bleomycin, doxorubicin, mitomycin-C, and mithramycin all show some cytoxic effects on normal respiratory epithelium, and a severe pulmonary reaction is induced with bleomycin and cyclophosphamide.[64, 66, 67] Squamous cell carcinoma is particularly sensitive to bleomycin, but use of the drug is limited by the severe epithelial injury that occurs in the lung (Figs. 4–50 and 4–51).

Combination chemotherapy is often used in the treatment of leukemia, of testicular or mediastinal germ cell tumors, and of lung and other tumors, especially when single-agent therapy has failed to cause significant reduction in tumor size. Such therapies often produce unique and bizarre cell changes in sputum (Figs. 4–52 and 4–53).

Corticosteroids

Primary pulmonary epithelial injury through use of corticosteroids has not been observed in our laboratory.

EMPHYSEMA

Emphysema is defined as an exaggerated dilatation of the pulmonary air spaces distal to the terminal bronchioles with ultimate destruction of their walls.[4] The condition results from progressive injury and disruption of the elastic fibers that control the relaxation and contraction of the alveolar ducts, alveolar sacs, and alveoli.[87, 119] A decrease in the serum glycoprotein α_1-protease inhibition factor can occur from a genetic deficiency but mainly appears to be produced by air pollution and especially cigarette smoking.[76, 79] A deficiency

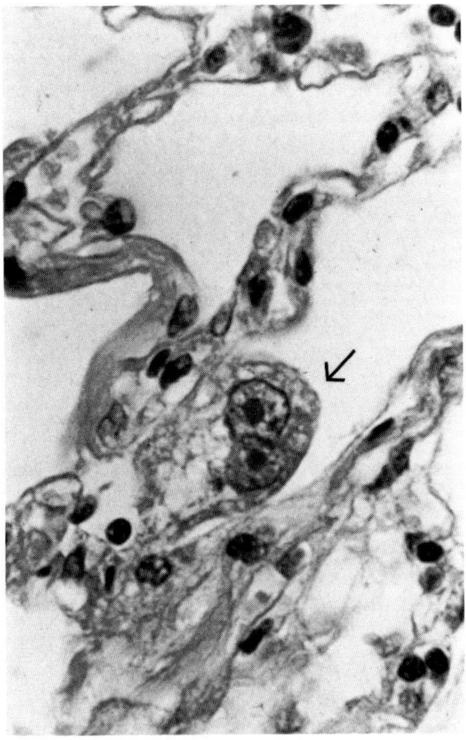

Figure 4–51. Biopsy of the lung (same case as Figure 4–50) revealed interstitial edema, some fibrosis, enlargement of type II pneumocytes, and prominence of nucleoli *(arrow)*. Cyclophosphamide produces similar interstitial fibrosis. (Hematoxylin-eosin, ×265)

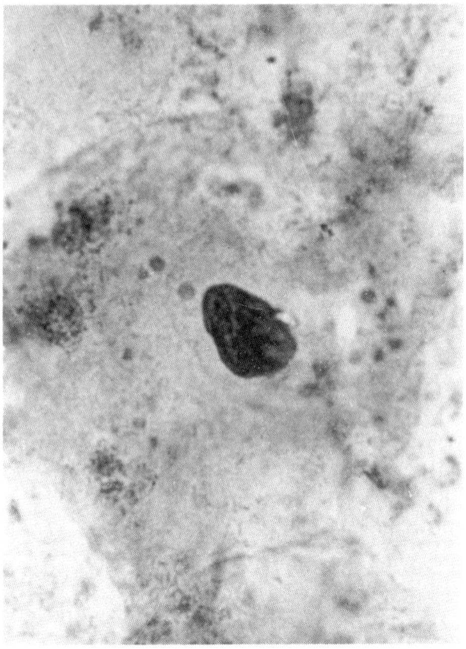

Figure 4–52. Combined chemotherapy. An atypical, hyperchromatic squamous cell nucleus with abnormal chromatin and swollen, pale, barely visible cytoplasm. (Papanicolaou, ×425)

or reduction of the α_1-protease inhibitor enzyme results in an increase in protease activity. Uninhibited protease activity is mediated by alveolar macrophages and directly destroys the elastic fibers in the walls of the small air spaces.[79, 88] Elastase found in granulocytes has similar properties, and together these enzymes destroy the elastic fibers of the small air chambers and produce emphysema.[76, 107, 122]

Cytologically there are few diagnostic findings on which to base a definitive diagnosis.

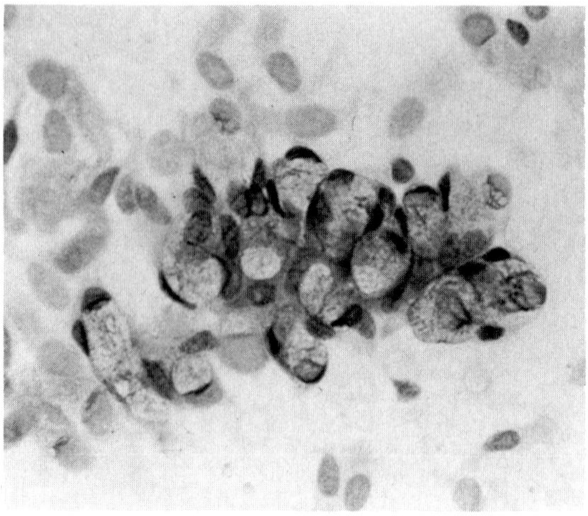

Figure 4–54. Case 14. Emphysema. Sputum specimen: goblet cell metaplasia in a relatively clean background. (Papanicolaou, ×425)

In emphysema, a spectrum of changes is seen that overlaps with those in bronchiectasis and chronic obstructive pulmonary disease. Goblet cell metaplasia may be found in the emphysematous lung and in chronic obstructive pulmonary disease, and it is frequently seen in the sputum of patients with these disorders.

Case Study 14. *A 58-year-old man, a heavy smoker, developed a squamous cell carcinoma below the tragus of the right ear. It was excised with margins free of residual carcinoma but recurred within a year. The recurrent cancer was reexcised and local radiation therapy was given. Months later, a small nodule of metastatic squamous cell carcinoma was found in the right upper lobe and lobectomy was performed. The surgical specimen revealed marked emphysema in addition to the*

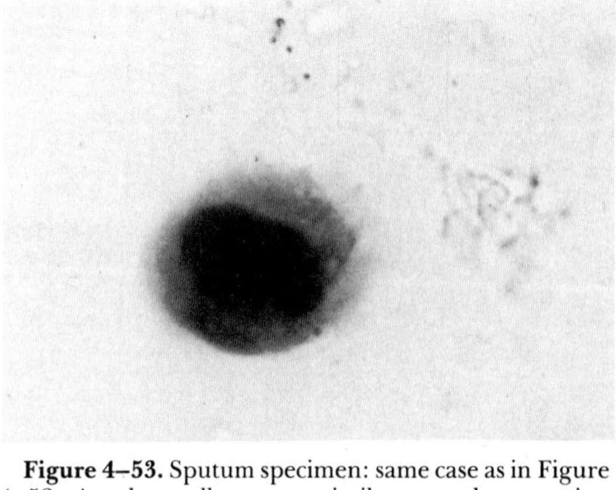

Figure 4–53. Sputum specimen: same case as in Figure 4–52. Another cell appears similar to a degenerating cell of squamous cell carcinoma. (Papanicolaou, ×425)

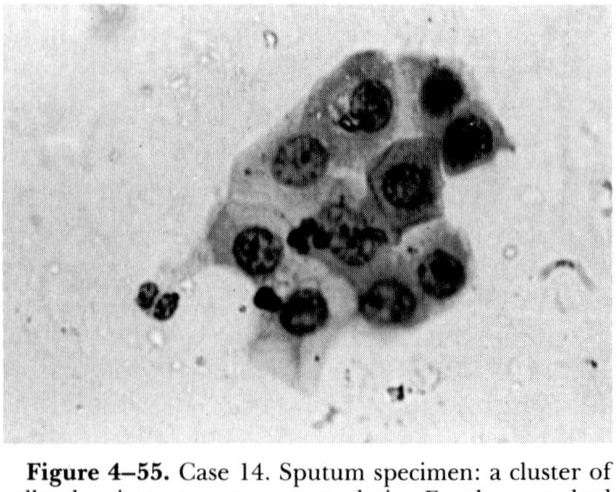

Figure 4–55. Case 14. Sputum specimen: a cluster of cells showing squamous metaplasia. Emphysema had been present for over 10 years. (Papanicolaou, ×425)

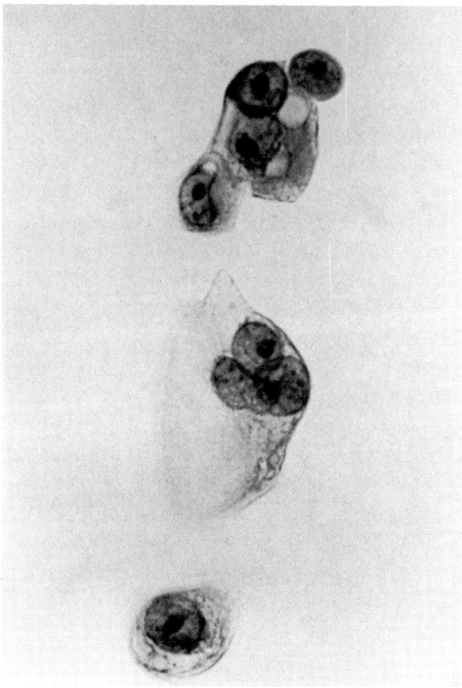

Figure 4–56. Case 14. Prominence of nucleoli and cell aggregation. Such aggregates are highly suggestive of adenocarcinoma and can readily lead to misdiagnosis. (Papanicolaou, ×425)

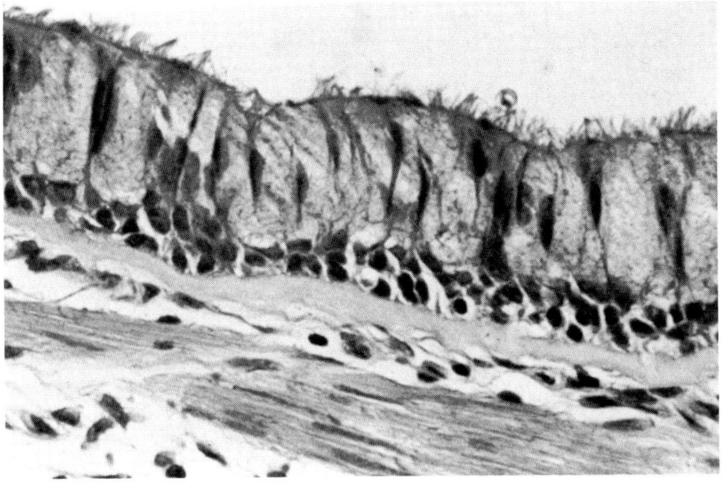

Figure 4–57. Case 14. Tissue section: goblet cell metaplasia in a large secondary bronchus, with reserve cell hyperplasia at the base of the epithelium. (Hematoxylin-eosin, ×265)

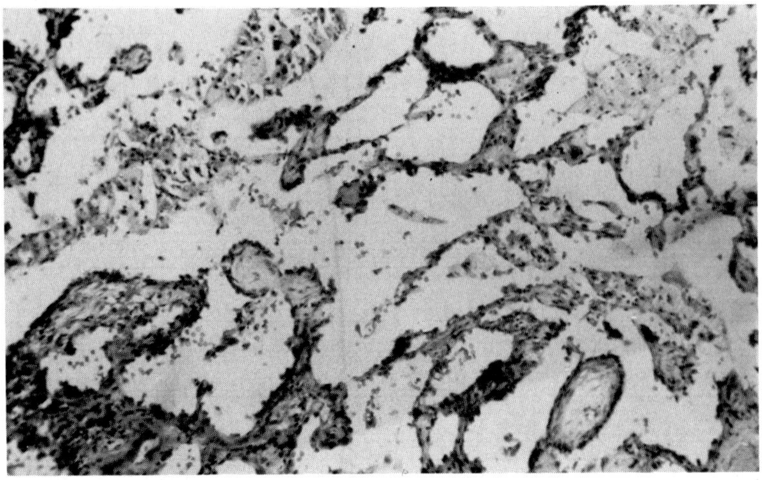

Figure 4–58. Case 14. Tissue section: a characteristic appearance in emphysema with interstitial septal thickening. Rupture and retraction of the septal walls and mild chronic inflammation were present focally. (Hematoxylin-eosin, ×165)

metastatic squamous cell carcinoma. Follow-up chest radiographs at 6 months and 1 year revealed extensive, progressive bullous emphysema but no evidence of recurrent carcinoma. Sputum examination was negative in nine specimens, but the tenth contained cells that were diagnosed as adenocarcinoma, and a subsequent specimen contained markedly suspicious cells. A more recent chest radiograph revealed no evidence of carcinoma and sputum samples at this time were also negative. The cell atypia found in the sputum samples of this emphysematous patient is shown in Figures 4–54 through 4–58.

BRONCHIECTASIS

Bronchiectasis is an irreversible dilatation of the bronchi or bronchioles, usually of the lower lobes, secondary to chronic necrotizing inflammation. A chronic cough associated with the production of large amounts of foul-smelling mucopurulent sputum is characteristic.[79] The condition appears to be a sequel to viral or bacterial pneumonia and often develops in association with bronchial compression or obstruction by tumor, foreign body, mucous impaction, or necrotizing pneumonia.[122] It is found in some patients with cystic fibrosis, in immunodeficiency disease such as hypogammaglobulinemia, and in Kartagener's syndrome (situs inversus, sinusitis, and bronchiectasis), which is associated with a lack of ciliary motility.[32]

The bronchi are dilated, often to a marked degree. Some are tubular or cylindrical, while others are saccular, and they contain a sup-

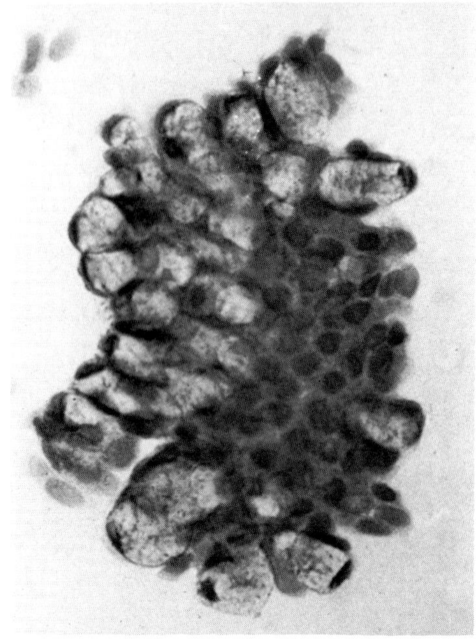

Figure 4–60. Case 15. Sputum specimen: a large aggregate of metaplastic goblet cells admixed with columnar cells. Some cells at the periphery resemble those of a signet-ring adenocarcinoma. (Papanicolaou, ×425)

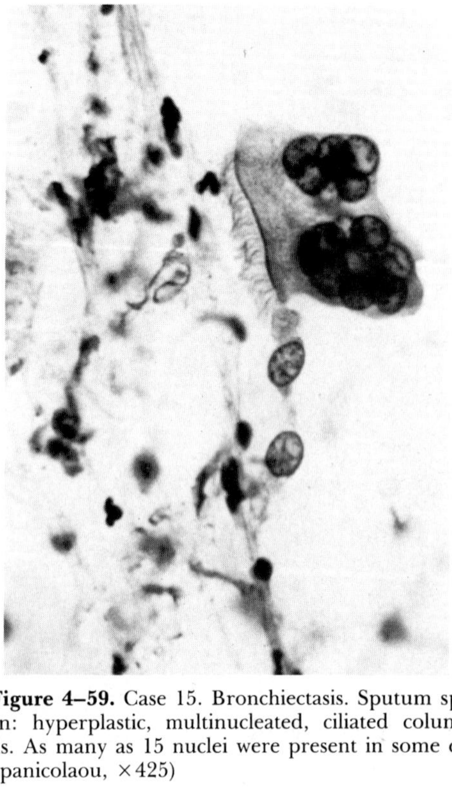

Figure 4–59. Case 15. Bronchiectasis. Sputum specimen: hyperplastic, multinucleated, ciliated columnar cells. As many as 15 nuclei were present in some cells. (Papanicolaou, ×425)

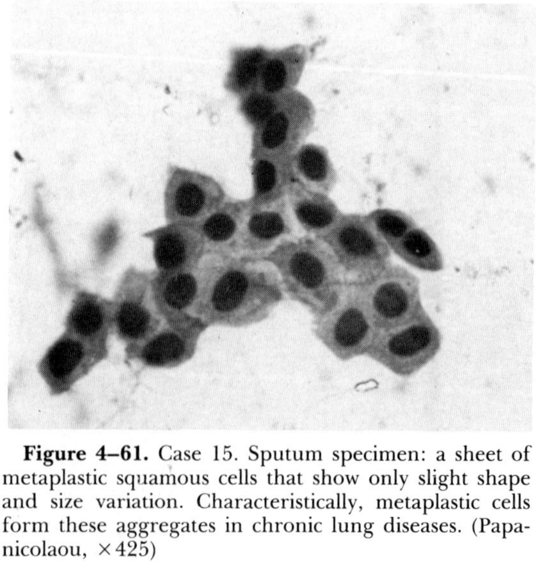

Figure 4–61. Case 15. Sputum specimen: a sheet of metaplastic squamous cells that show only slight shape and size variation. Characteristically, metaplastic cells form these aggregates in chronic lung diseases. (Papanicolaou, ×425)

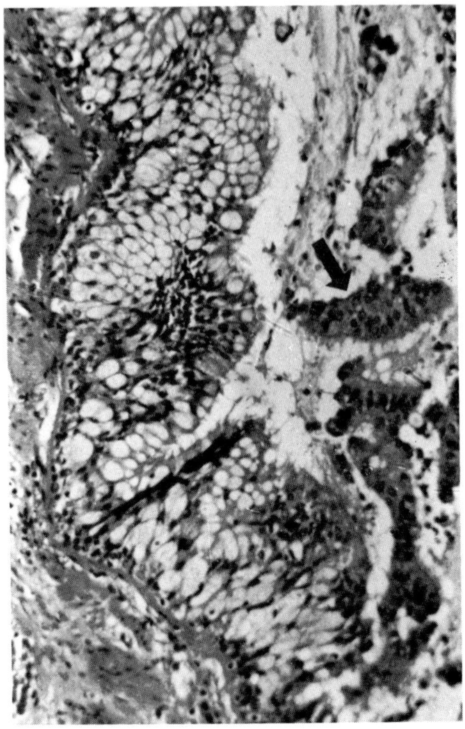

Figure 4–62. Case 15. Tissue section: marked shedding of large fragments of mucosa *(arrow)*, chronic inflammation, and a severe degree of goblet cell metaplasia and hyperplasia. (Hematoxylin-eosin, ×265)

purative exudate that on removal reveals areas of ulcerated or denuded mucosa. Histologically, severe acute and chronic inflammation is seen and fragments of desquamated epithelium lie in the bronchi. Cytologically, desquamated atypical epithelium or metaplastic squamous epithelium may be found in the purulent exudate.

Case Study 15. *A 69-year-old male with a long history of smoking two packs of cigarettes per day had a chronic productive cough and mild recurrent bouts of pneumonitis. At the time of hospitalization for pneumonitis, haziness adjacent to a major bronchus was detected on the chest radiograph, and cells suggestive of adenocarcinoma were present in the sputum. Bronchial brushings, washings, and a biopsy were obtained but showed no evidence of tumor (Figs. 4–59 through 4–62).*

AUTOIMMUNE DISEASE

Autoimmune disease is a consequence of the body's immune response to antigens produced in its own tissues. The concept was introduced early in the century and subsequently confirmed by immunologic studies of a number of disease entities. Blood dyscrasias, pemphigus vulgaris, rheumatoid disease, systemic lupus erythematosus, and Hashimoto's thyroiditis are but a few of the confirmed autoimmune diseases.[84] It is often difficult to establish the diagnosis because of the extremely sensitive reactions required and because of the formation of other innocuous interfering antibodies. The autoantibodies may be directed toward one organ as in Hashimoto's disease or toward many different tissues or organs.

Rheumatoid Pulmonary Nodules

Rheumatoid pulmonary nodules occur occasionally with rheumatoid arthritis.[31] Rheumatoid lesions may also be found in the heart, spleen, skin, vertebral column, salivary glands, and other organs.[48, 84] In all instances identification of the serum rheumatoid factor is diagnostic. In the lung, rheumatoid nodules show central acute necrosis with destruction of the walls of involved bronchioles and alveoli in the early acute phase. Neutrophils and macrophages lie within the necrotic areas. Later, macrophages surround the amorphous debris and edematous connective tissue. Peripheral to these are an admixture of lymphocytes, plasma cells, histiocytic giant cells, and reactive fibrous connective tissue. The giant cells are prominent in some areas and scanty in others.

Case Study 16. *A 38-year-old white woman developed a persistent cough occasionally productive of bitter-tasting phlegm. She was treated for 3 weeks with a cough suppressant and antibiotics but*

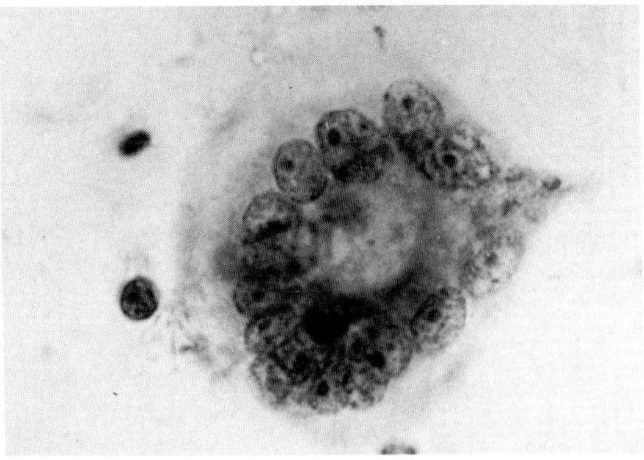

Figure 4–63. Case 16. Rheumatoid lung disease. An unusual finding in a sputum specimen of a multinucleated giant cell, possibly from a bronchiole in or adjacent to an area of necrosis. (Papanicolaou, ×425)

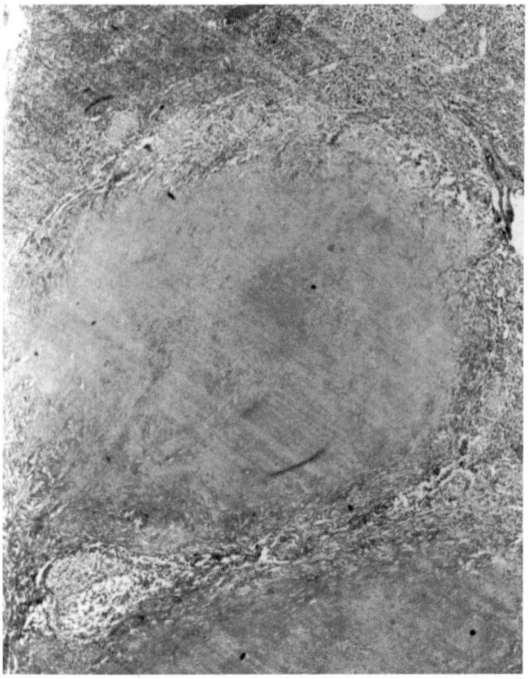

Figure 4–64. Case 16. Tissue section from patient with rheumatoid lung disease shows an area of necrosis surrounded by histiocytes and lymphocytes admixed with giant cells in the rheumatoid pulmonary nodule. (Hematoxylin-eosin, ×65)

did not improve. Finally a chest radiograph revealed two posterolateral subpleural nodules in the left lower lobe. They had not been present 5 months earlier in a chest radiograph taken during her annual physical examination. The larger nodule measured 3 cm, and the smaller one was 1.6 cm in diameter. They were interpreted as metastatic carcinoma by the radiologist. Careful workup revealed no evidence of an occult primary neoplasm. The larger lesion was removed by wedge resection and found to be a rheumatoid nodule. The patient admitted on further questioning that she had been taking analgesics for rheumatoid arthritis for the previous 3 years. Her rheumatoid factor was positive. The cytologic and histologic findings in this case of rheumatoid lung disease are shown in Figures 4–63 through 4–66.

Pemphigus

Pemphigus is an autoimmune disease of unknown etiology characterized by the appearance of successive crops of vesicles or bullae that often begin in the oral cavity as painful vesicles and spread to the skin. There

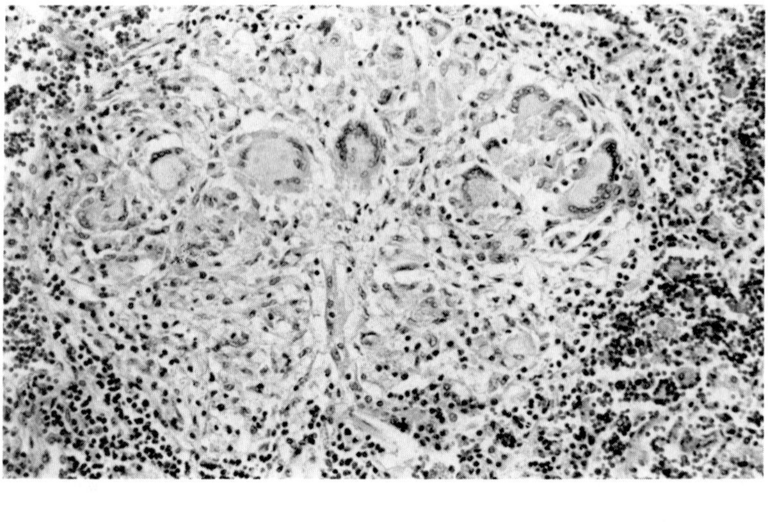

Figure 4–65. Case 16. Tissue section: low-magnification view showing part of the wall of the localized granulomatous reaction surrounding the area of central necrosis with numerous giant cells. (Hematoxylin-eosin, ×165)

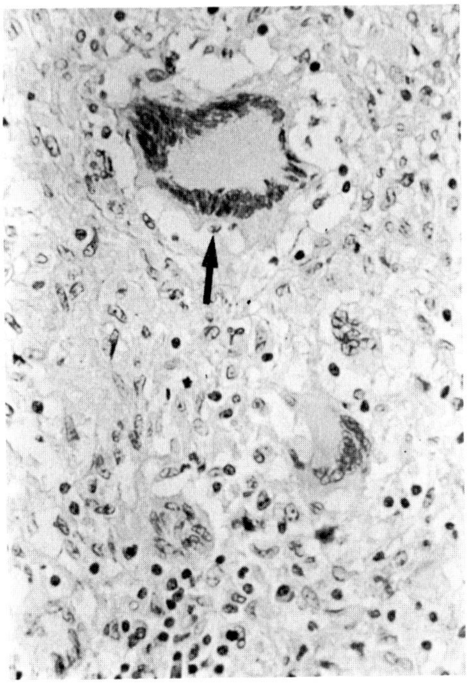

Figure 4–66. Case 16. Tissue section: higher-magnification view showing histiocytes, lymphocytes, edematous tissue, and a multinucleated giant cell *(arrow)* not dissimilar to the one in the sputum specimen in Figure 4–63. (Hematoxylin-eosin, ×265)

are many variants, but all are characterized by the presence of serum autoantibodies directed against intercellular epithelial antigens that are present in junctions between squamous epithelial cells.[41] The four most frequently encountered forms are pemphigus vulgaris, vegetans, foliaceus, and erythematosus. A specific IgG antibody has been detected that is directed against the intercellular binding proteins. Formation of the antibody–antigen complex results in acantholysis of the basal layer of the epithelium, separating it from the layers of epithelium above that level by an accumulation of serous fluid. In many patients there is no inflammatory response; in others, an inflammatory reaction, consisting of neutrophils, lymphocytes, plasma cells, and some eosinophils and macrophages, is present.[68] The most serious form of pemphigus is vulgaris. Pemphigus vegetans, a variant of pemphigus vulgaris, is characterized by the presence of verrucoid hypertrophic epithelial masses, acanthosis, and elongation of the dermal rete.

Case Study 17. *An 80-year-old woman went to see her local physician because she had been coughing and "spitting up" blood for 2 months. Examination revealed a crusted lesion at the base of the tongue. A biopsy specimen and three sputum samples were reported positive for cells of squamous cell carcinoma. A chest radiograph and tomograms of the chest were unremarkable. Further inquiry revealed that Novahistine had been prescribed because of the "spitting up" of blood. One week after*

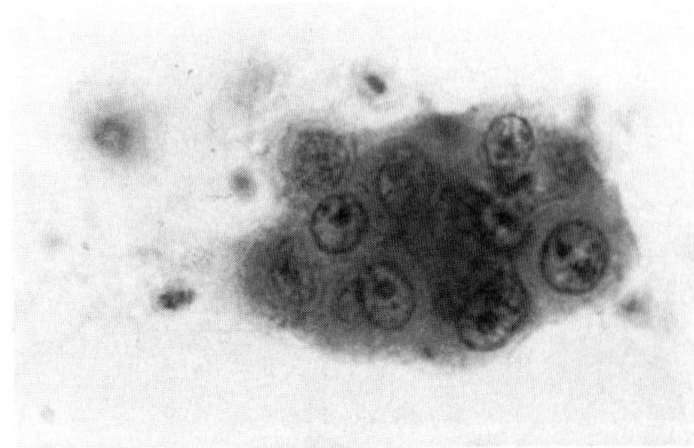

Figure 4–67. Case 17. Pemphigus vegetans. Sputum specimen: this cluster of atypical squamous epithelial cells shows nuclear enlargement, thickening of nuclear membranes, some loss of polarity, and prominence and irregularity of nucleoli. (Papanicolaou, ×425)

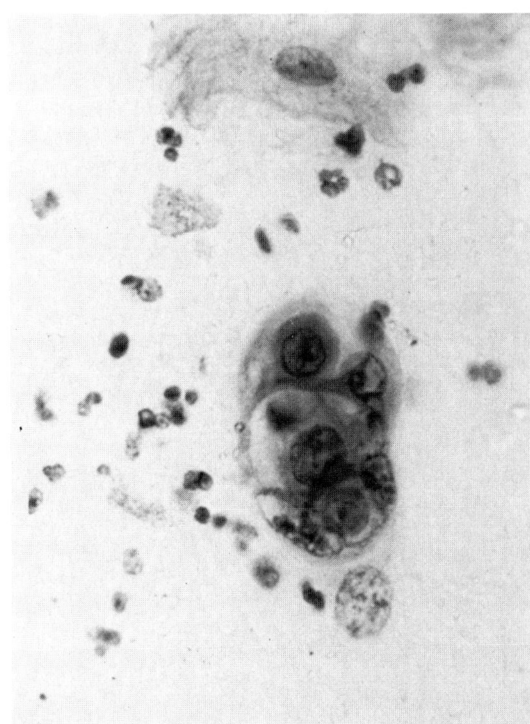

Figure 4–68. Case 17. Sputum specimen: another cluster of enlarged epithelial cells with molding and nuclear irregularity also suggesting malignancy. Such a cluster may be found in mucoepidermoid and squamous cell carcinomas. (Papanicolaou, ×425)

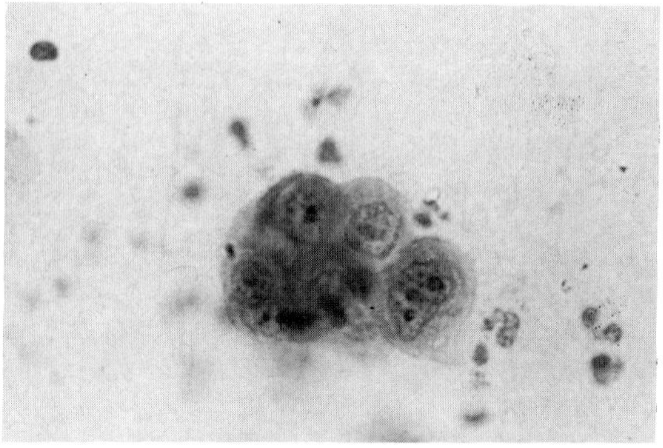

Figure 4–69. Case 17. Sputum specimen: a third cluster of cells in the sputum with cell enlargement, irregular nuclear borders, and prominence of nucleoli. The diagnosis of squamous cell carcinoma was reached by the contributing pathologist without any knowledge of the patient's history. (Papanicolaou, ×425)

beginning the Novahistine, vesicles developed beneath the breasts and in the axillary and inguinal areas. Because of her age and the diagnosis of oral cancer, she was admitted to a cancer center for further evaluation and treatment. A thorough review of her past medical history revealed no evidence of hypersensitivity, chronic illness, or heart or lung disease.

Oral examination revealed many crusted vesicles and a friable, white, granular, ulcerated mucosa that bled easily. There were no enlarged neck lymph nodes, and the chest was clear. The differential diagnosis was Stevens-Johnson syndrome versus pemphigus vegetans. The original oral biopsy specimen was reviewed, and the diagnosis was revised to marked epithelial atypia. The sputum smears were also reviewed: they revealed marked distortion and dysplasia but were not considered diagnostic of carcinoma. A biopsy specimen of an axillary skin lesion revealed the characteristic changes of pemphigus vegetans. The patient was treated with corticosteroids and made an uneventful recovery. Follow-up after 2 years revealed no evidence of squamous cell carcinoma. The cytologic atypia seen in the sputum and the representative lesion in the tissue biopsy specimen are shown in Figures 4–67 through 4–70.

CHEMICAL PNEUMONIAS

Oxygen Toxicity

Other than in controlled therapeutic hyperbaric regimens for cancer, exposure to high concentrations of oxygen may prove dangerous and even fatal. The type I alveolar pneumocytes and endothelial cells of small capillaries are severely damaged,[51] and ultimately interstitial fibrosis develops. The circumstances under which the condition may occur include delivery in obstetrical patients and the acute respiratory distress syndrome after elective surgery, usually for abdominal disease.[8, 27, 36, 114] Oxygen toxicity has also been reported with exposure to ozone and other gases, and it may be associated with shock that occurs in deep sea exploration for oil.[51, 56, 72] Kapanci and co-workers have induced the lesions of oxygen toxicity in monkeys and have shown that they may be reversible.[55]

Case Study 18. *A 24-year-old obstetrical patient para I, gravida II had a difficult, prolonged labor and was delivered of a cyanotic infant. During the last part of labor, the mother's blood pressure fell and at delivery she was in shock. She was immediately transferred to the emergency care center where fluids, blood, and 100% oxygen were administered. She was held in intensive care for 17 days but failed to respond and died. Autopsy revealed disseminated intravascular coagulation, and the lung tissues showed marked atypia of type*

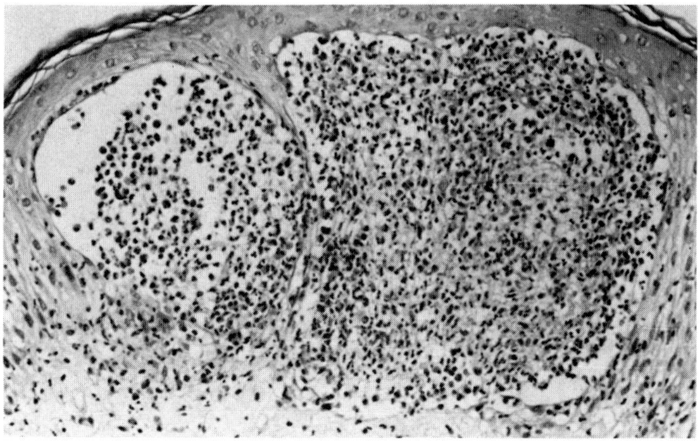

Figure 4–70. Case 17. Tissue section of skin beneath the breast showed characteristic findings of pemphigus vegetans. This section reveals an intraepithelial vesicle with an inflammatory exudate; elsewhere there was epithelial hyperplasia. (Hematoxylin-eosin, ×115)

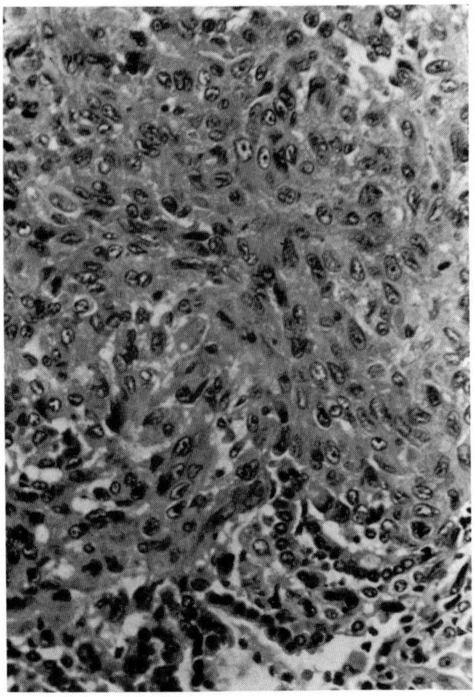

Figure 4–71. Case 18. Oxygen toxicity. Areas of interstitial reaction on right and reactive alveolar epithelial cells on the left secondary to 17 days of high-concentration oxygen therapy. (Hematoxylin-eosin, ×115)

I pneumocytes and interstitial edema with beginning fibrosis (Figs. 4–71 and 4–72).

Paraquat Poisoning

The herbicide paraquat dichloride is an effective weed killer, but it is also an exceedingly toxic chemical that affects the lung. Many fatal cases of exposure to it have been reported in the United States, Japan, and Great Britain.[69, 116] It is rapidly absorbed by the oral mucosa when ingested or through the skin. It is toxic to the liver and kidney but accumulates mainly in the skeletal muscles and lung. Lung injury begins early in the course of the illness. Cyanosis, dyspnea, and pulmonary edema are noted by the fourth day after absorption or ingestion. Respiratory failure occurs in 1 to 5 weeks.[69, 111] Examination of the pulmonary parenchyma at autopsy reveals alveoli filled with sloughed epithelium, hyaline membranes, macrophages, and debris. The changes are similar to those found in acute oxygen toxicity, described in the preceding case.[97] If the patient survives, fibroblastic proliferation occurs in the interstitial tissues of the lung and expands into alveoli, which become lined by reactive type II pneumocytes that become compressed and obliterated. Ultimately a honeycomb lung results. Spencer has demonstrated the paraquat lung 3 weeks after poisoning.[111]

Industrial Compounds

The rapid development of industrial organic compounds such as aromatic hydrocarbons, vinyl chloride, and chloromethyl methyl ether has proliferated beyond our ability to evaluate the biologic hazards that may ensue.[37, 86, 112] The number of compounds developed has doubled every 8 years since 1940, and the Environmental Protection Agency has catalogued 45,000 of them, but only about 15% have been evaluated.[126]

The aromatic hydrocarbons including benzo(a)pyrene, vinyl chloride, chloromethyl methyl ether, and *bis*-chloromethyl ether may produce lung cancers in experimental animals and probably possess the same potential for humans.[74, 103] Beryllium salts evoke an acute pulmonary reaction and may induce multiple chronic granulomas after the acute

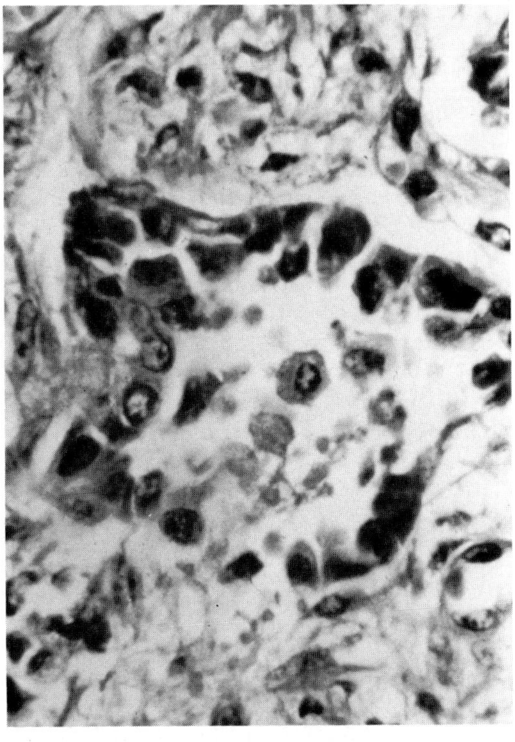

Figure 4–72. Case 18. Tissue section: note the markedly reactive and hyperchromatic epithelium lining an alveolus and swelling of the adjacent interstitial tissue. (Hematoxylin-eosin, ×425)

phase subsides. These are indistinguishable from the granulomas produced in sarcoidosis, but on fluorescence, beryllium crystals may be identified.

Obviously many subtle pulmonary reactions to industrial compounds go unrecognized, and the causes of minor reactions may not be identified.[112, 123] Such changes when seen at autopsy cannot always be explained pathologically, although a foreign substance might be detectable by microprobe analysis. The gathering and reliable recording of epidemiologic data contribute documentation of exposure to industrial compounds. As these data accumulate, more definitive assessment of the delicate and often undiagnosed changes found in the pulmonary parenchyma will become possible.[39]

MISCELLANEOUS CAUSES OF CELLULAR ATYPIA

Cellular atypias of moderate degree in sputa obtained after laryngectomy may be disturbing. These specimens should be reviewed with great caution.

Atypical cells are also associated with bronchopleural fistulas that develop postoperatively or in association with infections caused by *Histoplasma capsulatum, Mycobacterium tuberculosis, Hemophilus influenzae, Pseudomonas aeruginosa,* and other organisms. Fistulas may occur after instrumentation (improper insertion of a nasogastric tube) or after rupture of a subpleural bulla in an emphysematous patient.[22] The cells in sputum show a moderate degree of atypia with mild cell and nuclear enlargement and some granularity of the nuclear chromatin.[86] Awareness of the presence of the fistula usually enables the cytopathologist to interpret the cytologic changes with accuracy.[105–108]

REFERENCES

1. Aisner SC, Gupta LN, Prabodh K et al: Sputum cytology in pulmonary sarcoidosis. Acta Cytol 21:394, 1977
2. Allen AK, Fullmer CD: Primary diagnosis of pulmonary echinococcosis by the cytologic technique. Acta Cytol 16:212, 1972.
3. American Thoracic Society: Chronic bronchitis, asthmas and pulmonary emphysema. Statement by the committee on diagnostic standards for non-tuberculous respiratory disease. Am Rev Respir Dis 85:762, 1962.
4. Anderson WAD: Emphysema. In: Anderson's Pathology, 8th ed, vol 22, p 906. St. Louis, CV Mosby, 1985.
5. Anderson WAD: Radiation injury. In: Anderson's pathology, 8th ed, vol 6, p 239. St. Louis, CV Mosby, 1985.
6. Baker PD, Check EW: Proceedings of International Symposium on Opportunistic Fungus Infections. Lab Invest 11:1017, 1962.
7. Baker RD: Histoplasmosis in routine autopsies. Am J Clin Pathol 45:457, 1964.
8. Balentine JD: Pathology of Oxygen Toxicity. New York, Academic Press, 1983.
9. Bartlett JG, Gorbach S, Finegold S: The bacteriology of aspiration pneumonia. Am J Med 56:202, 1974.
10. Bedrossian CWM, Miller WC, Luna MA: Methotrexate-induced diffuse interstitial pulmonary fibrosis. South Med J 72:313, 1979.
11. Bell WR: Disseminated intravascular coagulation. Johns Hopkins Med J 146:289, 1980.
12. Bell WR, Simon TL: Current status of pulmonary thromboembolic disease: Pathophysiology, diagnosis, prevention and treatment. Am Heart J 103:239, 1982.
13. Bell WR, Simon TL, DeMets DL: The clinical features of submassive and massive pulmonary emboli. Am J Med 62:355, 1977.
14. Berkheiser SW: Bronchiolar proliferation and metaplasia associated with bronchiectasis, pulmonary infarcts and anthracosis. Cancer 12:499, 1959.
15. Berry FB: Lobar pneumonia: Analysis of 400 autopsies. Med Clin North Am 4:571, 1920.
16. Bode FR, Paré JA, Fraser RE: Pulmonary diseases in the compromised host: A review of clinical and roentgenographic manifestations in patients with impaired host defense mechanisms. Medicine 53:255, 1974.
17. Borrie J, Gwynne JF: Paraffinoma of lung: Lipid pneumonia. Thorax 28:214, 1973.
18. Butcher BT, Hendrick DJ: Occupational asthma. Clin Chest Med 4:43, 1983.
19. Campbell GD: Primary pulmonary cryptococcosis. Am Rev Respir Dis 94:236, 1966.
20. Cho SY, Choi HY: Opportunistic fungal infection among cancer patients. Am J Clin Pathol 72:617, 1979.
21. Colp CR, Cook WA: Successful treatment of pleural aspergillosis and bronchopleural fistula. Chest 68:96, 1975.
22. Culpepper JA, Veremakis C, Guntupalli K et al: Malpositioned nasogastric tube causing pneumothorax and bronchopleural fistula. Chest 81:389, 1982.
23. Dalen JE, Haffaiee CI, Alpert JS et al: Pulmonary embolism, pulmonary hemorrhage and pulmonary infarction. N Engl J Med 296:1431, 1977.
24. Dalen JE, Alpert JS: Natural history of pulmonary embolism. Prog Cardiovasc Dis 17:257, 1975.
25. Dalrymple ME, Gaulden ME, Kollmorgen GM et al: Medical Radiation Biology. Philadelphia, WB Saunders 1973, p. 190, p. 213.
26. Davis WC, Sasahara AA: Management of pulmonary embolism in the postoperative patient. Surg Clin North Am 48:869, 1968.
27. Davis WB, Rennards I: Oxygen toxicity. N Engl J Med 309:878, 1983.
28. Deppisch LM, Donowho EM: Pulmonary coccidioidomycosis. Am J Clin Pathol 58:489, 1972.

29. Donath J, Khan FA: Tuberculous and post-tuberculous bronchopleural fistula: Ten year clinical experience. Chest 86:697, 1984.
30. Dubois PJ, Myerowitz RL, Allen CM: Pathoradiology correlation of pulmonary candidiasis in immunosuppressed patients. Cancer 40:1026, 1977.
31. Eisenberg H: The interstitial lung diseases associated with collagen vascular disorders. Clin Chest Med 3:564, 1982.
32. Eliasson R, Mossberg B, Cammer P et al: The immotile cilia syndrome—a congenital ciliary abnormality as an etiologic factor in chronic airway infections and male sterility. N Engl J Med 297:1, 1977.
33. Emmons CW, Binford CH, Utz JP: Immunology of the mycoses. In: Medical Mycology, 3rd ed. Philadelphia, Lea & Febiger, 1977.
34. Enders JF, McCarthy K, Mitus A et al: Isolation of measles virus at autopsy in cases of giant cell pneumonia without rash. N Engl J Med 261:875, 1959.
35. Fanta CH, Pennington JE: Fever and new lung infiltrates in the immunocompromised host. Clin Chest Med 2:19, 1981.
36. Fantone JC, Ward PA: Role of oxygen-derived free radicals and metabolites in leukocyte dependent inflammatory reactions. Am J Pathol 107:397, 1982.
37. Farber E: Chemical carcinogens. N Engl J Med 305:1379, 1981.
38. Feingold ML, Koss LG: Effect of long-term administration of busulfan. Arch Intern Med 124:66, 1969.
39. Frost JK, Erozan YS, Hollander DH et al: Pulmonary cytologic alterations in toxic environmental inhalation. Hum Pathol 4:521, 1973.
40. Gale AM, Kleitsch WP: Solitary pulmonary nodule due to phycomycosis (mucormycosis). Chest 62:752, 1972.
41. Graber P: Hypothesis: Autoantibodies and immune theories: An analytic review. Clin Immunol Immunopathol 4:453, 1975.
42. Grieco MH: Candidosis. In Grieco MH (ed): Infections in the Abnormal Host. New York, Yorke Medical Publishers, 1980, p 284.
43. Griffin M, Weiss JW, Leitch MB et al: Effects of leukotriene D on the airways in asthma. N Engl J Med 308:436, 1983.
44. Hector MF: Sputum cytology in two cases of Wegener's granulomatosis. J Clin Pathol 29:259, 1976.
45. Hensen PM, Fantone JC, Ward PA et al: Immune complex injury of the lung. Am Rev Respir Dis 124:738, 1981.
46. Hershfield ES: Tuberculosis in the world. Chest 176(suppl):805, 1979.
47. Hogg JC: Bronchial asthma. In Thurlbeck WM, Abell MR (eds): The Lung: Structure, Function and Disease, pp 180–191. Baltimore, Williams & Wilkins, 1978.
48. Hollingworth JW, Saykaly RJ: Systemic complications of rheumatoid arthritis. Med Clin North Am 61:217, 1977.
49. Hutchinson F: The molecular basis of radiation effects on cells. Cancer Res 26:2045, 1966.
50. Hutter RVP, Lieberman PH, Collins HS: Aspergillosis in a cancer hospital. Cancer 17:747, 1964.
51. Janoff A, Carp H: Proteases, antiproteases and oxidants: Pathways of tissue injury during inflammation. In Majno G, Cotran RS (eds): Current Topics in Inflammation and Infection, pp 62–82. Baltimore, Williams & Wilkins, 1982.
52. Jay SJ, Platt MR, Reynolds RC: Primary pulmonary sporotrichosis. Am Rev Respir Dis 115:1051, 1977.
53. Johanson WG Jr, Harris GD: Aspiration pneumonia, aerobic infections and lung abscess. Med Clin North Am 64:385, 1980.
54. Johns LE Jr, Garrison RG, White TG: Bronchopleurocutaneous fistula due to infection with *Histoplasma capsulatum*. Chest 63:638, 1973.
55. Kapanci YA, Weibel ER, Kaplan HP: Pathogenesis and reversibility of pulmonary lesions of oxygen toxicity in monkeys. Lab Invest 20:101, 1969.
56. Katzenstein AL, Bloor CM, Leibow AA: Diffuse alveolar damage: The role of oxygen, shock and related factors. Am J Pathol 85:209, 1976.
57. Kenney M, Abrams H, Eveland LK et al: Amebiasis: Unusual location in the lung. NY State J Med 75:1542, 1975.
58. Kenney M, Webber CA: Diagnosis of strongyloidiasis in Papanicolaou-stained sputum smears. Acta Cytol 18:270, 1974.
59. Kirschner RH, Esterly JR: Pulmonary lesions associated with busulfan therapy of chronic myelogenous leukemia. Cancer 27:1074, 1971.
60. Koss LG, Melamed MR, Mayer K: The effect of busulfan on human epithelia. Am J Clin Pathol 44:385, 1965.
61. Leff A, Lester TW, Addington WW: Tuberculosis: A chemotherapeutic triumph, but a persistent socioeconomic problem. Arch Intern Med 139:1375, 1979.
62. Lequesne LP: Relation between deep vein thrombosis and pulmonary embolism in surgical patients. N Engl J Med 291:1292, 1974.
63. Liebow AA: Pulmonary angiitis and granulomatosis. Am Rev Respir Dis 108:1, 1973.
64. Luna MA, Bedrossian CW, Lichtiger B et al: Interstitial pneumonitis associated with bleomycin therapy. Am J Clin Pathol 58:501, 1972.
65. Macher A: Histoplasmosis and blastomycosis. Med Clin North Am 64:447, 1980.
66. Mark GJ, Lehimgar-Zadeh A, Ragsdale BD: Cyclophosphamide pneumonitis. Thorax 33:89, 1978.
67. Martin EW: Hazards of Medication, vol 18, p 686. Philadelphia, JB Lippincott, 1978.
68. Masur H: Infections in immunologically abnormal patients. In Roberts RB (ed): Infectious Diseases: Pathogenesis, Diagnosis, and Therapy. Chicago, Year Book Medical Publishers, 1986.
69. Matthew H, Logan A, Woodruff MF: Paraquat poisoning—lung transplantation. Br Med J 3:759, 1968.
70. McCluskey RT, Feinberg O: Vasculitis in primary vasculitides, granulomatoses and connective tissue diseases. Hum Pathol 14:305, 1983.
71. McCollun SM: Ova of the lung fluke *Paragonimus kellicotti* in fluid from a cyst. Acta Cytol 19:279, 1975.
72. McCord JM, Fridovich I: The biology and pathology of oxygen radicals. Ann Intern Med 80:122, 1978.
73. McFadden ER, Ingram RH: Exercise induced asthma: Observations on initiating stimulus. N Engl J Med 301:763, 1979.
74. Miller EC, Miller JA: Mechanism of chemical carcinogens. Annu Rev Biochem 4:315, 1980.
75. Min K-W, Gyorkey F: Interstitial pulmonary fibro-

sis, atypical epithelial changes and bronchiolar cell carcinoma following busulfan therapy. Cancer 22:1027, 1968.
76. Morse JO: Alpha-1-antitrypsin deficiency. N Engl J Med 299:1045, 1978.
77. Moser KM: Pulmonary Embolism, State of the Art (1976–1977). New York, American Lung Association, 1978.
78. Moser KM: Pulmonary embolism. Am Rev Respir Dis 115:829, 1977.
79. Mossberg B: Immotile cilia syndrome: Clinical features. Eur J Respir Dis 118(suppl):111, 1982.
80. Myerowitz RL: Localized and disseminated candidiasis. Invasive pulmonary and disseminated aspergillosis. In The Pathology of Opportunistic Infections With Pathogenetic, Diagnostic and Clinical Correlations, vol 10, pp 95–144; vol 11, pp 115–128. New York, Raven Press, 1983.
81. Nash G, Foley FD: Herpetic infection of the middle and lower respiratory tract. Am J Clin Pathol 54:857, 1970.
82. Oldenburger D, Maurer WJ, Efstathios B et al: Inhalation lipid pneumonia from burning fats. JAMA 222:1288, 1972.
83. Perlman LV, Lerner E, Desopo N: Clinical classification and analysis of 97 cases of lung abscess. Am Rev Respir Dis 99:390, 1969.
84. Petty TL, Wilkins M: The five manifestations of the rheumatoid lung. Dis Chest 49:75, 1966.
85. Pizzarello DJ, Whitcolski RL: Basic Radiation Biology, vol 9, p 56. Philadelphia, Lea & Febiger, 1975.
86. Plamenac G, Nikulin A, Pikula B et al: Cytologic changes of the respiratory tract of young adults as a consequence of air pollution and smoking. Acta Cytol 17:241, 1973.
87. Pratt PC: Pathology of adult respiratory distress syndrome. In Thurlbeck W, Abell MR (eds): The Lung: Structure, Function and Disease, p 43. Baltimore, Williams & Wilkins, 1978.
88. Reid L, Simon G, Zorab PA et al: The pathology of emphysema. Br J Dis Chest 61:190, 1967.
89. Reiner RR, Hoover R, Fraumeri JF et al: Acute leukemia after alkylating-agent therapy of ovarian cancer. N Engl J Med 297:177, 1977.
90. Reynolds HY (ed): Hypersensitivity Pneumonitis. Clin Chest Med 2:1, 1981.
91. Robbins SL, Cotran RS, Kumar V: Pulmonary embolism, pulmonary hemorrhage and pulmonary infarction. In: The Pathologic Basis of Disease, 3rd ed, vol 16, p 711. Philadelphia, WB Saunders, 1984.
92. Robbins SL, Cotran RS, Kumar V (eds): The Pathologic Basis of Disease, 4th ed. Philadelphia, WB Saunders, 1989, p. 389.
93. Rosen PP: Opportunistic infections in patients with neoplastic disease. Pathol Annu 11:255, 1976.
94. Rossman I: True incidence of pulmonary embolization and vital statistics. JAMA 230:1677, 1974.
95. Rosenow EC, Osmundson PJ, Brown ML: Pulmonary embolism. Mayo Clin Proc 56:161, 1981.
96. Rubin P, Casarett GW: Clinical Radiation Pathology, pp 850, 894, and 903. Philadelphia, WB Saunders, 1968.
97. Meunier F: Candidiasis. In Rubin RH (ed): Clinical Approach to Infection in the Compromised Host, 2nd ed. New York, Plenum Book Co, 1988.
98. Rubin R: Pneumonia in the immunocompromised host. In Fishman AP (ed): Update: Pulmonary Disease and Disorders, pp 1–26. New York, McGraw-Hill, 1982.
99. Sabiston DC: Pulmonary embolism. Surg Gynecol Obstet 126:1075, 1968.
100. Sabiston DC: Pathophysiology, diagnosis and management of pulmonary embolism. Am J Surg 138:384, 1979.
101. Samuelsson B: Leukotrienes: Mediators of immediate hypersensitivity reactions and inflammation. Science 220:568, 1983.
102. Sborbaro JA: Tuberculosis. Med Clin North Am 64:417, 1980.
103. Schottenfield D, Haas FJ: The workplace as a cause of cancer. Clin Bull 8:54, 1979.
104. Schuyler MR: Allergic bronchopulmonary aspergillosis. Clin Chest Med 4:15, 1983.
105. Schwartz RH, Hollick GE: Allergic bronchopulmonary aspergillosis with low serum immunoglobulin E. J Allergy Clin Immunol 68:290, 1981.
106. Schwartz J, Salfelder K: Blastomycosis: A review of 152 cases. Curr Top Pathol 65:165, 1977.
107. Snider GL: Pathogenesis of emphysema and chronic bronchitis. Med Clin North Am 65:647, 1981.
108. Snyder J: Histopathology of pulmonary lesions caused by atypical mycobacteria. J Pathol Bacteriol 90:65, 1965.
109. Sostman HD, Matthay RA, Putman CE: Cytotoxic pulmonary disease: Methotrexate-induced pneumonitis. Am J Med 62:608, 1977.
110. Spencer H: Chronic infective pneumonias. In: Pathology of the Lung, 4th ed, vol 7, p 261. New York, Pergamon Press, 1985.
111. Spencer H: Pathology of the Lung, 4th ed, vol 2, p 719. New York, Pergamon Press, 1985.
112. Subcommittee on Environmental Carcinogenesis, National Cancer Advisory Board: General criteria for assessing the evidence for carcinogenicity of chemical substances. JNCI 58:461, 1977.
113. Sullivan RJ Jr, Dowdle WR, Marine WM et al: Adult pneumonia in a general hospital. Arch Intern Med 129:935, 1972.
114. Suttorp N, Simon LM: Lung cell oxidant injury. J Clin Invest 70:342, 1982.
115. Theofilopoulos AN, Dixon FJ: Autoimmune diseases: Immunopathology and etiopathogenesis. Am J Pathol 108:321, 1982.
116. Timmerman RJ, Schroer JA: Lipid pneumonia caused by methenamine mandelate suspension. JAMA 225:1524, 1973.
117. Tsou E, Yeader H, Katz S: Later bronchopleural fistula and *Hemophilus influenzae* empyema complicating longstanding oleothorax: Report of two cases. Chest 74:573, 1978.
118. University of Texas MD Anderson Cancer Center: Cellular radiation biology. Eighteenth symposium on fundamental cancer research, Houston, 1964. Baltimore, Williams & Wilkins, 1965.
119. Wewers M, Bone RC: Emphysema and chronic bronchitis. Pulmonary Dis Rev 3:229, 1983.
120. Williams DM, Krick JA, Remington JS: Pulmonary infection in the compromised host: I. Am Rev Respir Dis 114:359, 1976.
121. Williams DM, Krick JA, Remington JS: Pulmonary infection in the compromised host: II. Am Rev Respir Dis 114:593, 1976.

122. Williams WD, Fajardo LE: Alpha-1-antitrypsin deficiency: A hereditary enigma. Am J Clin Pathol 61:311, 1974.
123. Williams WJ: Alveolar metaplasia: Its relationship to pulmonary fibrosis in industry and the development of lung cancer. Br J Cancer 11:30, 1956.
124. Willie SM, Snyder RN: The identification of *Paragonimus westermani* in bronchial washings: Case report. Acta Cytol 21:101, 1977.
125. Wilson C: Immunologic diseases of lungs and kidney. In Fishman AP (ed): Pulmonary Diseases and Disorders, p 699. New York, McGraw-Hill, 1980.
126. Wynder EL, Gori GB: Contribution of the environment to cancer incidence. JNCI 58:825, 1977.
127. Youmans GP: Tuberculosis, p 348. Philadelphia, WB Saunders, 1985.
128. Youmans GP, Patterson PY, Sommers HM: The Biologic and Clinical Basis of Infectious Diseases, vol 4, p 290. Philadelphia, WB Saunders, 1985.
129. Zinserling A: Peculiarities of viral and *Mycoplasma* infections of the respiratory tract. Virchows Arch 356:259, 1972.

Chapter

5

PREMALIGNANT LESIONS

The wide range of noxious agents that are capable of injuring the bronchial epithelium includes viruses, tobacco tars, toxic chemicals, and gases. They produce a series of cell alterations that are inconspicuous early in their development: at this stage the patient may be asymptomatic and the changes are reversible. With continued exposure, the epithelial damage is likely to increase in severity, and it can progress to malignant change.[4] Collectively, therefore, these alterations in the bronchial epithelium are referred to as premalignant lesions. Nettesheim and coworkers[21] described three stages in the response of the respiratory epithelium to carcinogens. An acute injury pattern was followed by a preneoplastic phase in which atypical changes in nuclei became detectable, leading to a truly dysplastic state with neoplastic cytologic features. Hyperplastic and dysplastic changes can also involve the endocrine cells of the respiratory passages.[7, 17, 27]

Preneoplastic changes can often be detected in cytologic specimens of sputa, and consequently they are significant criteria in screening programs for lung cancer. They are also encountered in bronchoscopic biopsy specimens procured because carcinoma was suspected clinically and are seen frequently in resection specimens in the immediate vicinity of carcinoma.

Mucous cell hyperplasia is an early response of the tracheal or bronchial epithelium to injury. It is seen in bronchiectasis and other forms of chronic pulmonary disease,[19] and in many patients with bronchogenic carcinoma. Amphicrine cells[5] containing mucous vacuoles as well as dense-core granules have been described in mucous cell hyperplasia and in the reserve cell hyperplasia that ensues if exposure to the irritant continues.[18] In basal or reserve cell hyperplasia (Figs. 5–1 and 5–2), the deepest stratum of the epithelium may become several layers thick. In foci of reserve cell hyperplasia, an occasional slightly enlarged polyhedral or

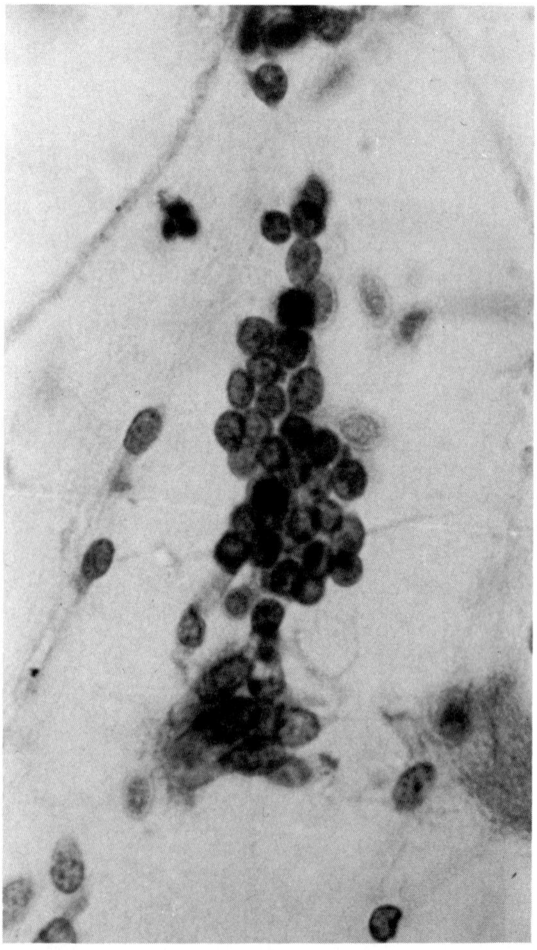

Figure 5–1. Reserve cell hyperplasia in a bronchial brushing specimen.

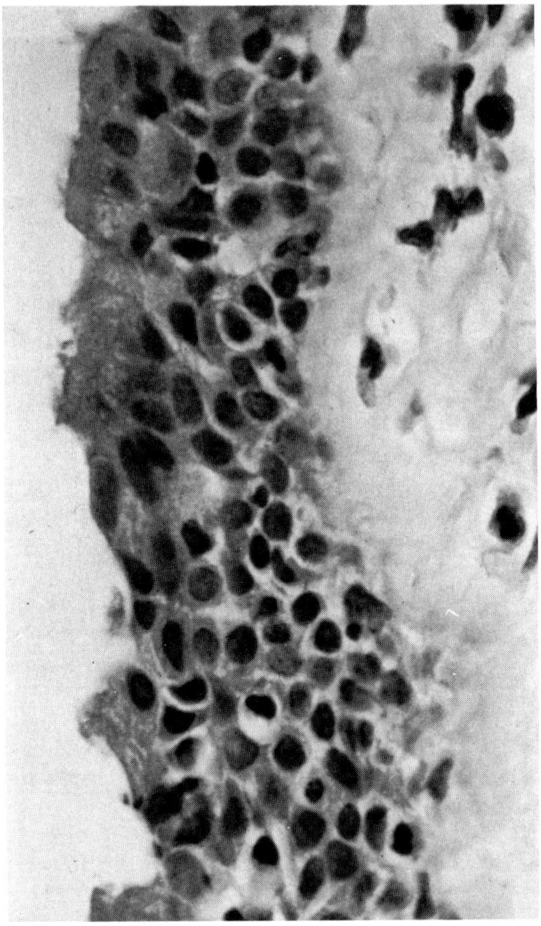

Figure 5–2. Tissue section showing reserve cell hyperplasia merging into squamous cell metaplasia.

oval cell with slight irregularity of the nuclear membrane and a recognizable nucleolus, but with little change in the nuclear chromatin, may be noted. Kierszenbaum[10] believed that this cell indicated a form of epithelial reactive change intermediate between reserve cell hyperplasia and squamous metaplasia, which he termed *transitional metaplasia.* The criteria are subtle, and this degree of splitting is not practical.

With the use of computer-assisted image analysis of cells in sputum specimens, the atypia status index (a numerical classification based on a weighted composite of morphometric markers identified in the digitized images) can be obtained. The values place cells in categories ranging from squamous metaplasia to carcinoma, and the cell atypia profile that can be constructed reflects the overall status of the patient's bronchial epithelium and can be used to diagnose and monitor epithelial atypias.[8] The procedure has potential in the evaluation of high-risk patients for the possible early detection of premalignant lesions.

SQUAMOUS METAPLASIA

Metaplasia, transformation of one form of differentiated adult tissue into another, was first described in the respiratory passages by Linberg, a Finnish pathologist, in 1935.[12] The columnar cells are converted into a stratified squamous type of epithelium (Figs. 5–3 and 5–4). Metaplastic epithelium is not ciliated, and consequently it is incapable of performing mucociliary transport. As a result, this protective mechanism is lost in areas where the change has occurred, and the altered mucosa is more susceptible to infections and to damage by carcinogens. The development and progression of metaplastic changes have been confirmed in experimental animal models. Sassy-Dobray and co-workers[24] observed it by applying the carcinogen benzo(a)pyrene to the tracheal mucosa of Syrian hamsters. Boutet and associates[3] instilled a nitrosamine compound into the trachea of hamsters and found that regenerating cells during the recovery phase to the initial acute injury were not ciliated and led to mucous cell hyperplasia followed by squamous cell metaplasia.

Endobronchial application of chemical carcinogens in dogs[2] induced a consistent sequence of mucosal changes beginning with squamous hyperplasia: squamous metaplasia occurred in 6 to 18 weeks and was followed

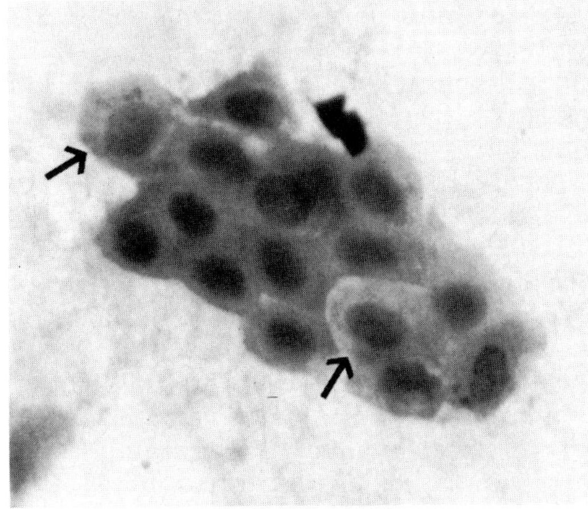

Figure 5–3. Squamous metaplasia in sputum. A small sheet of metaplastic cells is shown. The cells indicated by the arrows are separated from their neighbors by slender clefts.

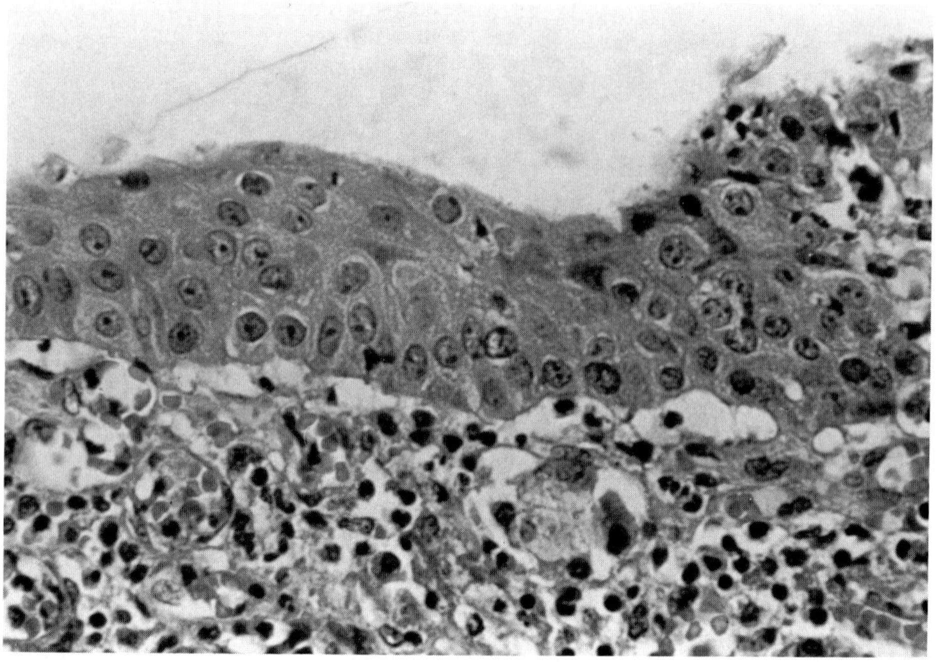

Figure 5–4. Tissue section showing squamous metaplasia that has replaced the entire epithelium.

by progressive squamous atypia. Submucosal injection of methylcholanthrene every 2 to 3 weeks produced cancers at preselected sites within 2 years of first exposure. Four regimens in 58 dogs caused 31 cancers, including five T1 or T2 tumors confined to the lung and 17 metastasizing carcinomas. The interval until invasive cancer developed varied with the regimen employed: methylcholanthrene was the most efficient carcinogen, producing invasive cancer in about 20 months.

An association between squamous metaplasia and smoking was demonstrated by Mathe and colleagues[13] in a study on 144 heavy smokers (125 males and 19 females) who voluntarily underwent bronchoscopy with systematic biopsies at ten sites in the bronchial tree. A significant correlation was observed between the degree of metaplasia and the number of cigarettes smoked. The incidence of metaplasia was distinctly lower in women than men in the series. It is not known whether metaplastic squamous epithelium is invariably capable of reverting to normal epithelium, but experimental studies have shown that this can occur.[25, 26, 28] It is well established that squamous metaplasia can be a forerunner of the development of malignancy. The incidence of squamous metaplasia associated with primary and metastatic tumors in the lung was investigated by Tsuchiya and associates,[31] who found it in 83% of male lungs containing primary squamous cell or small cell carcinoma, but in only 43% of the lungs of both sexes with adenocarcinoma or metastatic tumors. Remarkably extensive squamous metaplasia diffusely involving the terminal bronchioles and alveoli throughout the lungs of two patients treated for lung carcinoma was reported by Miyamoto and colleagues.[15]

The mechanism of the process that gives rise to squamous metaplasia is not thoroughly understood. Initially, it was believed that a direct transformation to metaplastic epithelium occurred after repeated injury to the normal surface epithelium. However, electron microscopic studies have shown that the metaplastic cell is derived from both mucus cells and reserve cells that proliferate and alter their pattern of differentiation.[1, 29] The use of markers to determine the phenotypes of cells in premalignant processes is described by Trump and associates.[30]

Saccomanno and co-workers[23] accumulated a database of 9,817 men in their studies on the incidence of, and mortality rates from, lung cancer among uranium workers of the Colorado plateau during the period from 1960 to 1980. Squamous metaplasia was followed in succession by mild, moderate, and severe dysplasia, and ultimately by carcinoma *in situ*. Mild dysplasia required approximately 6 years to progress to carcinoma *in situ*. With continued exposure, invasive cancer developed in untreated patients in approximately 3.2 additional years. If the uranium miners smoked cigarettes, the probability of their developing invasive cancer increased considerably.

In cytologic preparations, cells of squamous metaplasia are round or polyhedral instead of the usual columnar respiratory cells, and they tend to occur in small sheets or clusters. Cell and nuclear size are approximately equal to those of parabasal cells of the squamous epithelium of the oral cavity. The cytoplasm is more basophilic than that of normal respiratory epithelium. Nuclei are central and round to oval, and the chromatin has a "ground glass" appearance. A small nucleolus is often visible.

DYSPLASIA AND CARCINOMA *IN SITU*

While squamous metaplasia is easily recognized histologically, the subtle transition from squamous metaplasia to mild dysplasia (squamous metaplasia with mild atypia) can be more difficult to detect and assess. To some extent, the subjective impressions of the pathologist enter into the analysis and account for interobserver and intraobserver variability. In addition, differences in the techniques used to process and stain the smears or sections render it difficult to precisely define criteria for distinguishing between squamous metaplasia and mild dysplasia.

Histologic and cytologic features that are used to separate squamous metaplasia and mild dysplasia are variation in the size of the cells and their nuclei within an area of squamous metaplasia and alterations in the nuclear/cytoplasmic ratio. The degree of cytoplasmic basophilia is also helpful, although it is not as obvious in cytologic smears as in tissue sections. Some variation in the nuclear chromatin may also be detected, reflected in cytologic preparations in the size and number of the chromatin particles.

DNA studies have shown that cells of squamous metaplasia without atypia show only diploid values by flow cytometry.[20] However, as dyskaryosis increases in severity, diploid values become decreased and tetraploid values increase. The changes appear to be proportional to the degree of severity of the dysplasia.

The distinctions between moderate and severe dysplasia and between severe dysplasia and carcinoma *in situ* are often difficult, and interpretation varies with the experience of the pathologist and the criteria that are believed to be important. However, a precise assessment should be sought from cytologic preparations because they sample the bronchial epithelium more extensively than a small biopsy; the findings from the latter may not be representative of changes in a more peripheral or other unsampled area. The onus is on the pathologist since precancerous intraepithelial changes cannot be detected by radiologic examination. Even small invasive cancers less than 1 cm in diameter are often not recognized with standard radiologic procedures. Patients with all degrees of dysplasia should be considered to be at high risk and ought to be carefully monitored. The importance of early recognition of dysplasia and carcinoma *in situ* cannot be overemphasized since it may be possible to reverse these precursor lesions. Cytologic examination of sputa is currently the most feasible means with which to evaluate the number of smokers who are at high risk for the development of lung cancer. During the first 10 years of the Mayo Lung Project,[32] 68 radiologically

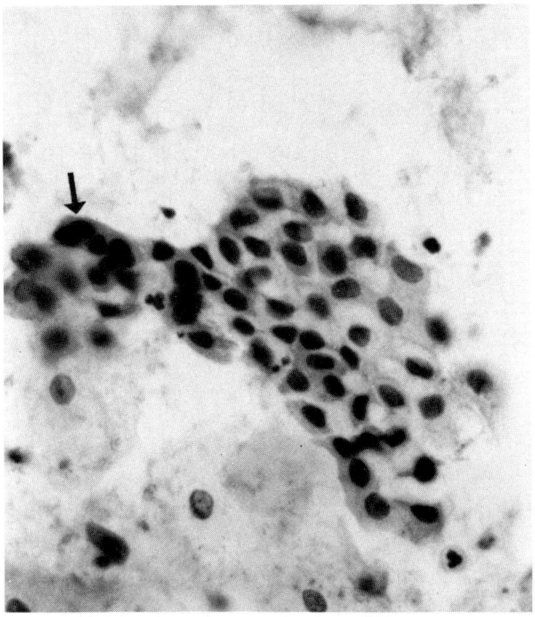

Figure 5–5. Squamous metaplasia in sputum with early dysplastic changes *(arrow)*.

occult lung cancers were detected and resected and 23 were *in situ* lesions.

The diagnostic significance of a cytologic diagnosis of severe dysplasia on sputum samples was assessed by Risse and associates[22] in a group of 46 patients. Follow-up showed no evidence of the development of cancer in 25 patients (54%) and a malignant process in 21 (46%). The authors advocate that a cytodiagnosis of severe dysplasia on sputum specimens be considered an indication for bronchoscopy with brushings of all suspicious areas of the mucosa and segmental bronchial washings. They further recommend that if a malignant process is not discovered, sputum examinations should be repeated at 3-month intervals.

It is difficult to provide precise, reproducible criteria for the different grades of dysplasia. The alterations are essentially ones of degree with blurred separation of the named categories. Some of the features described below for the different grades of dysplasia and carcinoma *in situ* in the bronchial epithelium apply to cytologic preparations.

In mild dysplasia (Figs. 5–5 and 5–6), the epithelium may be thickened, and minimal variations in cell and nuclear size without loss of polarity are apparent. In moderate dysplasia (Figs. 5–7 and 5–8), the cells are distinctly basophilic and pleomorphism of cells and nuclei can be seen with increase in the nuclear/cytoplasmic ratio and some loss of polarity. In severe dysplasia (Figs. 5–9 and 5–10), greater degrees of variation in cell and nuclear size and shape are found with nuclear/cytoplasmic ratios as high as 80%, marked hyperchromasia with clumped chromatin is seen in smears, and many nuclear profiles are irregular. In carcinoma *in situ* (Figs. 5–11 through 5–13), the nuclear/cytoplasmic ratio is particularly high and may in fact be greater than in cells of well-differentiated or moderately differentiated invasive

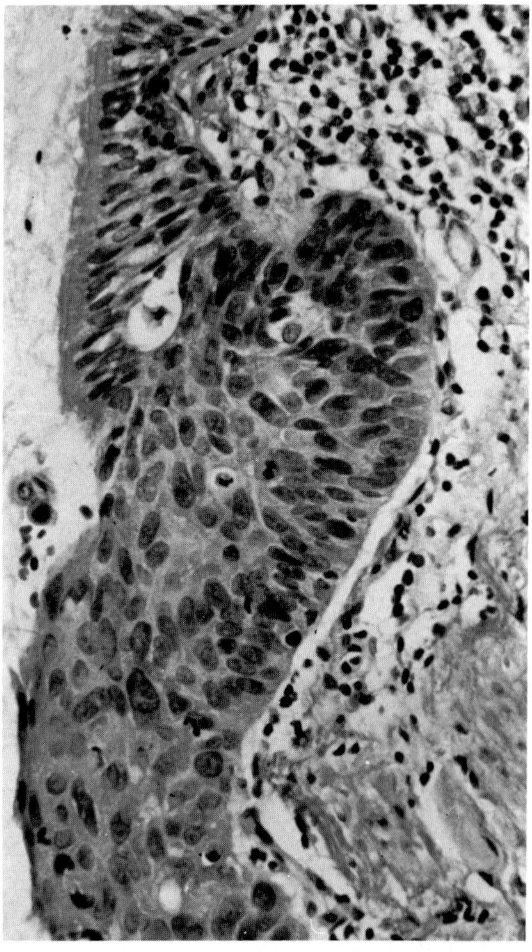

Figure 5–6. Tissue section showing an area of mildly dysplastic epithelium merging with normal respiratory epithelium.

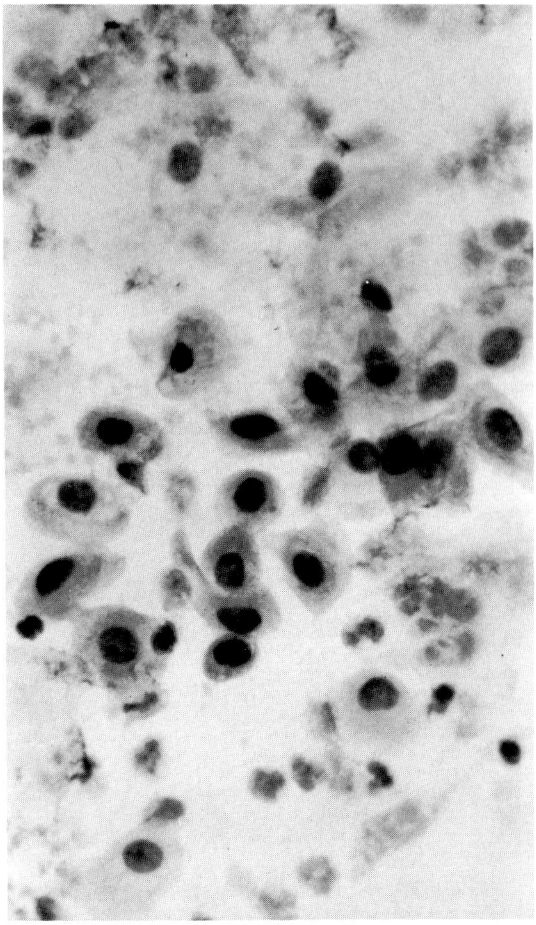

Figure 5–7. Sputum specimen: a loose collection of moderately dysplastic epithelial cells with some nuclear pleomorphism.

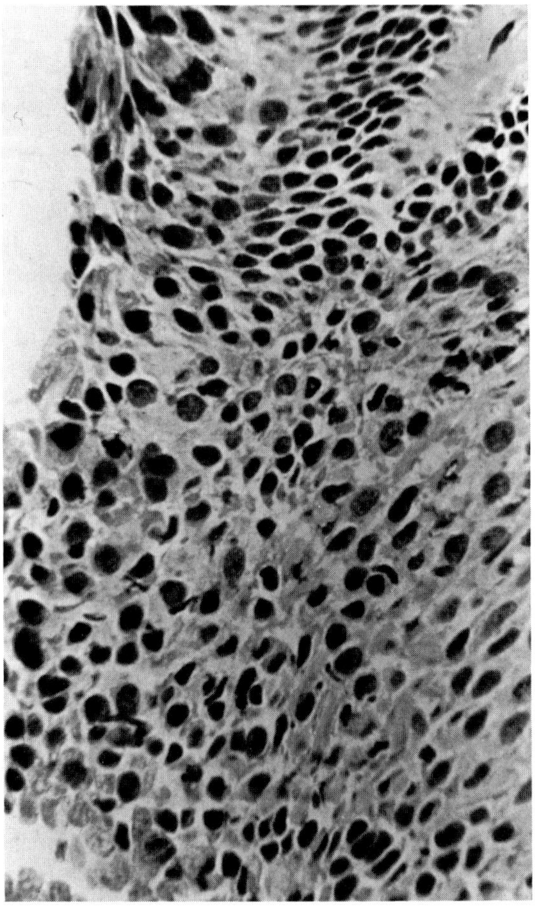

Figure 5–8. Tissue section showing moderate dysplasia overlying reserve cell hyperplasia.

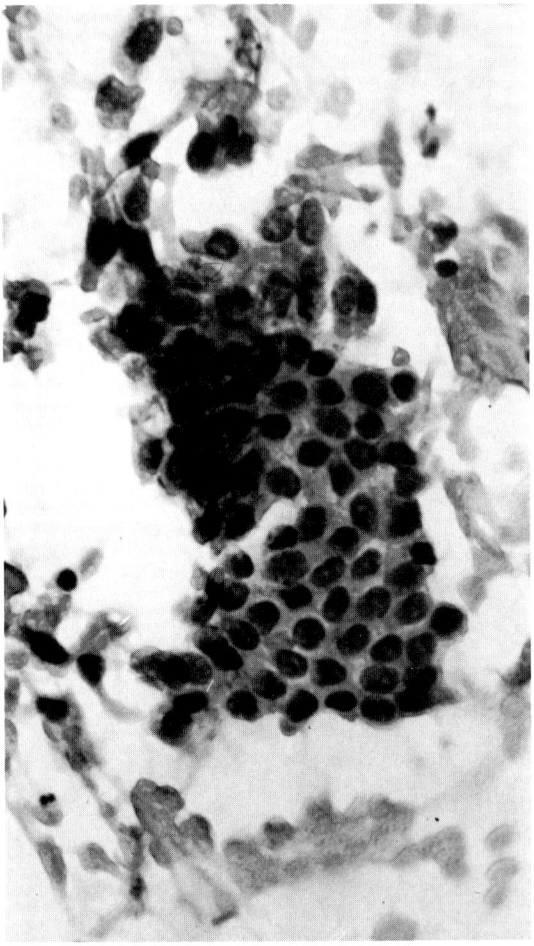

Figure 5–9. A clump of cells in sputum showing high nuclear/cytoplasmic ratios and dense, hyperchromatic nuclei, consistent with severe dysplasia.

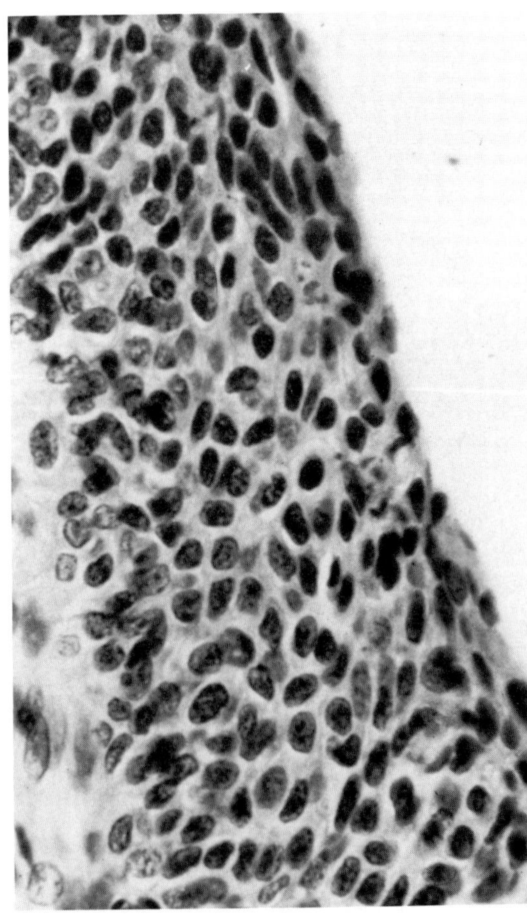

Figure 5–10. Severe dysplasia. Tissue section showing full-thickness involvement by the dysplastic process.

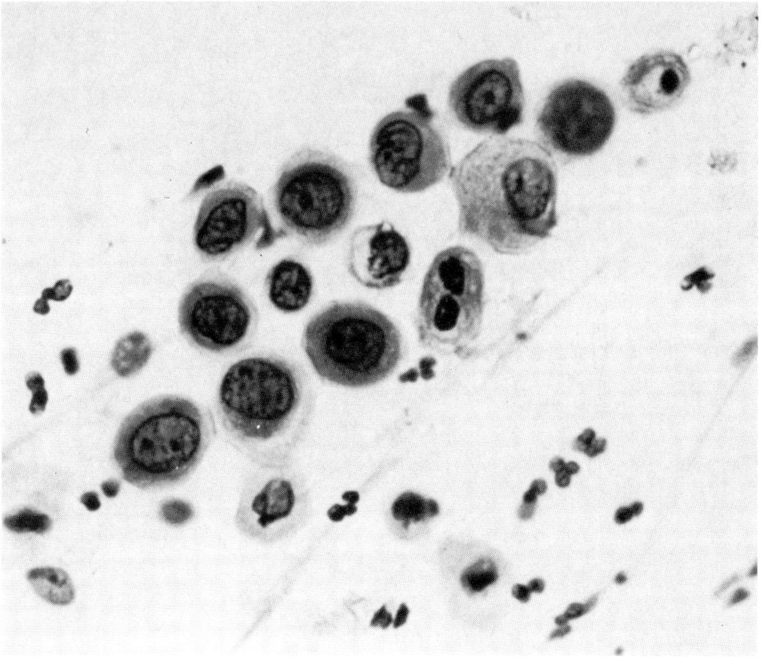

Figure 5–11. Cells of carcinoma *in situ* in a bronchial brushing specimen.

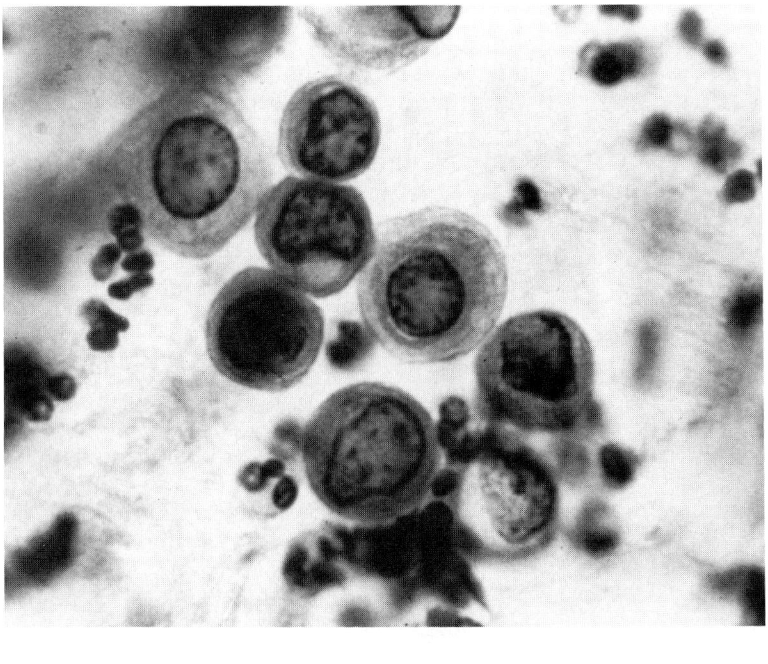

Figure 5–12. Cells from the same case as Figure 5–11 at higher magnification.

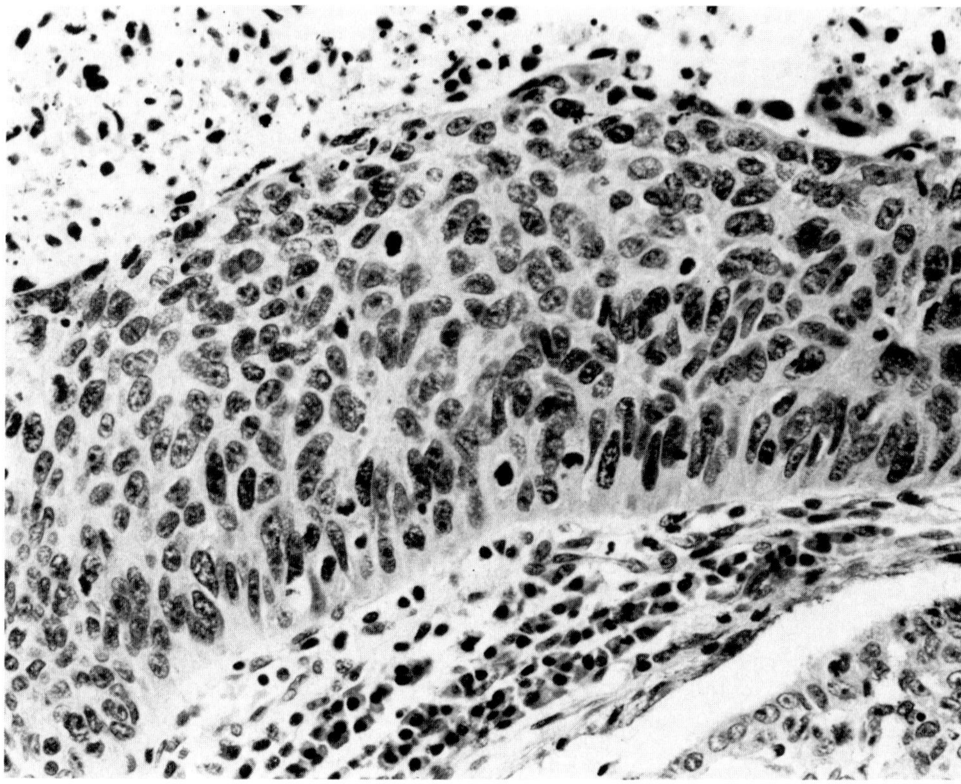

Figure 5–13. Tissue section showing carcinoma *in situ*. The full thickness of the epithelium is involved. The cells show considerable nuclear pleomorphism with coarse chromatin clumping, prominent nucleoli, and loss of polarity.

squamous cell carcinoma. As a result, it may be impossible to distinguish these categories on the basis of single cells in cytologic preparations. However, cells in small aggregates occur in sputum, and tissue fragments are frequently present in bronchial brushings. Prominent nucleoli are found in many of the cells. Occasionally, the cells of carcinoma *in situ* become spindle shaped and suggest sarcoma, and immunostaining for keratin may be required to confirm that they are epithelial. Papanicolaou-stained smears are generally fixed in alcohol, and this type of fixation lends itself to destaining and restaining with the immunoperoxidase techniques. Ultrastructural features of carcinoma *in situ* and microinvasive squamous cell carcinoma are described by Imai and colleagues.[9]

RETINOIDS

On the basis of animal experiments and the responses observed in patients with dermatologic and head and neck cancer, it is known that squamous metaplasia, dysplasia, and carcinoma *in situ* may be prevented and perhaps cured if homologues of vitamin A are administered.[6, 16] When the lesions appear in patients who are deficient in vitamin A, they may be reversed with the use of adequate doses of the retinoid compounds. Studies performed on organ cultures of rodent respiratory epithelium suggest that retinoids may be useful for the treatment of early precancerous changes in the bronchi.[11] In a study of 40 volunteers who were heavy smokers, Misset and co-workers[14] found a significant reduction of squamous metaplasia following 6 months of retinoid administration. The problem of determining which patients with preneoplastic changes are likely to progress to invasive cancer is one that requires additional investigation. Retinoid deficiency, hormonal imbalance, excessive exposure to carcinogens, altered immunocompetence, and genetic predisposition probably play important roles.

REFERENCES

1. Becci PJ, McDowell EM, Trump BF: The respiratory epithelium: IV. Histogenesis of epidermoid metaplasia and carcinoma *in situ* in the hamster. JNCI 61:577, 1978.
2. Benfield JR, Hammond WG, Paladugu RR et al: Endobronchial carcinogenesis in dogs. J Thorac Cardiovasc Surg 92:880, 1986.
3. Boutet M, Montminy L, Castonguqy A: Cellular changes induced by the tobacco-specific carcinogen 4-(N-nitrosomethylamino)-1-(3-pyridyl)-1-butanone in the respiratory tract of Syrian golden hamsters. IARC Sci Publ 84:438, 1987.
4. Carter D: Squamous cell carcinoma of the lung: An update. Semin Diagn Pathol 2:226, 1985.
5. Chejfec G, Capella C, Solcia E et al: Amphicrine cells, dysplasias, and neoplasias. Cancer 56:2683, 1985.
6. Goodman DS: Vitamin A and retinoids in health and disease. N Engl J Med 310:1023, 1984.
7. Gould VE, Linnoila RI, Memoli VA et al: Neuroendocrine components of the bronchopulmonary tract: Hyperplasia, dysplasias, and neoplasms. Lab Invest 49:519, 1983.
8. Greenberg SD, Spjut HJ, Estrada RG et al: Morphometric markers for the evaluation of preneoplastic lesions in the lung: Diagnostic evaluation by high-resolution image analysis of atypical cells in sputum specimens. Anal Quant Cytol Histol 9:49, 1987.
9. Imai T, Saito Y, Nagamoto N et al: Electron microscopic observations in *in situ* and microinvasive bronchogenic squamous cell carcinoma. J Pathol 156:241, 1988.
10. Kierszenbaum AL: Bronchial metaplasia: Observations on its histology and cytology. Acta Cytol 9:365, 1965.
11. Lasnitzki I, Bollag W: Prevention and reversal by a nonpolar arotinoid (Ro 15-0778) of 3,4-benzpyrene– and cigarette smoke condensate–induced hyperplasia and metaplasia of rodent respiratory epithelium grown *in vitro*. Eur J Cancer Clin Oncol 23:861, 1987.
12. Linberg K: Uber die Formale Genese des Lungerkreboes. Helsingfors, Mercator Trycken Aktiebolaget, 1935.
13. Mathe G, Santelli G, Gouveia J et al: Correlation of bronchial epidermoid metaplasia with level of tobacco consumption in heavy smokers. Cancer Detect Prev 9:79, 1986.
14. Misset JL, Mathe G, Santelli G et al: Regression of bronchial epidermoid metaplasia in heavy smokers with etretinate treatment. Cancer Detect Prev 9:167, 1986.
15. Miyamoto T, Morita S, Tsunemoto H et al: Acute squamous metaplasia of the whole lung after combined radiation and chemotherapy in advanced lung cancer. Gan No Rinsho 33:89, 1987.
16. Moon C, McCormick DL, Metha RG: Inhibition of carcinogenesis by retinoids. Cancer Res 43(suppl)24:695, 1983.
17. Mosca L, Ceresoli A, Anzanello E et al: Neuroendocrine structures in normal and diseased human lung. Appl Pathol 4:147, 1986.
18. Muller KM, Fisseler-Eckhoff A: What's new in lung tumor heterogeneity? Pathol Res Pract 184:108, 1988.
19. Nagai A, West WW, Thurlbeck WM: The National Institutes of Health Intermittent Positive-Pressure Breathing trial: Pathology studies: II. Correlation between morphologic findings, clinical findings, and evidence of expiratory air-flow obstruction. Am Rev Respir Dis 132:946, 1985.
20. Nasiell M, Kato H, Auer G et al: Cytomorphological grading and Feulgen DNA-analysis of metaplastic and neoplastic bronchial cells. Cancer 41:1512, 1978.
21. Nettesheim P, Klein-Szanto JP, Yarita T: Experimental models for the study of morphogenesis of lung cancer. In Shimosato Y, Melamed MR (eds): Morphogenesis of Lung Cancer, p 132. Boca Raton, FL, CRC Press, 1982.
22. Risse EK, Vooijs GP, van Hof MA: Diagnostic significance of "severe dysplasia" in sputum cytology. Acta Cytol 32:629, 1988.
23. Saccomanno G, Yale C, Dixon W et al: An epidemiological analysis of the relationship between exposure to Rn progeny, smoking and bronchogenic carcinoma in the U-mining population of the Colorado Plateau—1960–1980. Health Phys 50:605, 1986.
24. Sassy-Dobray G: Possibilities of early diagnosis of bronchogenic carcinoma. Acta Cytol 10:351, 1975.
25. Schreiber H, Saccomanno G, Martin DH et al: Sequential cytologic changes during development of respiratory tract tumors induced in hamsters by benzo(a)pyrene-ferric oxide. Cancer Res 34:689, 1974.
26. Schreiber H, Bibbo M, Wied GL et al: Bronchial metaplasia as a benign or premalignant lesion. Acta Cytol 23:496, 1979.
27. Shimosato Y: Pathology of early lung cancer. Gan No Rinsho 34:1373, 1989.
28. Topping DC, Griesemer RA, Nettesheim P: Quantitative assessment of generalized epithelial changes in tracheal mucosa following exposure to 7,12,dimethylben(a)anthracene. Cancer Res 39:4823, 1979.
29. Trump BF, McDowell EM, Glavin F et al: The respiratory epithelium: III. Histogenesis of epidermoid metaplasia and carcinoma *in situ* in the human. JNCI 61:563, 1978.
30. Trump BF, McDowell EM, Shamsuddin AK et al: Preneoplasia and neoplasia of the bronchus, esophagus, and colon: The use of markers in determining phenotypes and classification. Monogr Pathol 26:101, 1985.
31. Tsuchiya E, Kitagawa T, Oh S et al: Incidence of squamous metaplasia in large bronchi of Japanese lungs: Relation to pulmonary carcinomas of various subtypes. Jpn J Cancer Res 78:559, 1987.
32. Woolner LB, Fontana RS, Cortese DA et al: Roentgenographically occult lung cancer: Pathologic findings and frequency of multicentricity during a 10-year period. Mayo Clin Proc 59:453, 1984.

Chapter

6

ADENOCARCINOMA

INCIDENCE

The incidence of adenocarcinoma of the lung has been increasing in the United States. The progressive rise in the total number of cases of lung cancer has been accompanied by a relative increase in the percentage of adenocarcinomas, particularly in women, and a decline in the frequency of squamous cell carcinoma. The changing figures may be influenced to some extent by enhanced sophistication in diagnosis as a result of pathologists' attaching greater concern to the subclassification of lung tumors and using ancillary techniques to determine the subtype of poorly differentiated tumors.

Squamous cell carcinoma used to be accepted as the common type of lung cancer in the United States, but in 1977, Vincent and co-workers[191] drew attention to an increase in adenocarcinoma in their review of cases at Roswell Park Memorial Institute. Valaitis and colleagues[187] supported this observation in a study of 219 patients at a Chicago hospital. In the Lung Cancer Study Group report of 1,121 classified tumors,[116] adenocarcinoma and squamous cell carcinoma were almost equal in incidence, and nearly half of the lung cancers in the population screened in New York City were adenocarcinomas.[106]

Johnston and colleagues[65] reported relative frequencies and changes in morphologic patterns as they were documented in histologic and cytologic specimens obtained from 2,580 patients with lung cancer diagnosed and treated at Duke University Medical Center over a 15-year period. During the first 5 years, the relative frequency of acinar adenocarcinoma was 18.6% and that of bronchioloalveolar adenocarcinoma was 3.5%, while squamous cell carcinoma made up 43.1%, undifferentiated large cell carcinoma, 22.5%, small cell carcinoma, 11.6%, and adenosquamous carcinoma, 0.7%. During the second and third 5-year periods, squamous cell carcinoma continued as the most common tumor but its incidence declined to 35.7%, while acinar adenocarcinoma became the second most common type at 22% and replaced squamous cell carcinoma as the most frequent primary lung cancer in women. In a study of lung cancer in elderly patients, Teeter and associates[177] found that the proportion of patients with adenocarcinoma decreased with increasing age, as did the figures for small cell carcinoma, while the percentage of squamous cell carcinoma rose.

The incidence of adenocarcinoma is clearly different between the sexes, although there are variations in the reported figures. Valaitis and colleagues[187] noted an increase of adenocarcinomas in men but did not find a relative change in the percentage of adenocarcinomas in women. Dodds and co-workers[27] examined the incidence trends by histologic type in western Washington state between 1974 and 1981 and found that the rate of increase of adenocarcinoma was higher among women (86%) than men (54%). However, Wu and associates[201] found an increase of adenocarcinoma in men in Los Angeles County over a 10-year period, and while all lung cancer types had increased in women, the smallest increase was shown by adenocarcinoma.

Similar trends to those occurring in the United States have been noticed in some other countries. Adenocarcinoma is the most frequent lung carcinoma in Japan. Watanabe and co-workers[196] analyzed 4,419 cases from the records of the Japanese National Cancer Center through the period 1966 to 1985.

The proportions of the different histologic types remained relatively unchanged in men, approximately 40% of the tumors being squamous cell carcinomas and one third adenocarcinomas. However, among women in the study, an increase in adenocarcinoma from 52% to 69.1% was seen while the occurrence of squamous cell carcinoma decreased from 21% to 11.4%. Morita and associates[114] reported that adenocarcinoma was found in 34% of cases in a group of Japanese men, with squamous cell carcinoma occurring in 33%. In women, 55% of tumors were adenocarcinomas and 18% were squamous cell carcinoma. A comparison of the histopathology of resected lung cancer in women in hospitals in Hong Kong and Japan[183] revealed some striking differences. Adenocarcinoma made up 90.9% in Japan as against 68.8% in Hong Kong, and 50% of the adenocarcinomas in Japan were classified as bronchioloalveolar adenocarcinomas compared with only 17% in Hong Kong. Gao and colleagues[44] noted a high rate of adenocarcinoma among women in Shanghai. Hanai and co-workers[55] compared 14,521 cases of lung cancer in the Osaka cancer registry in Japan with 29,859 in the northwest region of England and found a higher proportion of adenocarcinoma in Osaka (36% in men, 62% in women) than in the English cases (12% in men, 19% in women).

Adenocarcinoma, like other types of lung carcinoma, is uncommon in young patients, and there are conflicting reports on its behavior in this age group. Larrieu and associates[90] reviewed 101 patients between the ages of 18 and 40. There were 65 men and 36 women; 87% smoked and 50% had a strong family history of malignancy. Thirty-nine patients had adenocarcinoma, 29 had squamous cell carcinoma, and 18 had small cell carcinoma. Eighty-six patients presented with stage III disease as against only 9 with stage I disease and 6 with stage II disease. In contrast, Roviaro and co-workers[144] found no significant difference in patients younger than the age of 45 with regard to clinical picture, operability, histologic type, or prognosis. Komatsu and colleagues[85] reported a 6-cm well-differentiated adenocarcinoma in a 24-year-old woman and provided information on 14 patients younger than the age of 40 among 154 with lung cancer: in this group, 6 women and 2 men had adenocarcinomas. The young women with lung carcinoma were mostly nonsmokers, and it was the impression of the authors that they had a better prognosis than the men in the same age range.

Adenocarcinoma was the diagnosis in 45% of 60 Chinese patients with primary lung cancer between the ages of 17 and 39 from a series of 1,645 cases.[26] Thirty-five were male and 25 were female, and 60% of the lesions were stage III. The survival rates in these younger patients were similar to that of lung cancer overall. In a group of 76 Chinese patients younger than the age of 40,[181] 59.2% had adenocarcinomas, and while many had advanced disease, they did not as a whole have significantly poorer resectability or prognosis than older patients. However, the 19 patients (25%) who were younger than age 30 had a more virulent course.

In contrast to squamous cell carcinoma, adenocarcinoma of the lung does not appear to have a strong relationship with smoking.[182] Most of the 672 female Chinese patients with adenocarcinoma reported by Gao and colleagues[44] were lifelong nonsmokers. Anton-Culver[2] observed that adenocarcinoma was the most common cell type among women smokers and nonsmokers, whereas squamous cell carcinoma predominated in both male smokers and nonsmokers.

The relationship between lung cancer and occupation, adjusted for smoking, was studied in a series of 4,431 white men from Missouri.[205] Excess risk of developing adenocarcinoma was observed among many *a priori* suspected high-risk occupations including carpenters, furniture makers, plumbers, printers, and welders.

CLINICAL FEATURES

Most bronchogenic adenocarcinomas arise peripherally and form discrete oval or irregular masses. The majority are between 2.0 and 5.0 cm in diameter when they are resected, but a few are smaller and many are larger. The peripheral tumors are frequently asymptomatic in contrast to central lesions, which can give rise to obstructive effects. An asymptomatic peripheral lesion on a chest radiograph is the presentation in almost half of the patients who are found to have bronchioloalveolar adenocarcinoma, and the patient may be followed for months before the diagnosis is made. Others have chest pain, weight loss, cough with increased mucus, dyspnea, and, infrequently, hemoptysis. A peripheral adenocarcinoma may cause a pleural effusion. Unusual symptoms are occasionally reported in association with bronchogenic adenocarcinoma, including the myasthenic syndrome,[140] Raynaud's phenomenon,[199] ectopic ACTH syndrome,[119] acanthosis nigricans, and the Leser-Trélat sign.[61]

Radiologic Appearance

A variety of changes may be seen on the chest radiograph, including a solitary peripheral, or less often a central, mass; multiple peripheral nodules; or features that are considered indicative of bronchioloalveolar adenocarcinoma. To an experienced radiologist, a hazy bilateral upper lobe infiltrate may suggest the diagnosis of bronchioloalveolar adenocarcinoma. The so-called rabbit ear sign is produced by strands of tumor extending to the pleural surface; it can be seen in 57% of cases,[152] but it has also been described in some infectious processes and hence is not specific. In the later stages, a diffuse pneumonic type of spread can involve much of a lobe.

Computed tomographic findings on 30 patients with solitary bronchioloalveolar adenocarcinoma were reviewed by Kuhlman and colleagues.[86] Common features were the peripheral or subpleural location of the mass in 25 cases, pseudocavitation (18 cases), heterogeneous attenuation (17 cases), irregular margins forming a star pattern (22 cases), and pleural tags (21 cases). Using these computed tomographic criteria, four independent observers tried to identify cases of bronchioloalveolar adenocarcinoma among a larger sample of lung carcinomas and benign lesions by categorizing a series of test cases into four probability categories. Although the bronchioloalveolar adenocarcinomas were correctly ranked in the two highest probability categories 75% of the time (in 45 of 60 cases), there was considerable overlap with other lung lesions and particularly with other adenocarcinomas and undifferentiated large cell carcinomas.

Multiple Primary Tumors

The incidence of multiple primary lung adenocarcinomas in apparently operable patients is higher than the literature might be considered to indicate.[103, 108] In 62 consecutive lung resections for primary adenocarcinoma, 12 patients (19%) were found to have two or more adenocarcinomas.[108] As the authors note, the more careful the pathologic examination, the more likely is the discovery of a second primary tumor. At least half of the multiple primary lesions found in Japanese who were nonsmokers were adenocarcinomas.[171]

If more than one large nodule is present, the possibility that more than a single tumor type may be present should be investigated by fine-needle aspiration biopsies. The fourth report of triple malignant lung neoplasms was the case of a patient who had a central bronchial carcinoid and peripheral small cell carcinoma in the right middle lobe and a peripheral adenocarcinoma in the right middle lobe.[68]

Behavior

Peripheral adenocarcinomas spread to lymph nodes frequently, and even tumors smaller than 3 cm show lymph node involvement in 50% of cases. Lymph nodes involved by a well-differentiated papillary adenocarcinoma are not always enlarged and may not be detected by radiography.[156] Libshitz and co-workers[91] found a higher prevalence of mediastinal lymph node metastases in patients with adenocarcinoma compared with squamous cell carcinoma and a much higher frequency of mediastinal metastases without lobar or hilar involvement in patients with adenocarcinoma. The presence of mediastinal lymph node involvement is a contraindication to surgical resection as the primary treatment of adenocarcinoma: among 57 patients who were operated on for adenocarcinoma, 19 with mediastinal lymph node metastases underwent potentially curative pulmonary resections combined with complete mediastinal node dissection, and the 5-year survival was nil.[145]

More than 50% of lung cancers invade branches of the pulmonary arterial system,[84, 88] and the arterial invasion is followed by thrombosis, organization by granulation tissue, and scarring. Kolin and colleagues[84] did not find a correlation with the histologic type or grade of the tumors, or the lymph node status at the time of surgery, and postulated that the greater resistance of systemic arteries to infiltration by carcinoma can be attributed to the higher blood pressure in the lumen, which results in a steep pressure gradient through the wall that successfully opposes the advance of the cancer. However, embolic carcinomatosis in which small arteries and arterioles are filled with tumor is more common in adenocarcinoma than squamous cell carcinoma, and adenocarcinoma has a greater propensity for extrathoracic dissemination, especially to the brain. Differences have not been documented between adenocarcinoma and undifferentiated large cell carcinoma.[20] In a group of 259 patients with inoperable adenocarcinoma,[164] brain metastases were diagnosed in 25 patients before entry into protocol and in 37 during treatment and brain autopsy was positive in 44% of the patients in whom it was performed. Patients younger than the age of 60 had a somewhat higher overall frequency of brain metastases than older patients. Patients with good performance status, and those responding to chemotherapy during treatment had a greater risk of developing brain metastases. Median survival after onset of brain metastases was 73 days. Meningeal carcinomatosis may be diagnosed by cerebrospinal fluid cytology.[21] The Lung Cancer Study Group generated survival characteristics for 1,121 patients who underwent apparent complete resection of non–small cell lung carcinomas and were subsequently entered into various protocols.[116] In this study, a high level of consistency in classification was achieved through the use of criteria designed to minimize intraobserver variability. The outcome for patients with adenocarcinoma was poorer than for those with squamous cell carcinoma in every TNM subset, and the differences in survival according to these major cell types were significant overall but not in the TNM subsets in stage III disease. In a series of 273 unselected patients with lung cancer from Sweden,[127] the 5-year survival for patients with adenocarcinoma was 11.7% compared with 7.5% for squamous cell carcinoma. Undifferentiated large cell carcinomas, which are often lumped with adenocarcinoma, made up 3.8% of the total. In a study of tumor cell type versus staging,[50] resected stage I adenocarcinomas had a survival of 38% at 5 years compared with 23% for squamous cell carcinomas.

Bronchioloalveolar adenocarcinomas may have a slightly improved survival compared with other adenocarcinomas, but they are by definition and selection differentiated tumors and might therefore be anticipated to behave better than a mixture of all grades. Keikkila and co-workers[74] examined the relationship of the growth rate of adenocarcinomas to prognosis following surgery in 26 patients, 12 with pure bronchioloalveolar adenocarcinoma, 7 with mixed forms, and 4 with adenocarcinoma only. The mean doubling times for the three groups were 300.1 days, 288.4 days, and 224.6 days, respectively. The mixed tumors had a poorer prognosis than the pure bronchioloalveolar adenocarcinomas, and there was no evidence of a correlation between tumor doubling times and regional lymph node metastases or patient survival. Brolly and associates[13] reported five patients with uninodular bronchioloalveolar adenocarcinoma whose disease ran a protracted course (14.5 and 11.5 years in two patients who died, and 7.5, 12, and 12.5 years in three who were still alive). Recurrence after an interval of 19 years has been recorded.[1]

GROSS APPEARANCE

The cut surface is pale gray to white, and it glistens if mucin is present. A desmoplastic reaction is often associated with the proliferating tumor, which then has a firm, fibrous consistency. Invasion of the bronchial cartilage was found in 26% of 229 cases[73] and occurred in 25% of the adenocarcinomas. Endobronchial growth can occur: Kodama and colleagues[82] reported five well-differentiated papillary adenocarcinomas with a predominantly endobronchial polypoid growth within large bronchi. Cavity formation is relatively rare in adenocarcinomas although foci of central necrosis are frequently seen, particularly in the larger tumors. Rarely, the cavity is the locus of a fungal infection. McGregor and associates[105] reported the fifth case of aspergilloma within a cavitating lung adenocarcinoma. Pritchard and co-workers[137] described two adults with large peripheral lung cysts, present for 9 and 12 years, that contained bronchioloalveolar adenocarcinoma. Hurley and co-workers[63] reported similar findings.

Bronchioloalveolar adenocarcinomas develop in the periphery of the lung, and they are more frequent in the upper lobes. There is usually some puckering of the overlying pleura. The tumor may be a solitary mass or form several nodules that can simulate metastatic disease, or it can grow as a lacy, diffuse process. The latter is often referred to as the pneumonic type because its margins are not easily defined, but the cut surface is more nodular than in lobar pneumonia. Mucus is present in most bronchioloalveolar adenocarcinomas, and it can be copious in the well-differentiated, tall columnar form.

The pleura covering a peripheral adenocarcinoma is usually puckered, and the pleura is thickened if it is being infiltrated by the tumor. Harwood and colleagues[56] described six cases of peripheral lung carcinoma with extensive pleural involvement that produced partial to total encasement of the lung, mimicking a mesothelioma, and suggested the term *pseudomesotheliomatous carcinoma of the lung.* Two additional cases were reported by Lin and co-workers.[93]

Adenocarcinomas are often associated with subpleural scars.[14] The scarring was formerly attributed to a variety of causes, including old infarcts, healed pnumonitis or granulomas, or trauma, but there were many instances in which evidence of a previous cause for lung damage could not be obtained, and it is currently believed that the fibrosis is elicited by the proliferating neoplastic cells. The roles of atelectasis and infarction in the formation of the scars are still controversial.[83, 87] Some idea of the frequency of scar adenocarcinoma is obtained from Auerbach and associates in their review of 1,186 lung cancers,[4] among which 82 (7%) peripheral tumors were related to scars: 72% of the scar cancers were adenocarcinomas, 18% were squamous, and there was no small cell carcinoma. Kung and colleagues[88] examined 49 consecutive specimens of lung cancer from surgery or autopsy, from 40 men and 9 women, and pleural puckering and central pigmentation in 22 of the tumors were adjudged to justify a designation of scar cancer. Nineteen tumors were peripheral, and 17 of them were adenocarcinomas.

Shimosato and associates[153] list the reasons why most fibrotic foci accompanying adenocarcinoma are formed after tumor development. Adenocarcinoma often develops without fibrosis, and the quantity of fibrosis is usually less in smaller tumors and more extensive in larger tumors. Central fibrosis is not infrequently seen in metastatic foci from a primary lung adenocarcinoma, and metastatic adenocarcinomas in the lung can also develop central scars. Retrospective studies of chest radiographs show gradual convergence of bronchi and pulmonary arteries toward the center of tumors, with development of pleural indentation after the tumor shadow has appeared. When there is unilateral lung damage because of previous chronic lung disease, adenocarcinoma is found almost equally in the damaged and healthy sites, whereas squamous cell carcinoma tends to develop in the healthy lung.

The experimental work of Madri and Carter[99] provided support for the concept that the fibrosis associated with lung adenocarcinoma is a host response. Type III collagen was assessed qualitatively by immunofluorescence within the lung tumors and in nonneoplastic lung tissue. The continuing presence of type III collagen in the scar was documented, and a decrease in type III and increase in other types of collagen in fibrosed lung parenchyma some distance from the tumor indicated a later, more mature stage of the fibrotic process. The findings were consistent with the notion that the desmoplasia in and around lung tumors is not mature and represents an active, continuing process.

LIGHT MICROSCOPY

The many histologic faces of bronchogenic adenocarcinoma occur in part because the tumors arise at different levels of the respiratory tree where prototypic cells, those from which regeneration occurs after injury, vary in their developmental potential. A particular tumor may thus reflect the architecture and cell population of main to subsegmental bronchi, bronchial glands, terminal or respiratory bronchioles, or acini, and its cells may show to varying degrees features of nonciliated, ciliated columnar, goblet, bronchial gland, or Clara cells or type 2 pneumocytes. The variety of mucin that the cells produce varies greatly, from none to extensive quantities that fill the cytoplasm, but for the amount to be assessed with reasonable accuracy a mucin stain must be performed. Changes in the histologic appearance of adenocarcinomas occur with loss of differentiation, and differences among the tumors may also reflect the heterogeneity of non–small cell lung cancer.[41] In some adenocarcinomas, reflections of the fetal lung structure may be perceived.[81, 118]

The all encompassing term *adenocarcinoma* consequently lacks specificity, and attempts have been made to make the diagnosis more clinically relevant by identifying subtypes and by assessing the level of differentiation and assigning a histologic grade. Histochemical and immunocytochemical findings contribute to the subclassification of adenocarcinomas, as does electron microscopy, but to be useful and reproducible throughout the world, the criteria must be applicable to conventional hematoxylin-eosin–stained sections with the addition of histochemical stains for mucin. No current classification based exclusively on tumor cell type as assessed by light microscopy is completely reproducible with different observers.

Subtyping has generally defined three histologic types—acinar, papillary, and bronchioloalveolar—but there is overlap among them. Acinar and papillary adenocarcinomas are often intermixed and can probably be combined as a single group for practical purposes, and bronchioloalveolar adenocarcinoma is not often a pure tumor. It has been referred to as an entity with a spectrum of morphology that overlaps related forms, because other patterns of adenocarcinoma are often present.[143] The revised World Health Organization (WHO) classification[200] lists four categories of adenocarcinoma: acinar, papillary, and bronchioloalveolar adenocarcinomas, and solid carcinoma with mucus formation. Other groupings have been suggested. Edwards and associates[31] reviewed 106 resected lung adenocarcinomas and grouped them by cell morphology and site as parenchymal adenocarcinoma (67%), bronchial adenocarcinoma (13%), and adenocarcinoma of uncertain origin (20%). A precise grouping based on cell type is best achieved by using electron microscopy, although it is clearly not suitable for routine work. Shimosato and colleagues[153] subdivided 50 well-differentiated adenocarcinomas into five categories based on cell type: bronchial surface epithelial cell, goblet cell, bronchial gland cell, nonciliated bronchiolar (Clara) cell, and type II pneumocyte. The Clara cell tumors were the most common type and were peripheral tumors, while most of the tumors of the first three types arose from the main to the segmental bronchi.

In a study of 259 consecutive patients with inoperable stage III lung adenocarcinoma, the significance of subtyping prior to treatment was evaluated by Sorensen and associates[165]: 130 (50%) had acinar adenocarcinomas, 23 (9%) had papillary adencarcinomas, 13 (5%) had bronchioloalveolar adenocarcinomas, and 32 (12%) had solid carcinomas with mucus production. In 56 patients (22%), subtyping was not possible because of cytologic preparations or insufficient material. Bronchioloalveolar adenocarcinoma had the longest median duration of response to chemotherapy (47 weeks), time to progression (33 weeks), and median survival (40 weeks). Corresponding values for solid carcinoma with mucus formation were 8, 12, and 22 weeks. Acinar and papillary adenocarcinomas were intermediate. Forty-six percent of patients with bronchioloalveolar adenocarcinoma were alive at 1 year, compared with 16% to 22% for the other subtypes. Sorensen and Olsen[166] subsequently reported similar studies on a group of 137 patients with radically resected stage I or II adenocarcinomas: 57% were acinar tumors; 12%, papillary; 18%, bronchioloalveolar; and 14%, solid with mucin production. Patients with bronchioloalveolar adenocarcinoma had the longest median survival (44 months), and the shortest was for patients with solid carcinoma with mucus formation (median, 10 months).

Adenocarcinomas can be subdivided from their light microscopic appearance into well, moderately and poorly differentiated forms, basing the grading on the predominant pattern. The histologic criteria for subtyping adenocarcinomas include the degree of gland formation, regularity of the glandular architecture, cytologic features of the lining cells, presence of stratification, presence and extent of solid areas, level of mitotic activity, and occurrence and amount of necrosis. The grading gains precision when stains for mucin are performed. Once the tumors become less differentiated, grading is to some degree subjective, and artifactual change can influence the decision. Grading is of relatively little value when the assessment is from a small biopsy specimen, as more thorough sampling often reveals. Attempts at histologic grading are not reliable with metastases or after treatment. In a review of 2,260 lung adenocarcinomas at the M.D. Anderson Cancer Center (Lukeman JM, unpublished study), 5% were pure well-differentiated adenocarcinomas, 70% were moderately differentiated, and 25% were poorly differentiated. It was found in this study that survival data have little relevance to histologic grade. The poorly differentiated adenocarcinomas, especially when they contained foci of undifferentiated large cells and giant cells, had an especially poor prognosis with rapid death. Grading is thus poorly reproducible and inadequate since it relates poorly to the biologic activity of the tumors. Newer diagnostic modalities are badly needed to resolve the current problems and provide a means to correlate the microscopic appearance with the clinical course and survival. Takise and coworkers[175] studied histopathologic prognostic factors in small (under 2 cm) peripheral adenocarcinomas and found that the pathologic stage, lymph node involvement, and pleural involvement were the major prognostic determinants.

An acinar pattern is the most common type, particularly in central tumors. The better differentiated tumors form orderly glands (Fig. 6–1) lined by tall columnar cells that have a regular array of basal nuclei. Varying quantities of mucin may be demonstrated within the cytoplasm with appropriate stains. Small protrusions into the lumen are the earliest sign of a papillary architecture (Fig. 6–2). Acini can be numerous but small (Fig. 6–3). Papillary adenocarcinomas are usually formed by uniform columnar to cuboidal cells forming a single layer on a core of fibrous connective tissue. Stratification and intermingling of columnar and cuboidal cells are early indications of loss of differentiation (see Fig. 6–2), and a further stage is the intermingling of acini lined by cuboidal cells with solid areas (Fig. 6–4). Solid adenocarcinomas are poorly differentiated tumors, but a suggestion of gland formation may be detected within some of them (Figs. 6–5 through 6–8). It may be difficult to perceive the glandular nature of the tumor in a small biopsy specimen, and the task is easier if mucin-forming cells are evident (Fig. 6–9). Alcian blue–periodic acid–Schiff (PAS) is a useful mucin and glycogen stain: the PAS stains both glycogen and hyaluronic acid, and the alcian blue stains acid mucopolysaccharides as well as hyaluronic acid. A solid adenocarcinoma may be composed largely of signet-ring cells (Fig. 6–10).[78] Small cell adenocarcinomas occur, but they are uncommon. They are composed of nests and cords of relatively small cells with high nuclear/cytoplasmic ratios, and they may therefore resemble small cell undifferentiated carcinomas.

Scroggs and colleagues[150] described the

Text continued on page 111

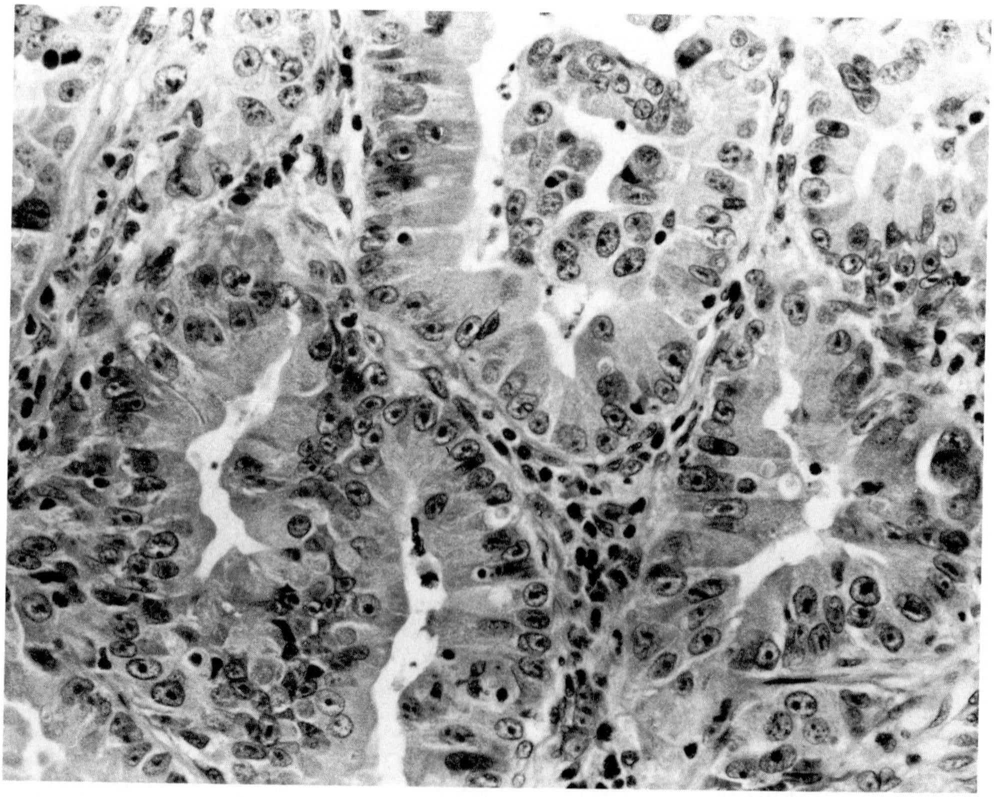

Figure 6–1. Adenocarcinoma, well differentiated. Columnar cells line a scanty stroma containing chronic inflammatory cells.

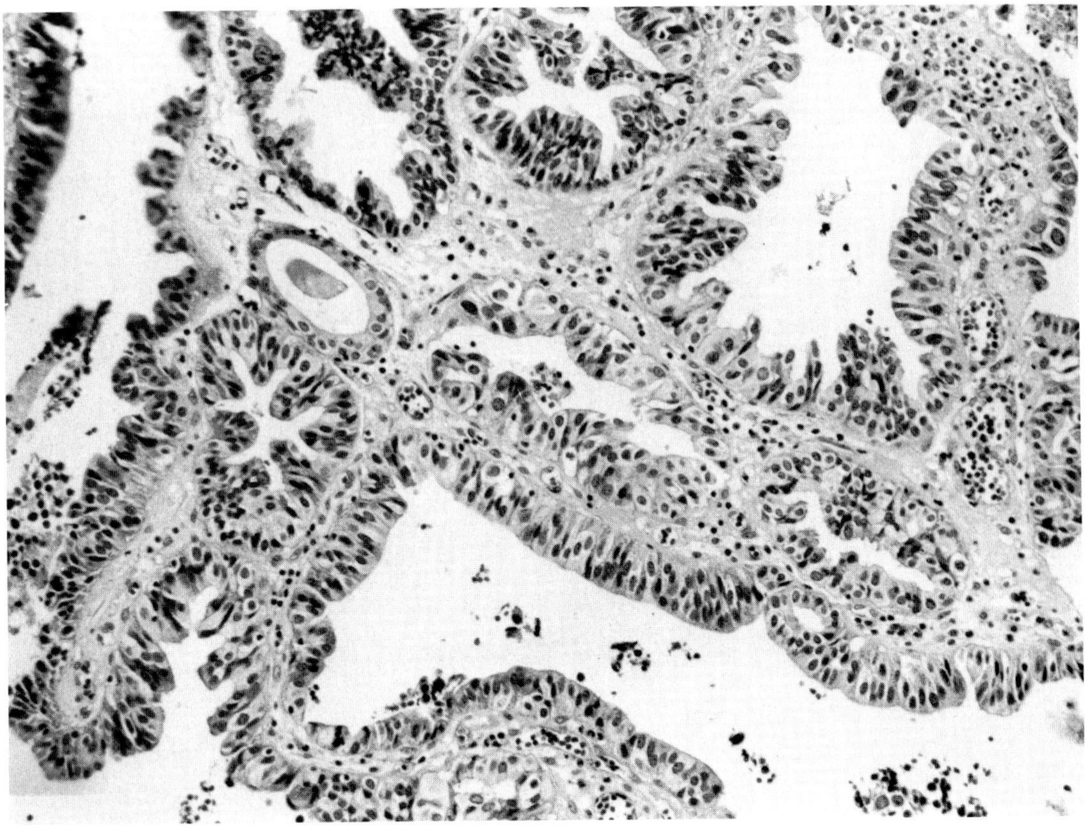

Figure 6–2. Adenocarcinoma, moderately differentiated. Some stratification and early formation of papillary structures is occurring.

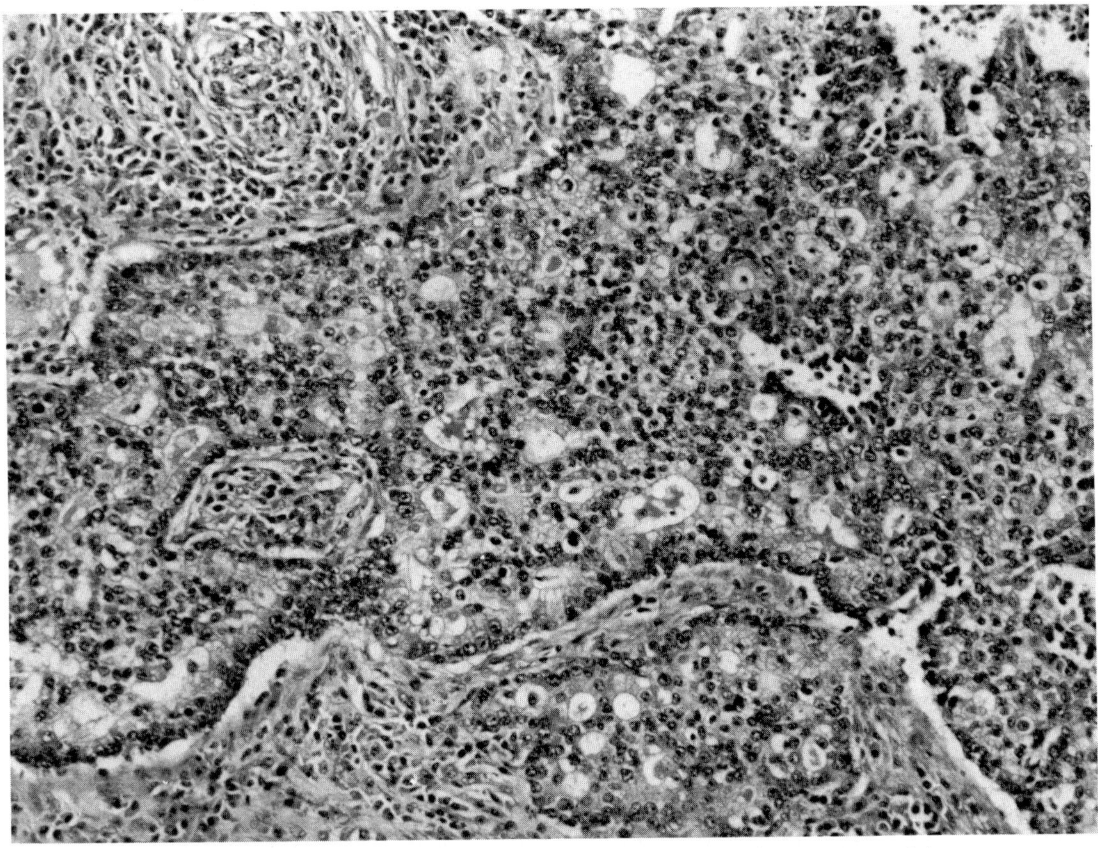

Figure 6–3. Adenocarcinoma, moderately differentiated, with many small acini.

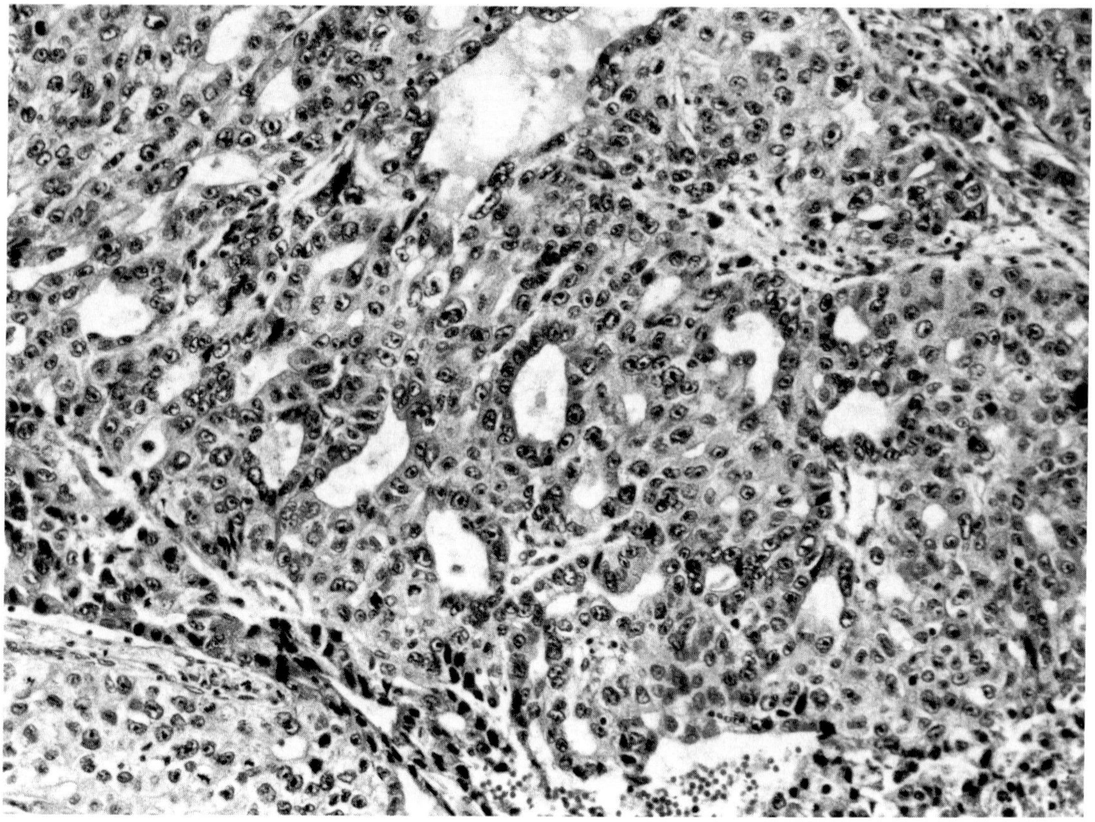

Figure 6–4. Adenocarcinoma, moderately differentiated, composed of a mixture of glands and solid areas.

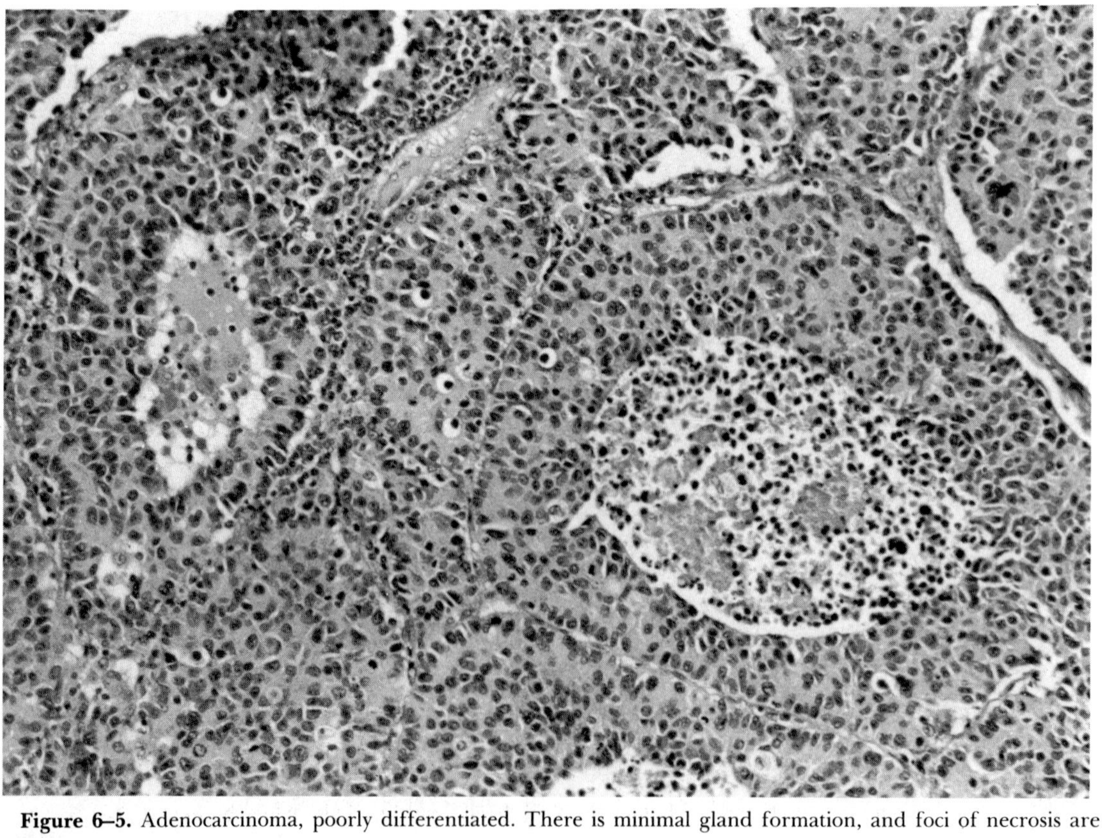

Figure 6–5. Adenocarcinoma, poorly differentiated. There is minimal gland formation, and foci of necrosis are present.

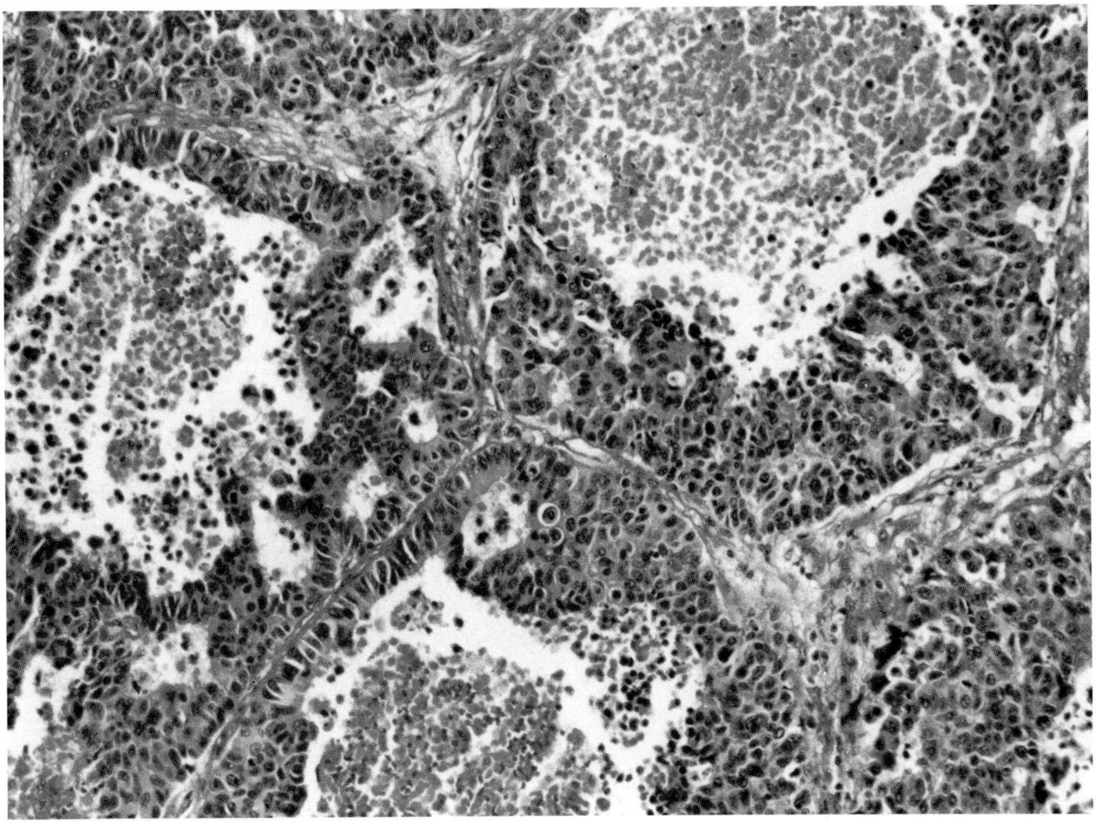

Figure 6–6. Adenocarcinoma, poorly differentiated. Single and stratified columnar cells form occasional glands and they surround spaces with necrotic tumor.

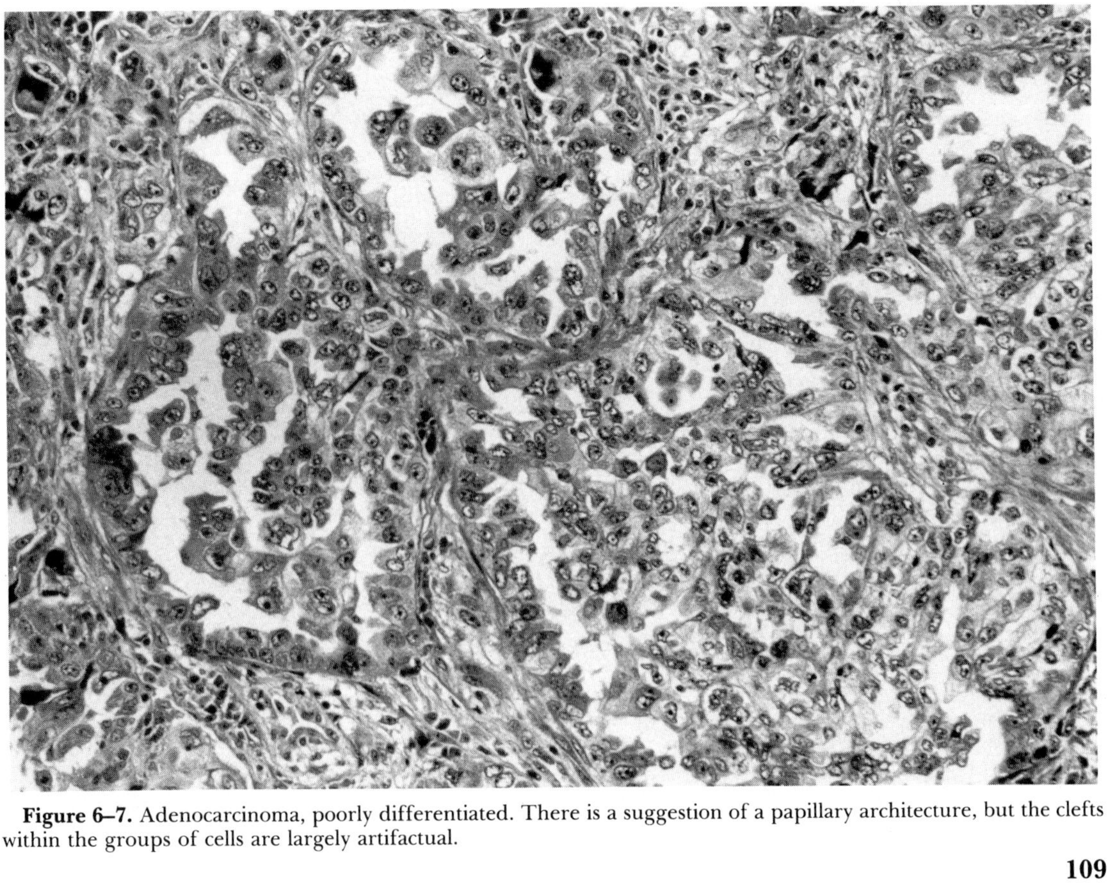

Figure 6–7. Adenocarcinoma, poorly differentiated. There is a suggestion of a papillary architecture, but the clefts within the groups of cells are largely artifactual.

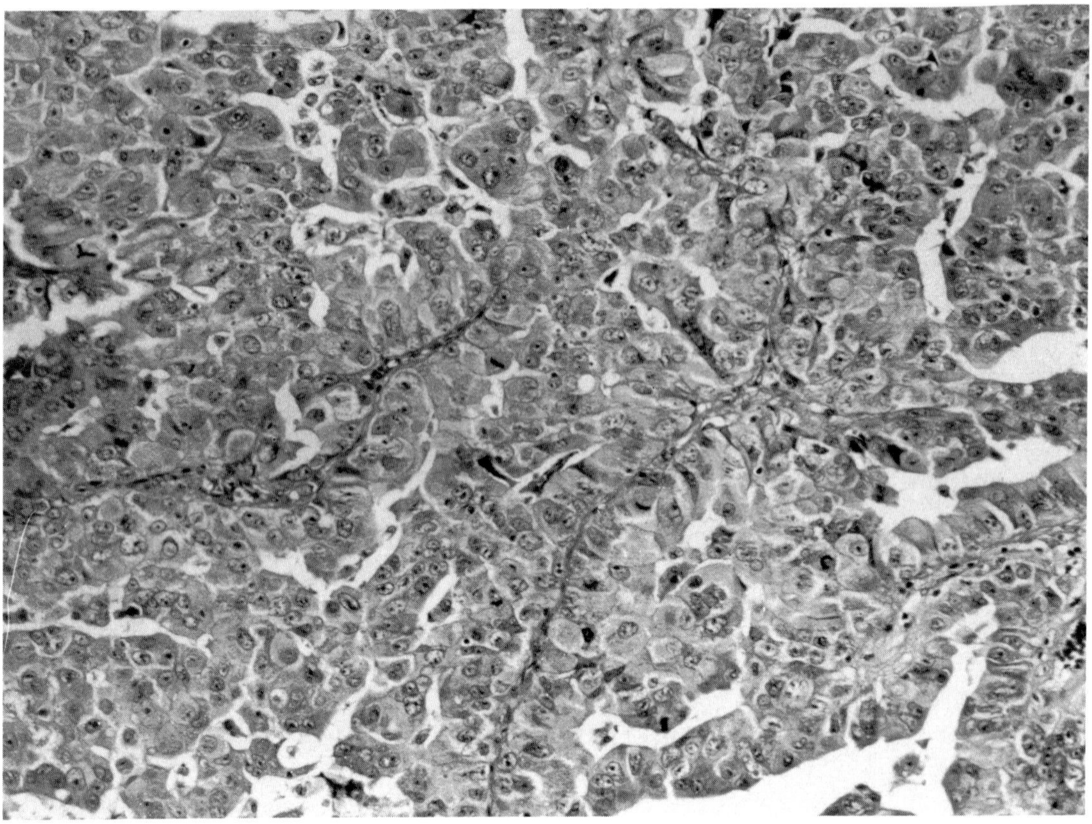

Figure 6–8. Adenocarcinoma, poorly differentiated. This was predominantly a solid tumor, but gland formation can be identified.

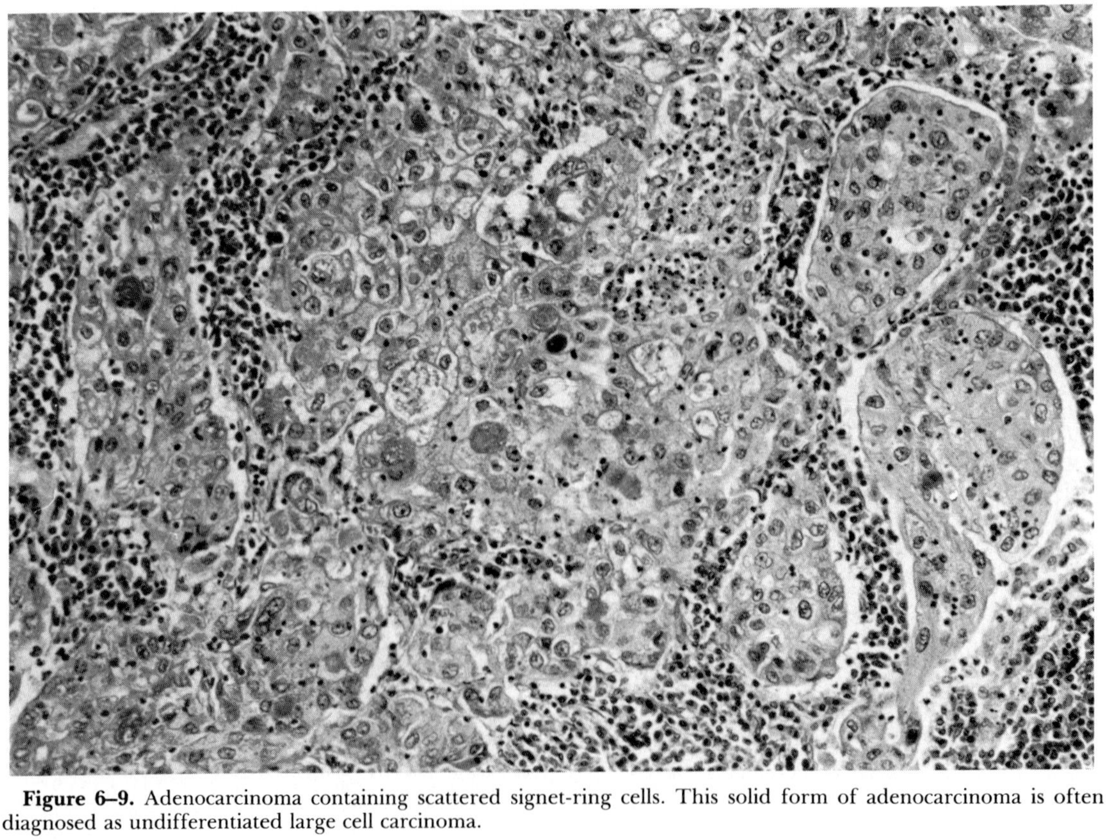

Figure 6–9. Adenocarcinoma containing scattered signet-ring cells. This solid form of adenocarcinoma is often diagnosed as undifferentiated large cell carcinoma.

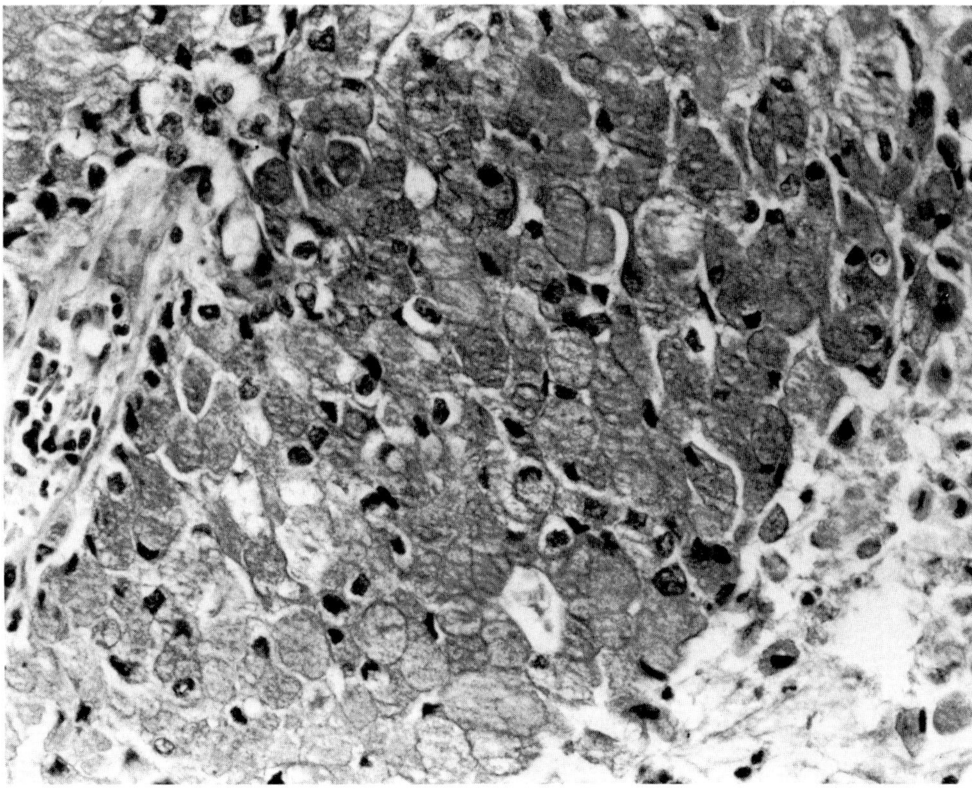

Figure 6–10. Adenocarcinoma entirely composed of mucin-filled signet-ring cells.

presence of intracytoplasmic eosinophilic globules in six adenocarcinoma. The globules stained brightly with the PAS stain with diastase and were homogeneous ultrastructurally. They were seen particularly in the vicinity of necrosis, and the authors postulate that they might represent secretory glycoprotein that accumulates in the cells in the area of tumor cell injury. Nakanishi and colleagues[121] found large intracytoplasmic bodies in 27 of 105 surgically resected lung tumors, including 13 adenocarcinomas. Sasou and associates[148] reported two adenocarcinomas containing crystals and psammoma bodies; histochemical stains suggested that mucopolysaccharides were a component of the crystals and the psammoma bodies.

Histiocytic cells may be present in varying numbers in lung adenocarcinomas, and S-100 protein–positive cells containing Langerhans' granules are relatively common, particularly in bronchioloalveolar carcinomas. Nakajima and co-workers[120] found S-100 protein–positive Langerhans' cells in various lung tumors, and especially in bronchioloalveolar adenocarcinomas of the type II alveolar cell type, but they were not found in goblet cell–type adenocarcinomas. Hammar[51] found Langerhans' cells in 80% to 93% of 66 lung adenocarcinomas and 17% of squamous cell carcinomas. The number varied from few to many. They were most numerous in bronchioloalveolar adenocarcinomas and were sometimes almost as frequent as the tumor cells. Furukawa and co-workers[43] found S-100 protein–positive cells in 77% of 40 cases and used the designation T-zone histiocytes to separate the cells from histiocytes containing nonspecific cross-reacting antigen and lysozyme. It is possible that the antigen-presenting function of the cells is a host response to the tumor. In support of this view is the finding that the patients tend to have longer survival when there is a dense infiltrate of the cells. Furukawa and co-workers[43] did not find a similar prognostic relationship with macrophages. Tumor-infiltrating lymphocytes are often seen in non–small cell lung cancers, and they are a heterogeneous population composed of T cells, B cells, monocytes, and natural killer cells in frequencies similar to those found in peripheral blood.[136]

Small foci of necrosis (see Figs. 6–5 and

6–6) are a further indication of dedifferentiation, as are variability in the size and shape of the cells and their nuclei. Distinction of a solid adenocarcinoma (Fig. 6–11) from undifferentiated large cell carcinoma is based on the absence in the latter of intracellular mucin or gland formation and may require electron microscopy for confirmation: this is discussed further in Chapter 8. Extensive necrosis is a feature of the poorly differentiated adenocarcinomas, and the cells bordering the zones of necrosis may display irregular stratification (Fig. 6–12). Even in a predominantly solid tumor with marked cytologic atypic and mitotic activity, the nuclear features and a suggestion of gland formation may indicate adenocarcinoma (Fig. 6–13). In the solid tumors, the cells are commonly in broad sheets with interspersed areas of necrosis, but they may also form cords or small clusters (Fig. 6–14).

Solid clear cell carcinomas whose cells are forming mucin are poorly differentiated adenocarcinomas. The cells may be uniform (Fig. 6–15) or show varying degrees of pleomorphism (Fig. 6–16). Clear cytoplasm can be seen in any type of lung carcinoma other than the pure small cell form. It generally is confined to areas of a particular tumor and varies in degree: some cells may be totally clear, while others are intermediate between these and cells with granular cytoplasm. The clarity can result from a number of factors, including degenerative change with swelling of the cytoplasm from influx of fluid. Mucin may create a clear appearance, as does lipid, although generally when cells contain many lipid droplets, they are visible in hematoxylin-eosin preparations as small vacuoles.

According to Katzenstein and co-workers,[72] glycogen is a common histochemical finding in clear cell carcinomas of the lung. They studied 348 consecutive cases of lung carcinoma to determine the incidence of clear cell tumors and found that clear cells were common in all types except small cell carcinoma. Fourteen cases (4%) contained over 50% of clear cells, and of these, ten showed foci of

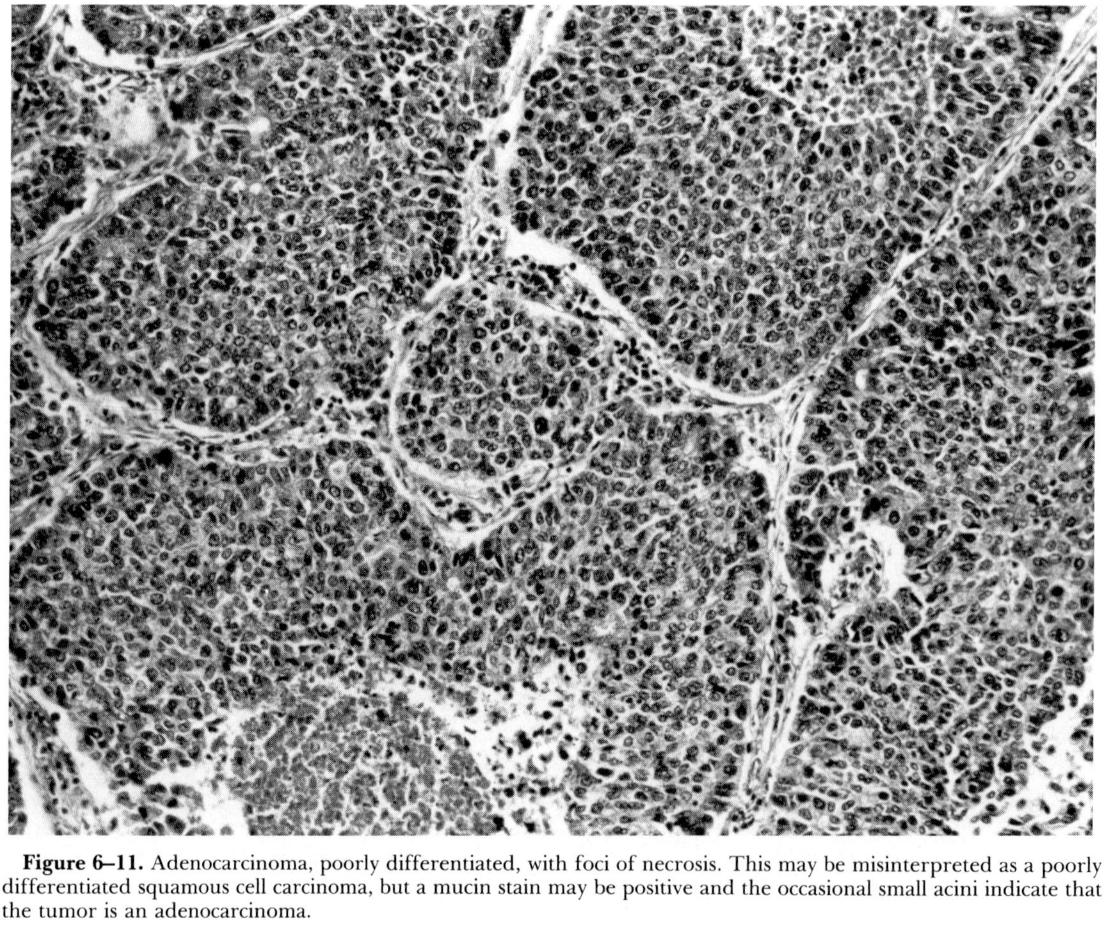

Figure 6–11. Adenocarcinoma, poorly differentiated, with foci of necrosis. This may be misinterpreted as a poorly differentiated squamous cell carcinoma, but a mucin stain may be positive and the occasional small acini indicate that the tumor is an adenocarcinoma.

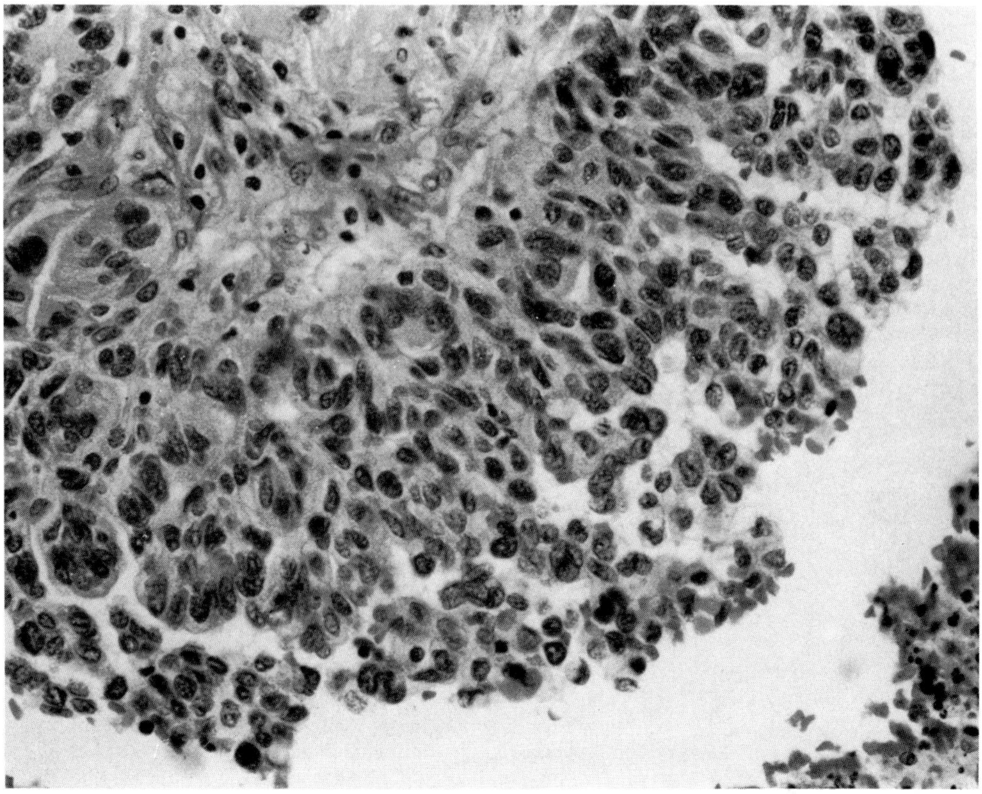

Figure 6–12. Adenocarcinoma, poorly differentiated, showing a focus of uneven stratification.

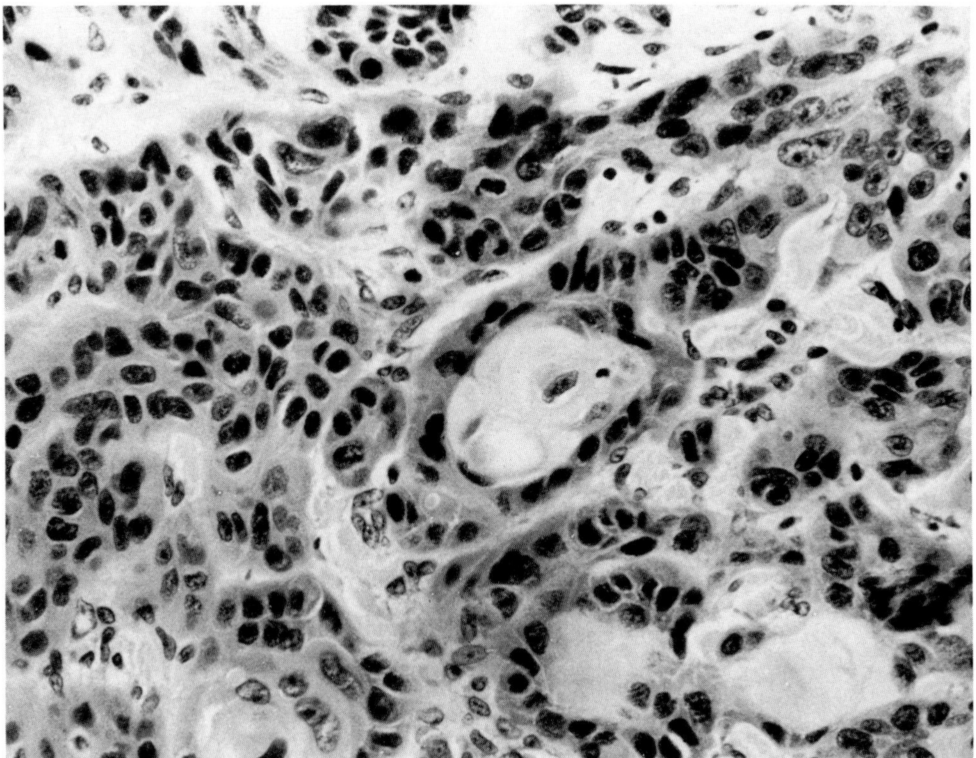

Figure 6–13. Adenocarcinoma, poorly differentiated. Although a glandular pattern can be discerned, much of the tumor was composed of solid groups of cells and there is considerable nuclear pleomorphism.

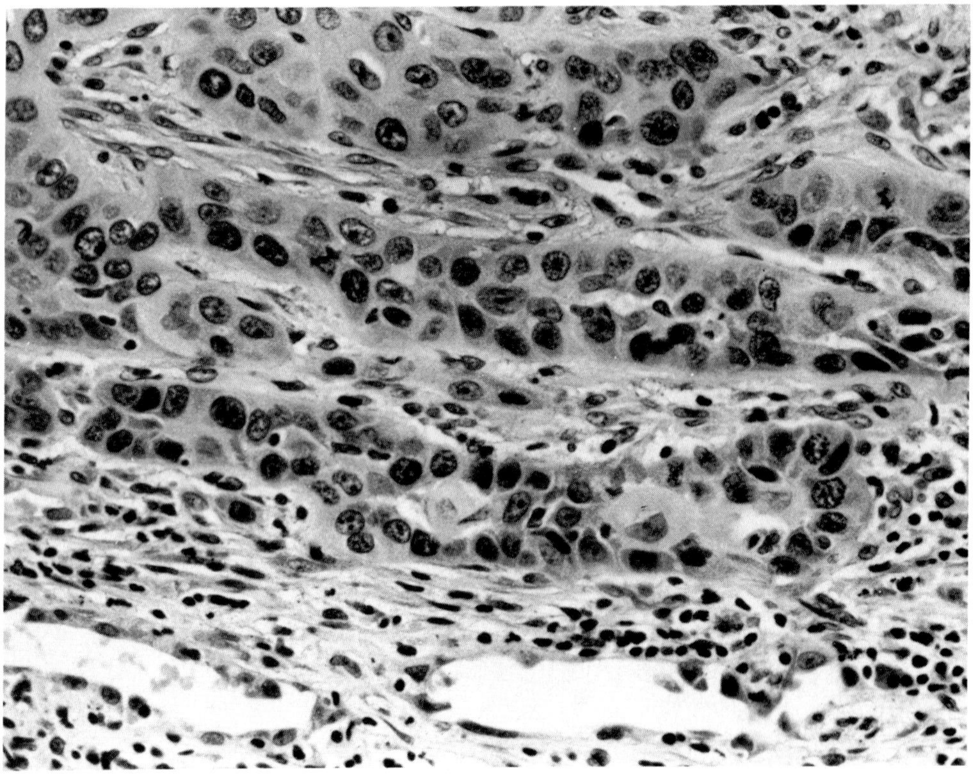

Figure 6–14. Adenocarcinoma, poorly differentiated. A moderate degree of nuclear pleomorphism is present within the solid cords of cells. In a fine-needle aspiration biopsy specimen, the pleomorphic cells might be interpreted as squamous cell carcinoma.

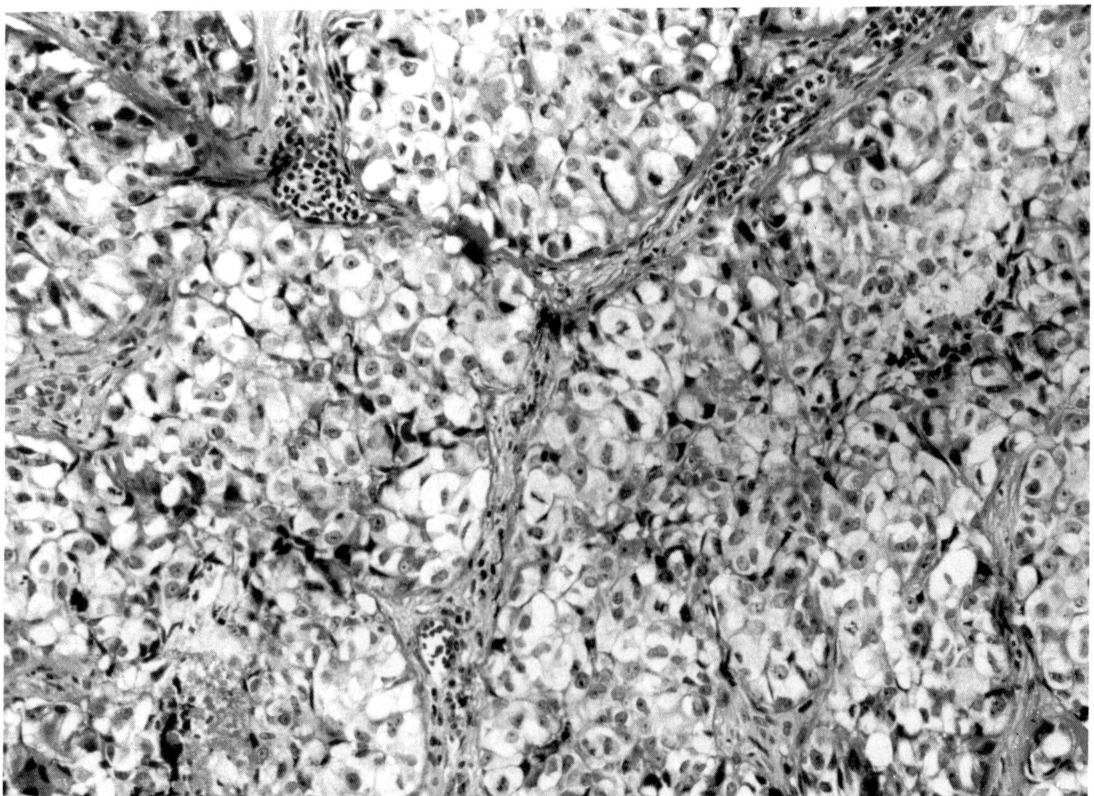

Figure 6–15. Adenocarcinoma composed of solid aggregates of cells with clear cytoplasm. This clear-cell pattern may also be seen in some squamous cell carcinomas.

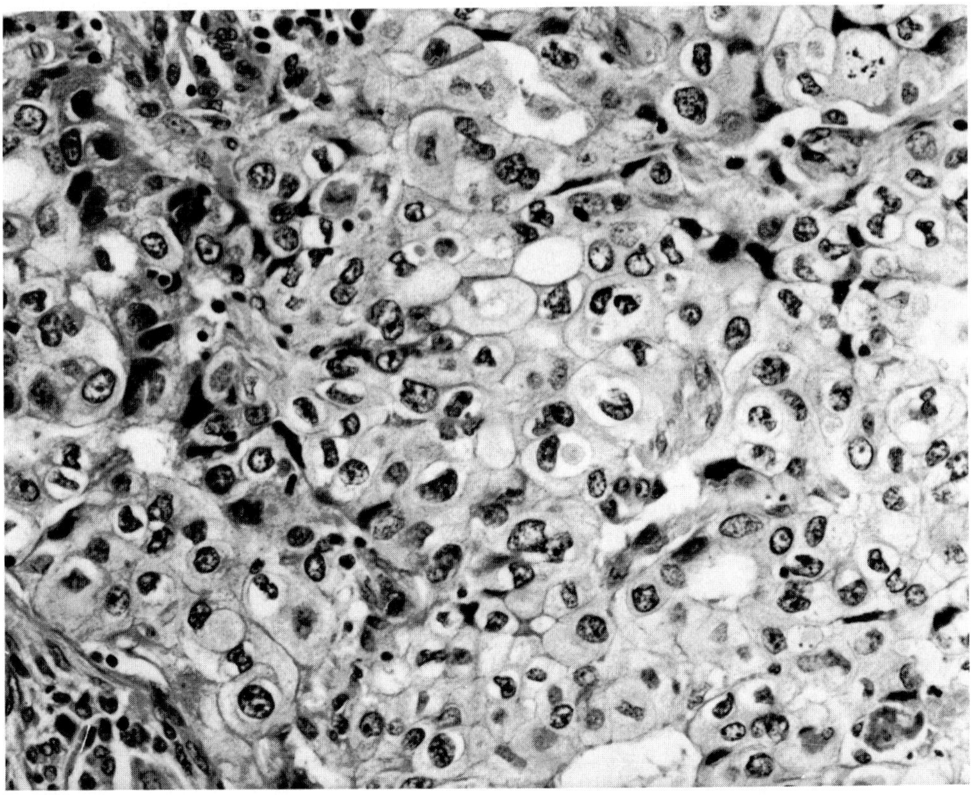

Figure 6–16. Adenocarcinoma. Some cells have clear cytoplasm. Many of the nuclei have irregular profiles, and some cells have a squamoid appearance.

squamous differentiation and four showed gland formation. Clear cell change did not influence behavior. Only one tumor fulfilled the WHO criteria for clear cell carcinoma, and the authors consider that clear cell carcinoma should not constitute a defined category and that the tumors should instead be classified according to the major WHO categories. Edwards and Carlile[29] studied six clear cell carcinomas by electron microscopy: three were adenocarcinoma, two were squamous cell carcinoma, and one was an undifferentiated large cell carcinoma. The clear cytoplasm was due to glycogen.

Metastatic renal cell adenocarcinoma, and the rare benign clear cell tumor of the lung (see Chapter 11), enter into the differential diagnosis of a clear cell lung neoplasm. Katzenstein and colleagues[71] analyzed 44 renal cell carcinomas metastatic to the lung. In 27 patients, the metastasis occurred after the primary renal neoplasm had been resected, while 19 had lung lesions before the kidney tumor was detected. Metastases may occur a long time after the resection of the renal adenocarcinoma, with intervals up to 28 years and an average period of around 16 years.

Bronchioloalveolar Adenocarcinoma

This variant of bronchogenic adenocarcinoma was described in 1876 by Mallassez.[101] The patient was a 47-year-old woman with a multinodular tumor. The tumor has had many names over the years,[30] but the term *bronchioloalveolar adenocarcinoma* coined by Liebow[92] has proved to be appropriate in the light of immunocytochemical and ultrastructural studies. Bronchioloalveolar adenocarcinomas are well-differentiated tumors that develop in the peripheral lung, distal to the bronchi. The tumor spreads along the existing framework of the distal air spaces, and as it does so, collagen is deposited in the alveolar septa. Continued proliferation of the cells results in the formation of intraluminal papillary fronds that protrude into the alveoli or into larger spaces as parts of the framework are disrupted. In a typical example, a single layer of columnar cells coats connective tissue papillae (Fig. 6–17). Spread of the tumor using the distal air spaces for support is characteristic (Fig. 6–18), but breakdown of areas of the lung structure produces larger spaces that become filled with mucinous se-

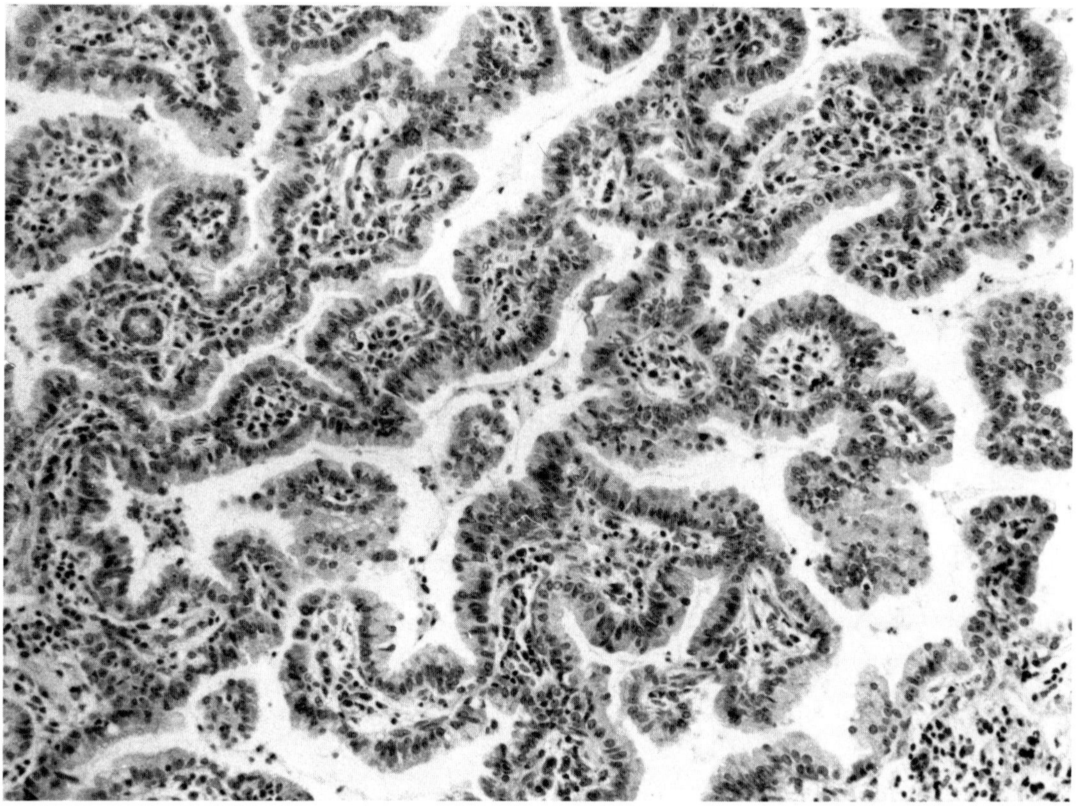

Figure 6–17. Bronchioloalveolar adenocarcinoma. The connective tissue cores are covered by a single layer of columnar cells. A lymphocytic infiltration is often present in the connective tissue stroma.

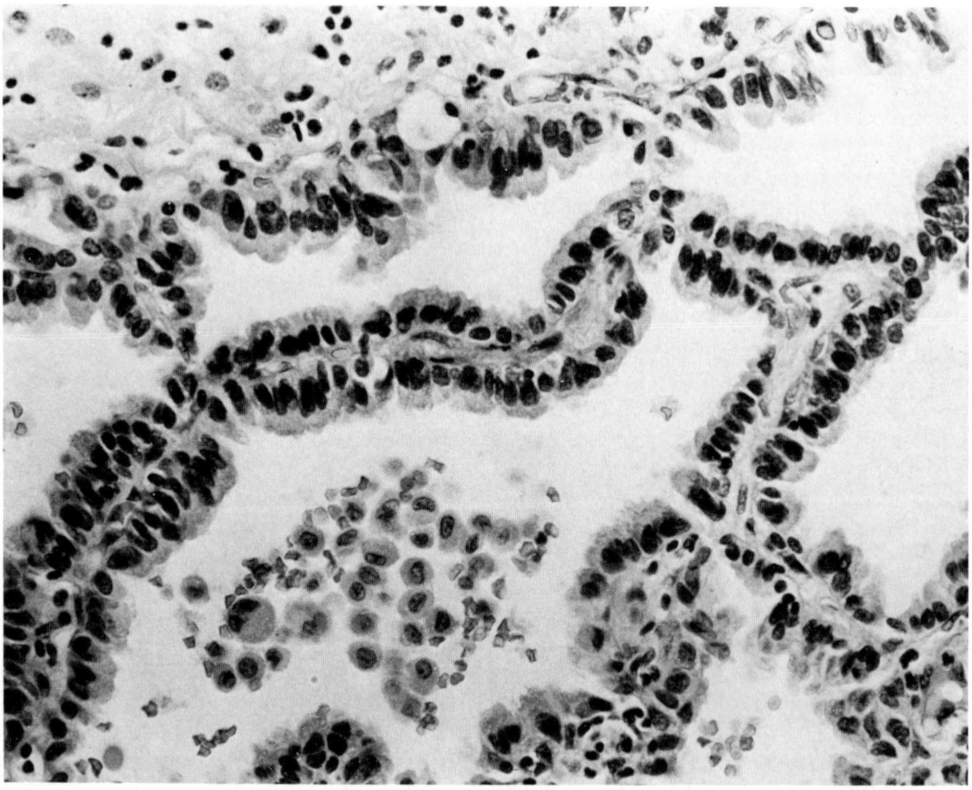

Figure 6–18. Bronchioloalveolar adenocarcinoma at higher magnification than the tumor in Figure 6–17. Slender strands of connective tissue are covered by simple columnar epithelium. The cells show minimal pleomorphism.

cretion (Fig. 6–19); small clusters of tumor cells are often seen floating within these little mucinous seas (Fig. 6–20), where they can be mixed with alveolar macrophages.

Mucin can usually be demonstrated in bronchioloalveolar adenocarcinoma cells, but it varies in quantity. When it is sparse, the mucin accumulates in the apical cytoplasm. In other tumors, mucin diffusely fills the cells (Fig. 6–21). The delicate fronds of a papillary tumor composed of mucinous cells are shown in Figure 6–22. Manning and colleagues[102] reviewed 34 cases of bronchioloalveolar adenocarcinoma and found two distinct pathologic types. In one group of nine cases, mucus production was evident grossly and microscopically and these tumors were likely to be multicentric. The second type (25 cases) contained less mucus and was frequently solitary. The patterns were prognostically significant: the 5-year survival was 26% for the mucus-rich type and 72% for the tumors with lesser amounts of mucus. Axiotis and associates[5] also described two forms of bronchioloalveolar adenocarcinoma, one mucinous type growing along the unaltered alveolar framework and eliciting a B-lymphocytic response and a nonmucinous type inducing desmoplasia and eliciting a Langherans cell and T-lymphocytic response. There is a colloid form of bronchioloalveolar adenocarcinoma that produces large amounts of mucus that can obstruct airways and cause electrolyte depletion from continued expectoration.[59] Glycogen can also be plentiful in the cells of a bronchioloalveolar adenocarcinoma.[157]

Because of the spread of the tumor through the alveolar spaces, small foci separated in a section by regions of uninvolved lung are a common finding (Fig. 6–23). Tall slender columnar cells clinging to the alveolar wall are evidence that the description of lepidic spread is appropriate (Fig. 6–24). At the edge of a bronchioloalveolar adenocarcinoma it can become difficult to distinguish tumor cells from the hyperplastic type II pneumocytes that are invariably present at this location and which may form a broad band encircling the tumor (Figs. 6–25 and 6–26). The cells of a bronchioloalveolar adenocar-

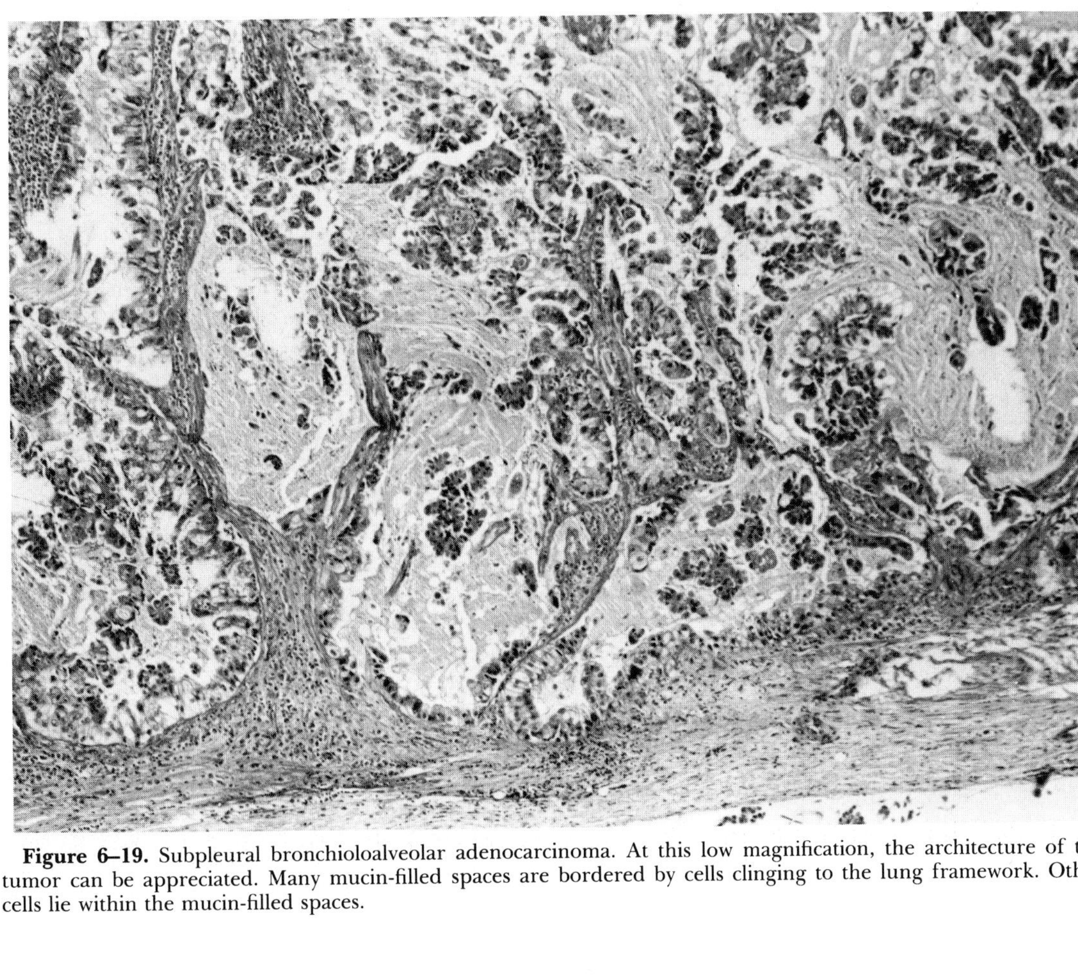

Figure 6–19. Subpleural bronchioloalveolar adenocarcinoma. At this low magnification, the architecture of the tumor can be appreciated. Many mucin-filled spaces are bordered by cells clinging to the lung framework. Other cells lie within the mucin-filled spaces.

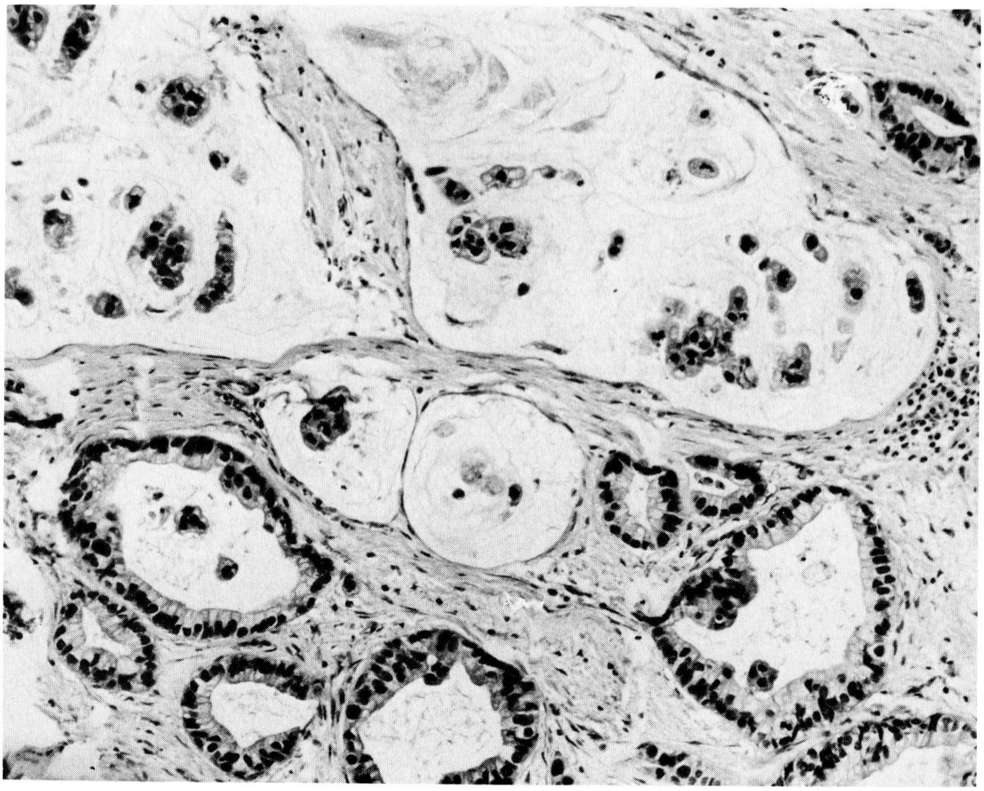

Figure 6–20. Bronchioloalveolar adenocarcinoma. Small nests of tumor cells float within the mucinous secretion.

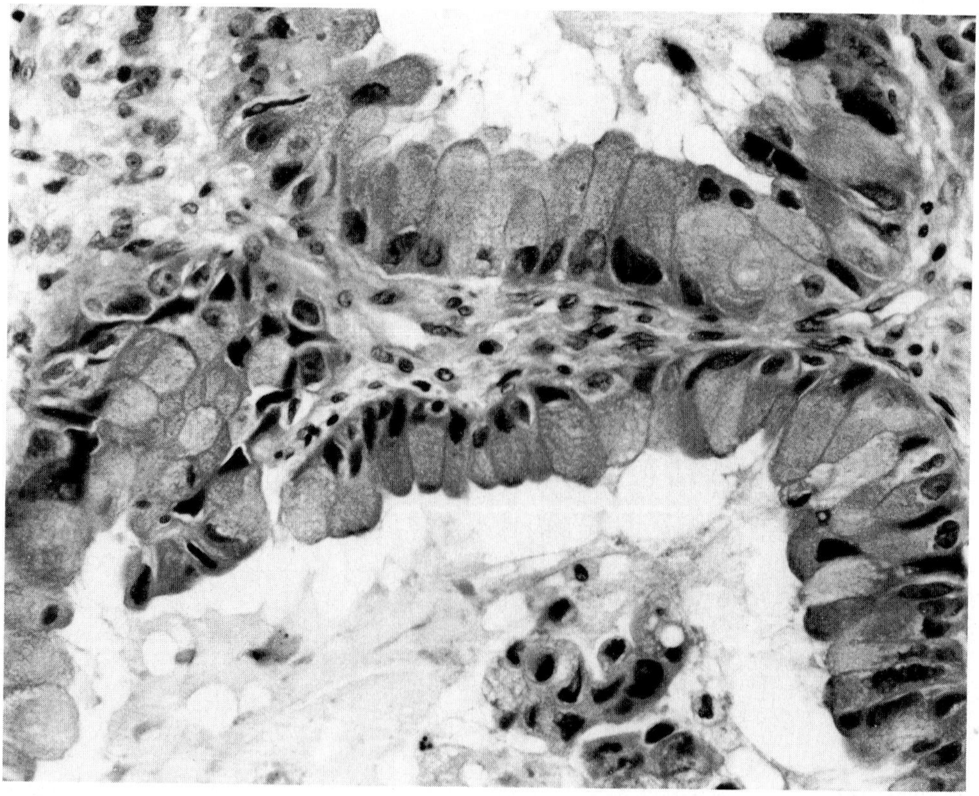

Figure 6–21. Bronchioloalveolar adenocarcinoma. The cells in this mucinous variant are tall columnar, and their cytoplasm is filled with mucin. Nuclei lie mostly at the base of the cells.

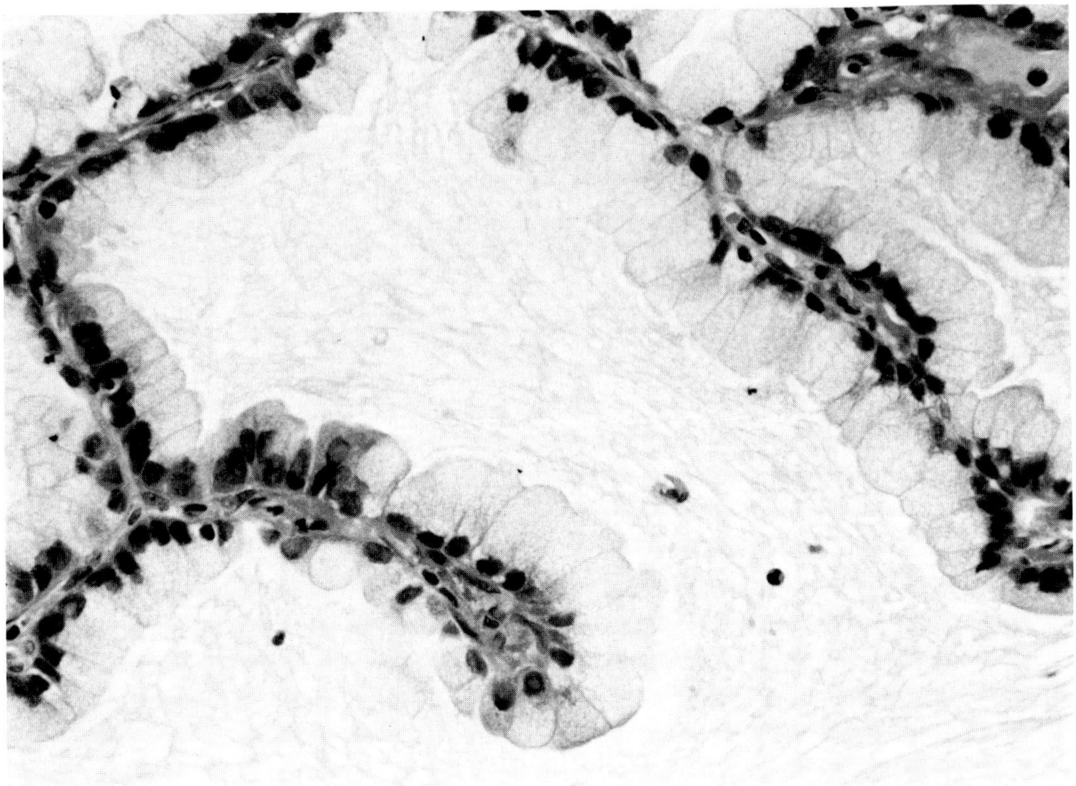

Figure 6–22. Bronchioloalveolar adenocarcinoma showing the often delicate papillary architecture with thin fibrovascular cores.

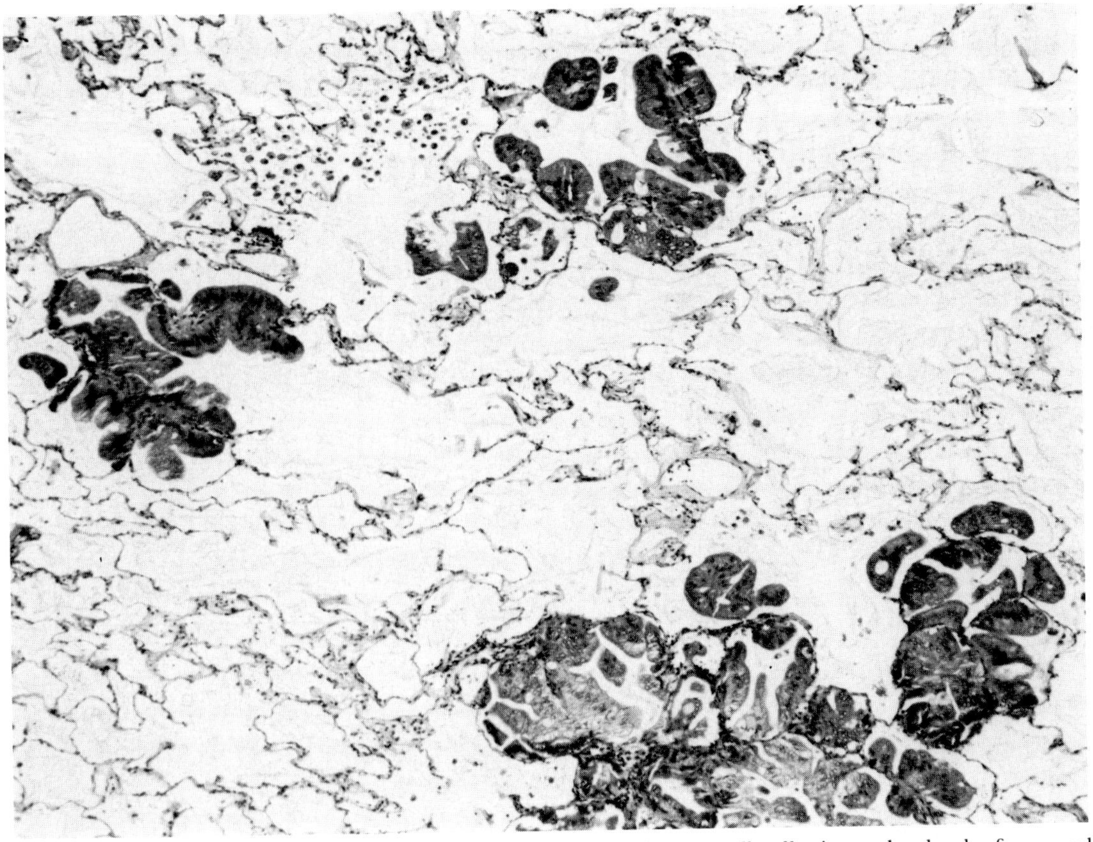

Figure 6–23. Bronchioloalveolar adenocarcinoma. Small clusters of tumor cells adhering to the alveolar framework are separated by zones of uninvolved alveoli.

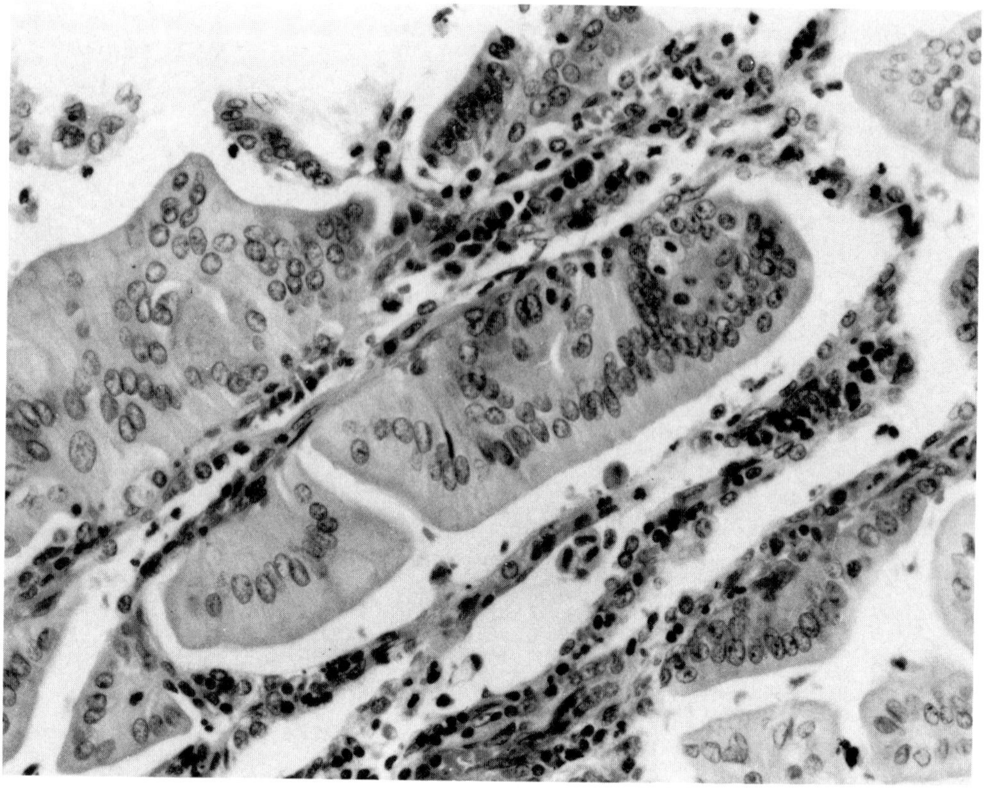

Figure 6–24. Bronchioloalveolar adenocarcinoma. Discrete foci of tall slender cells adhere to the alveolar walls in the classic lepidic pattern.

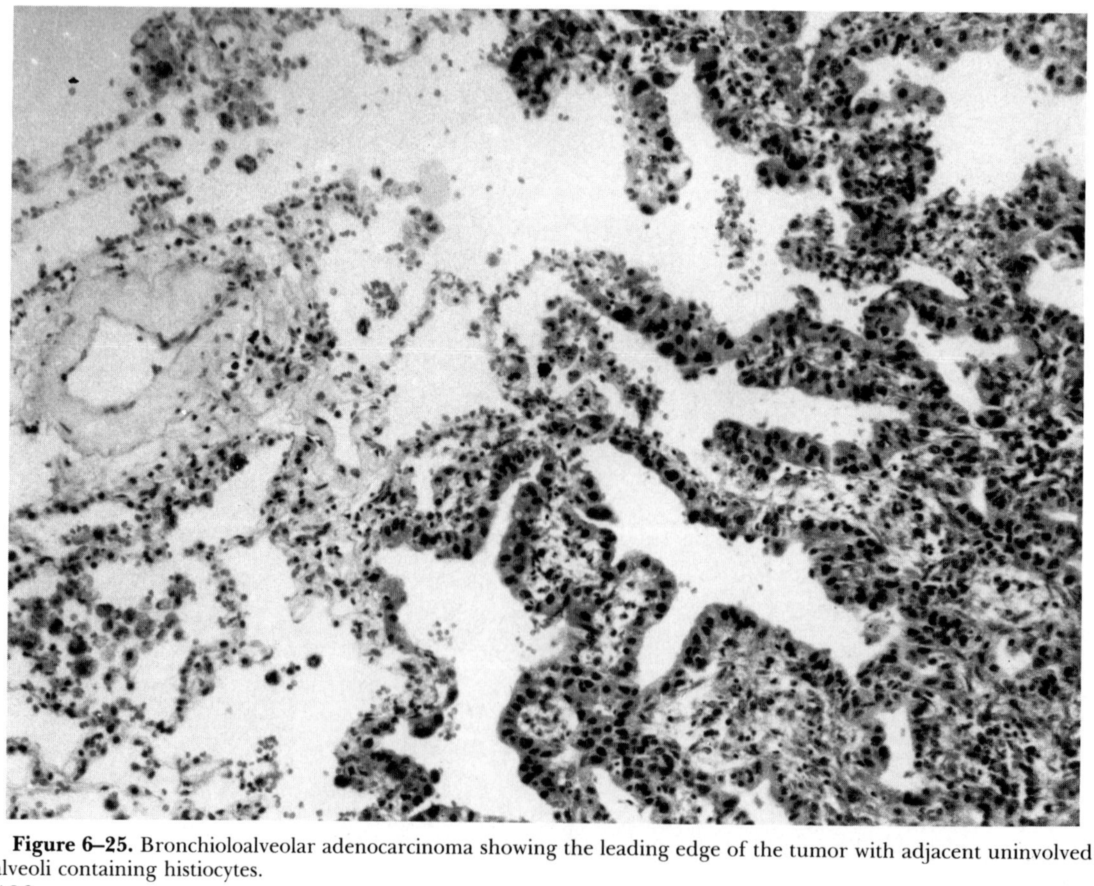

Figure 6–25. Bronchioloalveolar adenocarcinoma showing the leading edge of the tumor with adjacent uninvolved alveoli containing histiocytes.

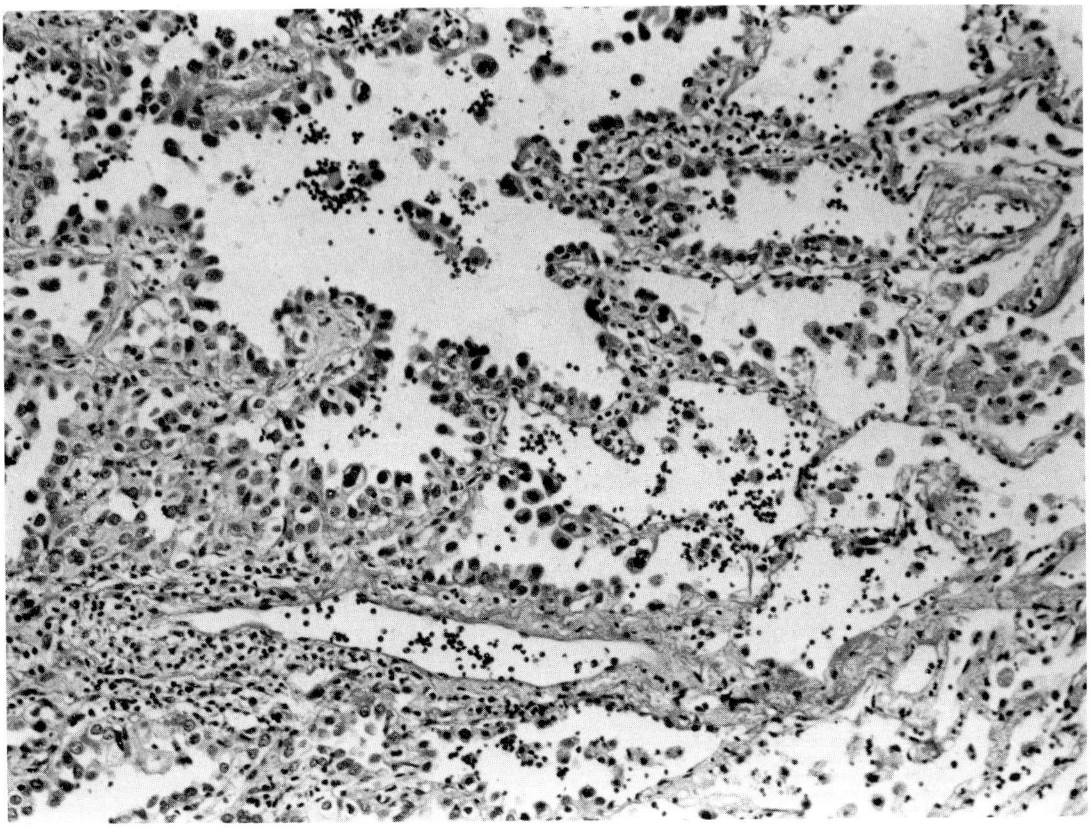

Figure 6–26. Bronchioloalveolar adenocarcinoma. Particularly at the periphery of the carcinoma, distinction between neoplastic cells and hyperplastic pneumocytes can be difficult.

cinoma are often variable in height, some projecting farther than their neighbors into the alveolar lumen (Figs. 6–27 and 6–28). The cells have been described as having a hobnail appearance. Nuclear inclusions may be seen, but they are more readily identified by electron microscopy. Psammoma bodies are occasionally present.[147, 186]

The variations in the microscopic appearance of these tumors are partly due to their formation by different cell types. Ultrastructural studies have shown that the Clara cell predominates, but type II pneumocytes, mucin-rich cells, and ciliated cells can also be present in the tumors. Some of the variation in histologic patterns and cytologic features is consequent on loss of differentiation. Variation in height of the lining cells, stratification among the columnar cells, distortion of the architectural pattern, increased mitotic activity, small solid clusters, and giant cells are sometimes seen in areas of an otherwise typical tumor. However, it becomes increasingly difficult to identify a dedifferentiating adenocarcinoma as bronchioloalveolar in type.

There are many adenocarcinomas that show features of a typical acinar or papillary adenocarcinoma in their central areas but have a bronchioloalveolar adenocarcinoma pattern toward their margin. The opposite also occurs: an unequivocal bronchioloalveolar adenocarcinoma may contain foci of typical glands in a fibrous stroma. Because of these variations, and the frequency with which a lung carcinoma is diagnosed from scanty material, the consensus of diagnosis of bronchioloalveolar adenocarcinoma is relatively poor. Elson and associates[34] reviewed 131 tumors with a bronchioloalveolar adenocarcinoma pattern and only 39 showed a pure pattern in histologic sections. In 76 tumors a dominant bronchioloalveolar adenocarcinoma pattern was accompanied by foci of acinar adenocarcinoma with fibrosis, and 16 tumors had only a focal BAC pattern. Of 115 tumors with at least a dominant bronchioloalveolar adenocarcinoma pattern, 51 showed predominantly mucinous differentiation and 64 were largely nonmucin-producing tumors. Roggli and colleagues[143] noted that tumors with bronchioloalveolar

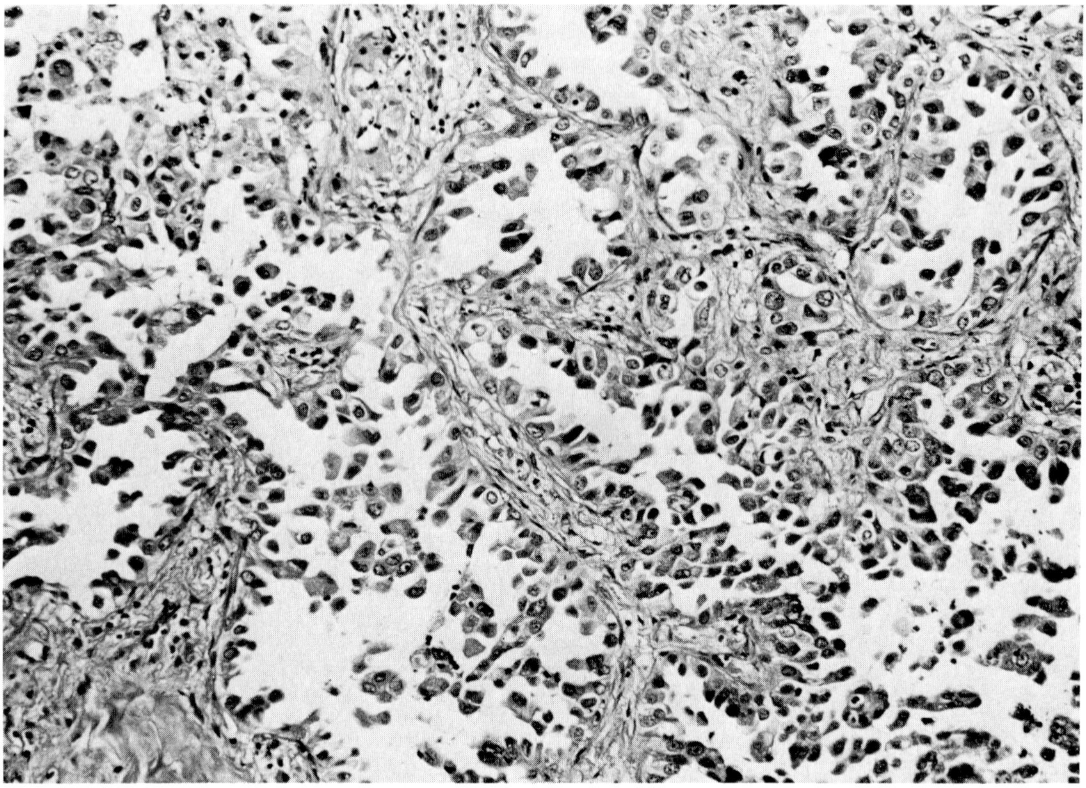

Figure 6–27. Bronchioloalveolar adenocarcinoma. The cells lining the spaces are quite variable in height, creating a ragged appearance. This pattern is generally an indication of Clara cell differentiation.

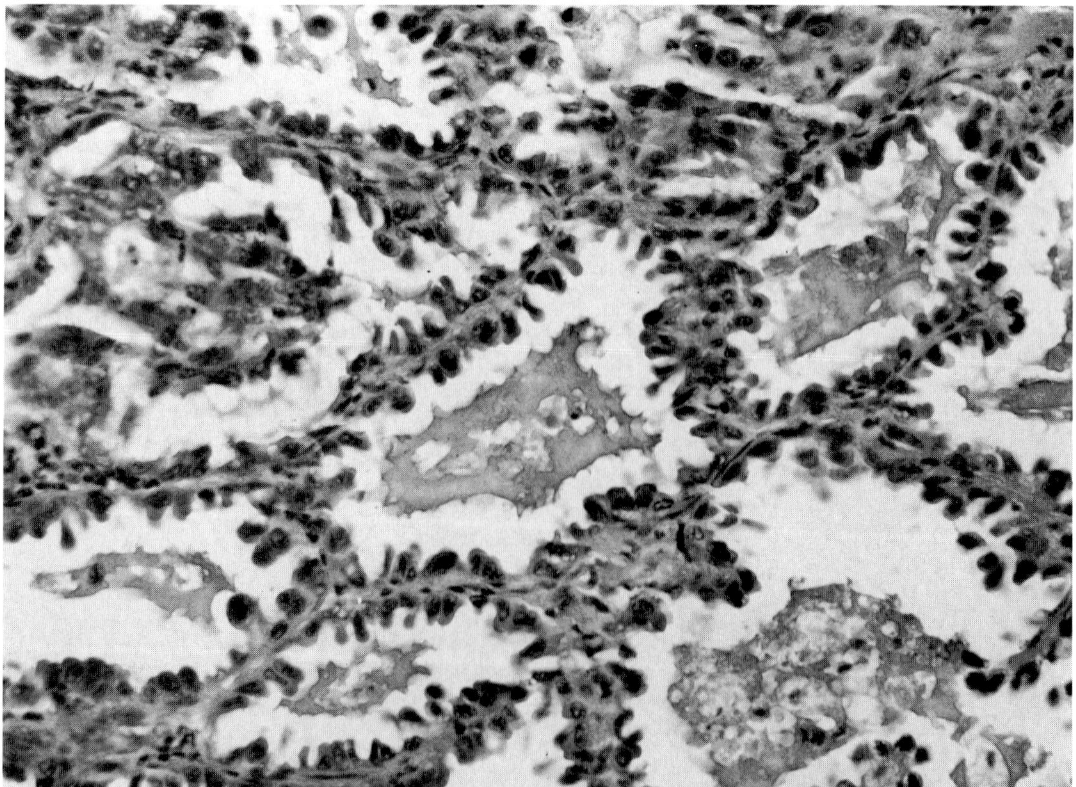

Figure 6–28. Bronchioloalveolar adenocarcinoma demonstrating marked irregularity in height and shape of the single layer of cells.

adenocarcinoma features almost always also contained other patterns of adenocarcinoma.

A similar lung lesion occurs in certain animals. Scarratt and co-workers[149] reported a bronchioloalveolar adenocarcinoma forming numerous firm nodules throughout both lungs of a cow. The best known animal model is jaagsiekte in sheep.[57, 206] The disease in sheep is infectious, and histologically there is a proliferation of pneumocytes within alveoli followed by the development of a malignant tumor that is histologically similar to the human bronchioloalveolar adenocarcinoma. The condition was studied most in South Africa, but cases have been reported in other countries, including North and South America. Its viral etiology is established, but the relationship if any with human bronchioloalveolar adenocarcinoma has not been clarified.

Sarcomatoid Adenocarcinoma

Small or large areas of an adenocarcinoma may be composed of diffuse sheets of spindle cells (Fig. 6–29). Usually architecture is not evident within these areas, but some organization into bundles can occur and distinction from a sarcoma is then a problem. With adequate material, foci of glandular differentiation may be found, and immunostaining for keratin is usually helpful in the analysis of sarcomatoid carcinomas.[62] Electron microscopy is of limited value since the cells tend to lose specific fine structural features with sarcomatoid transformation.

Neuroendocrine Differentiation

About 10% of non–small cell lung carcinomas have neuroendocrine differentiation, and the finding is most common in adenocarcinomas followed by large cell carcinomas; it is rarely seen in squamous cell carcinomas.[94] An abbreviated designation is "nsclc with ne features." They cannot be identified by conventional light microscopy but they contain cells that are immunoreactive for neuroendocrine markers (neuron-specific enolase, chromogranin, and individual neuropeptides). The clinical significance is not known.

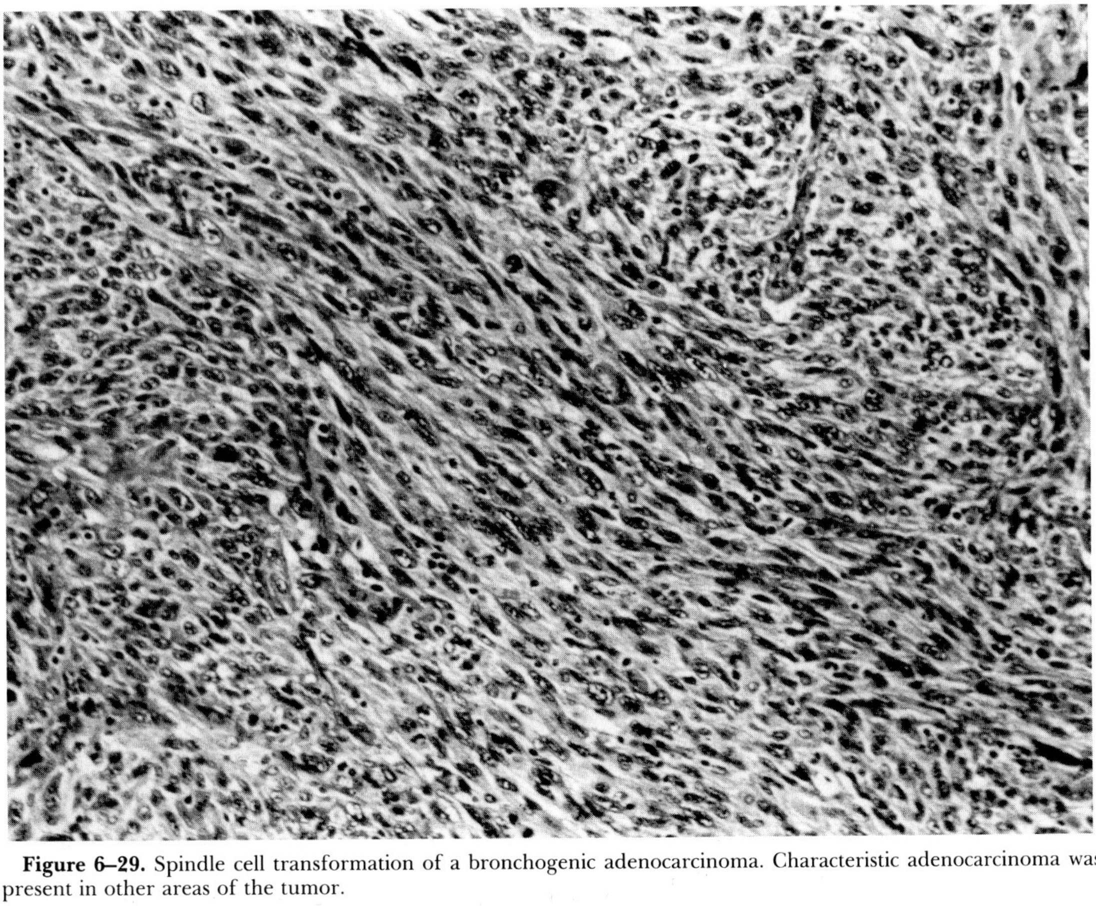

Figure 6–29. Spindle cell transformation of a bronchogenic adenocarcinoma. Characteristic adenocarcinoma was present in other areas of the tumor.

Adenosquamous Carcinoma

In an adenosquamous carcinoma,[58] zones of squamous cell carcinoma are present in company with areas of adenocarcinoma. The two parts may be clearly separate although contiguous (Fig. 6–30), in contrast to the intimate admixture and transitional forms seen in a mucoepidermoid carcinoma. Usually the two components are relatively well differentiated: if one or the other is poorly differentiated, the diagnosis can not be made with confidence. Adenosquamous carcinomas make up more than 2% of primary lung carcinomas, and they are usually bulky peripheral tumors. Cytology preparations may show only one component. The diagnosis will be higher with extensive sampling and careful mucin staining and higher still if electron microscopy is performed; but the small areas examined at the ultrastructural level can convey a misleading impression of the structure of the tumor as a whole, and correlation with the results of light microscopy is essential.

The close approximation of differentiated squamous and adenocarcinoma cells is shown at the ultrastructural level in Figures 6–31 and 6–32. However, it is not always easy to be certain, from electron microscopy of a small number of cells of a lung carcinoma, whether the tumor should be designated an adenocarcinoma or squamous cell carcinoma. This is illustrated in Figure 6–33, where numerous filopodia protrude into clefts between neighboring cells: the appearance suggests adenocarcinoma, but it can also be seen in a pseudoglandular (adenoid) variant of squamous cell carcinoma. The number of desmosomes and presence of tonofilaments are also not absolute criteria, although more are present in squamous cells. In Figure 6–34, the tumor cells have these properties, but they also contain electron-lucent aggregates of mucin and a small number of dense-core granules.

Between 1974 and 1985 at the University of Chicago, 20 of 873 patients (2.3%) with lung cancer had well-differentiated adenosquamous carcinomas.[122] Patients with stage I disease were amenable to operation, and 60% (3 of 5) were free of disease from 1 to 6 years later. However, stage II tumors (14

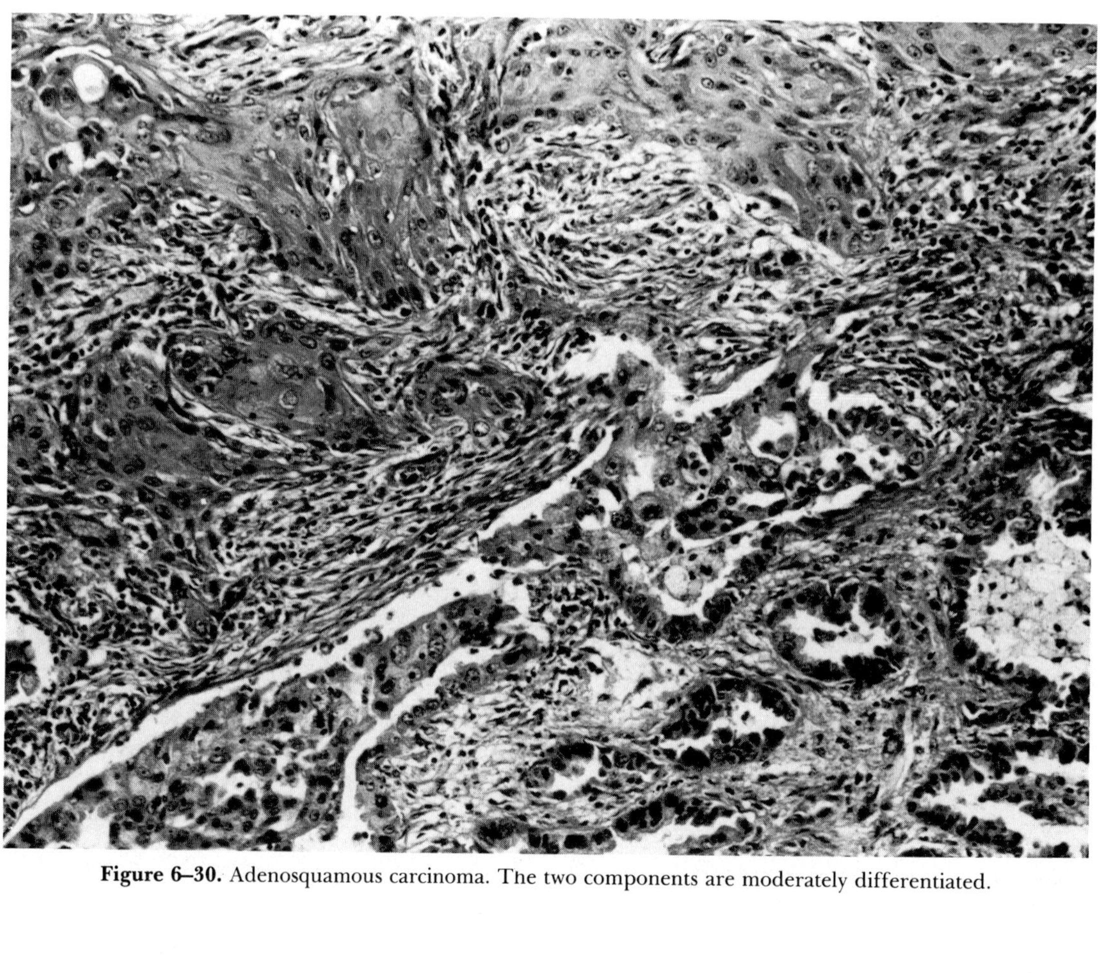

Figure 6–30. Adenosquamous carcinoma. The two components are moderately differentiated.

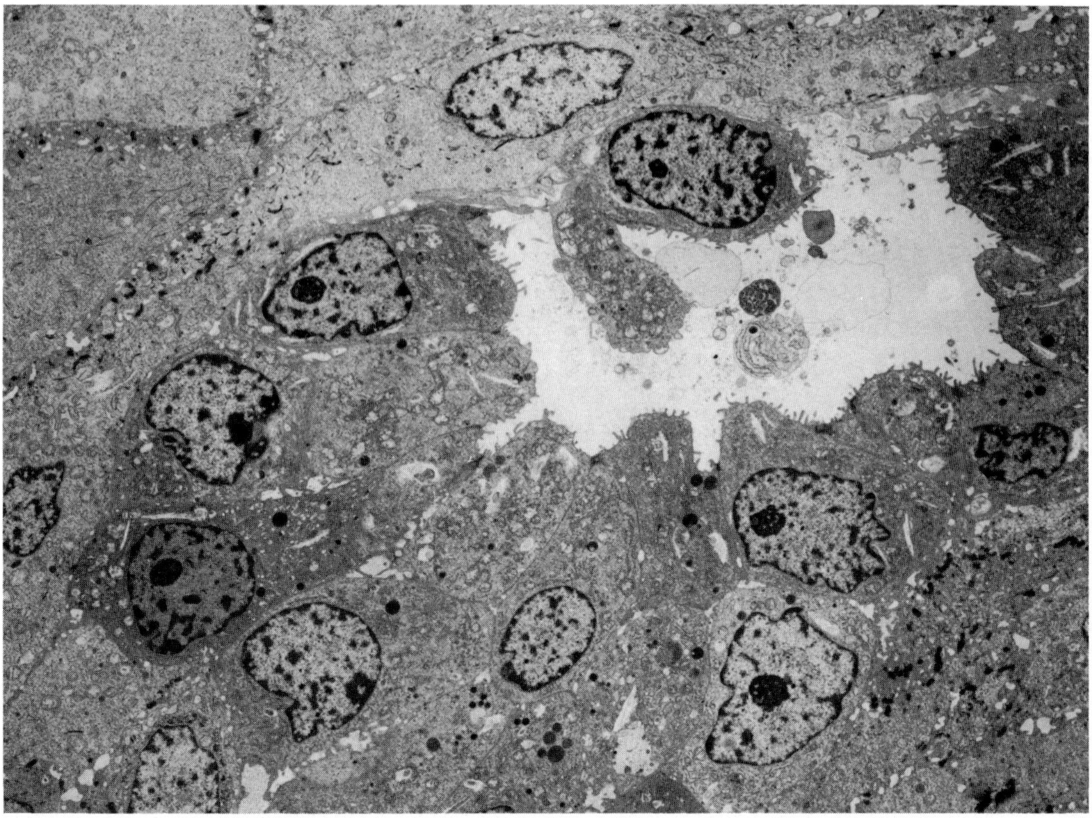

Figure 6–31. Adenosquamous carcinoma. Adenocarcinoma cells containing a few dense-core granules surround a lumen into which microvilli project. The adenocarcinoma cells are contiguous with squamous carcinoma cells joined by numerous desmosomes. (×3,000)

patients) showed highly aggressive behavior with rapid progression, and the median survival for patients with stage III tumors was 5 months. Fitzgibbons and co-workers[39] reported seven cases of adenosquamous carcinoma, which made up 0.6% of the 1,125 primary cancers examined. The tumors were from 1.3 to 5.5 cm, and five were peripheral. Three of five resected specimens contained regional lymph node metastases. Five patients died of their disease within 2 years of diagnosis, and two were short-term survivors.

CYTOLOGY

Since most adenocarcinomas occur in the periphery of the lung, sputum cytology is not as frequently positive as with squamous cell carcinomas. Bronchoscopic biopsy specimens may also be negative, but the yield from fine-needle aspiration is high.

Adenocarcinomas display more uniformity in their nuclear and cytoplasmic features than squamous cell carcinomas. Well-differentiated adenocarcinomas tend to exfoliate cells in small fragments rather than individually,[36] and in cytologic preparations the cells are consequently often cohesive with community cell borders (Fig. 6–35). The nuclei are round to ovoid with smooth profiles and thin nuclear membranes, and the chromatin is fine and granular. Nucleoli vary in size with the degree of differentiation, but they can be prominent in well-differentiated adenocarcinomas (Fig. 6–36). Hyperchromasia and irregularities in chromatin distribution are not as obvious in adenocarcinomas as in squamous cell carcinomas,[36] but they can be perceived as the tumors dedifferentiate. The cells of the tumor shown in Figure 6–37 show some attempt at cohesion, but they and their nuclei vary in shape. An increase in the nuclear/cytoplasmic ratio parallels the loss of differentiation, but because of the variation in any particular tumor, assessment based on a small number of cells in a cytologic preparation may not be as accurate as the information obtained from a tissue specimen. A suggestion of acinar formation may never-

Text continued on page 130

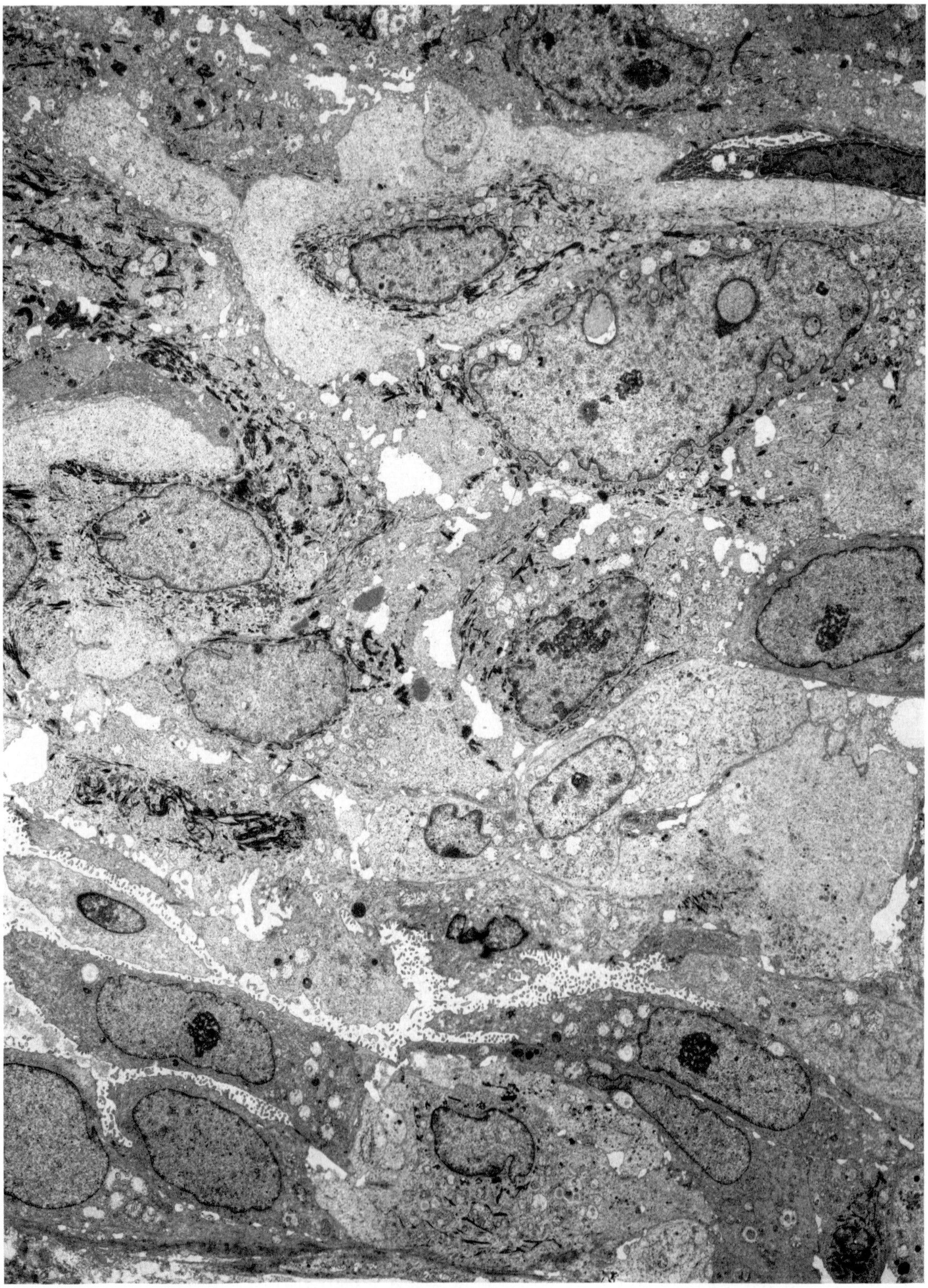

Figure 6–32. Adenosquamous carcinoma. A glandular lumen is present. The lining cells merge with squamous cells containing cytokeratin filaments and pleomorphic nuclei with large nucleoli. (×3,600)

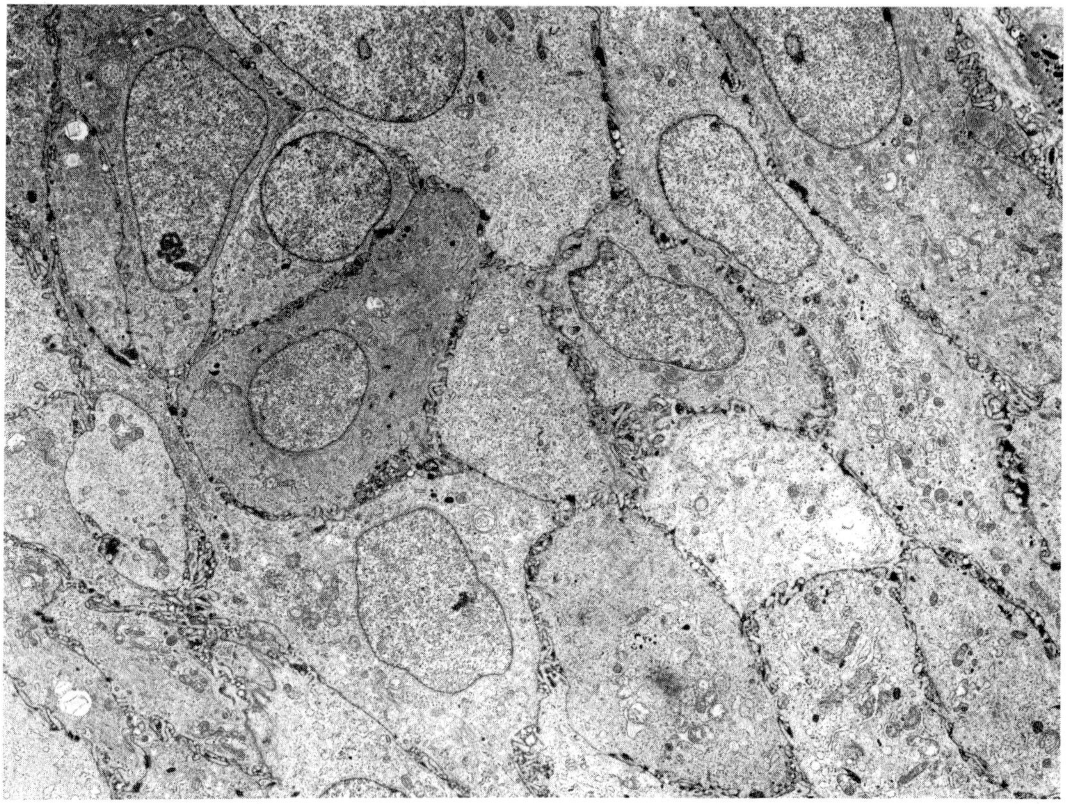

Figure 6–33. A poorly differentiated bronchogenic carcinoma had a squamous appearance by light microscopy. At the ultrastructural level there are many microvilli between the cells, an appearance that is more suggestive of adenocarcinoma though it can also be seen in an adenoid (pseudoglandular) variant of squamous carcinoma. (×3,750)

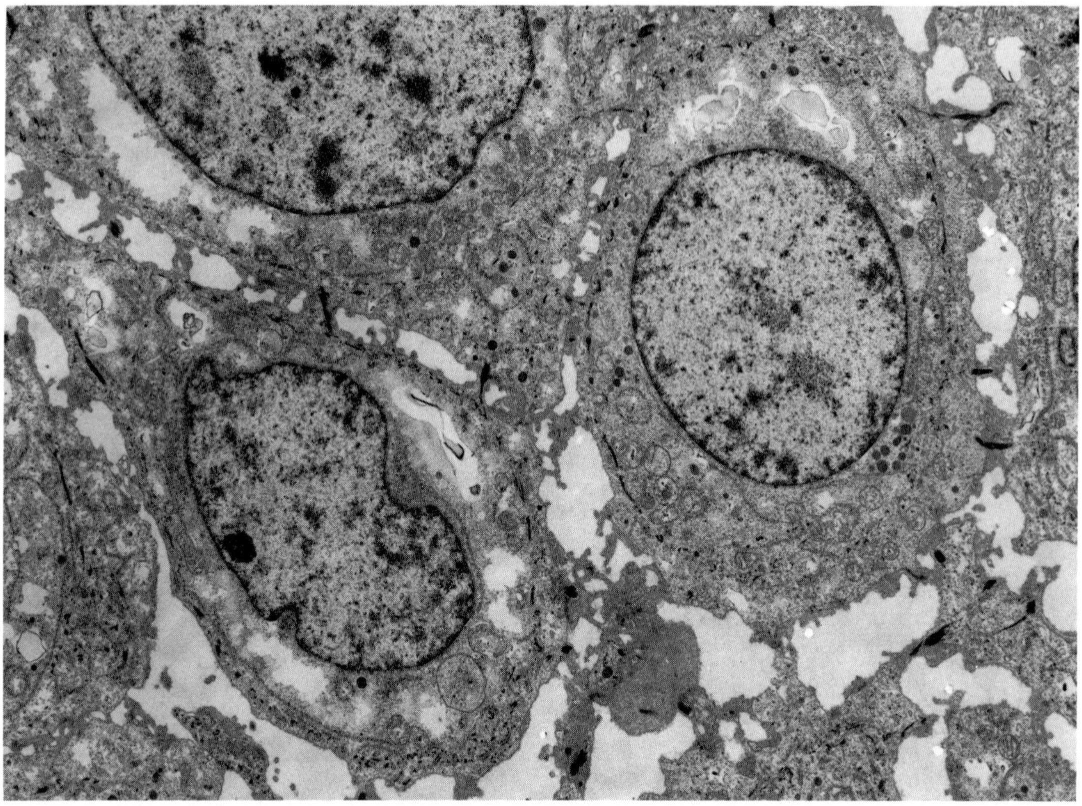

Figure 6–34. Poorly differentiated bronchogenic carcinoma. The tumor cells are separated by slender clefts bridged by protrusions of cytoplasm linked by desmosomes with tonofilaments. The cytoplasm contains electron-lucent secretory material and a few dense-core granules. The tumor thus has squamous and glandular features, a common finding by electron microscopy in non–small cell lung carcinomas. (×5,100)

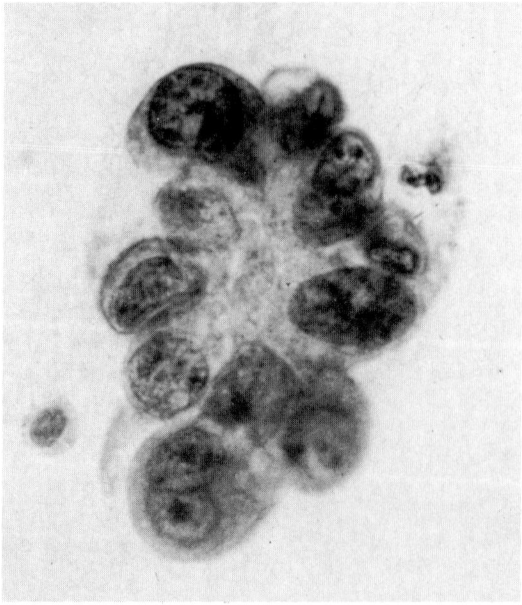

Figure 6–35. Adenocarcinoma, well differentiated. A small cluster of cells from a fine-needle aspirate. Nuclear membranes are thin. Secretory vacuoles can be seen in the cytoplasm.

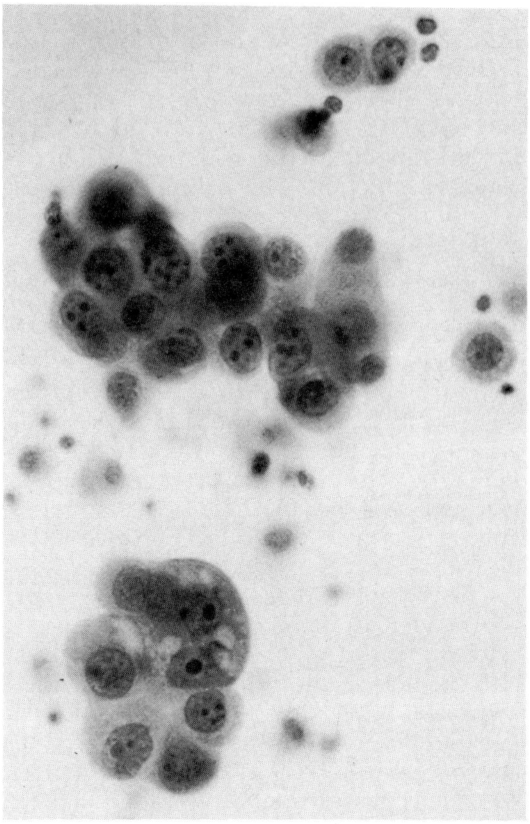

Figure 6–36. Adenocarcinoma, well differentiated. A nest of cells from a fine-needle aspirate. The cells have ovoid nuclei with smooth profiles, prominent nuclei, and vacuolated cytoplasm.

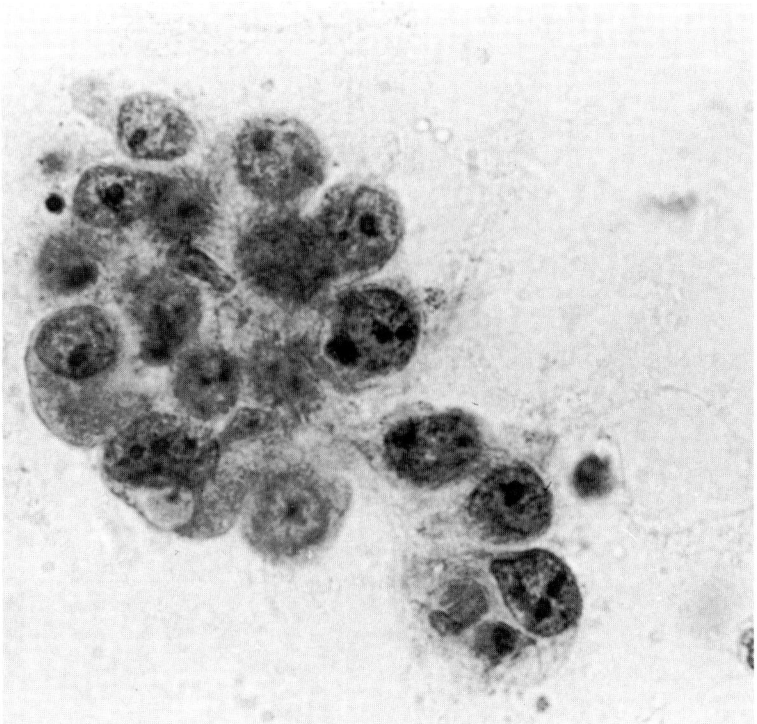

Figure 6–37. Adenocarcinoma, moderately differentiated. The cells are closely cohesive, but the cells and their nuclei vary in shape. The nuclear/cytoplasmic ratio is higher than in the cells in Figures 6–35 and 6–36.

theless be detected within a small group of cells (Fig. 6–38). The appearance of the cytoplasm is quite variable and is influenced by whether the tumor is mucin forming. Fine vacuoles (Fig. 6–39) may be evident; or if mucin is abundant, the cells can have a signet-ring configuration. The grouping of the cells may suggest a bronchioloalveolar adenocarcinoma (Fig. 6–40), but the arrangement in this figure is also seen in classic adenocarcinomas. The scanty cytoplasm of a poorly differentiated adenocarcinoma can suggest a small cell carcinoma, but the size of the nuclei and chromatin pattern and the often prominent nucleoli will indicate that the tumor is an adenocarcinoma (Fig. 6–41). If the carcinoma has cells with clear cytoplasm in histologic preparations, the cytoplasm may appear almost transparent in cytologic smears (Fig. 6–42).

The distinctive histology of bronchioloalveolar adenocarcinoma may be perceived in cytologic preparations,[159, 167, 168, 176] particularly in fine-needle aspiration biopsy specimens. Lozowski and co-workers[95] found that in experienced hands the diagnostic accuracy approached 100%, while adequate sputum specimens provided an 82% diagnostic yield. Sixty-six percent of 275 patients with bronchioloalveolar adenocarcinoma at the Toronto General Hospital were diagnosed by fine-needle aspiration biopsy.[176] Elson and colleagues[34] reviewed cytologic material from 111 patients with tumors that had a complete or partial bronchioloalveolar pattern and found that 60% were positive. Tumor cells were present in 45% of adequate sputum specimens, 27% of bronchoscopy biopsy specimens, and 83% of fine-needle aspirates. The

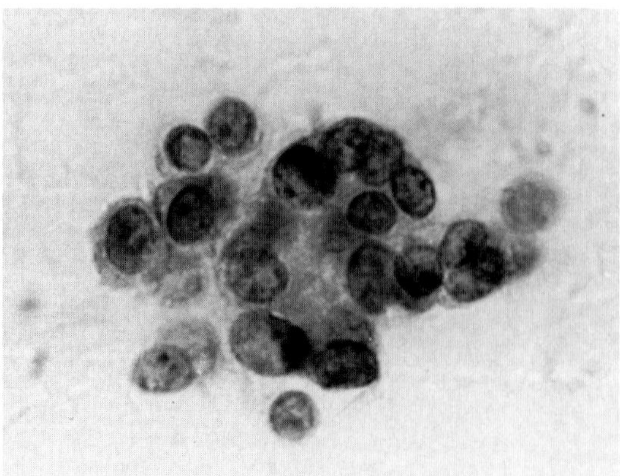

Figure 6–38. Adenocarcinoma, moderately differentiated. A loosely cohesive cluster of cells with a vague suggestion of an acinar arrangement.

typical finding in bronchioloalveolar adenocarcinomas is the presence of three-dimensional morula-like clusters of cells along with small groups and individual cells (Figs. 6–43 and 6–44). The cells usually appear more or less round, and of medium size, with sharply etched round nuclei that contain a single nucleolus. The single cells are not different from those of other adenocarcinomas, and the diagnosis depends on identifying the papillary architecture. Elson and colleagues[34] noted a significant degree of overlapping in the cytologic features of mucinous and nonmucinous tumors.

IMMUNOCYTOCHEMISTRY

Immunofluorescent techniques are now of proven value in diagnostic pathology, but when they were being developed a number of limiting factors had to be overcome. The need for special equipment, the requirement that frozen sections had to be used, and the frequent difficulties that were experienced in attempting to correlate the fluorescent images with conventional histology obstructed the use of immunohistochemistry in routine tumor diagnosis. The development of conjugated and unconjugated enzymatic histochemical techniques that can be used on sections of routinely processed tissues, and the availability of hybridoma-produced monoclonal antibodies, allowed the rapid growth and widespread use of immunohistochemistry in diagnostic histopathology and cytology that has been witnessed during the past decade. At the present time, a large number of antibodies directed against a wide variety of cell products, such as hormones, enzymes, oncofetal antigens, and other tumor markers, are being used in the diagnosis and classification of various tumors.[97] What is more important is that some of them can be identified and quantitated in the serum and then contribute not only to establishing the diagnosis but also to assessing the prognosis and to monitoring during the follow-up.

A number of molecular markers have been described that are specific for certain cell types or routes of differentiation, and they have proven useful in the identification and characterization of primary and metastatic tumors. Among these markers, certain components of the cytoskeleton, particularly intermediate filaments and actins, are currently

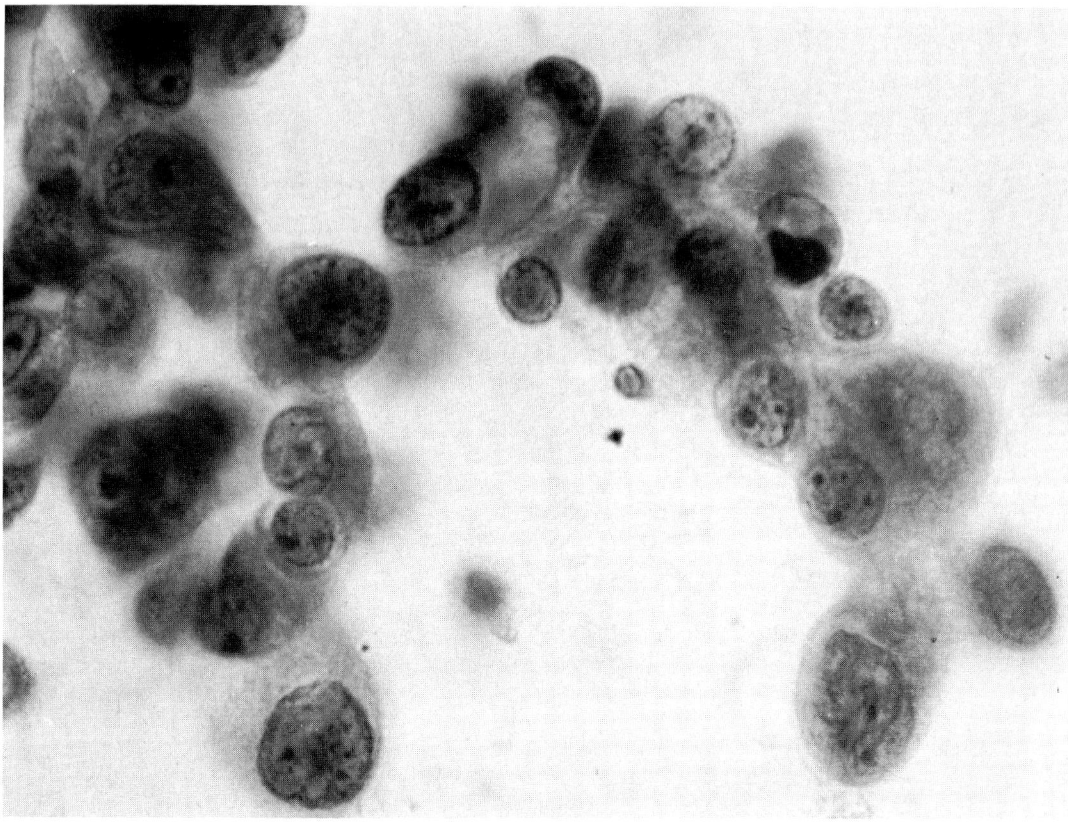

Figure 6–39. Adenocarcinoma, moderately differentiated. Some variation in nuclear size is evident, and multiple nucleoli are present in several cells. The cytoplasm is thin and contains vacuoles.

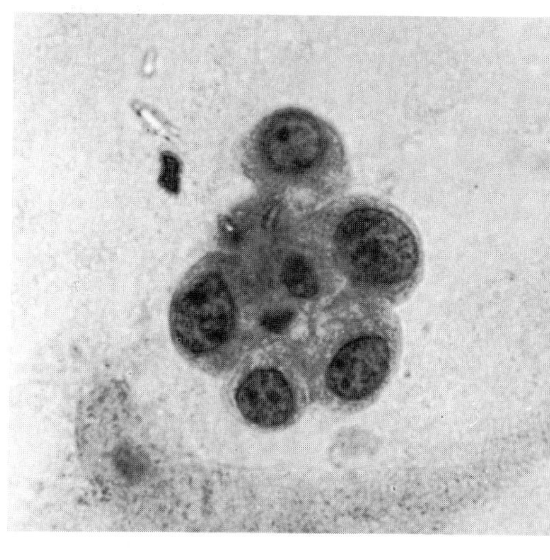

Figure 6–40. Adenocarcinoma, moderately differentiated. The nuclei have smooth profiles, thin nuclear membranes, and large nucleoli. This arrangement may be noted in bronchioloalveolar as well as classic forms of adenocarcinoma.

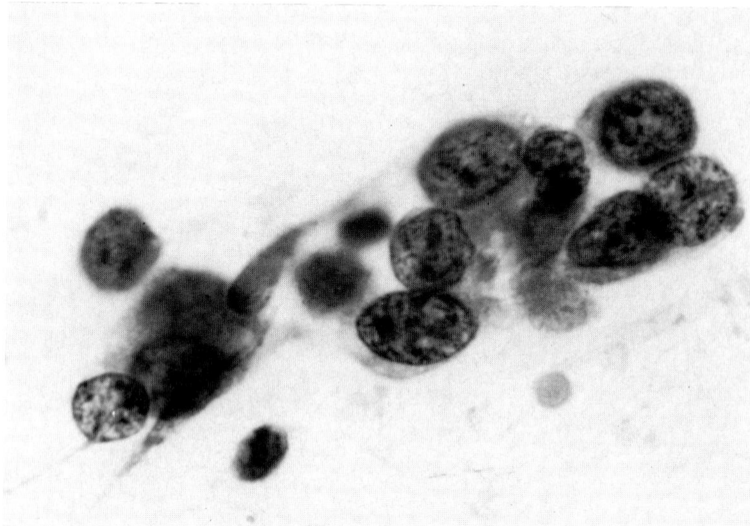

Figure 6–41. Adenocarcinoma, poorly differentiated. There is prominent clumping of the chromatin and variation in nuclear size. The cytoplasm is barely visible. This pattern should be carefully examined to avoid confusing it with undifferentiated small cell carcinoma.

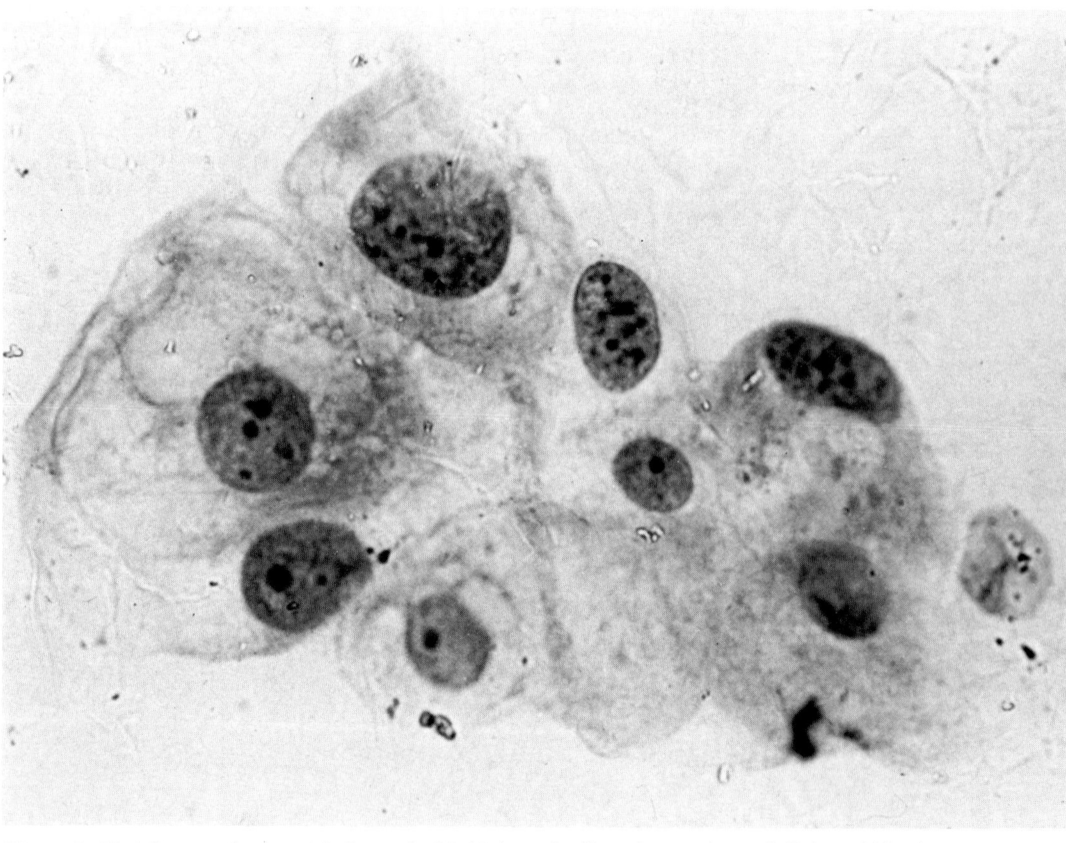

Figure 6–42. Adenocarcinoma with clear cells. Multiple nucleoli can be seen in nuclei lying within almost transparent cytoplasm.

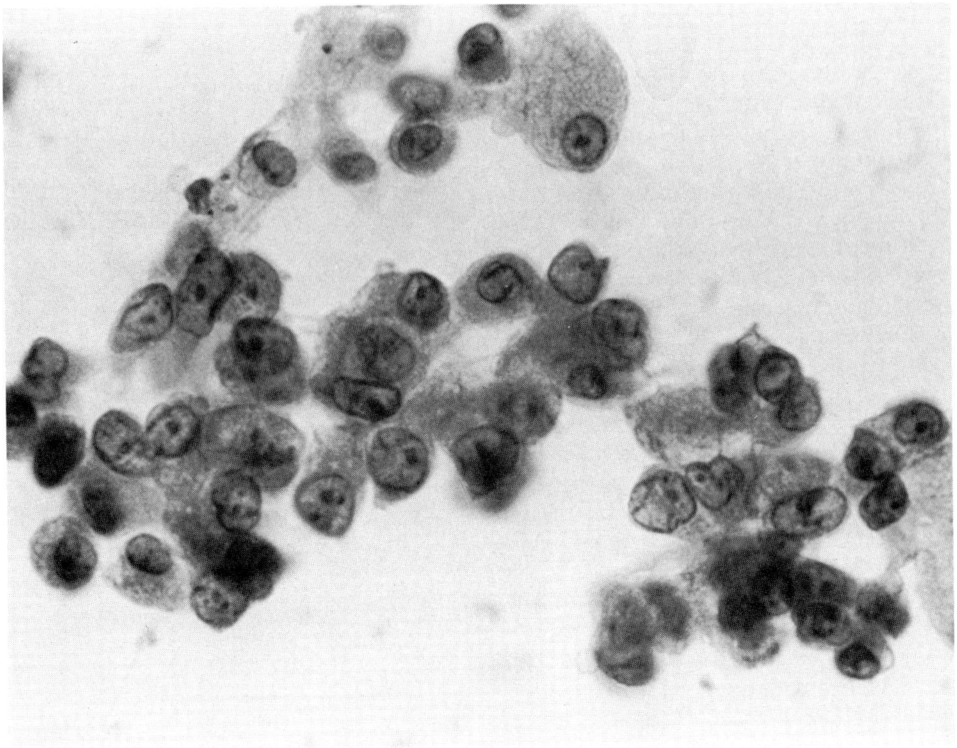

Figure 6–43. Bronchioloalveolar adenocarcinoma. The papillary pattern is apparent. Nucleoli can be seen, but they are not particularly large.

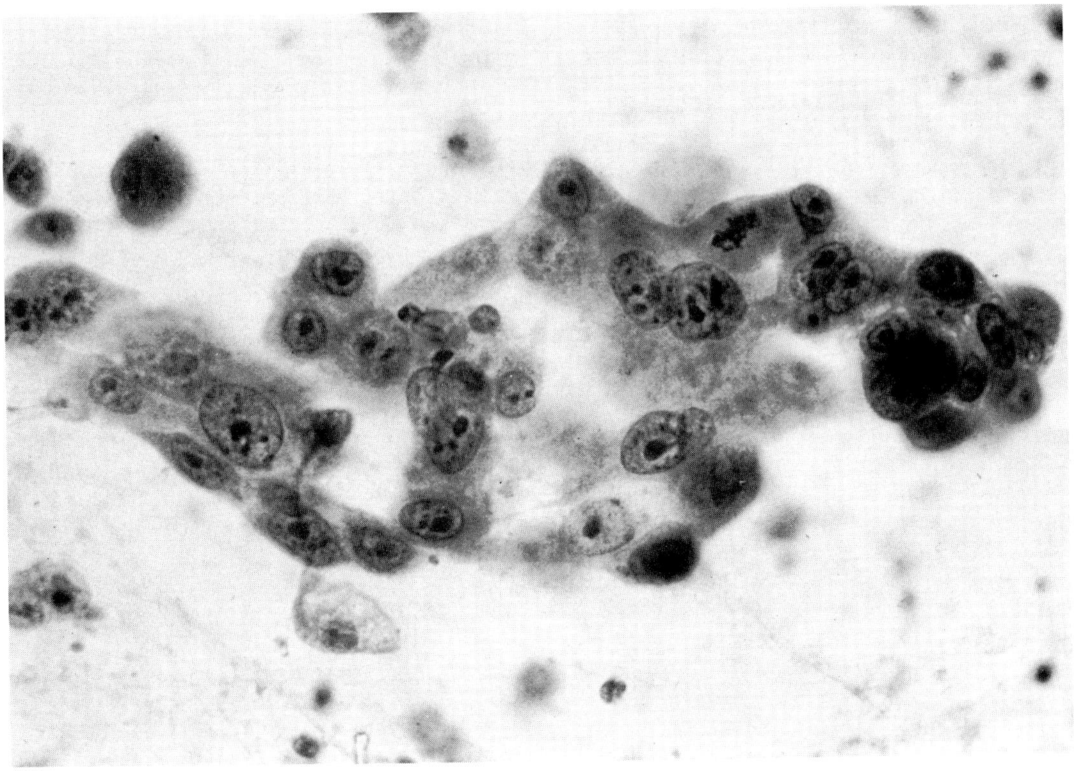

Figure 6–44. Bronchioloalveolar adenocarcinoma. As in Figure 6–43, a papillary grouping can be identified. Many of the nucleoli are larger, however. A characteristic papillary group lies at the edge of the aggregate of cells.

being successfully employed in the histopathologic diagnosis of a variety of tumors.[46-48, 132, 184, 188] Intermediate filaments are filamentous proteins that are ultrastructurally recognized as straight or slightly curved filaments that are 8 to 10 nm in diameter. They are thus intermediate in thickness between two other cytoskeletal components: the 6-nm actin microfilaments and the 25-nm microtubules. Biochemical and immunologic studies have shown that the IFs are formed from different subunit proteins and can be classified into five types whose expression is related to cellular differentiation. The vimentin type of intermediate filament is typical of mesenchymal cells and its derived tumors, melanomas and other nonepithelial neoplasms.[46, 48, 132] Desmin is characteristically present in muscle cells and most tumors derived from these cells.[132] Glial fibrillary acidic protein is found in glial cells and gliomas.[132, 134] Neurofilaments are differentiation markers that are diagnostic of neural cells and some types of neuroendocrine tumors.[107, 134] Finally, cytokeratin filaments are typical of epithelial cells and carcinomas.[19, 48, 132]

The cytokeratin filaments are unique among the intermediate filaments because of the high degree of diversity of their polypeptide subunits. Double-diffusion gel electrophoresis has been used to identify 19 subclasses ranging from 48 to 68 kd.[19, 112, 132] In human tissue, eight type II cytokeratins (Nos. 1–8 Moll's Catalog[112] and 11 type I cytokeratins (Nos. 9–19) have been identified (Table 6–1). They always are expressed as pairs of one basic and one acid cytokeratin polypeptide molecule forming defined complexes of coiled-coil α-helices that assemble into protofilaments that are 25 nm in diameter.[42] A given epithelial cell contains at least one cytokeratin pair.[19, 110] Because existing evidence indicates that the expression of cytokeratin polypeptides is tightly correlated with differentiation, the identification of a specific combination of cytokeratin patterns could distinguish between glandular and squamous differentiation without regard to morphologic features.[19, 111] This differentiation-dependent expression permits subdivision of cytokeratin polypeptides into two groups, those cytokeratins that are typical of simple, one-layered epithelia like hepatocytes and the glandular epithelium of the small intestine and colon (Nos. 7 and 8 of type II, and 18 and 19 of type I) and those characteristic of, but not exclusive to, stratified squamous epithelia (Nos. 1–6 of type II and Nos. 9–17 of type I).[19, 112] Fifteen types of cytokeratin polypeptides have so far been identified in human carcinomas.[112]

Table 6–1. Molecular Weights of the 19 Known Human Cytokeratin Polypeptides

Cytokeratin No.	Molecular Weight (kd)
1	68
2	65.5
3	63
4	59
5	58
6	56
7	54
8	52.2
9	64
10	56.5
11	56
12	55
13	54
14	50
15	50
16	48
17	46
18	45
19	40

Using immunofluorescence and two-dimensional gel electrophoresis of cytoskeletal preparations from microdissected tissue obtained from human lungs, Blobel and associates[9] found that alveolar cells contain cytokeratin polypeptides Nos. 7, 8, 18, and 19, which are also characteristic of simple epithelia. In contrast, bronchial epithelium showed the basic cytokeratin No. 5 and small amounts of No. 6, and acidic polypeptides Nos. 15 and 17, in addition to components Nos. 7, 8, 18, and 19. Antibodies that recognized simple epithelia stained only the ciliated and goblet cells of bronchi, while the basal cells were unstained (Figs. 6–45 and 6–46). The latter stained with antibodies that are highly selective for certain cytokeratins present only in stratified epithelia, and these antibodies did not react with alveolar or bronchial cells.

The cytokeratin pattern of carcinomas of the respiratory tract displays certain similarities to that of the normal lung. All adenocarcinomas of the lung reveal a simple epithelium-type cytokeratin pattern (Nos. 7, 8, 18, and 19). That of squamous cell carcinoma is, however, complex and appears dominated by a stratified epithelium-type cytokeratin pattern, especially Nos. 5 and 6. These tu-

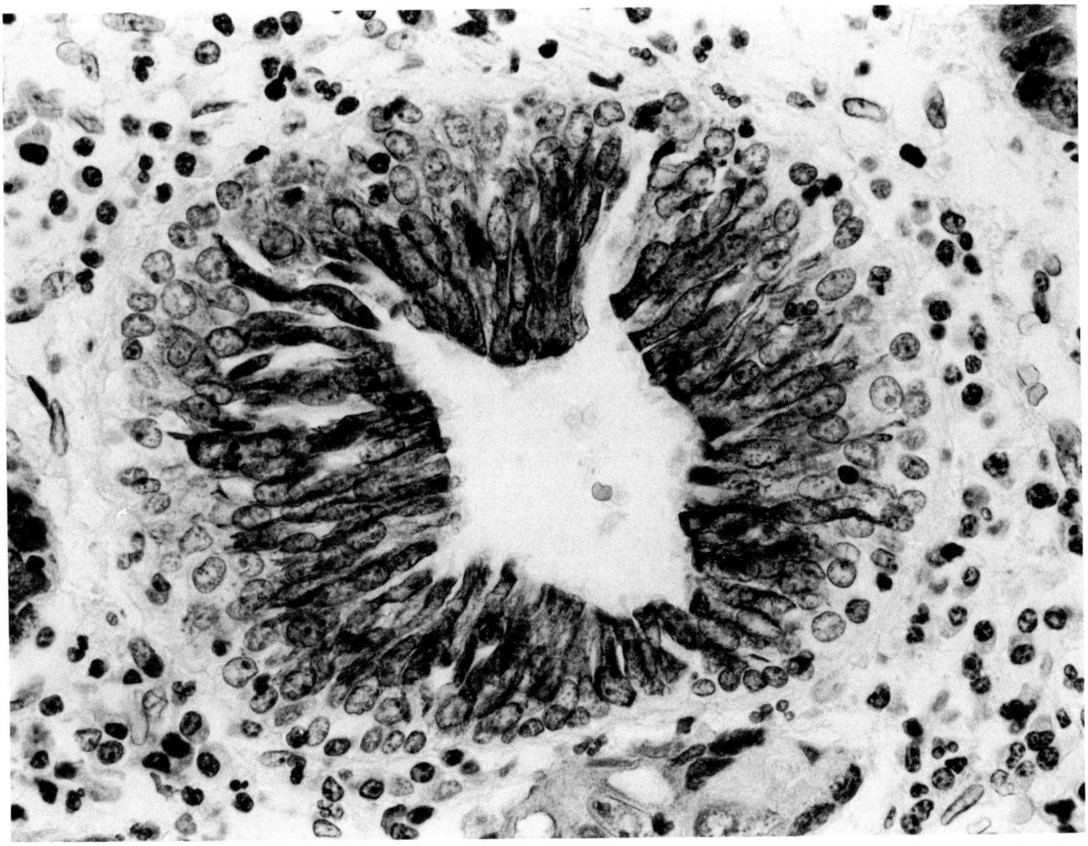

Figure 6–45. Reserve cell hyperplasia in bronchus. Immunostaining with antibody 35βH11 directed against low-molecular-weight keratin proteins stains the columnar cells but not the underlying reserve cells.

mors may also contain substantial amounts of simple epithelium-type cytokeratins and minor amounts of cytokeratin No. 13. Studies[9, 110, 111] indicate that the identification of a simple epithelium keratin pattern in a bronchogenic carcinoma is evidence of its glandular origin, while a mixed simple and squamous epithelium-type cytokeratin pattern provides support for the diagnosis of squamous cell carcinoma.

Several well-characterized monoclonal antibodies that react specifically with cytokeratins of simple epithelia or squamous epithelia are available and can be commercially obtained. Examples of these types of antibodies include AE_1, 35βH11, CAM5.2, and CK1-CK4, which recognize cytokeratins of simple epithelia, and AE_3 and 34βE12, which react with cytokeratins of squamous epithelia.[24, 46, 100, 123, 172] Although these antibodies react weakly or falsely negative with formaldehyde fixation, it is possible to obtain good immunostaining results with proteolytic enzymatic predigestion of the paraffin-embedded sections.[131] When possible, however, unfixed frozen sections, or methacarn- or alcohol-fixed paraffin sections, are to be preferred for the best results.

Immunohistochemical staining for cytokeratins can facilitate the distinction of a poorly differentiated bronchogenic squamous cell carcinoma from adenocarcinoma but provides no help in distinguishing between adenocarcinoma and bronchioloalveolar adenocarcinoma. In the limited number of tumors studied by Blobel and associates,[9] and by Moll and Franke,[111] the same cytokeratin pattern was demonstrated in adenocarcinoma and its bronchioloalveolar variant.

If inflammatory disease involving the epithelial tissues is not present, elevated serum carcinoembryonic antigen (CEA) levels may indicate the presence of a carcinoma originating from the gastrointestinal tract, the pancreas, the biliary system, the breast, or the lung.[124] Complete excision of the tumor shows a good correlation with a fall in the serum CEA level to the normal range, and, correspondingly, tumor recurrence is usually marked by rising serum CEA levels.[40, 169] It

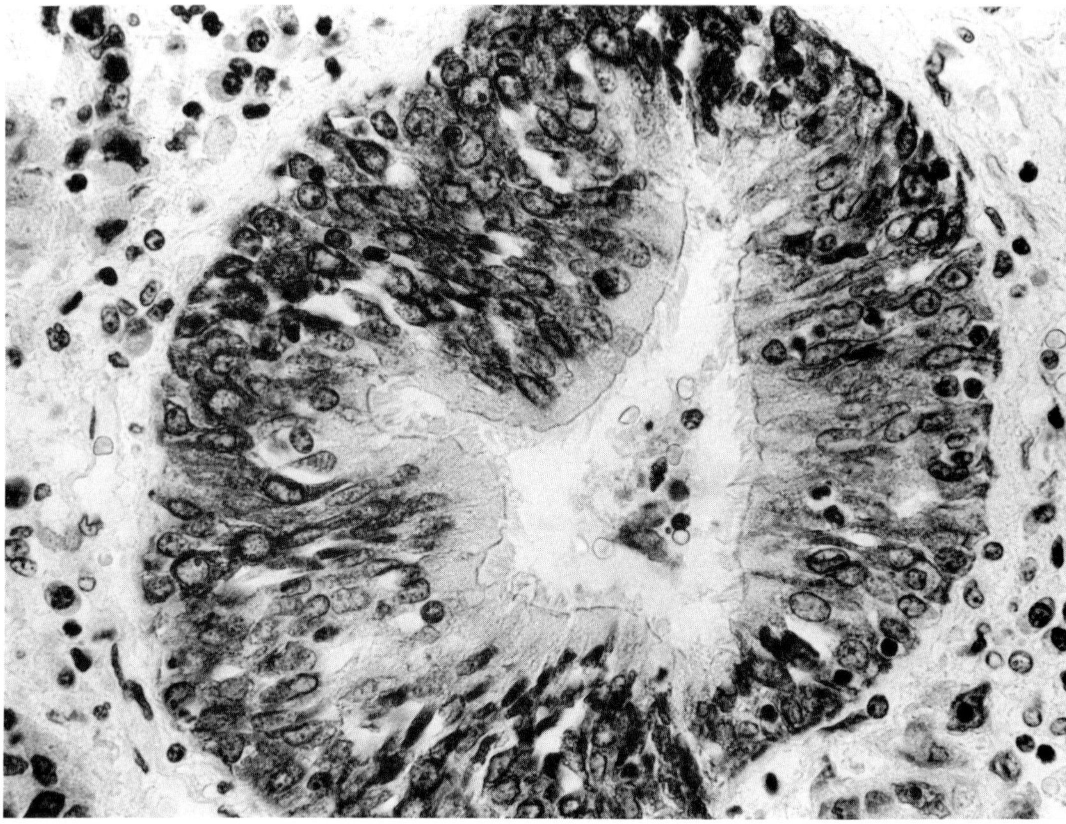

Figure 6–46. Reserve cell hyperplasia in bronchus. Immunostaining with antibody 34βE12 directed against high-molecular-weight keratin proteins stains the reserve cells strongly.

has also been shown that CEA concentration, measured at the time of diagnosis, can be related to the prognosis of many malignant tumors, including lung carcinomas[170]; and, although it is apparent that the plasma CEA assay does not possess sufficient sensitivity or specificity for cancer screening and cancer diagnosis, there is general agreement that the regular and sequential assay of plasma CEA is one of the best noninvasive methods for postoperative surveillance of patients in order to monitor the effectiveness of drug therapy and as a predictor of recurrence in patients with colorectal,[151] breast,[117] or lung cancer.[154, 193] It has been found in some carcinomas that the circulating CEA concentrations are related to the stage of the disease,[40] and rising titers of CEA appear most frequently in association with hepatic metastases.[96] Although these observations suggest that the CEA serum levels reflect the extent of the disease, the fact that serum CEA levels show a great variability from patient to patient during the same stage of the disease indicate that the relationship between them and the extent of tumor involvement is influenced by a number of other factors, such as the degree of necrosis and vascularization within the tumor or impairment of the liver's ability to adequately clear the circulation of CEA.[79]

All histologic types of lung carcinomas can be associated with elevated serum CEA levels, but bronchogenic adenocarcinoma more frequently shows elevated values than other types (Table 6–2). Although some authors[79] have indicated that better differentiated tumors tend to express CEA more often than anaplastic ones, Brockmann and colleagues,[12] in a study of different subtypes of bronchogenic adenocarcinomas, were unable to correlate the intensity of the immunostaining for CEA with the degree of tumor differentiation. Since CEA is expressed in a wide variety of tumors in addition to all types of bronchogenic carcinoma, its value in the histologic classification of lung carcinomas is very limited. The variation in the frequency with which CEA has been demonstrated using immunohistochemical methods in dif-

Table 6–2. Results of Immunocytochemical Demonstration of Carcinoembryonic Antigen in Different Histologic Types of Lung Tumors*

Reference	Adenocarcinoma	Squamous Cell Carcinoma	Large Cell Carcinoma	Small Cell Carcinoma
Pascal[a], 1977	10/14 (71.4)	2/9 (22.2)		4/8 (50.0)
Goldenberg[b], 1978	5/16 (31.2)	12/50 (30.0)		
Hill[c], 1979	15/17 (88.2)	11/16 (68.7)		
Wang[d], 1979	12/12 (100)	1/1 (100)		
Said[e], 1983	6/6 (100)	5/8 (62.5)	9/13 (69.2)	
Sun[f], 1983	12/16 (75)	26/62 (41.9)	8/20 (40)	5/23 (21.7)
Okamura[g], 1984	36/39 (92.3)	16/26 (100)	2/5 (40)	1/3 (33.3)
Wachner[h], 1984	25/25 (100)	46/51 (90.1)	10/11 (90.9)	18/37 (46.8)
Kimura et al[i], 1985	15/17 (88.8)	9/10 (90)	11/16 (68.7)	14/24 (58.3)
Brockmann[j], 1987	76/80 (95)			
Total	212/242 (87.6)	128/223 (57.3)	40/65 (61.5)	49/110 (44.5)

*Percentages given in parentheses following number of patients studied.
[a] Arch Pathol Lab Med 101:568, 1977
[b] Cancer 42:1546, 1978
[c] Lehmann FG (ed), Carcinoembryonic Proteins, Vol. II, Elsevier, Holland, 1979
[d] Cancer 44:937, 1979
[e] Hum Pathol 14:70, 1983
[f] Cancer 52:1632, 1983
[g] Acta Pathol Jpn 34:1209, 1984
[h] Virchow Archiv [A] 402:415, 1984
[i] Tohuku J Exp Med 145:23, 1985
[j] J Cancer Res Clin Oncol 113:379, 1987

ferent series of lung carcinomas (see Table 6–2) probably reflects the differences in specificity and sensitivity of the various CEA antibodies and immunocytochemical methods used. The main immunocytochemical application of CEA is to distinguish adenocarcinomas, which almost invariably are positive for CEA, from mesotheliomas, which are usually negative or weakly positive for this marker.[130, 133]

The technological advances in the generation of monoclonal antibodies have led to the recognition and study of a variety of new tumor markers. Among the monoclonal antibodies that have been generated using various cell lines and membrane fractions from different tissues, the KS1/9 monoclonal antibodies reported by Varki and co-workers[189] reacted with lung as well as other adenocarcinomas but not with squamous cell carcinomas, large cell carcinomas, or normal tissues. Monoclonal antibodies KM-93, generated by Shitara and associates,[155] and 44-3A6, developed by Radosevich and associates,[7, 138] which react with lung adenocarcinomas and large cell carcinomas in formalin-fixed, paraffin-embedded tissues but show weak or no reaction with small cell carcinomas, appear to have a potential application in the histopathologic classification of bronchogenic carcinomas. The 44-3A6-MoAb was also used successfully to detect glandular differentiation in destained cytology preparations that had been previously stained with the Papanicolaou method.[7] B72.3 is another monoclonal antibody that is becoming the subject of increasing interest for the immunocytochemical diagnosis of lung tumors.[66, 67] Because this antibody reacts with most adenocarcinomas of lung, breast, and ovary, but not with macrophages and mesothelial cells, it has been used to differentiate mesotheliomas of the pleura and peritoneum from adenocarcinomas involving these tissues.[130]

Bronchioloalveolar Adenocarcinoma

Pulmonary surfactant apoproteins are a heterogeneous group of proteins specific to the lung, and it is believed that their function is to stabilize the alveoli by reducing the surface tension of the alveolar interface.[77] Biochemical studies have demonstrated great heterogeneity in the apoprotein composition of the surfactant. It mostly consists of 30- to 40-kd proteins[69, 70, 76] but also contains moderate amounts of larger proteins (mainly 60 to 70 kd),[8, 198] and a minor content of smaller proteins (5 to 15 kd),[76, 173, 174, 204] which are believed to be the most important in reducing the surface tension of the alveoli.[174, 204] Although there is general agreement that surfactant apoproteins are mainly formed by type II pneumocytes,[6, 89, 194] there is some controversy as to whether Clara cells have the capacity to synthesize them. After an immunocytochemical study of patients with a variety of surfactant apoprotein disorders, Singh and co-workers[160] concluded that Clara cells do not have the capability of producing surfactant apoproteins. In a more recent study using antibodies against rat surfactant apoproteins and Clara cell antigen, the same authors were unable to demonstrate surfactant apoproteins in the Clara cells of spontaneous and chemically induced pulmonary tumors in mice.[195] However, Balis and colleagues[6] and Walker and associates[194] using polyclonal antibodies to a variety of surfactant-associated proteins, were able to demonstrate that both normal and proliferating type II pneumocytes and Clara cells synthesize, store, and secrete very similar, or the same group of, surfactant-associated proteins. In their studies, these authors were able to demonstrate surfactant protein reactivity in the rough endoplasmic reticulum, perinuclear cisternae, and Golgi complex; in multivesicular bodies and lamellar bodies in type II pneumocytes; and in the rough endoplasmic reticulum, Golgi complex, and secretory granules in the Clara cells. Their findings support the notion not only that Clara cells and type II pneumocytes are embryologically related cells but also that the Clara cell possesses the ability to synthesize surfactant apoproteins. The failure in earlier studies to demonstrate immunoreactivity for surfactant apoproteins in Clara cells may have been due to differences in the antibodies and techniques used in the different laboratories.

Bronchioloalveolar adenocarcinoma represents a heterogeneous group of lung carcinomas composed of ciliated cells, mucin-secreting cells, Clara cells, and type II pneumocytes. Using a polyclonal antibody to surfactant apoproteins, Singh and co-workers[162] were the first to identify a subset of bronchioalveolar adenocarcinomas that reacted with this antibody, and they designated the tumors carcinomas of type II pneumocytes. Following this report, some investigators[23, 37] provided evidence that certain bronchioloalveolar adenocarcinomas are derived from type II pneumocytes because of similarities of the ultrastructural and immunocytochemical characteristics of their cells with those of normal type II pneumocytes. Other authors[64, 207] indicated that some bronchioloalveolar carcinomas display ultrastructural features of Clara cells, and they introduced the term *Clara cell adenocarcinoma* for these neoplasms. Although none of the Clara cell carcinomas studied by Singh and co-workers[161, 163] using a polyclonal antibody showed any staining of surfactant apoproteins, other investigators[25, 109] have been able to demonstrate immunoreactivity for surfactant apoproteins in these tumors (Fig. 6–47). In a recent study, Mizutani and associates[109] found surfactant apoproteins in the cytoplasm and/or nuclear inclusion bodies in 36 of 75 primary nonmucinous adenocarcinomas of the lung, but not in other histologic types nor in any of the metastatic tumors to the lung that were studied. Typical adenocarcinomas of type II pneumocytes were excluded from the series. The findings from this and other studies[25] indicate that surfactant apoproteins are good markers with which to distinguish adenocarcinomas from other histologic types of lung cancer and that they are also helpful for the identification of metastatic tumors in the lung.

Although the origin and function of Clara cells remain uncertain, Evans and colleagues[38] have suggested that the Clara cells are one of the progenitors for the regeneration that occurs in the lungs of rats exposed to nitrous oxide. Since type II pneumocytes and Clara cells have a common embryogenesis, it would be reasonable to assume that normal and neoplastic Clara cells may retain a certain capacity for synthesis of surfactant apoproteins. Although one report[163] has indicated that subclassifying nonmucinous adenocarcinomas of the lung as apoprotein positive or apoprotein negative has no clinical or prognostic significance, more studies with a larger number of patients and well-characterized antibodies are needed before a definite conclusion can be reached.

ELECTRON MICROSCOPY

A characteristic feature of glandular differentiation in lung carcinomas at the ultrastructural level[33, 52-54, 75, 103, 139, 158] is the presence of lumens bordered by cells with apical microvilli (Figs. 6–48 and 6–49). Adjacent cells may be connected by junctional complexes. These findings are also readily identified in small groups of adenocarcinoma cells recovered by fine-needle aspiration (Fig. 6–50). A variant composed of cells ultrastruc-

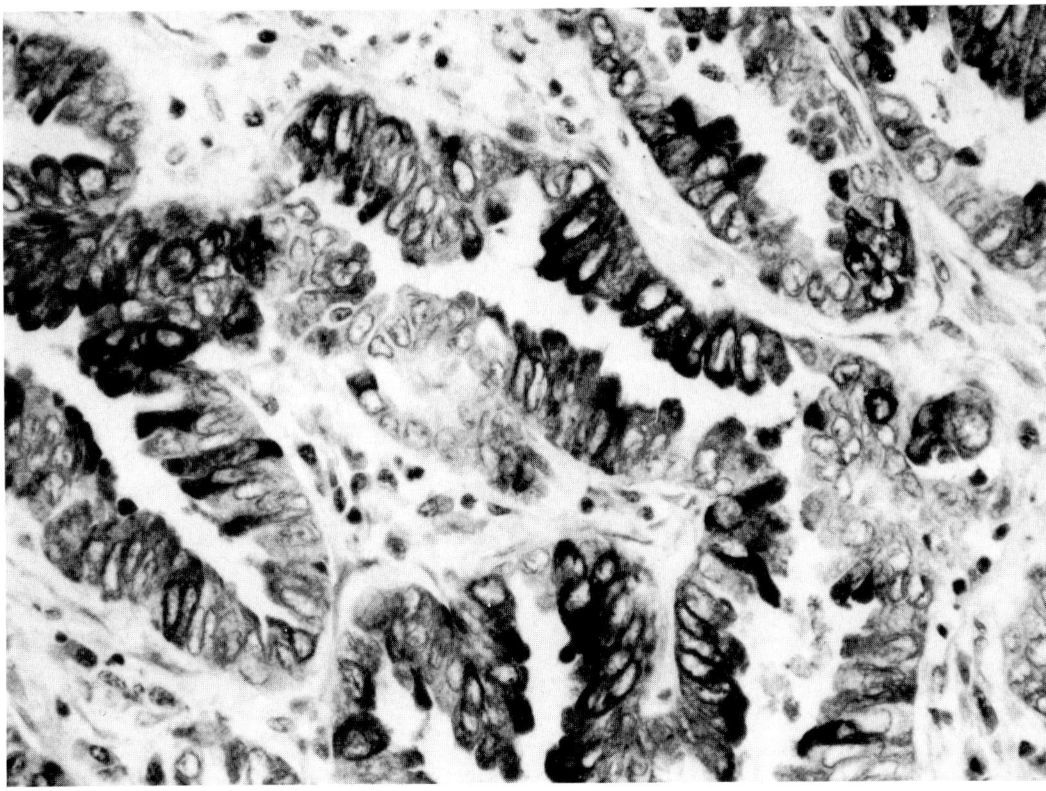

Figure 6–47. Bronchioloalveolar adenocarcinoma reacting against surfactant.

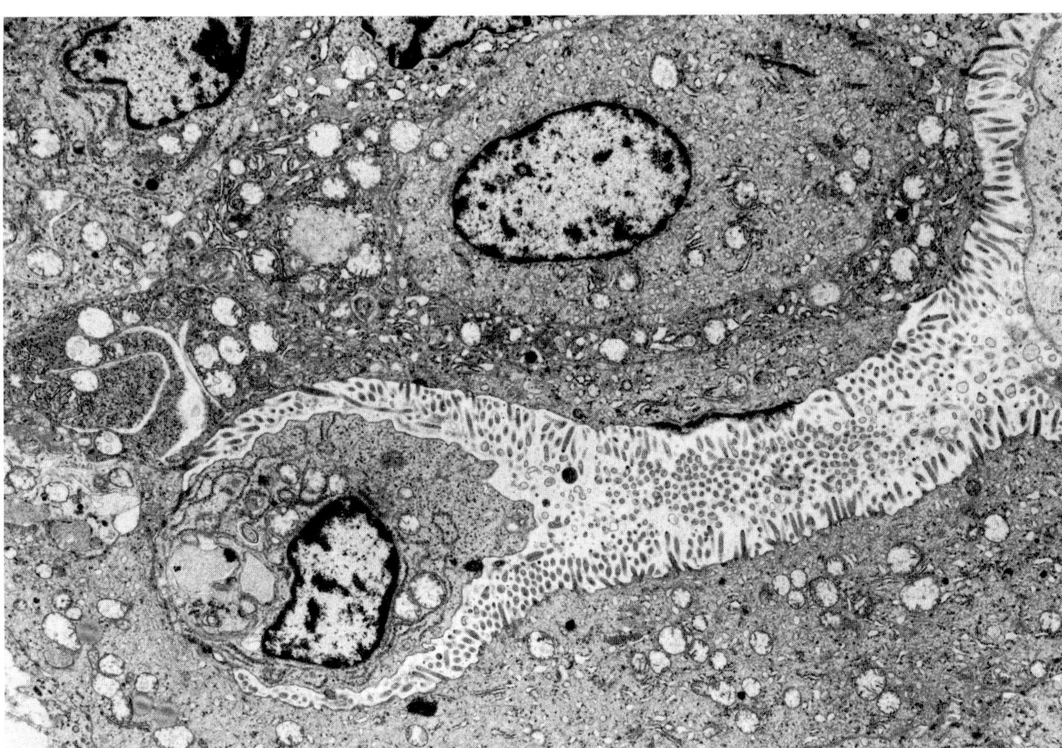

Figure 6–48. Adenocarcinoma, well differentiated. The electron micrograph shows many microvilli protruding from the apical surfaces of the cells into a slender lumen. (×5,200)

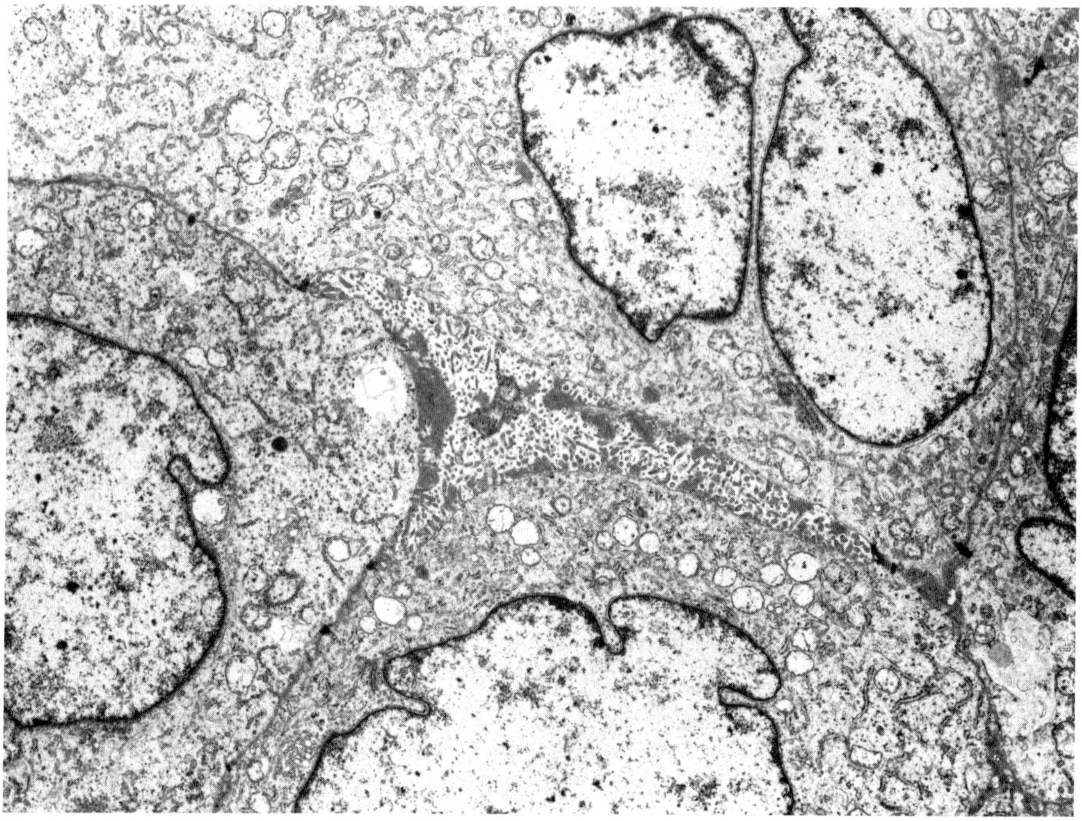

Figure 6–49. Adenocarcinoma, moderately differentiated. A small lumen surrounded by three tumor cells contains microvilli and some amorphous material. A few desmosomes can be identified. The cells have moderate numbers of mitochondria and cisternae. (×5,300)

turally related to the epithelial cells occurring in the terminal lung lobule was considered by Muller-Hermelink and colleagues[118] to represent an early stage in lung differentiation, and they referred to it as lung adenocarcinoma of fetal type.

With progressive loss of differentiation, acini become smaller but the number of microvilli does not relate to differentiation; small lumens in tumors that appear solid by light microscopy may contain many microvilli (Figs. 6–50 through 6–52). The tumor in Figure 6–53 was called a large cell undifferentiated carcinoma by light microscopy and it was mucin negative, but occasional tiny acini containing microvilli betrayed its glandular nature. A small acinus in an aspirated cell is shown in Figure 6–54. In a poorly differentiated adenocarcinoma, the cell surfaces may be devoid of microvilli but they may be seen lining a small intracytoplasmic lumen (Fig. 6–55). This appearance is common in breast carcinoma but is also occasionally seen in lung adenocarcinomas. The number of microvilli in the tumor shown in Figure 6–56 approach the minimum: they are sparse and sandwiched between neighboring cells. While this alone can only suggest adenocarcinoma, the tumor does not have squamous features and was considered to be a virtually undifferentiated adenocarcinoma at the ultrastructural level; by light microscopy it appeared to be an undifferentiated large cell carcinoma.

In Figure 6–57, some microvilli are squashed between apposed cells but there is also infolding of the cell membranes, an adenocarcinoma feature. Concentric arrays of slender cisternae (Fig. 6–58) are seen in occasional adenocarcinomas. The tumor in Figure 6–59 is clearly an adenocarcinoma because of the lumen formation and sparse microvilli, but the cells also show the considerable numbers of mitochondria and other organelles that may populate adenocarcinoma cells, and in addition they show small dense-core granules in the apical cytoplasm that indicate some form of secretory product.

Text continued on page 146

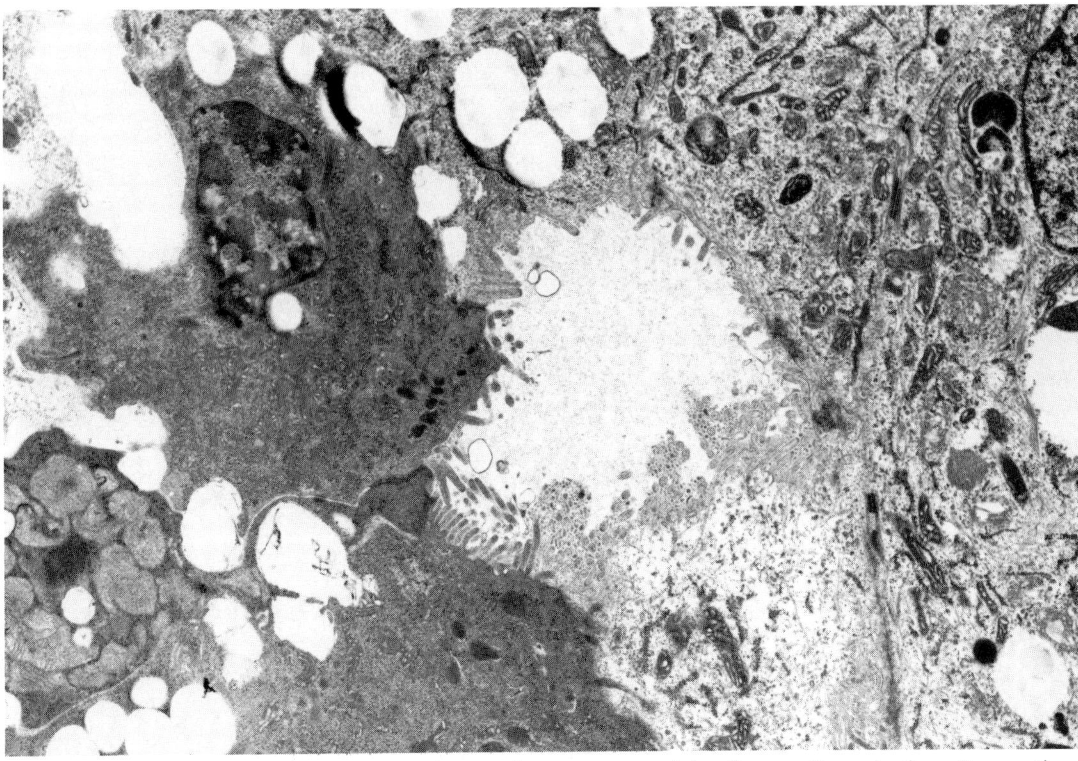

Figure 6–50. Cells of a bronchogenic adenocarcinoma recovered by fine-needle aspiration. Preservation is acceptable. The clear spaces in the cytoplasm are lipid droplets. A lumen containing microvilli is present at the center of the figure. (×3,900)

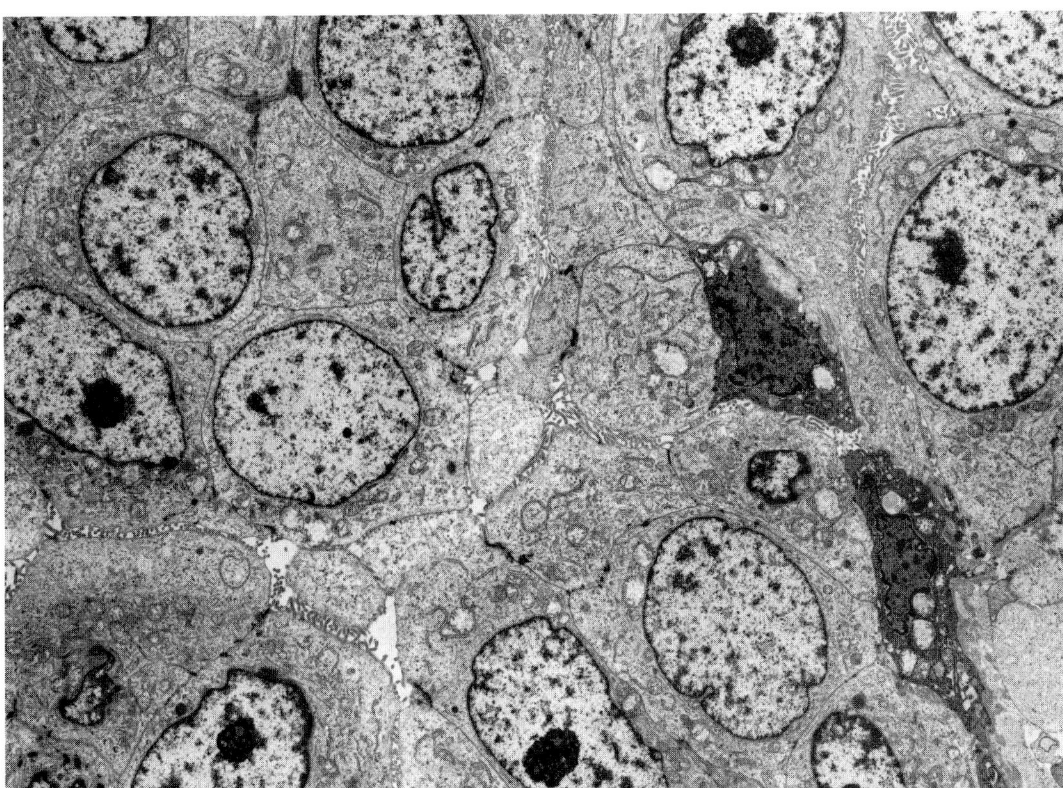

Figure 6–51. Adenocarcinoma, poorly differentiated. By light microscopy this was a solid carcinoma. At the ultrastructural level, tiny lumens containing microvilli are revealed. (×3,750)

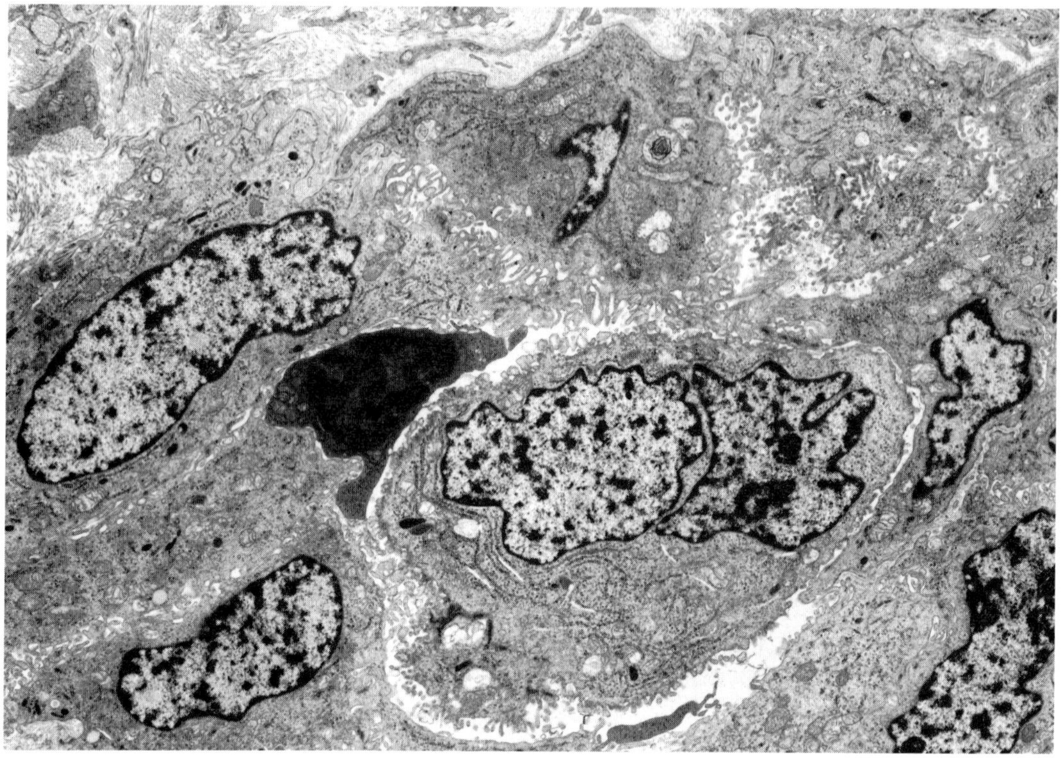

Figure 6–52. Adenocarcinoma, poorly differentiated. The cells are losing cohesion, and microvilli are present on many of the free surfaces. (×5,250)

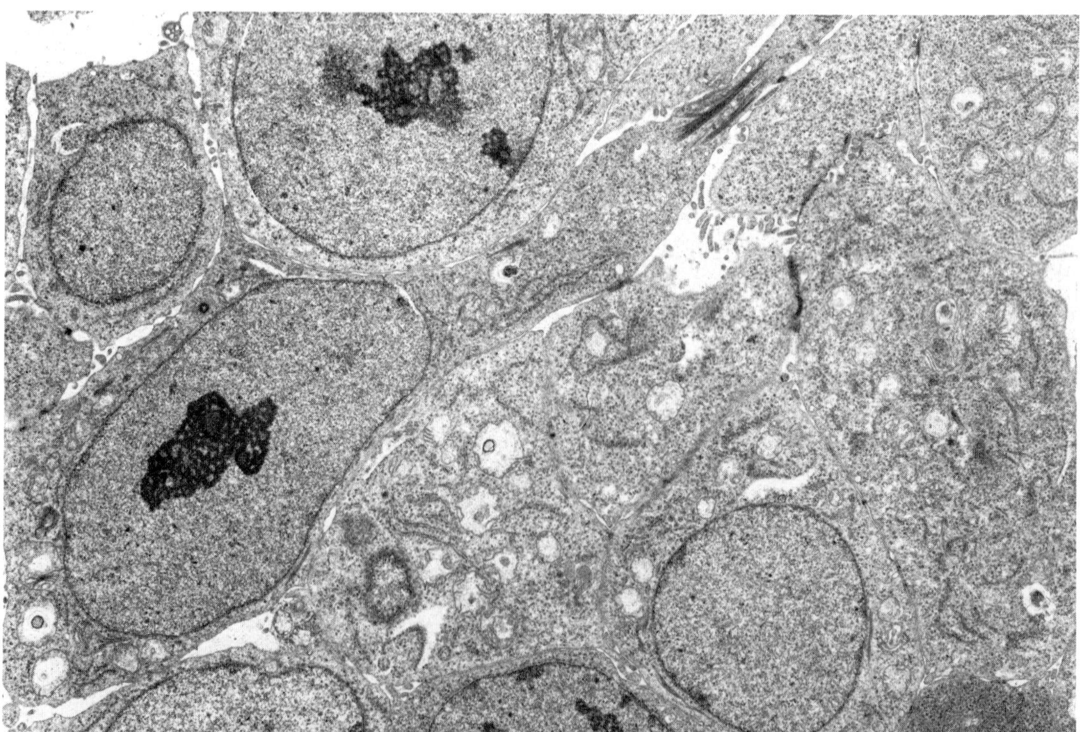

Figure 6–53. Adenocarcinoma, poorly differentiated. By light microscopy, this tumor was diagnosed as an undifferentiated large cell carcinoma. Minimal glandular differentiation could be detected by electron microscopy. Cell junctions are sparse, but a few tonofilament bundles can be seen. (×4,100)

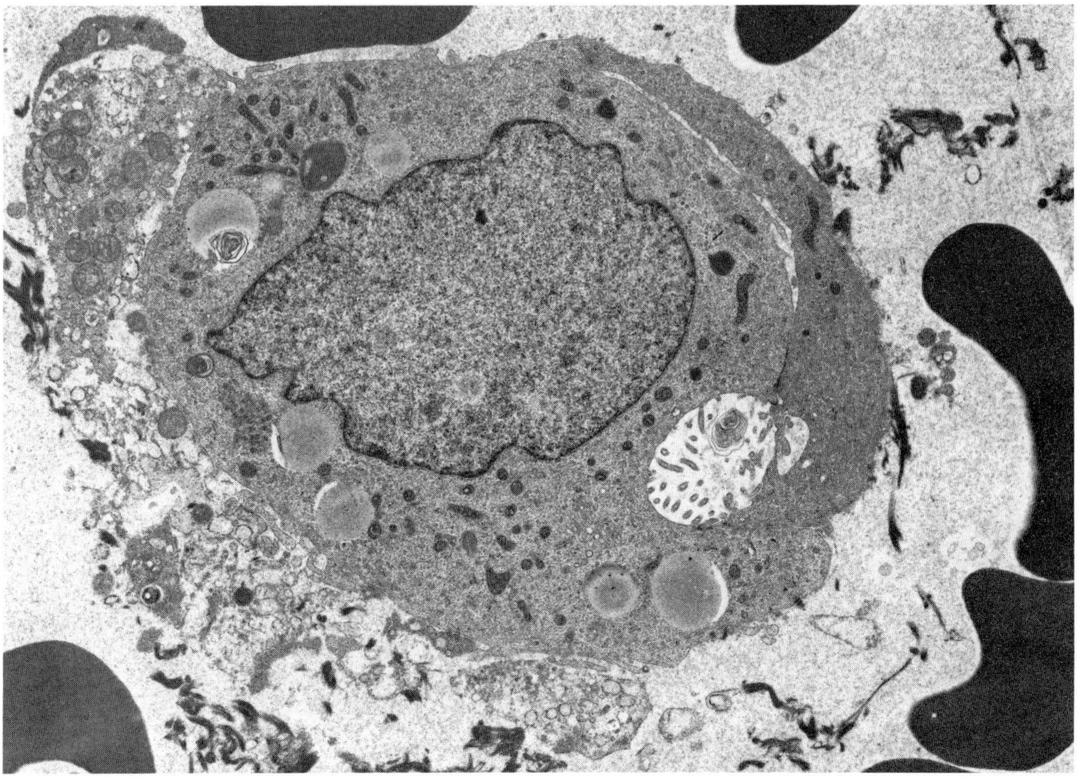

Figure 6–54. An occasional acinar lumen established the diagnosis of adenocarcinoma in this fine-needle aspiration biopsy. (×6,700)

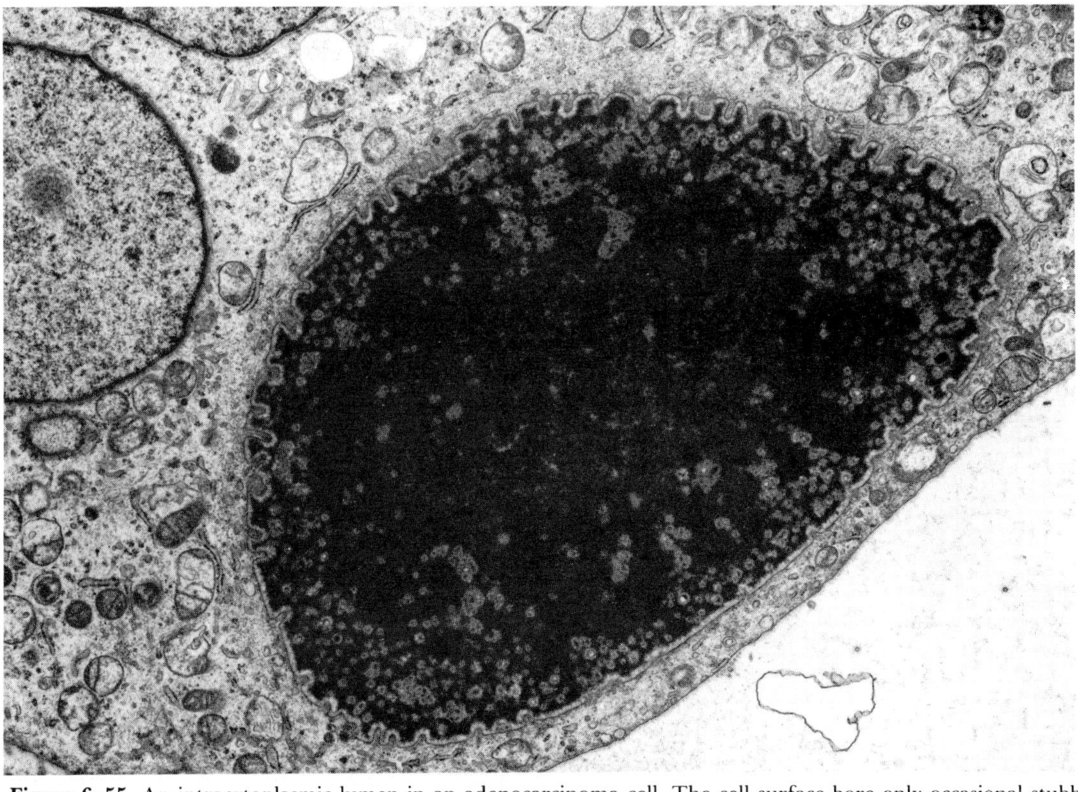

Figure 6–55. An intracytoplasmic lumen in an adenocarcinoma cell. The cell surface bore only occasional stubby microvilli, whereas they are relatively numerous within the lumen. (×9,600)

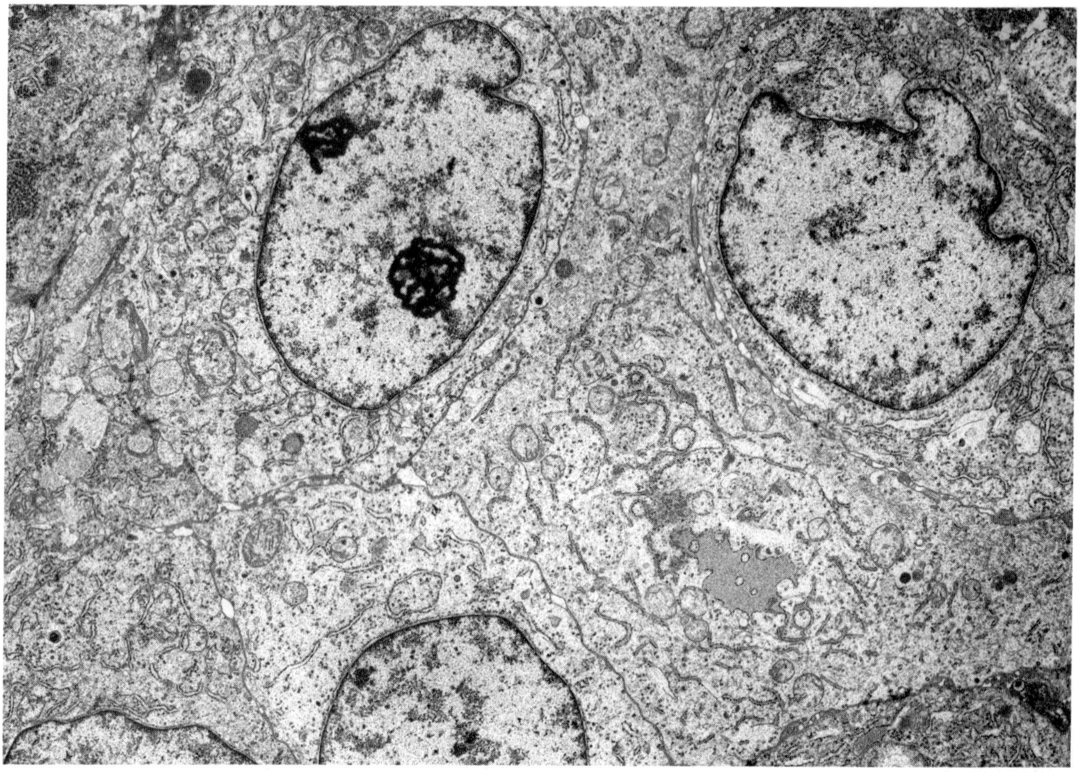

Figure 6–56. Adenocarcinoma, poorly differentiated. The tumor is virtually undifferentiated, and would be considered so by light microscopy, but a few microvilli can be seen within slender clefts that separate neighboring cells. Nuclei are ovoid with relatively smooth profiles. The cytoplasm contains numerous slender cisternae and sparse mitochondria. (×5,100)

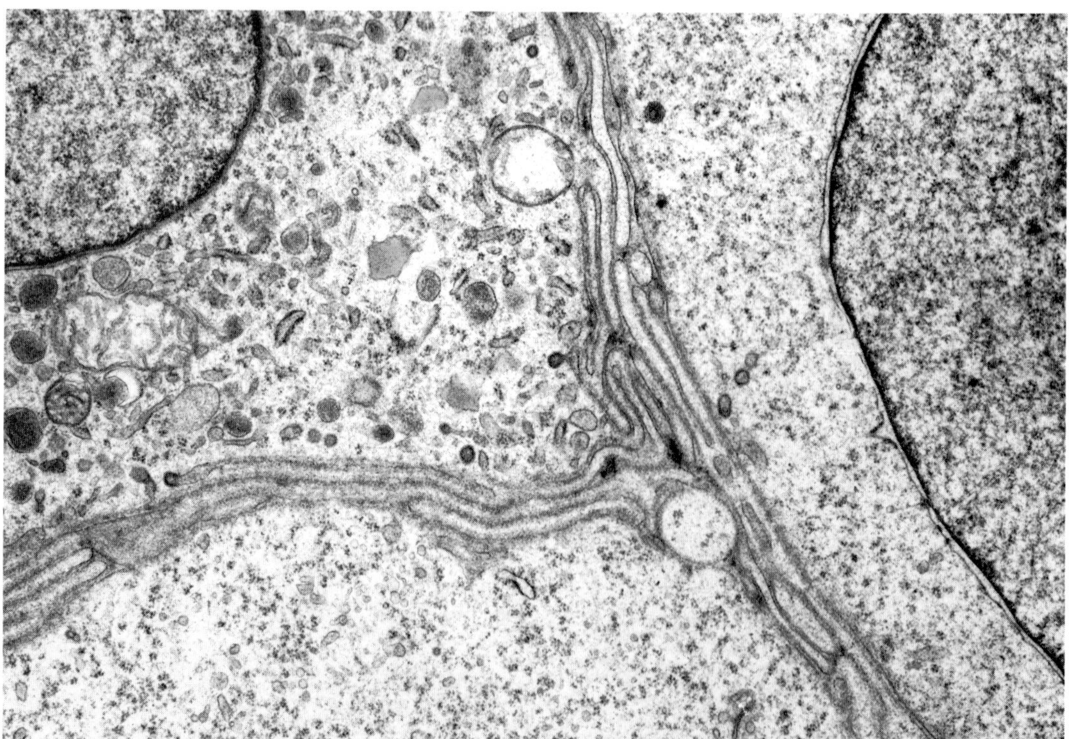

Figure 6–57. Adenocarcinoma, poorly differentiated. Infolding of the cell membranes and sandwiched microvilli indicate that the tumor is an adenocarcinoma. The dense bodies are probably lysosomes. (×13,200)

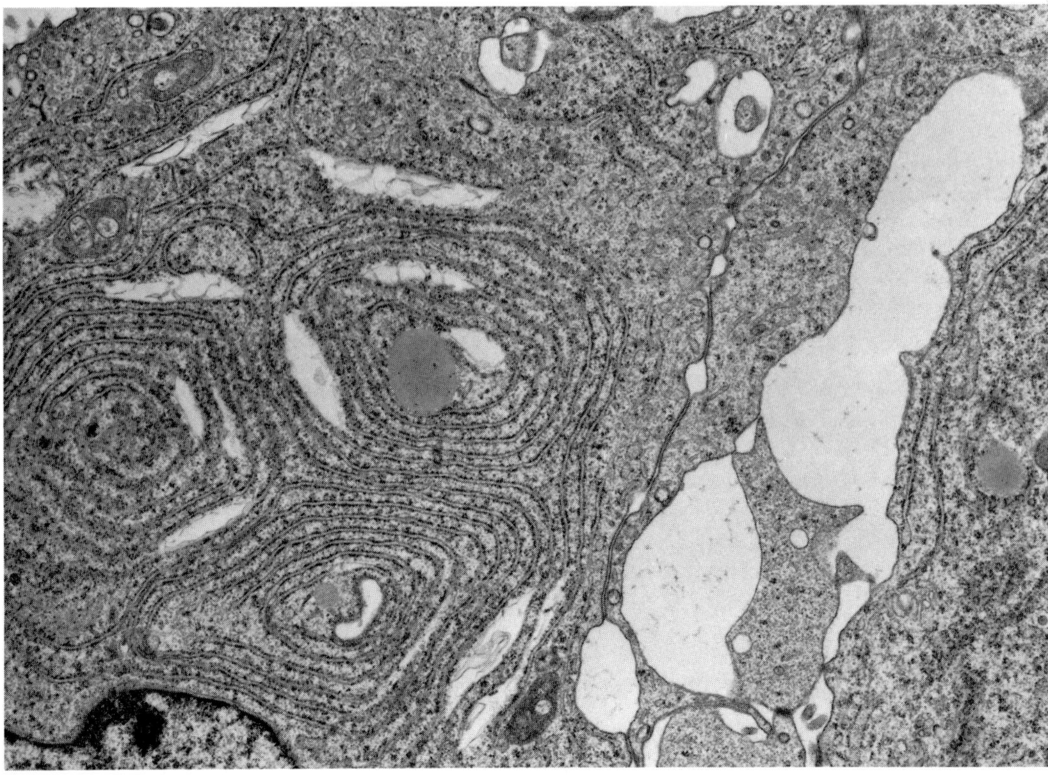

Figure 6–58. Concentric cisternae of endoplasmic reticulum in a moderately differentiated adenocarcinoma. (×7,700)

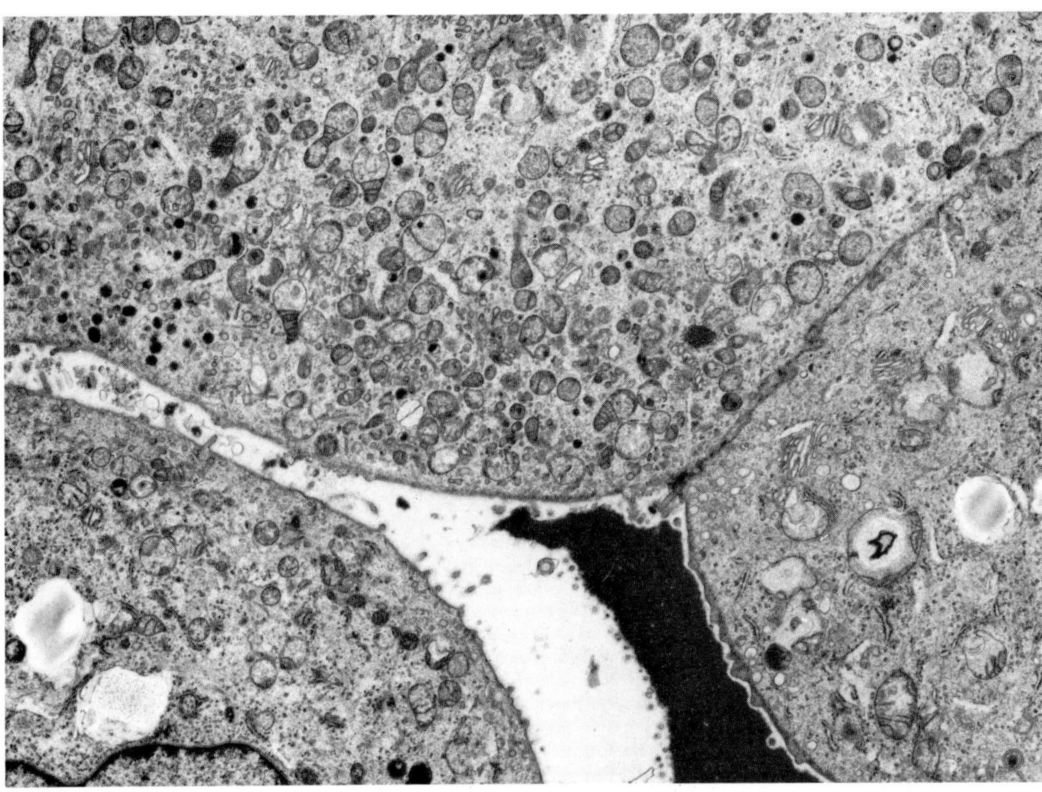

Figure 6–59. Small dense-core granules of endocrine caliber in the apical cytoplasm of cells of a moderately differentiated adenocarcinoma. (×6,400)

The large granules in the cells in Figure 6–59 are more like lysosomes. Mucin droplets can have a dense core (Fig. 6–60), or the mucin may occupy electron-lucent zones within the cytoplasm (Fig. 6–61) and may be present only in scattered cells (Fig. 6–62).

An occasional lung carcinoid has a glandular pattern. Ohtsuki and colleagues[129] reported an atypical carcinoid in a 67-year-old man with secretory granules measuring on average 220 nm in scattered cells associated with marked elevation of the serum α-fetoprotein level. Ultrastructurally, electron-dense material similar to the hyaline bodies of yolk sac tumors was observed. The authors argue that the case is comparable to the mixed adenocarcinomas and carcinoid tumors, which occasionally occur in the digestive tract. Two lung carcinoids with glandular features were diagnosed by fine-needle aspiration biopsy by Pilotti and co-workers.[135]

Bronchioloalveolar Adenocarcinoma

The fine structure of bronchioloalveolar adenocarcinoma cells has been described on many occasions[10, 11, 17, 18, 37, 45, 49, 113, 115, 146] and is shown in a low-magnification electron micrograph in Figure 6–63. A single layer of columnar cells rests on a basal lamina that separates the cells from the subjacent stroma. Although the nuclei are at different levels within the cells, it is clear that there is no stratification. Mucin may be present in bronchioloalveolar adenocarcinoma cells and, if scanty, occupies the apical cytoplasm, where it can form diffuse electron-lucent areas (Fig. 6–64). The apical cytoplasm of the cells often projects above the level of the junctional complexes that join adjacent cells (Figs. 6–65 and 6–66), and microvilli are more numerous between these apical caps than on their tips. Occasionally the surface is more irregular (Fig. 6–67).

Dense granules are a common finding in bronchioloalveolar adenocarcinoma cells, and they may be present in every cell of a tumor. They tend to concentrate in the apical cytoplasm and may be largely confined to the apical caps when they are present (Figs. 6–65 and 6–66). The granules are distinctly larger than endocrine granules and are comparable in size and appearance to the granules seen

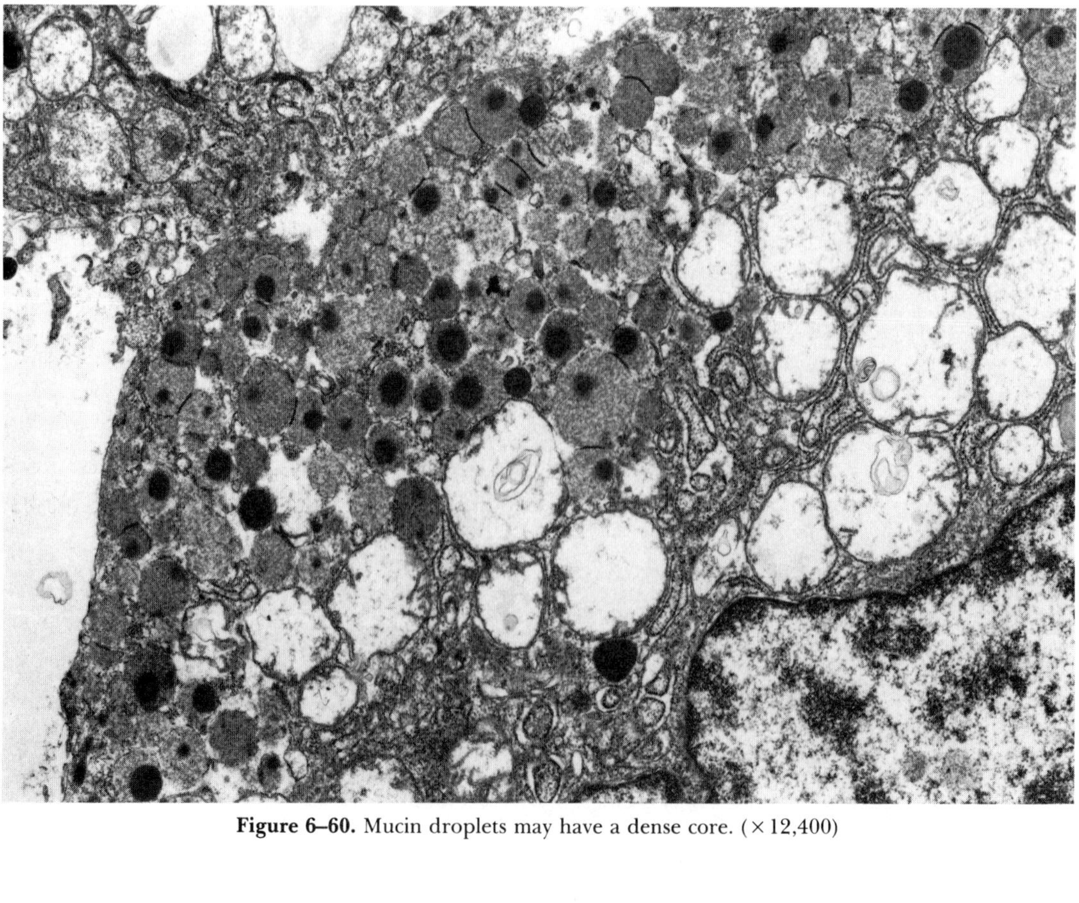

Figure 6–60. Mucin droplets may have a dense core. (×12,400)

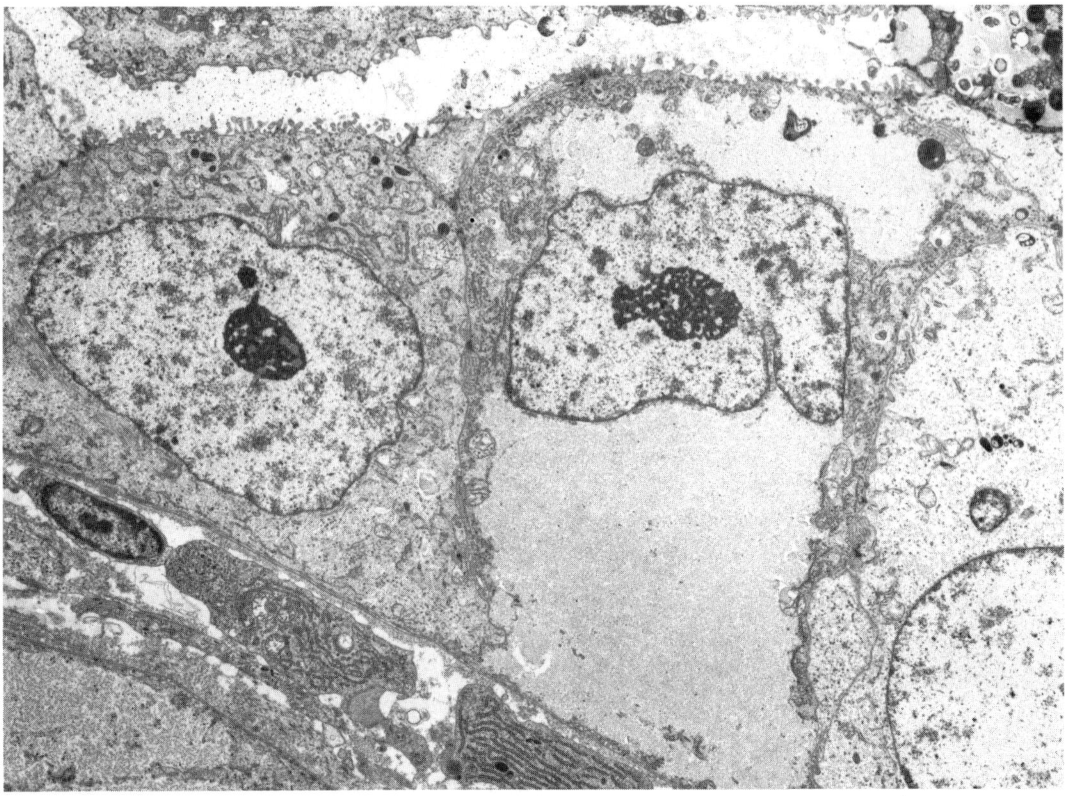

Figure 6–61. Mucopolysaccharide may accumulate as diffuse electron-lucent material. (×5,600)

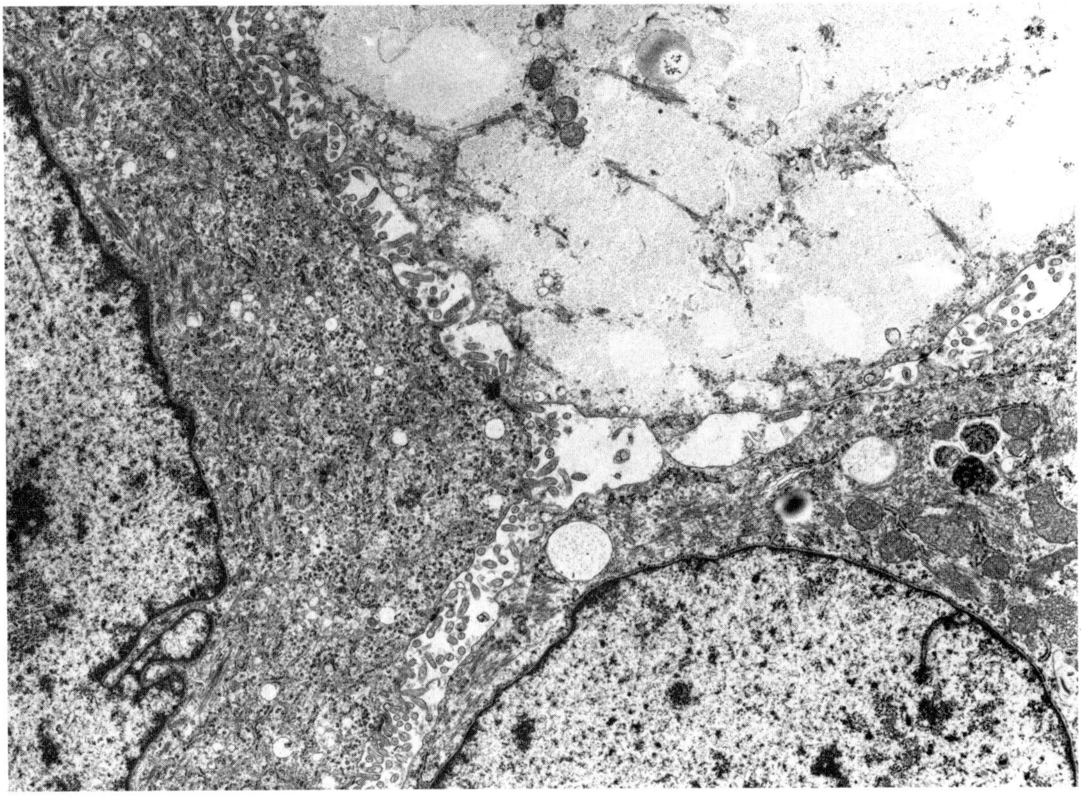

Figure 6–62. In this adenocarcinoma, only scattered cells contained electron-lucent material. (×8,000)

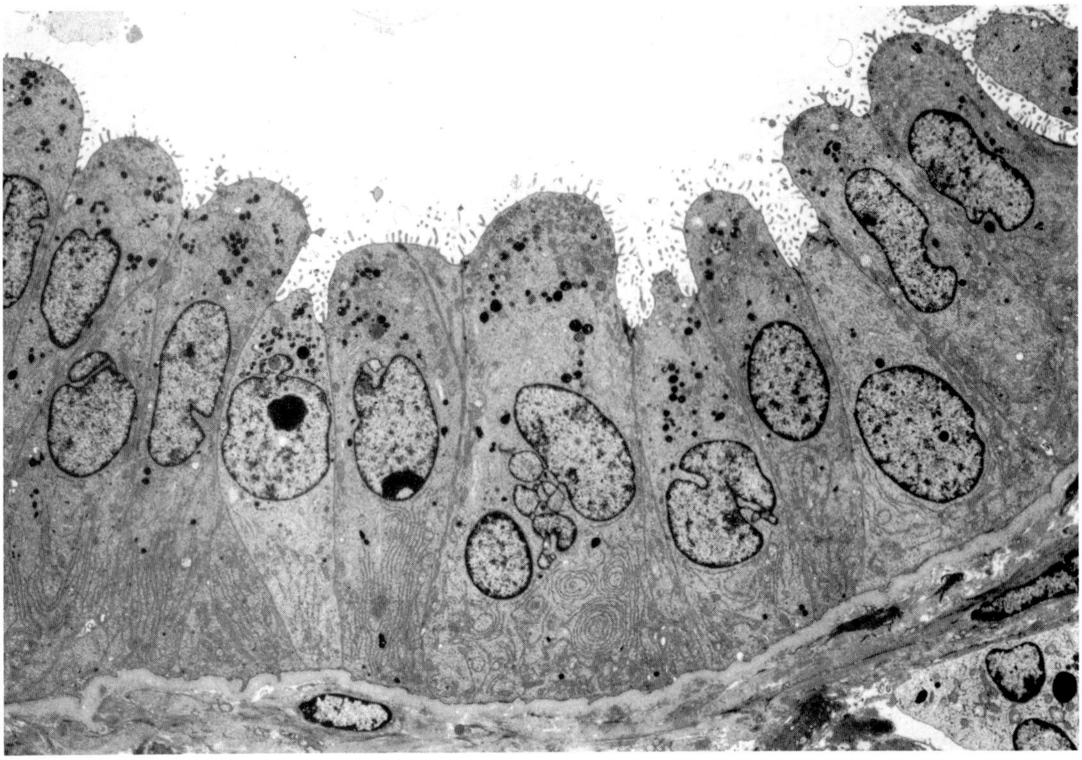

Figure 6–63. Bronchioloalveolar adenocarcinoma. In this low-magnification electron micrograph, the single row of columnar tumor cells rests on a basal lamina. Nuclei are at varying heights within the cells. (×2,300)

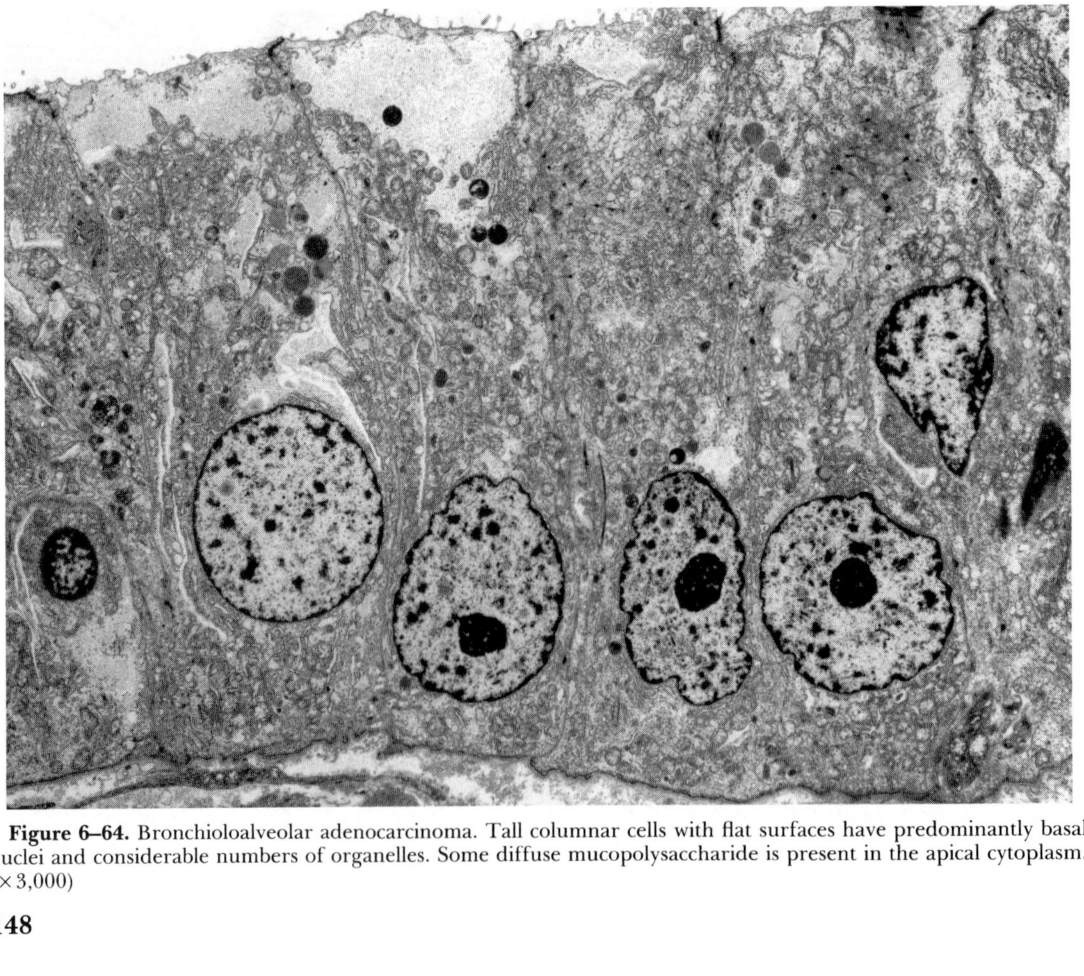

Figure 6–64. Bronchioloalveolar adenocarcinoma. Tall columnar cells with flat surfaces have predominantly basal nuclei and considerable numbers of organelles. Some diffuse mucopolysaccharide is present in the apical cytoplasm. (×3,000)

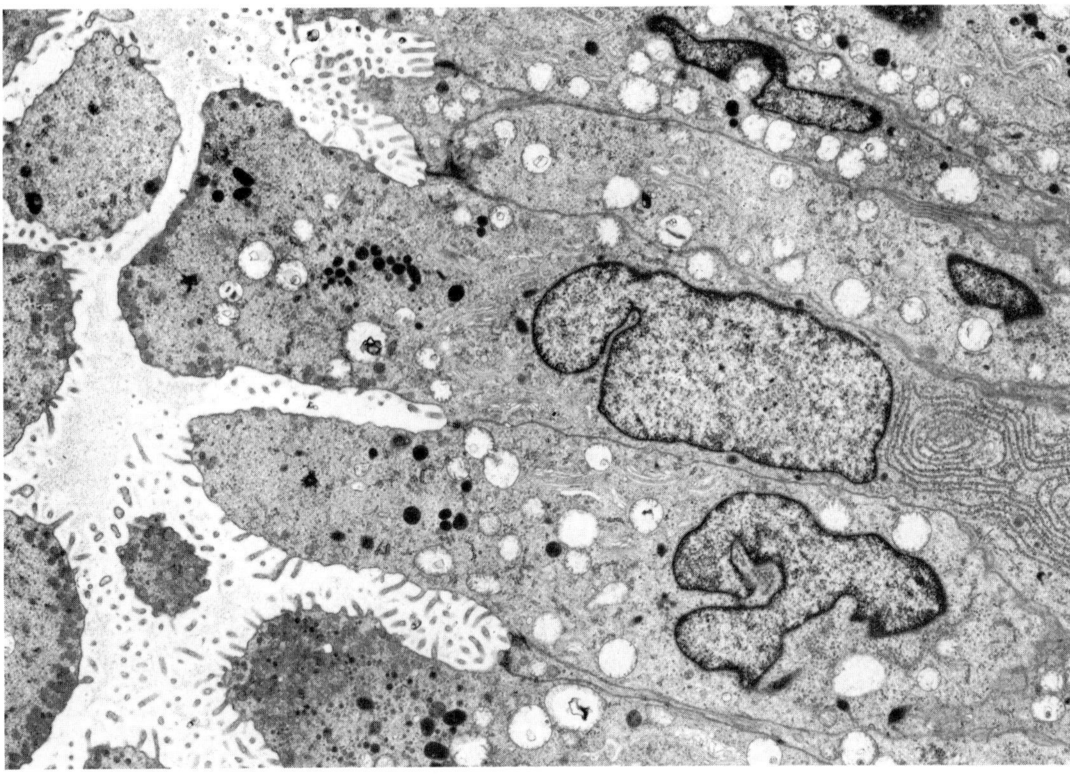

Figure 6–65. Bronchioloalveolar adenocarcinoma. The apical cytoplasm protrudes into the lumen, and most of the dense granules are congregated in this area of the cell. (×5,000)

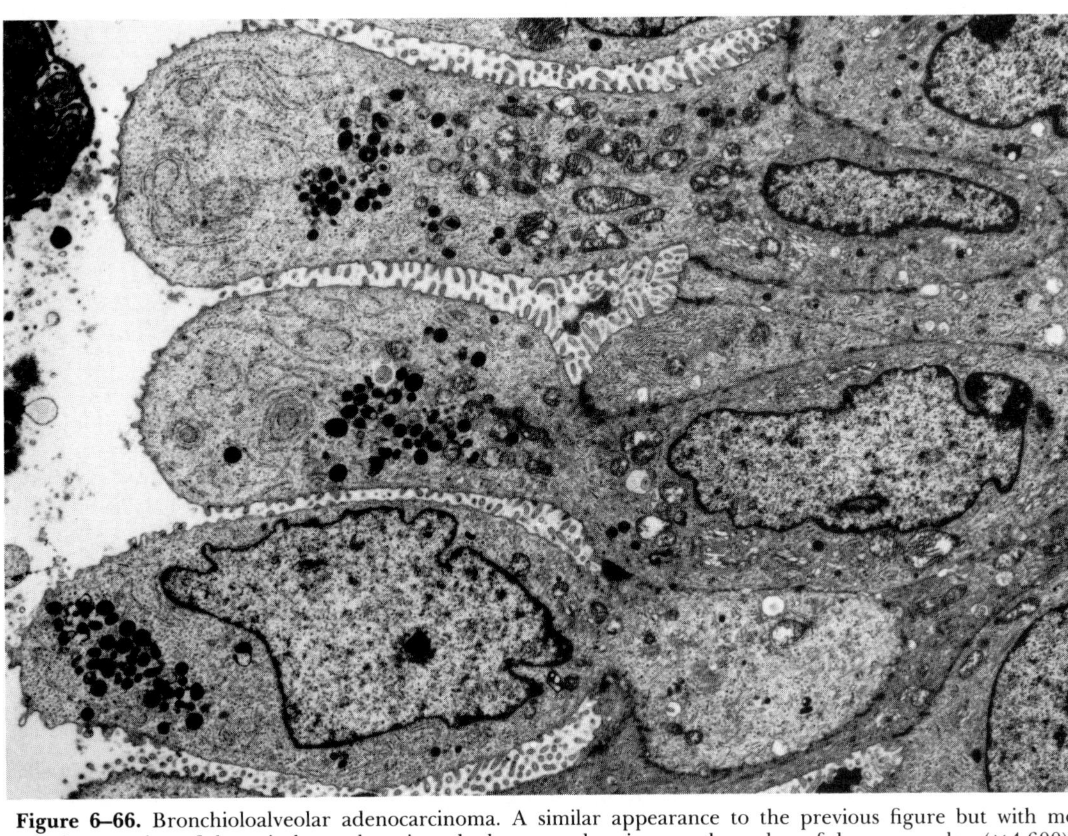

Figure 6–66. Bronchioloalveolar adenocarcinoma. A similar appearance to the previous figure but with more marked protrusion of the apical cytoplasm into the lumen and an increased number of dense granules. (×4,600)

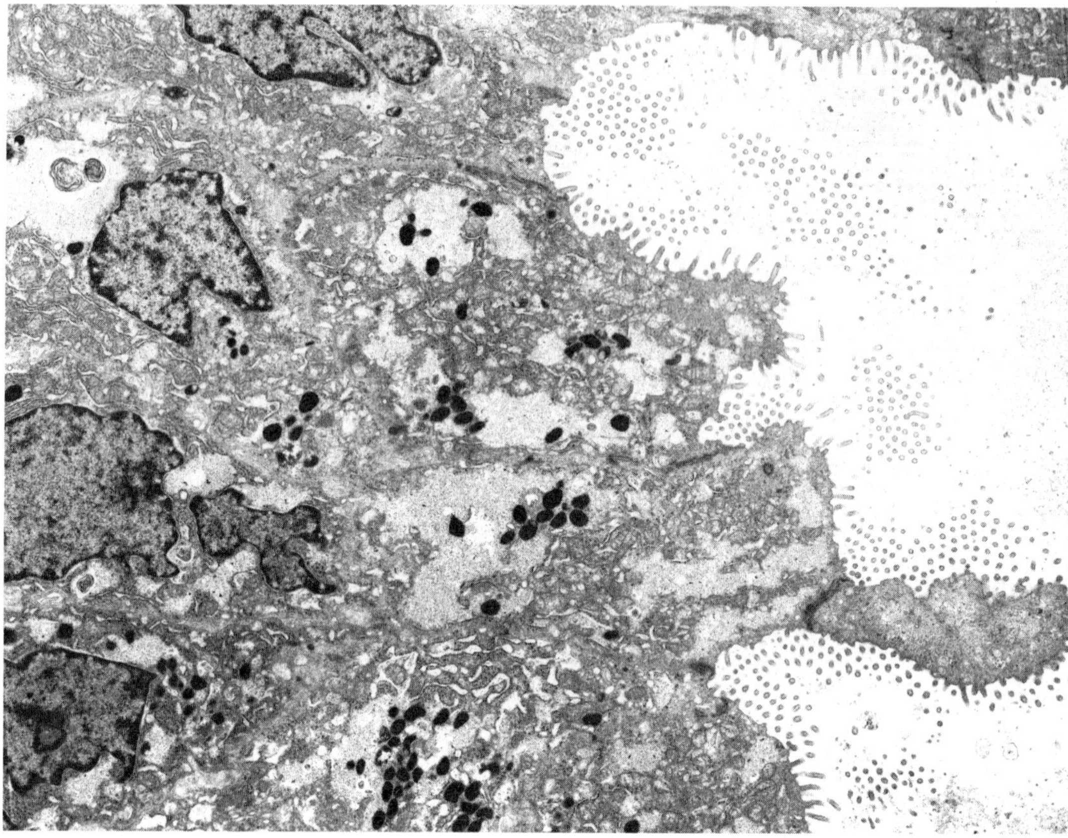

Figure 6–67. Bronchioloalveolar adenocarcinoma. The apical surface of the rows of cells in this tumor was quite irregular. (×5,300)

in the nonciliated bronchiolar (Clara) cell.[22] This appearance in a bronchioloalveolar adenocarcinoma indicates Clara cell differentiation. It is in our experience by far the most common ultrastructural appearance in bronchioloalveolar adenocarcinoma cells, either alone or with mucin, and it may be present in every cell, or there may be a mixture of cells with more mucin or with lamellar bodies indicative of type II pneumocyte differentiation. Bronchioloalveolar adenocarcinomas containing only type II cells have been recorded, but they are uncommon. Horie and associates,[60] in eight cases, found cells with features of totipotential bronchioloalveolar cells and differentiation to type II pneumocytes, Clara cells, and ciliated epithelial cells. Eimoto and colleagues[32] studied the ultrastructure of 20 well-differentiated adenocarcinomas including bronchioloalveolar adenocarcinoma, and the latter group was made up of five cases of Clara cell type, two cases of type II pneumocyte type, and four cases of mixed cell type. Bronchioloalveolar adenocarcinoma may have few or no granule-containing cells and more mucin (Figs. 6–68 and 6–69), which again tends to accumulate in the apical cytoplasm. Ogata and coworkers[128] reported that Clara cell granules were found in two acinar and four solid carcinomas in addition to papillary adenocarcinomas. These authors believed that the number of granules was related to the degree of tumor differentiation, and they consider that most peripheral adenocarcinomas have the potential for Clara cell differentiation regardless of whether they show histologic features of bronchioloalveolar adenocarcinoma.

The presence of microfilament cores in microvilli is a feature of cells of the gastrointestinal tract and their adenocarcinomas, but it has been observed in lung tumors (Fig. 6–70).[28, 54] It therefore cannot be used as a criterion to distinguish primary from metastatic adenocarcinomas in the lung. Engstrand and associates[35] examined 70 consecutive solitary lung cancers, including 42

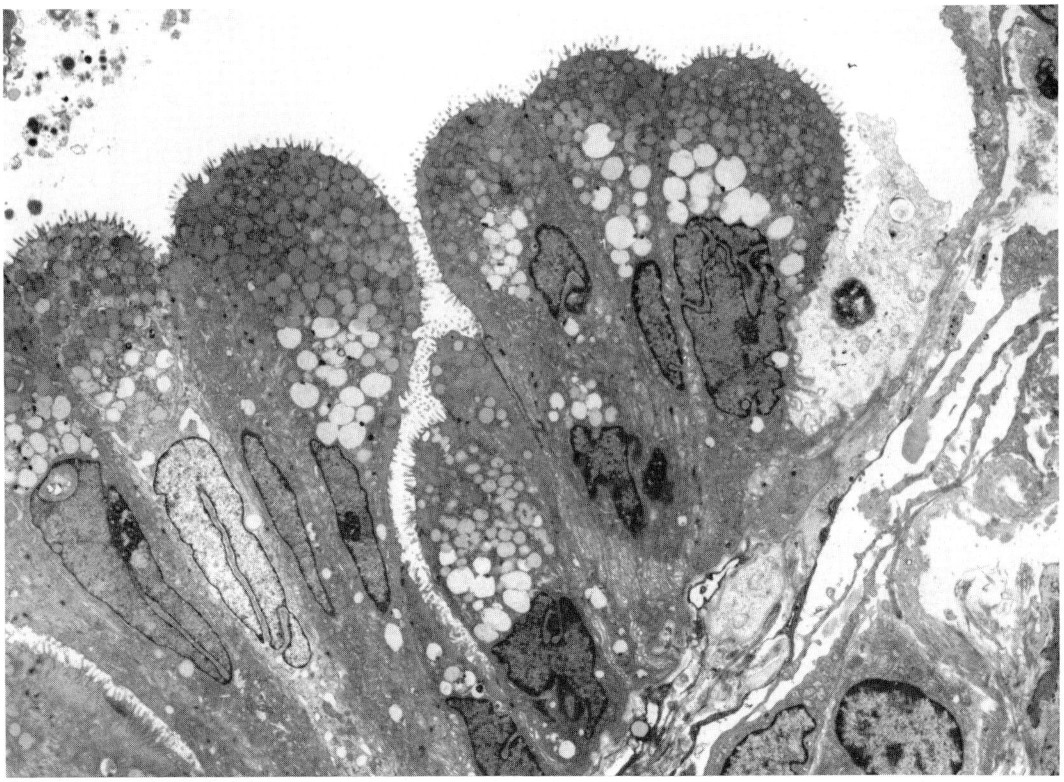

Figure 6–68. Bronchioloalveolar adenocarcinoma. The margin of a cluster of tumor cells attached to the alveolar surface. There is marked irregularity of the nuclear membrane. (×3,150)

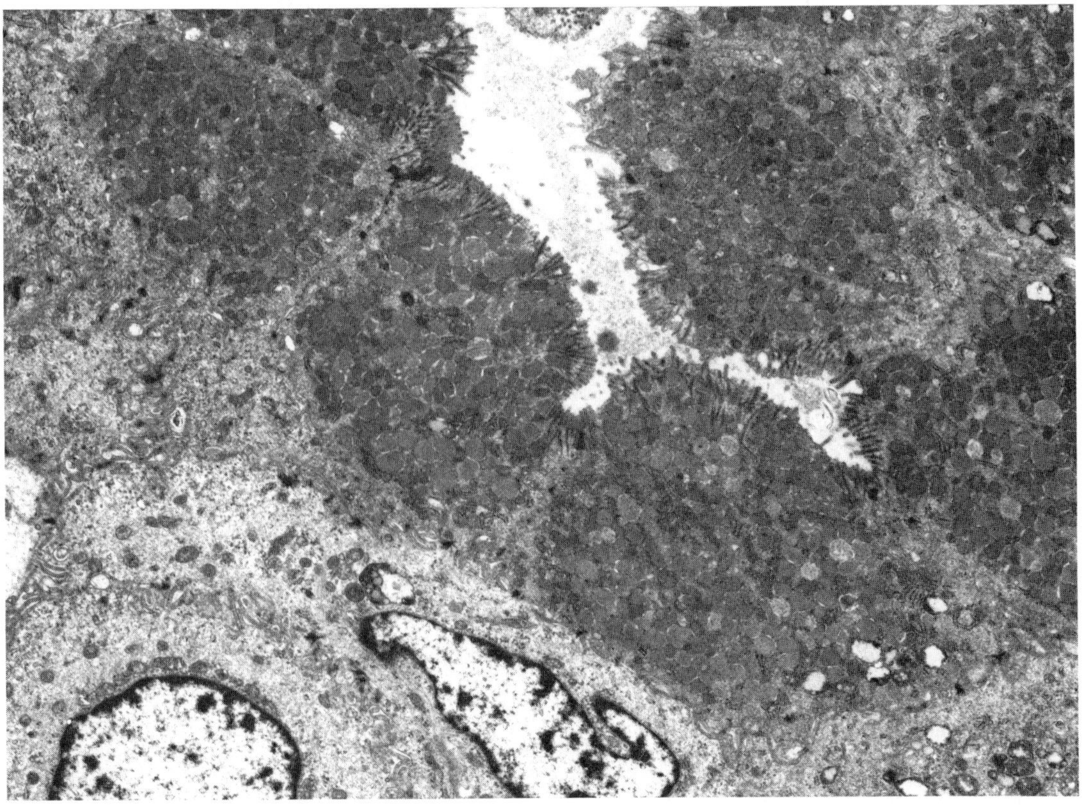

Figure 6–69. Bronchioloalveolar adenocarcinoma. Marked accumulation of mucin droplets in the apical cytoplasm of the tumor cells. (×5,600)

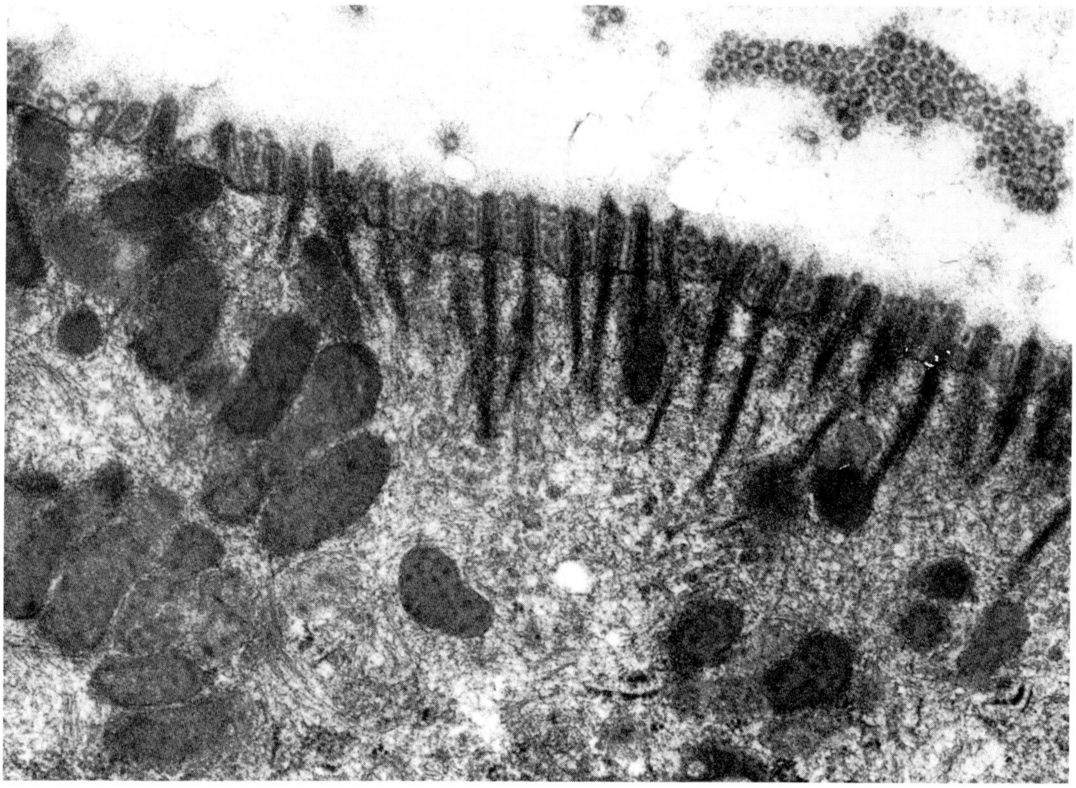

Figure 6–70. Bronchioloalveolar adenocarcinoma. The microvilli contain cores of actin filaments, and glycocalyceal bodies are present. (×30,000)

adenocarcinomas, 13 bronchioloalveolar adenocarcinomas, and 11 adenosquamous carcinomas. Of these, 19 (13 adenocarcinomas, 4 bronchioloalveolar adenocarcinomas, 2 adenosquamous carcinomas) contained cell surface microvilli with microvillous core rootlets and/or glycocalyceal bodies. On subsequent clinical follow-up, three were found to be metastatic colon carcinomas, but the remaining 16 were presumed to be primary lesions.

The nature of the nuclear inclusions in cells of some bronchioloalveolar adenocarcinomas has been clarified by electron microscopy (Figs. 6–71 and 6–72).[180, 185] They are formed of a complex of anastomosing tubules created by elaborate reduplication of the inner layer of the nuclear envelope. We find that they are only present in occasional tumors. They can also be seen in metastases, and they may stain for the apoprotein portion of surfactant. Nuclear inclusions were present in some of the cells of each of the eight cases of papillary adenocarcinoma studied by Horie and associates[60]; and the inclusions had tubular, granular, crystalline, and homogeneously dense structures.

Dedifferentiation in a bronchioloalveolar adenocarcinoma is difficult to assess because this tumor can coexist with a typical acinar adenocarcinoma. However, the ultrastructural finding of dense granules of Clara cell caliber is an indication of bronchioloalveolar adenocarcinoma differentiation. These granules can be found in some tumors diagnosed by light microscopy as acinar adenocarcinomas or even as poorly differentiated or undifferentiated large cell carcinomas (Figs. 6–73 and 6–74). When they are only present in small numbers, it can be difficult to distinguish the granules from lysosomes, but their presence is an indication that complete separation of bronchioloalveolar adenocarcinomas and acinar adenocarcinomas is difficult by conventional light microscopy and that the tumors classified as bronchioloalveolar adenocarcinomas by light microscopy are the well-differentiated neoplasms.

When lamellar bodies are detected during ultrastructural evaluation of a bronchioloalveolar adenocarcinoma, the finding will suggest type II pneumocyte differentiation. In our experience, it is uncommon, but it un-

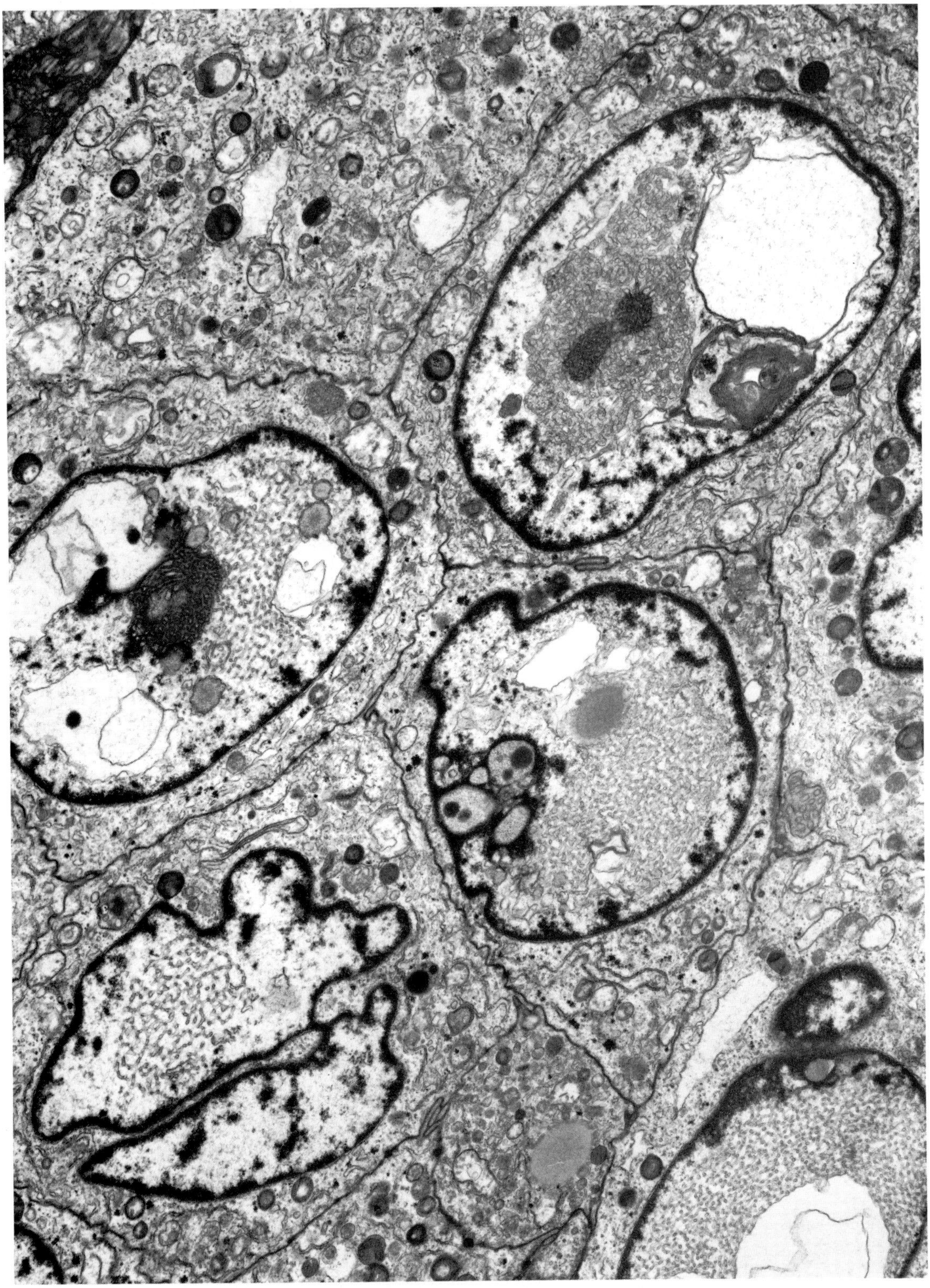

Figure 6–71. Bronchioloalveolar adenocarcinoma. The cells contain nuclear inclusions. (×9,600)

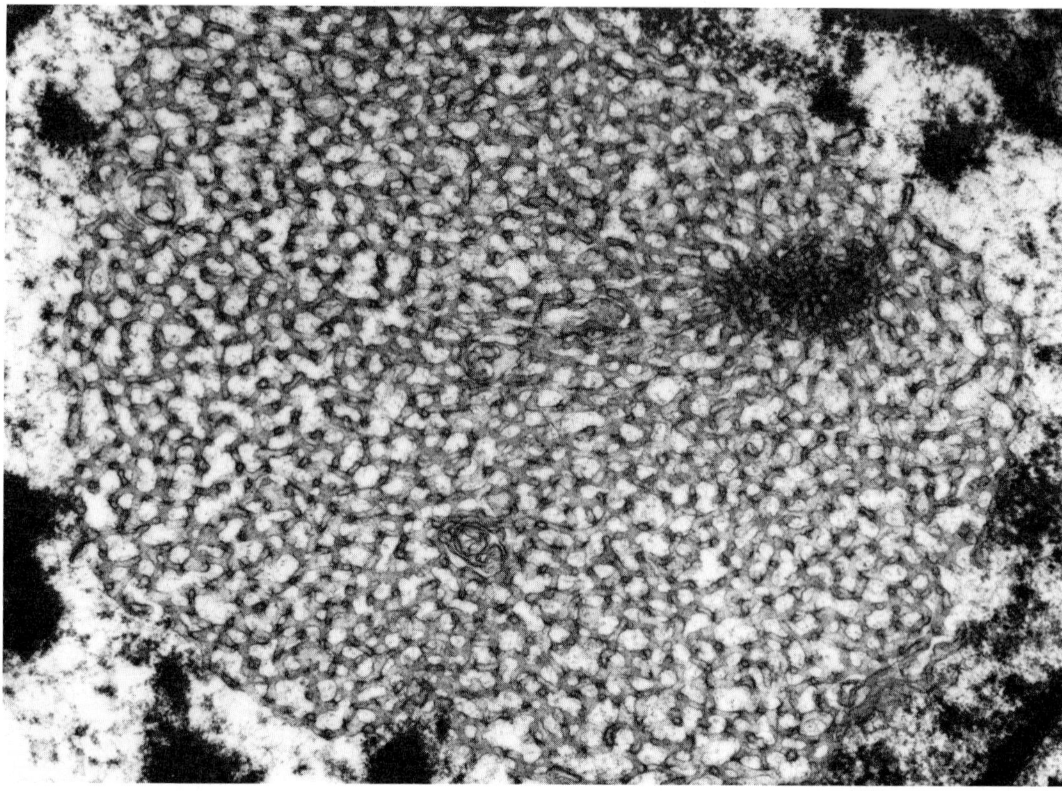

Figure 6–72. Bronchioloalveolar adenocarcinoma. The nuclear inclusions are formed of anastomosing tubules contiguous with the inner layer of the nuclear envelope. (×24,000)

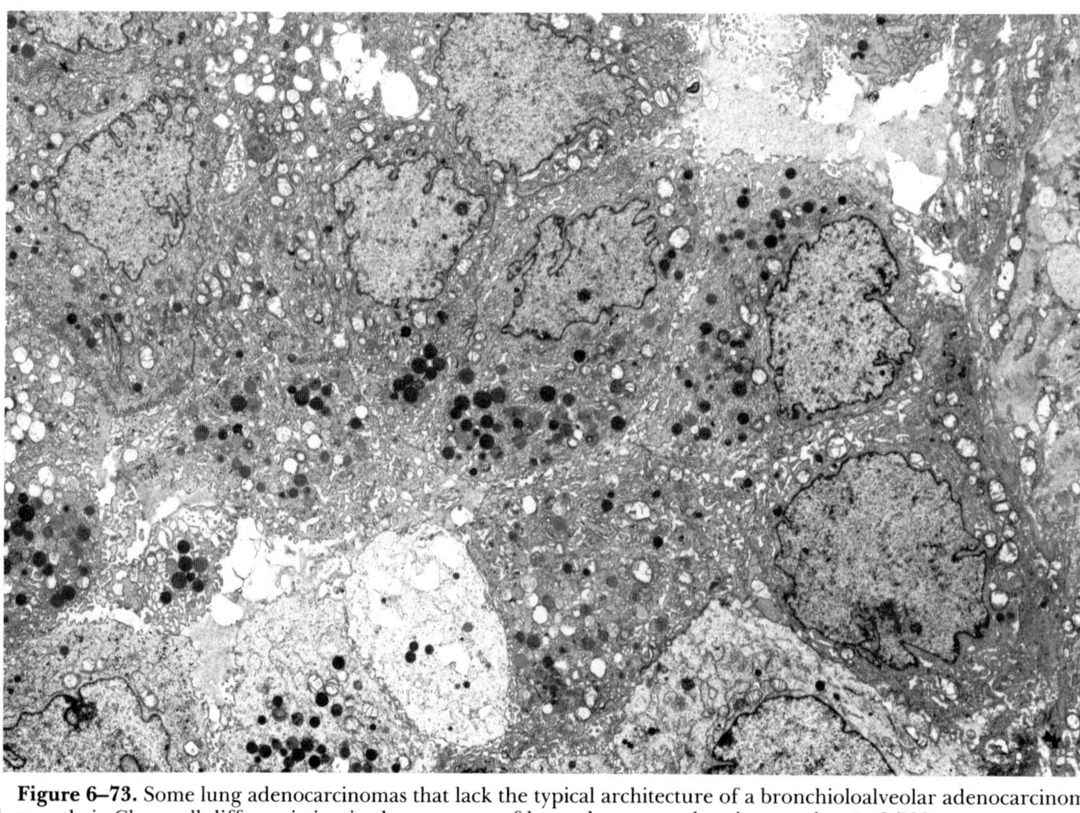

Figure 6–73. Some lung adenocarcinomas that lack the typical architecture of a bronchioloalveolar adenocarcinoma betray their Clara cell differentiation in the presence of large dense cytoplasmic granules. (×2,700)

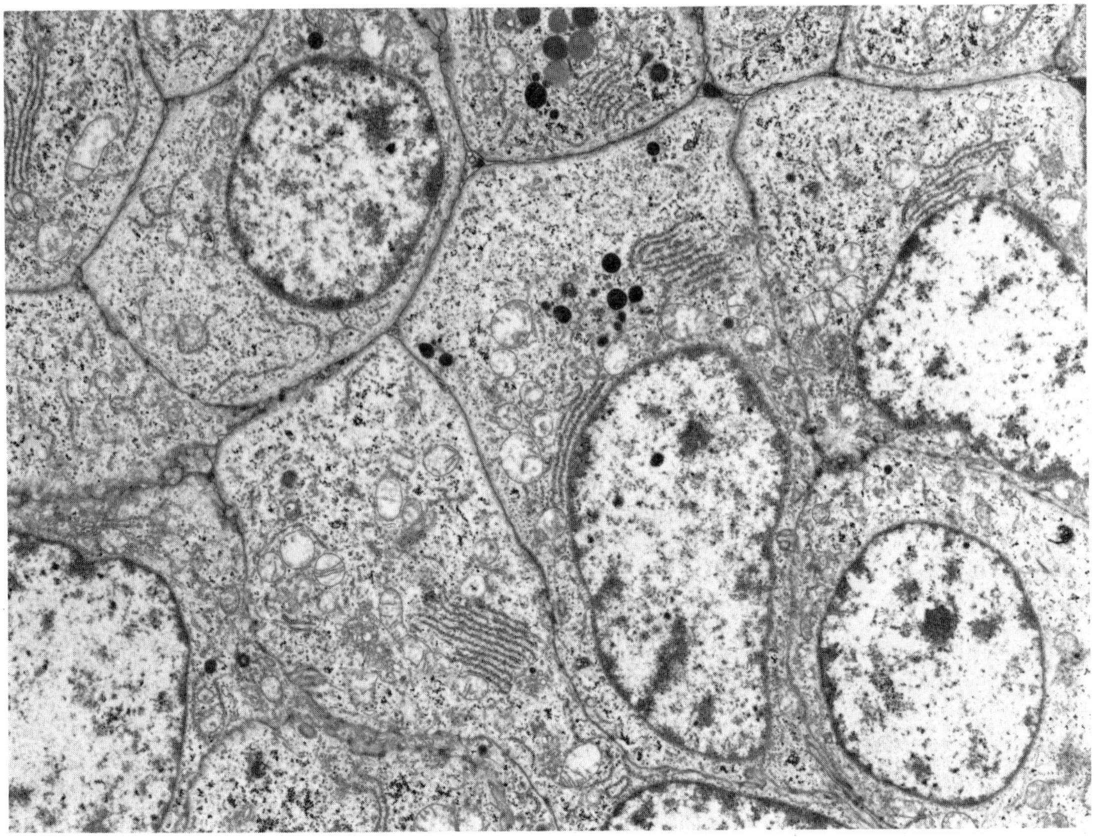

Figure 6–74. A small number of granules of this type is a common finding in lung adenocarcinomas. (×4,000)

doubtedly occurs and surfactant secretion by the tumor cells has been described at the ultrastructural level.[190] If the lamellar bodies are only present in an occasional cell or small group of cells, the possibility of entrapment (Fig. 6–75) should be kept in mind. When sections from the periphery of a bronchioloalveolar adenocarcinoma are examined with the electron microscope, large numbers of hyperplastic pneumocytes are likely to be seen (Fig. 6–76); again, they must not be confused with tumor cells. Careful correlation of the ultrastructural observations with light microscopy of 1-μm sections of the same plastic tissue blocks is indicated in these situations.

ANALYTICAL CYTOLOGY

A number of reports have indicated that flow cytometry and image analysis have potential in evaluating the prognosis of primary lung carcinomas. Fifty-four percent of the 101 tumors (including 22 adenocarcinomas) studied with flow cytometry by Tirindelli-Danesi and colleagues[179] showed evidence of more than one aneuploid cell line, but the incidence of this finding was statistically different in surgical cases where sampling of multiple sites from the primary tumor and lymph nodes was possible compared with material from a single site such as bronchial washings. Chassevent and co-workers[15] performed flow cytometry on 71 surgically resected lung cancers and 145 bronchoscopic biopsies. Abnormal DNA stem lines were frequently observed in the operated lung carcinomas (87%), and the mean DNA index was highest for adenocarcinoma. Asamura and co-workers[3] studied 46 stage I adenocarcinomas by flow cytometry and concluded that nuclear DNA content is a good predictor of prognosis, but that its prognostic contribution increases in more differentiated and smaller tumors, compared with less differentiated and larger tumors. Cibas and associates[16] compared tumor size and DNA distribution in 93 stage I adenocarcinomas and found no significant difference in sur-

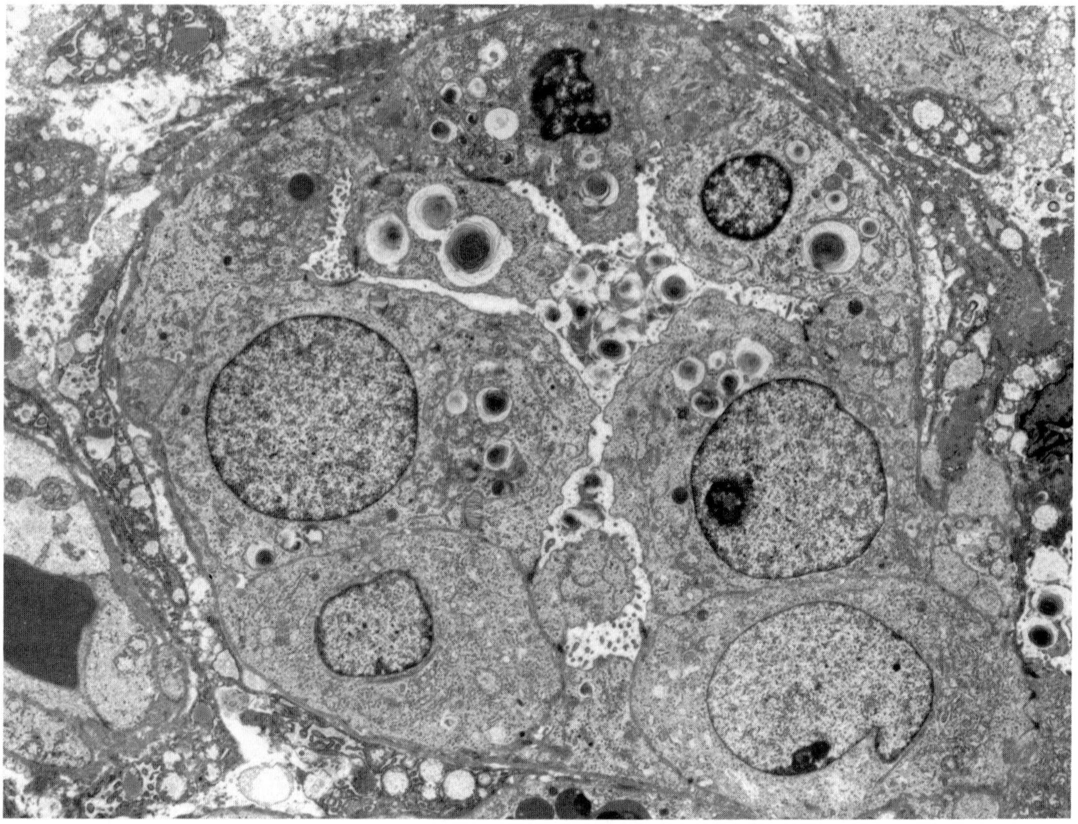

Figure 6–75. Lamellar bodies comparable to those seen in type II pneumocytes are an uncommon finding in bronchioloalveolar adenocarcinoma cells, and distinction from entrapped reactive pneumocytes can be difficult or impossible. (×3,600)

vival between patients with diploid (15%) and aneuploid (85%) tumors. However, patients with tumors smaller than 3 cm in diameter (the median was 2.5 cm) had a significantly better prognosis than those with larger tumors. Flow cytometry on 49 non–small cell tumors, including 14 adenocarcinomas, was reported by Teodori and co-workers.[178] The adenocarcinomas exhibited multiclonal cell populations with one to five aneuploid clones. Nishimiya and associates[125] assessed nuclear DNA in 4-μm sections of lung tumors from 58 patients who survived for at least 5 years. Twenty-five were adenocarcinomas, and some were composed of a majority of diploid cells, whereas in all the squamous cell carcinomas the majority of the cells had DNA values exceeding the normal tetraploid and or diploid region. The authors concluded that the DNA measurements do not add any significant prognostic information to that obtained by morphologic diagnosis.

In a morphometric comparison of the nuclei of adenocarcinoma cells with those of nonneoplastic cells, Kodama and colleagues[80] determined the mean nuclear areas in 10 well-differentiated adenocarcinomas and compared them with alveolar cuboidal cell hyperplasia, including some atypical examples. The mean and standard deviation of the nuclear areas in the adenocarcinomas were significantly larger than in the hyperplastic and atypical cells. The size range of adenocarcinoma nuclei overlaps those of squamous cell and undifferentiated large cell carcinomas.[98]

DIFFERENTIAL DIAGNOSIS

In histologic sections, lung adenocarcinoma can resemble colon adenocarcinoma and some primary lung adenocarcinomas may be analogous to the intestinal type of adenocarcinomas that occurs in the nasal cavity. It may then be difficult to distinguish between a primary lung adenocarcinoma and a metastasis, and the problem is a particularly difficult one if the patient has a history of colon cancer or when the decision has to be

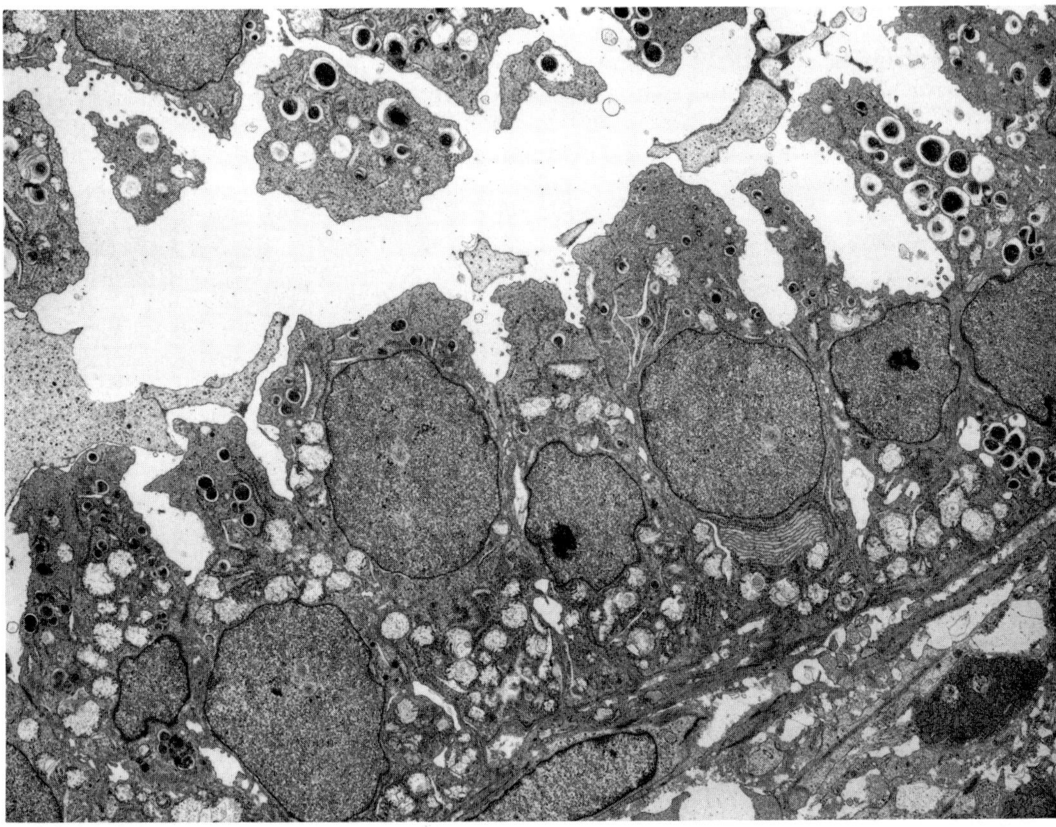

Figure 6–76. Reactive pneumocytes containing lamellar bodies at the periphery of a bronchioloalveolar adenocarcinoma. (×4,000)

based on evaluation of a frozen section. An educated guess may be the best the pathologist can offer, and the distinction is sometimes impossible. Nou and colleagues[126] examined the problem of excluding other tumors in the differential diagnosis of bronchial adenocarcinoma and found that the main nonbronchial tumors were colorectal and renal carcinomas, while the main misdiagnosed metastatic tumor was pancreatic carcinoma. These investigators advocate that the workup of patients for randomized therapy studies should include, in addition to a careful history and physical examination, renal, colorectal, and gynecologic studies, and the possibility of a pancreatic primary lesion should be excluded. They believe that the primary lesion may not be detected in 10% of patients.

CYTOGENETIC STUDIES

Cytogenetic studies have shown chromosome abnormalities in lung adenocarcinomas. Multiple structural aberrations have been found. Loss of heterozygosity on chromosome 3p was detected in primary[202] and metastatic[141] adenocarcinomas. Weston and associates[197] studied 54 non–small cell lung carcinomas, including 23 adenocarcinomas, and found that loss of heterozygosity was seen more often in squamous cell carcinoma than in adenocarcinoma, leading the authors to postulate that the frequent DNA sequence deletions seen in squamous cell carcinomas may reflect the mutagenic and clastogenic effects of tobacco smoke causing inactivation of putative tumor-suppressive genes.

BIOLOGIC STUDIES

Most biologic investigations on human lung tumors have focused on small cell carcinomas and carcinoids, but information on adenocarcinomas is accruing from experimental studies. Three recent reports are cited as examples.

Volm and colleagues[192] transplanted 49 lung adenocarcinomas into nude mice. Twenty-one (43%) showed growth, and 7 (14%) could be maintained by serial transplantation. There was no difference in the survival of the mice whether or not their tumors did grow in the first passage. On the other hand, the mice died significantly earlier if a tumor line could be established by serial transplantation.

Rodenhuis and associates[142] reported that Ras gene mutations (all K Ras) were present in 9 of 35 lung adenocarcinomas, and the adenocarcinomas with the mutations tended to be smaller tumors that were less likely to have metastasized to regional lymph nodes at the time of presentation.

The proliferative activity of lung adenocarcinomas has been studied in 52 tumors by Yoshida and co-workers[203] using *in vitro* labeling with bromodeoxyuridine and immunohistochemical staining with anti-BrdU monoclonal antibody. The labeling index values varied more in the adenocarcinomas than in squamous cell or small cell carcinomas examined as controls, and they were low for the goblet cell type and type II alveolar cell type, were intermediate for Clara cell type tumors, and showed wide variation in tumors of the bronchial surface epithelial cell type. The labeling index showed a correlation with the TNM classification, histologic differentiation, degree of nuclear atypia, and mitotic cell count, so it may be a useful prognostic factor.

REFERENCES

1. Adler JJ et al: Recurrence of bronchiolar carcinoma 19 years after resection. NY State J Med 83:1037, 1983.
2. Anton-Culver H, Culber BD, Kurosaki T et al: Incidence of lung cancer by histological type from a population-based registry. Cancer Res 48:6590, 1988.
3. Asamura H, Nakajima T, Mukai K et al: Nuclear DNA content by cytofluorometry of stage I adenocarcinoma of the lung in relation to postoperative recurrence. Chest 96:312, 1989.
4. Auerbach O, Garfinkel L, Parks VR: Scar cancer of the lung: Increase over a 21-year period. Cancer 43:636, 1979.
5. Axiotis CA, Jennings TA: Observations on bronchioloalveolar carcinoma with special emphasis on localized lesion: A clinicopathological, ultrastructural, and immunohistochemical study of 11 cases. Am J Surg Pathol 12:918, 1988.
6. Balis JU, Paterson JF, Paciga JE et al: Distribution and subcellular localization of surfactant-associated glycoproteins in human lung. Lab Invest 52:687, 1985.
7. Banner BF, Gould VE, Radosevich JA et al: Application of monoclonal antibody 44-3A6 in the cytodiagnosis and classification of pulmonary carcinomas. Diagn Cytopathol 1:300, 1985.
8. Bhattacharyya SN, Lynn WS: Structural characterization of a glycoprotein isolated from alveoli of

patients with alveolar proteinosis. J Biol Chem 254:5191, 1979.

9. Blobel GA, Moll R, Franke WW et al: Cytokeratins in normal lung and lung carcinomas: I. Adenocarcinomas, squamous cell carcinomas, and cultured cell lines. Virchows Arch [B] 45:407, 1984.
10. Bolen JW, Thorning D: Histogenetic classification of pulmonary carcinoma: Peripheral adenocarcinomas studied by light microscopy, histochemistry, and electron microscopy. Pathol Annu (part 1) 17:77, 1982.
11. Bonikos DS, Hendrickson M, Bensch KG: Pulmonary alveolar cell carcinoma: Fine structural and *in vitro* study of a case and critical review of this entity. Am J Surg Pathol 1:93, 1977.
12. Brockmann M, Brockmann I, Herberg U et al: Adenocarcinomas of the lung: Immunocytochemical findings (keratin/CEA). J Cancer Clin Res Oncol 113:379, 1987.
13. Brolly F, Schmitz C, Orion B et al: Uninodular bronchioloalveolar cancer: Apropos of 5 cases with a prolonged course. Rev Pneumol Clin 43:271, 1987
14. Cagle PT, Cohle SD, Greenberg SD: Natural history of pulmonary scar cancers: Clinical and pathologic implications. Cancer 56:2031, 1985.
15. Chassevent A, Berruchon J, Bertrand G et al: Flow DNA analysis in human lung cancer: Potentiality and limitations due to sampling methods. Biol Cell 58:121, 1986.
16. Cibas ES, Melamed MR, Zaman MB et al: The effect of tumor size and tumor cell DNA content on the survival of patients with stage I adenocarcinoma of the lung. Cancer 63:1522, 1989.
17. Clayton F: Bronchioloalveolar carcinomas: Cell types, patterns of growth, and prognostic correlates. Cancer 57:1555, 1986.
18. Clayton F: The spectrum and significance of bronchioloalveolar carcinomas. Pathol Annu 23:361, 1988.
19. Cooper D, Schermer A, Sun TT: Classification of human epithelia and their neoplasms using monoclonal antibodies to keratins: Strategies, applications, and limitations. Lab Invest 52:243, 1985.
20. Cox JD, Barber-Derus S, Hartz AJ et al: Is adenocarcinoma/large cell carcinoma the most radiocurable cancer of the lung. Int J Radiat Oncol Biol Phys 12:1801, 1986.
21. Csako G, Chandra P: Bronchioloalveolar carcinoma presenting with meningeal carcinomatosis: Cytologic diagnosis of cerebrospinal fluid. Acta Cytol 30:653, 1986.
22. Cutz E, Conen PE: Ultrastructure and cytochemistry of Clara cells. Am J Pathol 62:127, 1971.
23. Dairaku M, Sueishi K, Tanaka K et al: Immunohistological analysis of surfactant-apoprotein in the bronchioloalveolar carcinoma. Virchows Arch [A] 400:223, 1983.
24. Debus E, Moll R, Franke WW et al: Immunohistochemical distinction of human carcinomas by cytokeratin typing with monoclonal antibodies. Am J Pathol 114:121, 1984.
25. Dempo K, Satoh M, Tsuji S et al: Immunohistochemical studies in the expression of pulmonary surfactant apoproteins in human lung carcinomas using monoclonal antibodies. Pathol Res Pract 182:669, 1987.
26. Ding JA: Lung cancer in the young adult and results of surgical treatment. Chung Hua Chung Liu Tsa Chih 8:67, 1986.
27. Dodds L, Davis S, Polissar L: A population based study of lung cancer incidence trends by histologic type, 1974–81. JNCI 76:21, 1986.
28. Ebihara Y, Sagawa H: Mucin-producing bronchioloalveolar cell carcinoma: With special reference to a characteristic structure revealed by phosphotungstic acid–hematoxylin staining. Acta Cytol 30:643, 1986.
29. Edwards C, Carlile A: Clear cell carcinoma of the lung. J Clin Pathol 38:880, 1985.
30. Edwards CW: Alveolar carcinoma: A review. Thorax 39:166, 1984.
31. Edwards CW: Pulmonary adenocarcinoma: Review of 106 cases and proposed new classification. J Clin Pathol 40:125, 1987.
32. Eimoto T, Teshima K, Shirakusa T et al: Ultrastructure of well-differentiated adenocarcinomas of the lung with special reference to bronchioloalveolar carcinoma. Ultrastruct Pathol 8:177, 1985.
33. Elema JD, Keuning HM: The use of electron microscopy for the diagnosis of cancer in bronchial biopses. Hum Pathol 19:304, 1988.
34. Elson CE, Moore SP, Johnston WW: Morphologic and immunocytochemical studies of bronchioloalveolar carcinoma at Duke University Medical Center, 1968–1986. Anal Quant Cytol Histol 11:261, 1989.
35. Engstrand DA et al: Limitations of the usefulness of microvillous ultrastructure in distinguishing between carcinoma primary in and metastatic to the lung. Ultrastruct Pathol 11:53, 1987.
36. Erozan YS: Cytopathologic diagnosis of pulmonary neoplasms in sputum and bronchoscopic specimens. Semin Diagn Pathol 3:188, 1986.
37. Espinoza CG, Balis JU, Saba SR et al: Ultrastructural and immunohistochemical studies of bronchioloalveolar carcinoma. Cancer 54:2182, 1984.
38. Evans MJ, Shami SG, Cabral-Anderson LJ et al: Role of nonciliated cells in renewal of bronchial epithelium of rats exposed to NO_2. Am J Pathol 123:126, 1986.
39. Fitzgibbons PL et al: Adenosquamous carcinoma of the lung: A clinical and pathologic study of seven cases. Hum Pathol 16:463, 1985.
40. Fletcher RH: Carcinoembryonic antigen. Ann Intern Med 104:66, 1986.
41. Fraire AE, Roggli VL, Vollmer RT et al: Lung cancer heterogeneity: Prognostic implications. Cancer 60:370, 1987.
42. Franke WW, Schiller M, Hatzfeld M et al: Protein complexes of intermediate-sized filaments: Melting of cytokeratin complexes in urea reveals different polypeptide separation characteristics. Proc Natl Acad Sci USA 80:1713, 1988.
43. Furukawa T, Watanabe S, Kodama T et al: T-zone histiocytes in adenocarcinoma of the lung in relation to postoperative prognosis. Cancer 56:2651, 1985.
44. Gao YT, Blot WJ, Zheng W et al: Lung cancer among Chinese women. Int J Cancer 40:604, 1987.
45. Ghadially FN et al: Diagnostic ultrastructural markers in alveolar cell carcinoma. J Submicrosc Cytol 17:269, 1985.
46. Gown AM, Vogel AM: Monoclonal antibodies to human intermediate filament proteins: II. Dis-

tribution of filament proteins in normal human tissues. Am J Pathol 114:309, 1984.
47. Gown AM, Vogel AM: Monoclonal antibodies to human intermediate filament proteins of human cells: Unique and cross-reacting antibodies. J Cell Biol 95:414, 1982.
48. Gown A, Vogel AM: Monoclonal antibodies to human intermediate filament proteins: III. Analysis of tumors. Am J Clin Pathol 84:413, 1985.
49. Greenberg SD: Histopathology and ultrastructure of bronchioloalveolar carcinoma. In Shimosato Y, Melamed MR, Nettesheim P (eds): Morphogenesis of Lung Cancer, vol 1, p 121. Boca Raton, FL, CRC Press, 1982.
50. Greenberg SD, Fraire AE, Kinner BM et al: Tumor cell type versus staging in the prognosis of carcinoma of the lung. Pathol Annu 22:387, 1987.
51. Hammar S, Bockus D, Remington F et al: The widespread distribution of Langerhans cells in pathologic tissues: An ultrastructural and immunohistochemical study. Hum Pathol 17:894, 1986
52. Hammar SP: Adenocarcinoma and large cell undifferentiated carcinoma of the lung. Ultrastruct Pathol 11:263, 1987.
53. Hammar SP: The use of electron microscopy and immunohistochemistry in the diagnosis and understanding of lung neoplasms. Clin Lab Med 7:1, 1987.
54. Hammar SP: Common neoplasms. In Dail D, Hammar SP (eds): Pulmonary Pathology, p 727. New York, Springer-Verlag, 1988.
55. Hanai A, Whittaker JS, Tateishi R et al: Concordance of histological classification of lung cancer with special reference to adenocarcinoma in Osaka, Japan, and the North-West region of England. Int J Cancer 39:6, 1987.
56. Harwood TR, Gracey DR, Yokoo H: Pseudomesotheliomatous carcinoma of the lung. Am J Clin Pathol 65:159, 1976.
57. Hod I, Herz A, Zimber A: Pulmonary carcinoma (Jaagsiekte) of sheep: Ultrastructural study of early and advanced tumor lesions. Am J Pathol 86:545, 1977.
58. Holmes EC: Editorial: Adenosquamous carcinoma and the biology of lung cancer. Ann Thorac Surg 44:449, 1987.
59. Homma H, Kira S, Takashi Y et al: A case of alveolar cell carcinoma accompanied by fluid and electrolye depletion through production of voluminous amounts of lung liquid. Am Rev Respir Dis 111:857, 1975.
60. Horie A, Kotoo Y, Ohta M et al: Relation of fine structure to prognosis for papillary adenocarcinoma of the lung. Hum Pathol 15:870, 1984.
61. Horiuchi Y, Katsuoka K, Yoshimura H: Acanthosis nigricans and Leser-Trélat sign associated with squamous cell carcinoma and adenocarcinoma of the lung. Int J Dermatol 25:459, 1986.
62. Humphrey PA, Scroggs MW, Roggli VL et al: Pulmonary carcinomas with a sarcomatoid element: An immunocytochemical and ultrastructural analysis. Hum Pathol 19:155, 1988.
63. Hurley P et al: Bronchioloalveolar carcinoma arising in longstanding lung cysts. Thorax 40:960, 1985.
64. Jaques J, Currie W: Bronchioloalveolar carcinoma: A Clara cell tumor. Cancer 40:2171, 1977.
65. Johnston WW: Histologic and cytologic patterns of lung cancer in 2,580 men and women over a 15-year period. Acta Cytol 32:163, 1988.
66. Johnston WW, Szpak CA, Lottich SC et al: Use of monoclonal antibody (B72.3) as an immunocytochemical adjunct to diagnosis of adenocarcinoma in human effusions. Cancer Res 45:1894, 1985.
67. Johnston WW, Szpak CA, Lottich SC et al: Use of a monoclonal antibody (B72.3) as a novel immunohistochemical adjunct for the diagnosis of carcinomas in fine needle aspiration biopsy specimens. Hum Pathol 17:501, 1986.
68. Jung-Legg Y, McGowan SE, Sweeney KG et al: Synchronous triple malignant tumors of the lung: A case report of bronchial carcinoid, small cell carcinoma, and adenocarcinoma of the right lung. Am J Clin Pathol 85:96, 1986.
69. Katyal SL, Singh G: An immunological study of apoproteins of rat lung surfactant. Lab Invest 40:562, 1979.
70. Katyal SL, Singh G: Analysis of pulmonary surfactant apoproteins by electrophoresis. Biochem Biophys Acta 670:323, 1981.
71. Katzenstein A-L, Purvis RJ, Gmelich J et al: Pulmonary resection for metastatic renal adenocarcinoma: Pathologic findings and therapeutic value. Cancer 41:712, 1978.
72. Katzenstein A-L, Prioleau PG, Askin FB: The histologic spectrum and significance of clear-cell change in lung carcinoma. Cancer 45:943, 1980.
73. Kayser K, Ernst M, Stute H et al: Invasion of human lung carcinoma into cartilage of the bronchus. Invasion Metastasis 7:242, 1987.
74. Keikkila L, Mattila P, Harjula A et al: Tumour growth rate and its relationship to prognosis in bronchioloalveolar and pulmonary adenocarcinoma. Ann Chir Gynaecol 74:210, 1985.
75. Kimula Y: A histochemical and ultrastructural study of adenocarcinoma of the lung. Am J Surg Pathol 2:253, 1978.
76. King RJ, Klass DJ, Gikas EG et al: Isolation of apoproteins from canine surface active material. Am J Physiol 224:799, 1973.
77. King RJ: Pulmonary surfactant. J Appl Physiol 53:1, 1982.
78. Kish JK, Ro JY, Ayala AG et al: Primary mucinous adenocarcinoma of the lung with signet-ring cells: A histochemical comparison with signet-ring cell carcinoma of other sites. Hum Pathol 20:1097, 1989.
79. Kloppel G, Caselitz J: Epithelial tumor markers: Oncofetal antigens (carcinoembryonic antigen, alpha-fetoprotein, and epithelial membrane antigen) In Seifert G (ed): Current Topics in Pathology, Vol 77, Morphological Tumor Markers: General Aspects and Diagnostic Relevance, p 103. New York, Springer-Verlag, 1987.
80. Kodama T, Biyajima S, Watanabe S et al: Morphometric study of adenocarcinomas and hyperplastic epithelial lesions in the peripheral lung. Am J Clin Pathol 85:146, 1986.
81. Kodama T, Koide T, Shimosato Y et al: Six cases of well-differentiated adenocarcinoma simulating fetal lung tubules in pseudoglandular stage. Am J Surg Pathol 8:735, 1984.
82. Kodama T, Watanabe S, Shimosato Y et al: Endobronchial polypoid adenocarcinoma of the

lung: Histological and ultrastructural studies of five cases. Am J Surg Pathol 8:845, 1984.
83. Kolin A: Letter: Pulmonary scar cancers. Hum Pathol 20:605, 1989.
84. Kolin A, Koutoulakis T: Role of arterial occlusion in pulmonary scar cancers. Hum Pathol 19:1161, 1988.
85. Komatsu H et al: A lucky case of pulmonary adenocarcinoma in 24-year-old female and the clinical and pathological studies on the pulmonary carcinoma occurring in younger patients. J Jpn Assoc Thorac Surg 28:11, 1980.
86. Kuhlman JE, Fishman EK, Kuhajda FP et al: Solitary bronchioloalveolar carcinoma: CT criteria. Radiology 167:379, 1988.
87. Kung IT: Letter: Pulmonary scar cancers. Hum Pathol 20:605, 1989
88. Kung IT, Lui IO, Loke SL et al: Pulmonary scar cancer: A pathologic reappraisal. Am J Surg Pathol 9:391, 1985.
89. Kuroki Y, Dempo K, Akino T: Immunohistochemical study of human pulmonary surfactant apoproteins with monoclonal antibodies: Pathologic applications for hyaline membrane disease. Am J Pathol 124:25, 1986.
90. Larrieu AJ, Jamieson WR, Nelems JM et al: Carcinoma of the lung in patients under 40 years of age. Am J Surg 149:602, 1985.
91. Libshitz HI, McKenna RJ Jr, Mountain CF: Patterns of mediastinal metastases in bronchogenic carcinoma. Chest 90:229, 1986.
92. Liebow AA: Bronchioloalveolar carcinoma. Adv Intern Med 10:329, 1960.
93. Lin JI et al: Pseudomesotheliomatous carcinoma of the lung. South Med J 73:655, 1980.
94. Linnoila RI, Mulshine JL, Steinberg SM et al: Neuroendocrine differentiation in endocrine and nonendocrine lung carcinomas. Am J Clin Pathol 90:641, 1988.
95. Lozowski W, Hajdu SI: Cytology and immunocytochemistry of bronchioloalveolar carcinoma. Acta Cytol 31:717, 1987.
96. Mackay AM, Patel S, Carter S et al: Role of serial CEA assays in detection of recurrent and metastatic colorectal carcinoma. Br Med J 4:382, 1974.
97. Mackay B, Ordonez NG: The role of the pathologist in the evaluation of poorly differentiated tumors and metastatic tumors of unknown origin. In Greco FA, Oldham PC, Fer M (eds): Tumors of Unknown Origin and Poorly Differentiated Neoplasms. New York, Grune & Stratton, 1986.
98. Mackay B, Ordonez NG, Bennington JL et al: Ultrastructural and morphometric features of poorly differentiated and undifferentiated lung tumors. Ultrastruct Pathol 13:561, 1989.
99. Madri JA, Carter D: Scar cancers of the lung: Origin and significance. Hum Pathol 15:625, 1984.
100. Makin CA, Bobrow LG, Bodmer WF: Monoclonal antibody to cytokeratin for use in routine histopathology. J Clin Pathol 37:975, 1984.
101. Malassez L: Examin histologique d'un cas de cancer encephaloïde du poumon (epithelioma). Arch Physiol Nor Pathol 3:353, 1875.
102. Manning JT, Spjut HJ, Tschen JA: Bronchioloalveolar carcinoma: The significance of two histopathologic types. Cancer 54:525, 1984.
103. McElvaney G, Miller RR, Muller NL et al: Multicentricity of adenocarcinoma of the lung. Chest 95:151, 1989.
104. McGregor DH, Dixon A, McGregor DK: Adenocarcinoma of the lung: A comparative diagnostic study using light and electron microscopy. Hum Pathol 19:910, 1988.
105. McGregor DH, Papasian CJ, Pierce PD: Aspergilloma within cavitating pulmonary adenocarcinoma. Am J Clin Pathol 91:100, 1989.
106. Melamed MR, Flehinger BJ: Detection of lung cancer: Highlights of the Memorial Sloan-Kettering Study in New York City. Schweiz Med Wochenschr 117:1457, 1987.
107. Miettinen M: Synaptophysin and neurofilament proteins as markers for neuroendocrine tumors. Arch Pathol Lab Med 111:813, 1987.
108. Miller RR, Nelems B, Evans KG et al: Glandular neoplasia of the lung: A proposed analogy to colonic tumors. Cancer 61:1009, 1988.
109. Mizutani Y, Nakajima T, Morinaga S et al: Immunohistochemical localization of pulmonary surfactant apoproteins in various lung tumors: Special reference to non-mucus-producing lung adenocarcinomas. Cancer 61:532, 1988.
110. Moll R: Diversity of cytokeratins in carcinomas. Acta Histochem (Jena) vol. 34 (suppl.):37, 1987.
111. Moll R, Franke WW: Cytochemical cell typing of metastatic tumors according to their cytoskeletal proteins. In Lapis K, Liotta LA, Rabson AS (eds): Biochemistry and Molecular Genetics of Cancer Metastasis, p 101. New York, Martinus Nijhoff, 1986.
112. Moll R, Franke WW, Schiller DL et al: The catalog of human cytokeratins: Patterns of expression in normal epithelia, tumors and cultured cells. Cell 31:11, 1982.
113. Montes M, Binette JP, Chaudruy AP et al: Clara cell adenocarcinoma: Light and electron microscope study. Am J Surg Pathol 1:245, 1977.
114. Morita T, Sugano H: Lung cancer cases reported in the annual pathological autopsy cases in Japan (1958–1982), with special reference to the characteristics of lung cancer in Japan. Gan No Rinsho 34:416, 1988.
115. Morningstar WA, Hassan MO: Bronchioloalveolar carcinoma with nodal metastases: An ultrastructural study. Am J Surg Pathol 3:273, 1979.
116. Mountain CF, Lukeman JM, Hammar SP et al: Lung cancer classification: The relationship of disease extent and cell type to survival in a clinical trials population. J Surg Oncol 35:147, 1987.
117. Mughal AW, Hortobagyi GN, Fritsche HA et al: Serial plasma carcinoembryonic antigen measurements during treatment of metastatic breast cancer. JAMA 249:1881, 1983.
118. Muller-Hermelink HK, Kaiserling E: Pulmonary adenocarcinoma of fetal type: Alternating differentiation argues in favour of a common endodermal stem cell. Virchows Arch [A] 409:195, 1986.
119. Myers EA, Hardman JM, Worsham GF et al: Adenocarcinoma of the lung causing ectopic adrenocorticotrophic hormone syndrome. Arch Intern Med 142:1387, 1982.
120. Nakajima T, Kodama T, Tsumuraya M et al: S-100 protein–positive Langerhans' cells in various human lung cancers, especially in peripheral

adenocarcinomas. Virchows Arch [A] 407:177, 1985.

121. Nakanishi K, Kawai T, Suzuki M: Large intracytoplasmic body in lung cancer compared with Clara cell granule. Am J Clin Pathol 88:472, 1987.
122. Naunheim KS, Taylor JR, Skosey C et al: Adenosquamous lung carcinoma: Clinical characteristics, treatment, and prognosis. Ann Thorac Surg 44:462, 1987.
123. Nelson WG, Sun TT: The 50- and 58-K dalton keratin classes as molecular markers for stratified squamous epithelia: Cell culture studies. J Cell Biol 97:244, 1983.
124. Neville AM, Cooper EH: Biochemical monitoring of cancer: A review. Ann Clin Biochem 13:283, 1976.
125. Nishiyama K, Auer GU, Erhardt K et al: Nuclear DNA in histologic sections from squamous-cell carcinoma and adenocarcinoma of the lung. Anal Quant Cytol Histol 7:153, 1985.
126. Nou E: Bronchial adenocarcinoma: The value of attempts to exclude other primary tumors for randomized studies in epidemiologic material. Cancer 48:2121, 1981.
127. Nou E: The natural five-year course in bronchial carcinoma: Epidemiologic results. Cancer 53:2211, 1984.
128. Ogata T, Endo K: Clara cell granules of peripheral lung cancers. Cancer 54:1635, 1984.
129. Ohtsuki H, Midorikawa O, Okada H et al: Pulmonary atypical carcinoid tumor with marked alpha-fetoprotein production and features of adenocarcinoma differentiation. Pathol Res Pract 184:86, 1988.
130. Ordonez NG: The immunohistochemical diagnosis of mesothelioma: Differentiation of mesothelioma and lung adenocarcinoma. Am J Surg Pathol 13:276, 1989.
131. Ordonez NG, Manning JT Jr, Brooks TE: Effect of trypsinization on the immunostaining of formalin-fixed, paraffin-embedded tissues. Am J Surg Pathol 12:121, 1988.
132. Osborn N, Weber K: Tumor diagnosis by intermediate filament typing: A novel tool for surgical pathology. Lab Invest 48:372, 1983.
133. Otis CN, Carter D, Cole S et al: Immunohistochemical evaluation of pleural mesothelioma and pulmonary adenocarcinoma. Am J Surg Pathol 17:445, 1987.
134. Perentes E, Rubinstein LJ: Recent applications of immunoperoxidase histochemistry in human neuro-oncology. Arch Pathol Lab Med 111:796, 1987.
135. Pilotti S, Rilke F, Lombardi L: Pulmonary carcinoid with glandular features: Report of two cases with positive fine needle aspiration biopsy cytology. Acta Cytol 27:511, 1983.
136. Pisani RJ, Krco CJ, Wold WE et al: Lymphokine-activated killer (LAK) cell activity in tumor-infiltrating lymphocytes from non–small cell lung cancer. Am J Clin Pathol 92:435, 1989.
137. Pritchard MG, Brown PJ, Sterrett GF: Bronchioloalveolar carcinoma arising in longstanding lung cysts. Thorax 39:545, 1984.
138. Radosevich JA, Ma YX, Lee I et al: Monoclonal antibody 44-3A6 as a probe for a novel antigen found on human lung carcinomas with glandular differentiation. Cancer Res 45:5808, 1985.
139. Rainio P: Ultrastructure of neoplastic cells in different histologic subtypes of pulmonary adenocarcinoma. Pathol Res Pract 176:236, 1983.
140. Ramos-Yeo YL, Reyes CV: Myasthenic syndrome (Eaton-Lambert syndrome) associated with pulmonary adenocarcinoma. J Surg Oncol 34:239, 1987.
141. Rey JA, Bello MJ, de-Campos JM et al: Deletion 3p in two lung adenocarcinomas metastatic to the brain. Cancer Genet Cytogent 25:355, 1987.
142. Rodenhuis S, Slebos RJ, Boot AJ et al: Incidence and possible clinical significance of K-ras oncogene activation in adenocarcinoma of the human lung. Cancer Res 48:5738, 1988.
143. Roggli VL, Vollmer RT, Greenberg SD et al: Lung cancer heterogeneity: A blinded and randomized study of 100 consecutive cases. Hum Pathol 16:569, 1985.
144. Roviaro GC, Varoli F, Zannini P et al: Lung cancer in the young. Chest 87:456, 1985.
145. Rubinstein I, Baum GL, Bubis JJ et al: Prognosis of patients with adenocarcinoma of the lung and mediastinal lymph node metastases undergoing pulmonary resection. Respiration 47:70, 1985.
146. Saba SR, Espinoza CG, Richman AV et al: Carcinomas of the lung: An ultrastructural and immunocytochemical study. Am J Clin Pathol 80:6, 1980.
147. Salisbury JR, Darby AJ, Whimster WF: Papillary adenocarcinoma of lung with psammoma bodies: Report of a case derived from type II pneumocytes. Histopathology 10:877, 1986.
148. Sasou S, Takayama K, Iwasaki T et al: Crystals and psammoma bodies in adenocarcinoma of the lung. Gan No Rinsho 32:520, 1986.
149. Scarratt WK, Sponenberg DP, Collins TJ et al: Bronchiolar adenocarcinoma in a cow. J Am Vet Med Assoc 185:1549, 1984.
150. Scroggs MW, Roggli VL, Fraire AE et al: Eosinophilic intracytoplasmic globules in pulmonary adenocarcinomas: A histochemical, immunohistochemical, and ultrastructural study of six cases. Hum Pathol 20:845, 1989.
151. Shani A, O'Connell MJ, Moertel CG et al: Serial plasma carcinoembryonic antigen measurements in the management of metastatic colorectal carcinoma. Ann Intern Med 89:625, 1978.
152. Shapiro R, Wilson GL, Yesner R et al: A useful roentgen sign in the diagnosis of localized bronchioloalveolar carcinoma. AJR 114:516, 1949.
153. Shimosato Y, Kodama T, Kameya T: Morphogenesis of peripheral type adenocarcinoma of the lung. In Shimosato, Melamed MR, Nettesheim P (eds): Morphogenesis of Lung Cancer, vol 1, p 65. Boca Raton, FL, CR Press, 1982.
154. Shinkai T, Saijo N, Tominaga K et al: Serial plasma carcinoembryonic antigen measurement for monitoring patients with advanced lung cancer during chemotherapy. Cancer 57:1318, 1986.
155. Shitara K, Hanai N, Yashida H: Distribution of lung adenocarcinoma–associated antigens in human tissues and sera defined by monoclonal antibodies KM-52 and KM-93. Cancer Res 47:1267, 1987.
156. Sider L, Horejs D: Frequency of extrathoracic metastases from bronchogenic carcinoma in patients with normal-size hilar and mediastinal lymph nodes on CT. AJR 151:893, 1988.
157. Sidhu GS, Forrester EM: Glycogen-rich Clara cell-

type bronchioloalveolar carcinoma: Light and electron microscopic study. Cancer 40:2209, 1977.
158. Sidhu GS: The ultrastructure of malignant epithelial neoplasms of the lung. Pathol Annu 20 (part 1):235, 1985.
159. Silverman JF, Finley JL, Park HK et al: Fine needle aspiration cytology of bronchioloalveolar cell carcinoma of the lung. Acta Cytol 29:887, 1985.
160. Singh G, Katyal SL: Surfactant apoprotein in nonmalignant pulmonary disorders. Am J Pathol 101:51, 1980.
161. Singh G, Katyal S, Ordonez et al: Type II pneumocytes in pulmonary tumors. Arch Pathol Lab Med 108:44, 1984.
162. Singh G, Katyal SL, Torikata C: Carcinoma of type II pneumocytes: Immunodiagnosis of a subtype of bronchioloalveolar carcinomas. Am J Pathol 102:195, 1983.
163. Singh G, Scheithauer BW, Katyal L: The pathobiologic features of carcinomas of type II pneumocytes: An immunocytologic study. Cancer 57:994, 1986.
164. Sorensen JB, Hansen HH, Hansen M et al: Brain metastases in adenocarcinoma of the lung: Frequency, risk groups, and prognosis. J Clin Oncol 6:1474, 1988.
165. Sorensen JB, Hirsch FR, Olsen J: The prognostic implication of histopathologic subtyping of pulmonary adenocarcinoma according to the classification of the World Health Organization. Cancer 62:361, 1988.
166. Sorensen JB, Olsen JE: Prognostic implications of histopathologic subtyping in patients with surgically treated stage I or II adenocarcinoma of the lung. J Thorac Cardiovasc Surg 97:245, 1989.
167. Spriggs AI, Cole M, Dunnill MS: Alveolar cell carcinoma: A problem in sputum diagnosis. J Clin Pathol 35:1370, 1982.
168. Springmeyer SC, Hackman R, Carlson YY et al: Bronchioloalveolar cell carcinoma diagnosed by bronchoalveolar lavage. Chest 83:278, 1983.
169. Staab HJ, Brummendorf T, Arderer FA et al: Differentiation of disease recurrence in various primary malignancies using CEA slope analysis. Tumor Biol 6:157, 1985.
170. Stokes TC, Stevens JFS, Long P et al: Preoperative carcinoembryonic antigen and survival after resection of lung carcinoma. Br J Dis Chest 74:390, 1980.
171. Sugimura H, Watanabe S, Tsugane S et al: Case-control study on histologically determined multiple primary lung cancer. JNCI 79:435, 1987.
172. Sun TT, Eichner R, Nelson WG et al: Keratin classes: Molecular markers for different types of epithelial differentiation. J Invest Dermatol 81:1095, 1983.
173. Suzuki Y, Nakai E, Ohkata K: Experimental studies on the pulmonary surfactant reconstitution in surface-active material. J Lipid Res 23:53, 1982.
174. Takahashi A, Fujiwara T: Proteolipid in bovine lung surfactant: Its role in surfactant function. Biochem Biophys Res Commun 135:527, 1986.
175. Takise A, Kodoma T, Shimosato Y et al: Histopathologic prognostic factors in adenocarcinomas of the peripheral lung less than 2 cm in diameter. Cancer 61:2083, 1988.
176. Tao LC, Weisbrod GL, Pearson FG et al: Cytologic diagnosis of bronchioloalveolar carcinoma by fine-needle aspiration biopsy. Cancer 57:1565, 1986.
177. Teeter SM, Holmes FF, McFarlane MJ: Lung carcinoma in the elderly population: Influence of histology on the inverse relationship of stage to age. Cancer 60:1331, 1987.
178. Teodori L, Tirindelli-Danesi D, Mauro F et al: Non–small cell lung carcinoma: Tumor characterization on the basis of flow cytometrically determined cellular heterogeneity. Cytometry 4:174, 1983.
179. Tirindelli-Danesi D, Teodori L et al: Prognostic significance of flow cytometry in lung cancer: A five year study. Cancer 60:844, 1987.
180. Torikata C, Ishiwata K: Intranuclear tubular structures observed in the cells of an alveolar cell carcinoma of the lung. Cancer 40:1194, 1977.
181. Tsai CM, Perng RP, Huang WL: Lung cancer in young Chinese. Cancer Detec Prev 11:235, 1988.
182. Tsuchiya E, Oh S, Kitagawa T et al: The influence of smoking on the development of various subtypes of pulmonary carcinoma. Gan No Rinsho 33:27, 1987.
183. Tsuchiya E, Chan JK, Chan SH et al: Comparative histopathology of resected bronchial cancers of women in Hong Kong and Japan. Int J Cancer 41:661, 1988.
184. Tsukada T, Tippens D, Gordon D et al: HHF35, a muscle actin-specific monoclonal antibody: I. Immunocytochemical and biochemical characterization. Am J Pathol 126:51, 1984.
185. Tsumuraya M et al: Light and electron microscopic analysis of intranuclear inclusions in papillary adenocarcinoma of the lung. Acta Cytol 25:523, 1981.
186. Unterman DH, Reingold IM: The occurrence of psammoma bodies in papillary adenocarcinoma of the lung. Am J Clin Pathol 57:297, 1972.
187. Valaitis J, Warren S, Gamble D: Increasing incidence of adenocarcinoma of the lung. Cancer 47:1042, 1981.
188. Vandekerckhove J, Weber K: At least six different actins are expressed in higher mammals: An analysis based in the amino acid sequence of the aminotryptic peptide. J Mol Biol 126:783, 1978.
189. Varki NM, Reisfeld RA, Walker LE: Antigens associated with a human lung adenocarcinoma defined by monoclonal antibodies. Cancer Res 44:681, 1984.
190. Vazquez M, Sidhu GS: Surfactant production by neoplastic type II pneumocytes. Ultrastruct Pathol 12:605, 1988.
191. Vincent RG, Pickren JW, Land WW: The changing histopathology of lung cancer: A review of 1682 cases. Cancer 39:1647, 1977.
192. Volm M, Mattern J, Vogt-Schaden M et al: Flow cytometric analysis of primary lung carcinomas and their lymph node metastases. Anticancer Res 7:71, 1987.
193. Waakes TP, Abeloff MD, Woo KB et al: Carcinoembryonic antigen for monitoring patients with small-cell carcinoma of the lung during treatment. Cancer Res 40:4420, 1980.
194. Walker SR, Williams MC, Benson B: Immunocytochemical localization of the major surfactant apoproteins in type II cells, Clara cells, and alveolar macrophages of rat lung. J Histochem Cytochem 34:1137, 1986.

195. Ward JM, Singh G, Katyal SL et al: Immunocytochemical localization of the surfactant apoprotein and Clara-cell antigen in chemically induced and naturally occurring pulmonary neoplasms in mice. Am J Pathol 118:439, 1985.
196. Watanabe S, Tsugane S, Arimoto H et al: Trend of lung cancers in the National Cancer Center of Japan and comparison with that of Japanese pathological autopsy records. Jpn J Cancer Res 78:460, 1987.
197. Weston A, Willey JC, Modali R et al: Differential DNA sequence deletions from chromosomes 3, 11, 13, and 17 in squamous-cell carcinoma, large-cell carcinoma, and adenocarcinoma of the human lung. Proc Natl Acad Sci USA 86:5099, 1989.
198. Williams MC, Benson BJ: Immunocytochemical localization and identification of the major surfactant protein in adult rat lung. J Histochem Cytochem 29:291, 1981.
199. Wilmalaratna HS, Sachdeev D: Adenocarcinoma of the lung presenting with Raynaud's phenomenon, digital gangrene and multiple infarctions in the internal organs. Br J Rheumatol 26:473, 1987.
200. World Health Organization Histological Typing of Lung Tumors, 2nd ed. Am J Clin Pathol 77:123, 1982.
201. Wu AH, Henderson BE, Thomas DC et al: Secular trends in histologic types of lung cancer. JNCI 77:53, 1986.
202. Yokota J, Wada M, Shimosato Y et al: Loss of heterozygosity on chromosomes 3, 13, and 17 in small-cell carcinoma and on chromosome 3 in adenocarcinoma of the lung. Proc Natl Sci USA 84:9252, 1987.
203. Yoshida K, Morinaga S, Shimosato Y et al: A cell kinetic study of pulmonary adenocarcinoma by an immunoperoxidase procedure after bromodeoxyuridine labeling. Cancer 64:2284, 1989.
204. Yu SH, Possmayer F: Reconstitution of surfactant activity by using 6-kDa apoprotein associated with pulmonary surfactant. Biochem J 236:85, 1986.
205. Zahm SH, Brownson RC, Chang JC et al: Study of lung cancer histologic types, occupation, and smoking in Missouri. Am J Ind Med 15:565, 1989.
206. Zimber A et al: Heterotransplantation of experimentally induced sheep lung adenomatosis into nude mice. Res Vet Sci 36:122, 1984.
207. Zolliker AS, Jaques J: Clara cell carcinoma of the human lung. Hum Pathol 12:748, 1981.

Chapter

7

SQUAMOUS CELL CARCINOMA

Squamous cell carcinoma is the most common form of lung cancer in many countries. However, reports from the United States and Japan indicate that the relative frequencies of squamous cell carcinoma and adenocarcinoma have altered to the point where adenocarcinoma is more common, especially in women.

Figures vary among reported series, and they are influenced by the disposition of undifferentiated large cell carcinomas, which are often lumped with adenocarcinomas, by the diligence with which a search for glandular features is conducted including the use of mucin stains, by the amount and quality of the material available for study, and by the precision with which specific features are sought and recognized by reviewing pathologists. The Lung Cancer Study Group adopted stringent criteria for their review of 1,121 cases of apparently completely resected non–small cell carcinomas,[32] and 46% were squamous cell carcinomas. Collier and colleagues[9] reported a figure of 45% in their review of 4,117 lung resections. In a study of 2,580 patients with lung cancer at Duke University over a period of 15 consecutive years, Johnston[25] found that during the first 5 years, 43.1% were squamous cell carcinomas. In the second and third 5-year periods, it remained the most common tumor but declined to 35.7%. During this same time interval, adenocarcinoma of acinar type replaced squamous cell carcinoma as the most common lung cancer in women.

Similar findings have been reported from Japan. A large series of autopsied Japanese cases (28,303 men, 9,540 women) were reviewed by Morita and Sugano.[31] Squamous cell carcinoma made up 33% and adenocarcinoma 34%, but 55% of the lung cancers in women were adenocarcinomas while squamous cell carcinomas made up only 18%. As Carter[7] notes, squamous cell carcinomas make up a greater percentage of surgical cases than autopsy cases because of their slower growth and greater tendency to remain localized than the other cell types. Watanabe and associates[48] analyzed 4,419 surgical cases accrued during the 20-year period from 1966 to 1985 at the National Cancer Center Hospital in Japan. The proportions of histologic types in men remained relatively unchanged, about 40% being squamous cell carcinoma, but squamous cancer in women decreased from 21% to 11.4%.

Age and occupation affect the figures. Teeter and co-workers[44] studied 9,062 cases of lung cancer occurring between 1975 and 1984 in Kansas and western Missouri. The proportion of squamous cell carcinomas rose with increasing age, while those of adenocarcinoma and small cell lung carcinoma fell; and the number of cases with local disease at the time of diagnosis also increased with age. In men, this trend was significant for squamous cell carcinoma, and in women squamous cell carcinoma was the only type to show the trend to a significant degree. Tokudome[45] found that 75% of lung cancers in a group of male Japanese copper smelter workers were squamous cell tumors.

SITE AND PATTERN OF GROWTH

A majority of squamous cell carcinomas arise centrally from the major or segmental bronchi. Most central cancers are ulcerated growths that infiltrate through the mucosa into the surrounding lung parenchyma, but a central tumor occasionally forms a papillary endobronchial mass or a polypoid, sessile, or superficially spreading growth. A review of 34 endobronchial carcinomas[13] indicated that there is no significant difference in survival when these tumors are compared with the more common infiltrating, nonexophytic squamous tumors, although metastases to lymph nodes were encountered in only two patients in the series. Carter[7] reviewed 146 preclinical, asymptomatic squamous cell carcinomas and grouped them into three categories: 25% were carcinoma *in situ* without invasion, 42% showed early invasion, and 32% had extensive extrabronchial spread with or without lymph node metastases. The majority of clinically occult tumors are amenable to resection, and the survival figures are high.[7]

SYMPTOMS

Central squamous cell carcinomas vary considerably in size, but most are between 3 and 5 cm at the time they are detected. They give rise to symptoms relatively early because of their proximity to vital structures at the root of the lung. The symptoms are not specific. The most common is a nonproductive cough that is often ignored by the patient, especially if a heavy smoker. An increase in mucus secretion may also be disregarded if there is no accompanying hemoptysis. Many patients with invasive carcinoma are asymptomatic at the time of diagnosis, with the lesion being detected on a routine chest radiograph. More advanced tumors are associated with loss of appetite and weight and fatigue on exertion. Chest pain is a late symptom seen with large tumors. An endobronchial growth may produce obstructive pneumonitis and atelectasis.

DIAGNOSIS

Central squamous cell carcinomas can generally be diagnosed by cytologic examination of sputum, but bronchial washings and brushings, or endoscopic biopsy specimens, may be obtained for confirmation, and they are required when a sputum series is consistently negative. Most of the central lesions are amenable to transbronchial biopsy. Peripheral squamous cell carcinomas may be bulky masses 10 cm or larger, and these tumors tend to outgrow their blood supply. If they undergo central cavitation, they may then be indistinguishable from cavitary tuberculosis on radiography. If a bronchus is in communication with the cavity, hemoptysis may be an initial symptom. Percutaneous fine-needle aspiration biopsy will usually provide acceptable specimens of a peripheral mass for diagnosis, but in order to be diagnostic, the aspirate must contain viable tissue, which is more likely to be found at the periphery of the lesion. An aspirate from the center may only yield blood cells, necrotic debris, inflammatory cells, and clumps of bacterial or fungal organisms.

GROSS APPEARANCE

Squamous cell carcinoma arising in the lung forms a firm, gray-white mass. The appearance of the cut surface varies depending on the amount of hemorrhage and necrosis, and it may show evidence of cavitation. Like many adenocarcinomas, the infiltrating tumor can incite a desmoplastic response and the texture will then be firm and rubbery or even gritty. Foci of calcification occasionally occur. If the cut surface of a suspected squamous cell carcinoma has a glistening appearance and a mucoid consistency, it may turn out to be an adenocarcinoma or a combined adenosquamous carcinoma.

An unusual case of squamous cell carcinoma occurring in a 28-year-old woman who had juvenile laryngotracheal papillomatosis since the age of 2½ years was reported by Helmuth and Strate.[21] The carcinoma as well as randomly chosen papillomas excised over a period of years demonstrated positive nuclear staining for papillomavirus structural antigen.

LIGHT MICROSCOPY

The appearance of a bronchogenic squamous cell carcinoma in paraffin sections is influenced by the degree of differentiation, which can change dramatically from one area to another. A tumor in a small biopsy specimen may look quite different from the dominant pattern in the resected tumor. Small biopsy specimens are therefore not reliable for grading, and it is sometimes difficult to determine from a small or distorted biopsy specimen that a tumor is indeed a squamous cell carcinoma.

Squamous cell carcinoma grows in irregular lobules that typically are composed of intercommunicating solid nests of cells (Figs. 7–1 through 7–4). Maturation toward the center of a cell nest is accompanied by the accumulation of keratin within the cytoplasm of the swollen cells (see Fig. 7–1) or extracellularly as concentric whorls (see Fig. 7–2). Evidence of keratinization may be present throughout all but the peripheral layer of cells (see Fig. 7–3), or it may only be evident in scattered small foci (see Fig. 7–4) or be confined to individual cells. The cytoplasm of the keratin-forming cells has a filamentous character (Fig. 7–5) that becomes homogeneous as the cell degenerates into a structureless blob of dense keratin (Fig. 7–6).

The size and shape of the individual cells varies, but they are usually round to polygonal, with at least moderate quantities of cytoplasm. The nuclei tend to be irregular with coarsely clumped chromatin. Close apposition is usual, although dropout of many cells creates a fenestrated appearance. If there are areas of degeneration within well-demarcated nodules, the surrounding cells may simulate a poorly differentiated adenocarcinoma at low magnification (Fig. 7–7). Between adjacent cells, a slender gap is often visible, and it may be traversed by fine strands of cytoplasm, which constitute the so-called intercellular bridges (Figs. 7–8 and 7–9). Small thickenings corresponding to the sites of desmosomes can sometimes be made out on the connecting strands. The intercellular bridges are often conspicuous in cutaneous squamous cells and their tumors, and in contrast they are an inconsistent finding in bronchogenic squamous cell carcinomas, even the well-differentiated tumors. When the bridges cannot be identified, the squamous nature of a tumor may be suggested by uniform clefts separating neighboring cells (Fig. 7–10).

Some tumors produce abundant keratin, but others form little or none and the cytoplasm may then have an almost clear appear-

Text continued on page 172

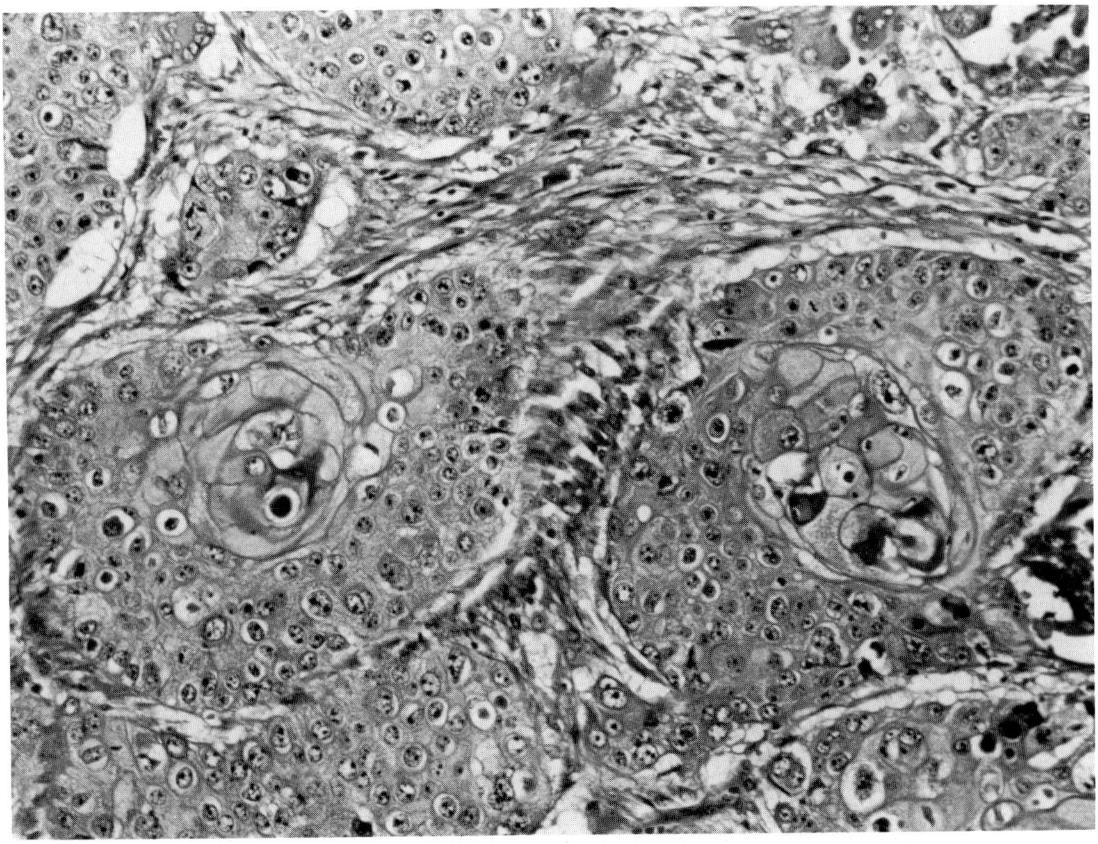

Figure 7–1. Nests of tumor cells from a well-differentiated squamous cell carcinoma.

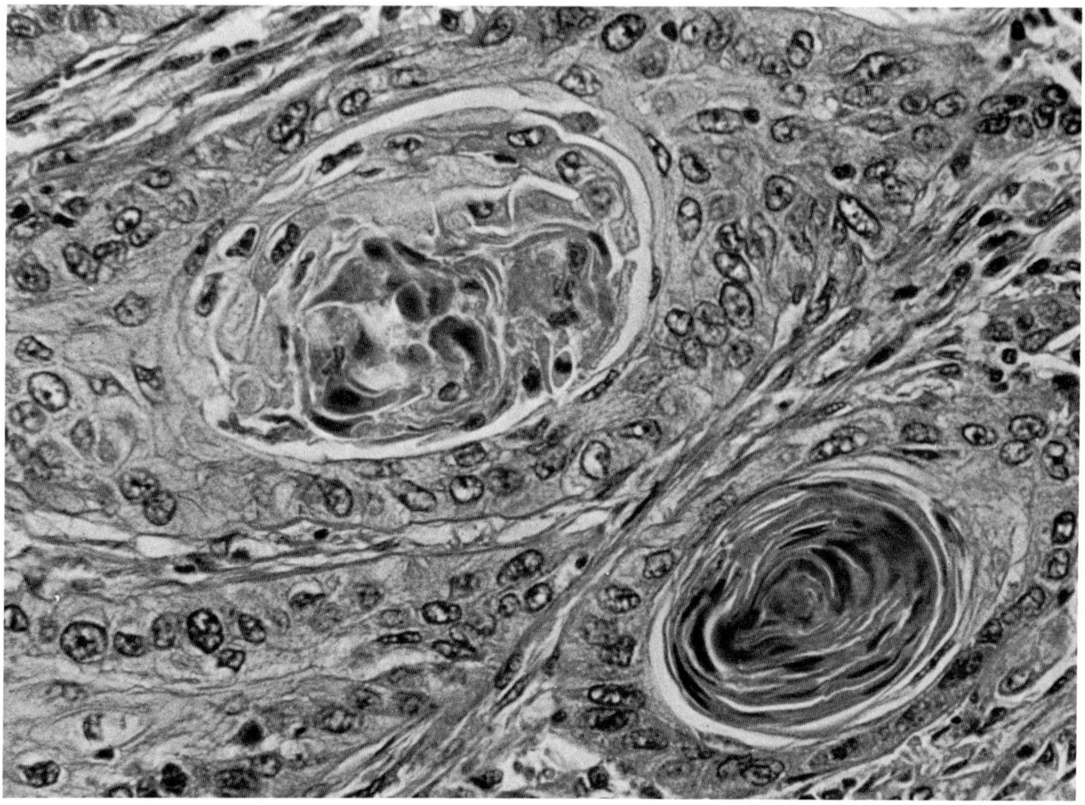

Figure 7–2. A concentric whorl of keratin is present. Another is in the process of formation.

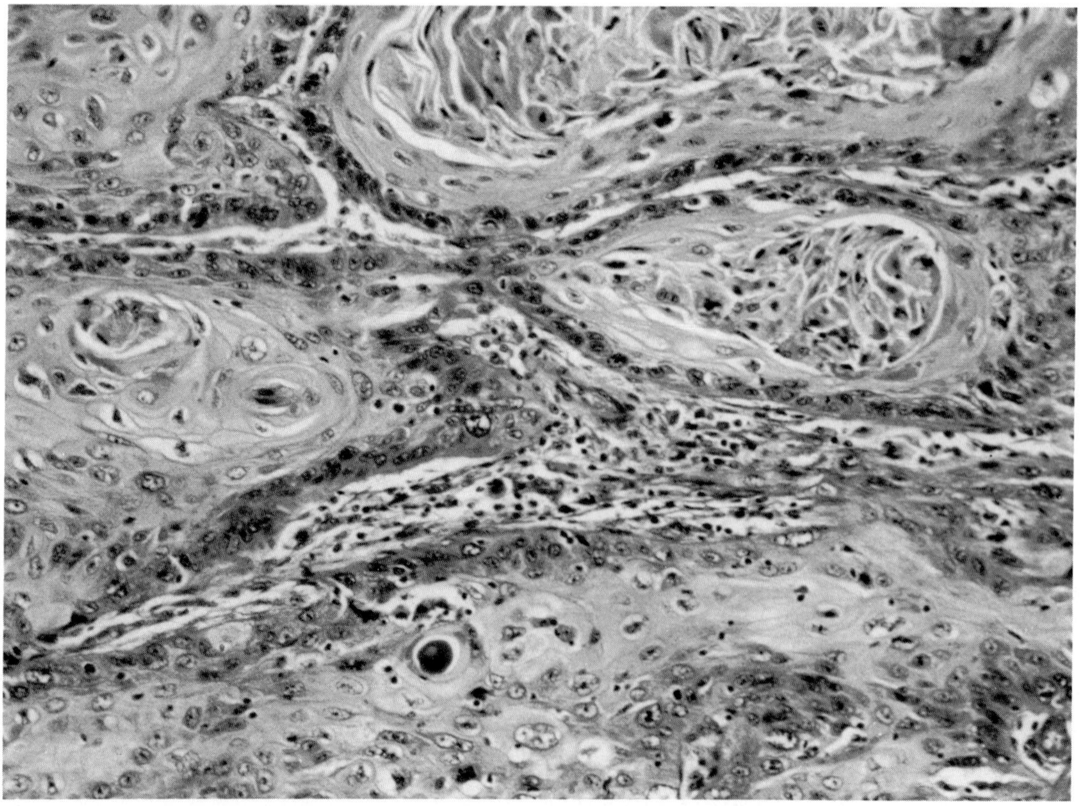

Figure 7–3. Keratinization is evident in all but the peripheral cells of this squamous cell carcinoma.

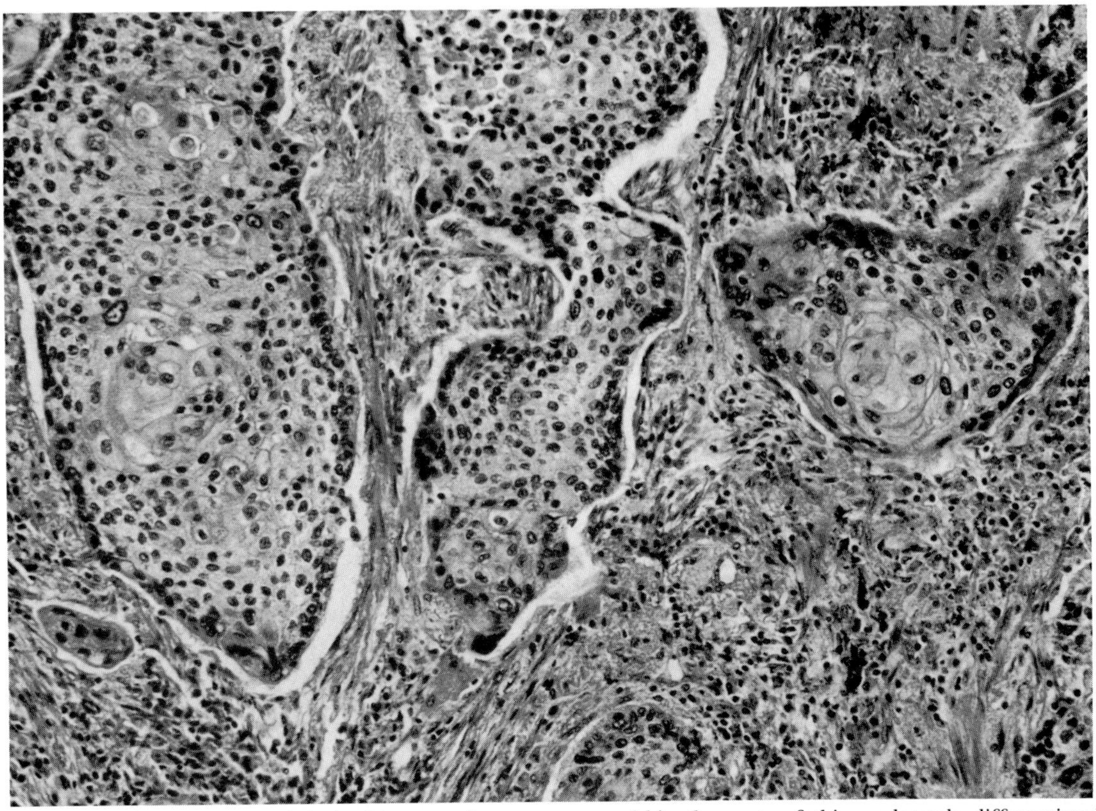

Figure 7–4. Scattered small foci of larger cells are present within the nests of this moderately differentiated squamous cell carcinoma.

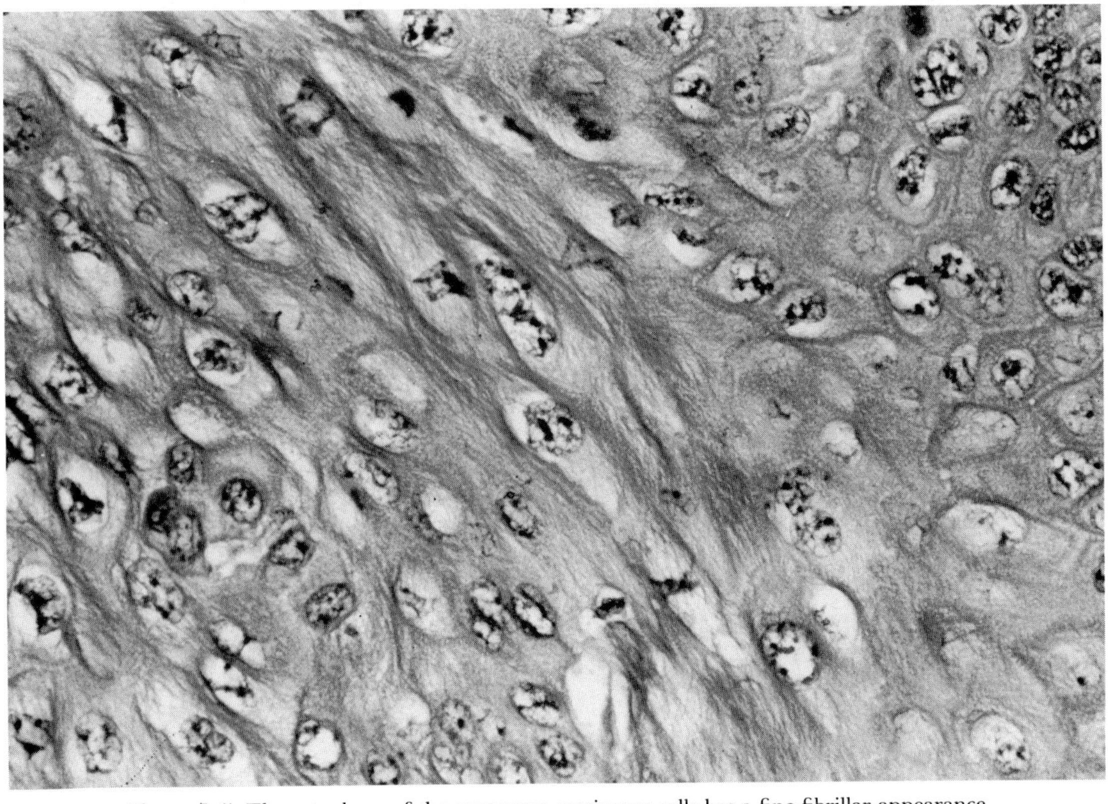

Figure 7–5. The cytoplasm of the squamous carcinoma cells has a fine fibrillar appearance.

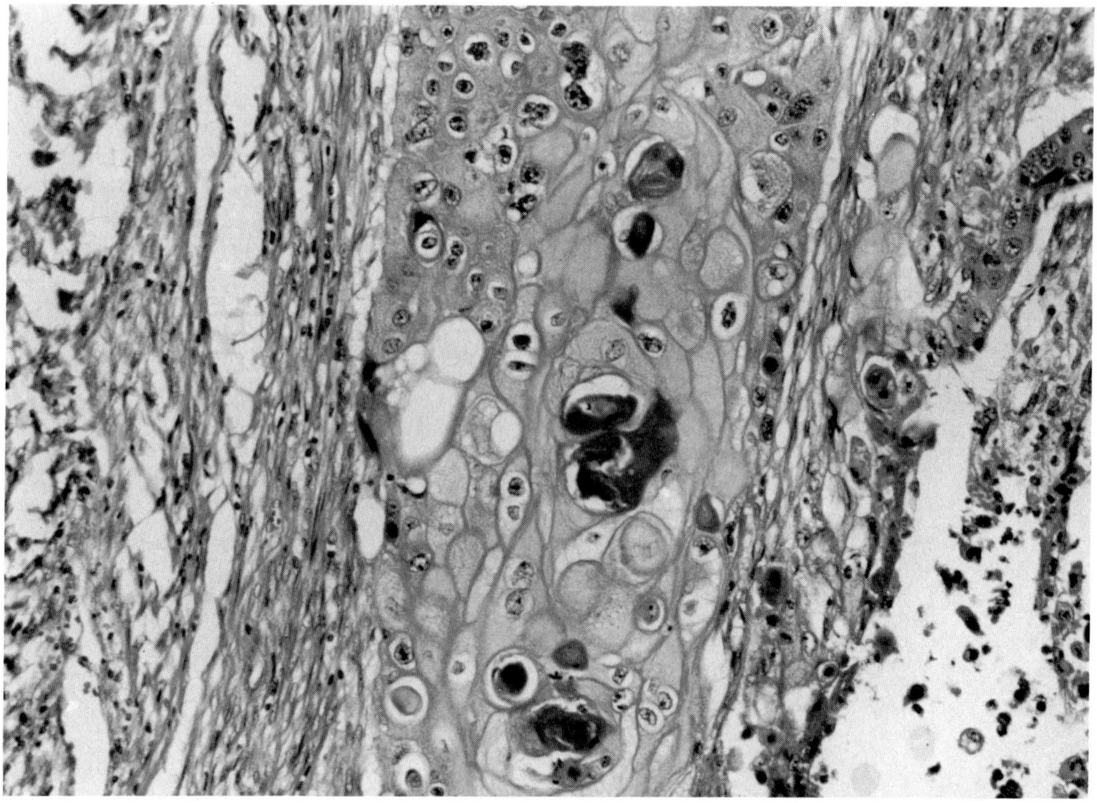

Figure 7–6. Structureless aggregates of dense keratin in a squamous cell carcinoma.

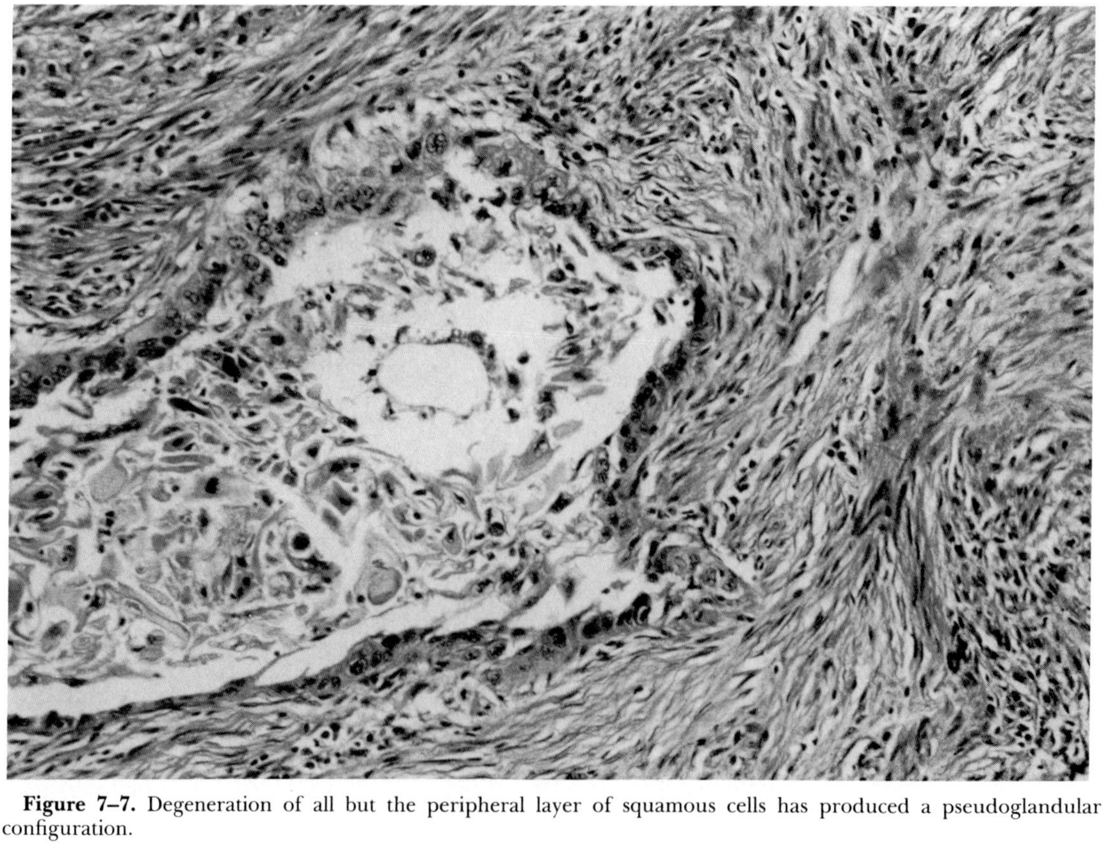

Figure 7–7. Degeneration of all but the peripheral layer of squamous cells has produced a pseudoglandular configuration.

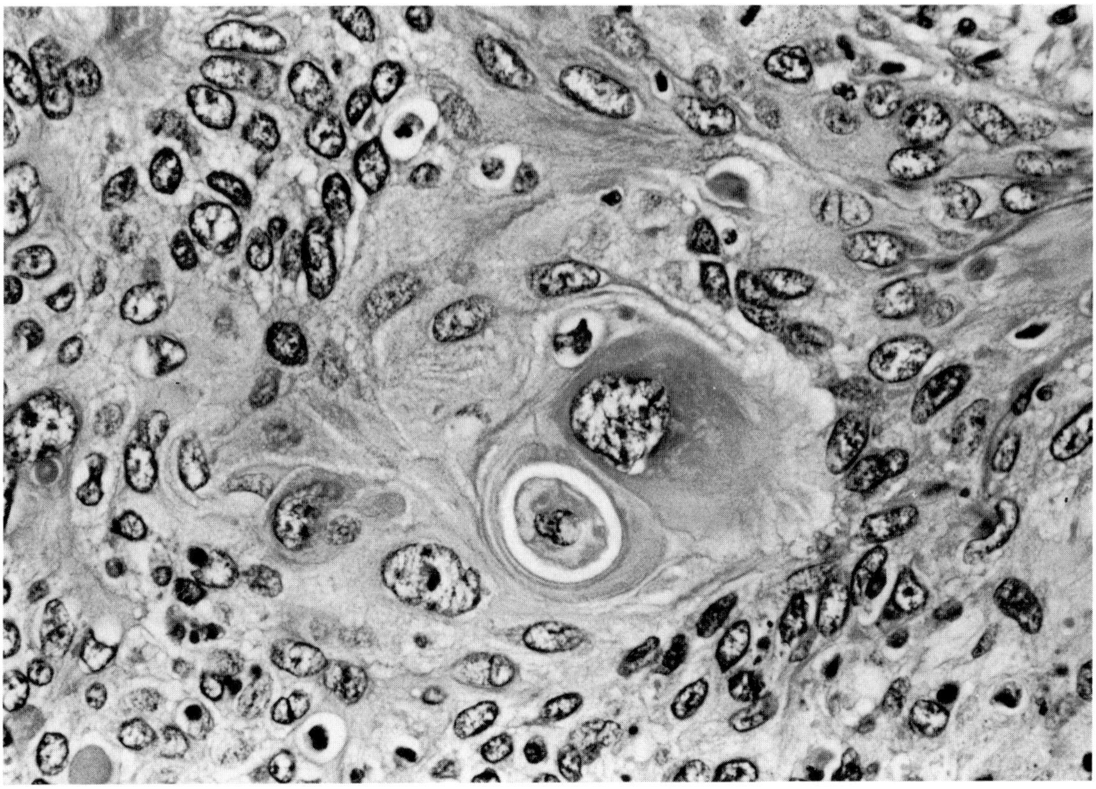

Figure 7–8. Intercellular bridges can be seen between the larger cells at the center of the figure.

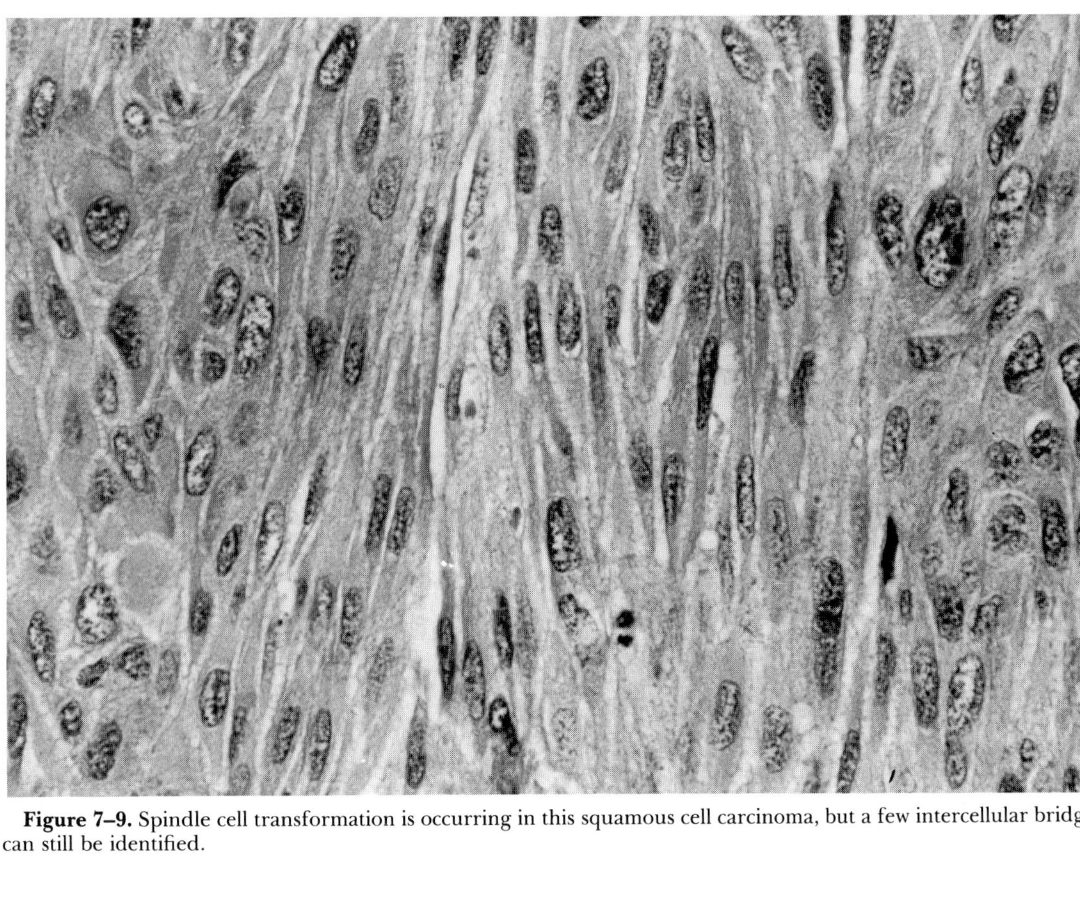

Figure 7–9. Spindle cell transformation is occurring in this squamous cell carcinoma, but a few intercellular bridges can still be identified.

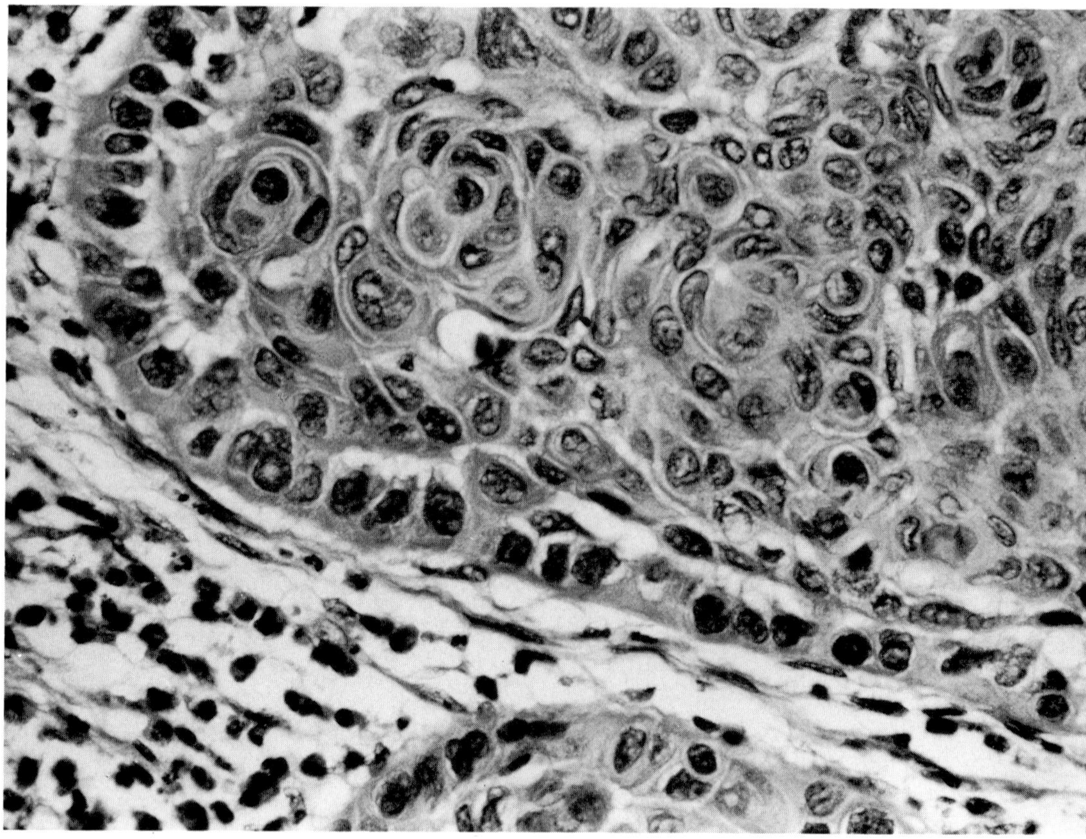

Figure 7–10. Many of the cells of this squamous cell carcinoma are separated by narrow clefts.

ance (Fig. 7–11). Marked variation in the degree of differentiation is common within a bronchogenic squamous cell carcinoma, and foci of keratinizing, well-differentiated cells are frequently juxtaposed to or intermingled with groups of poorly differentiated cells. In the absence of keratinization, it may be difficult to recognize that a poorly differentiated carcinoma is squamous in type. A tumor with varying degrees of differentiation should be graded on the basis of the predominant component. Thus, a squamous cell carcinoma that is mainly composed of well- or moderately differentiated cells but also contains small areas of poor differentiation should be designated a moderately differentiated tumor, and the presence of the poorly differentiated foci should be noted in the diagnosis or a comment.

Cell shape becomes more variable in dedifferentiating tumors (Figs. 7–12 through 7–14) and reaches an extreme degree in the foci of pleomorphic carcinoma that occasionally coexist with an otherwise more differentiated tumor (Fig. 7–15). The tumor cell nuclei in these figures demonstrate the increasing level of cytologic atypia that accompanies dedifferentiation. In a few poorly differentiated squamous cell carcinomas, many or all of the cells are small; and particularly in a biopsy specimen, distinction from a small cell undifferentiated carcinoma may not be possible (see Chapter 9). Small nests of keratinizing cells will provide a clue to the histogenesis, but the possibility of a combined variant of small cell carcinoma must be also considered. Necrosis within tumor nodules can create an impression of stratification, but the cells bordering the necrotic foci generally show little evidence of organization (Figs. 7–16 and 7–17).

The amount of stroma in lung tumors was assessed by Fisseler-Eckhoff and associates[16] in 60 totally excised peripheral neoplasms. Squamous cell tumors possessed 37% of fibrous tissue, contrasting to an average of 48% of stroma in adenocarcinomas and 30% in small cell carcinomas, and large squamous tumors showed a relative increase in the amount of stroma.

Text continued on page 176

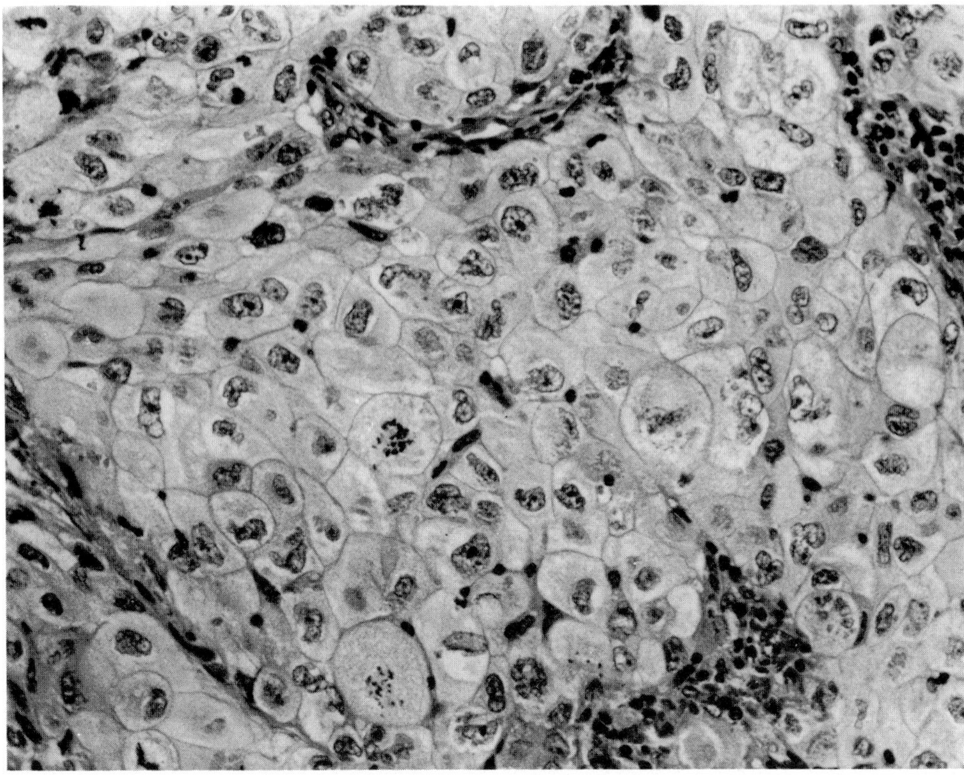

Figure 7–11. An area of a squamous cell carcinoma in which the cells have relatively clear cytoplasm.

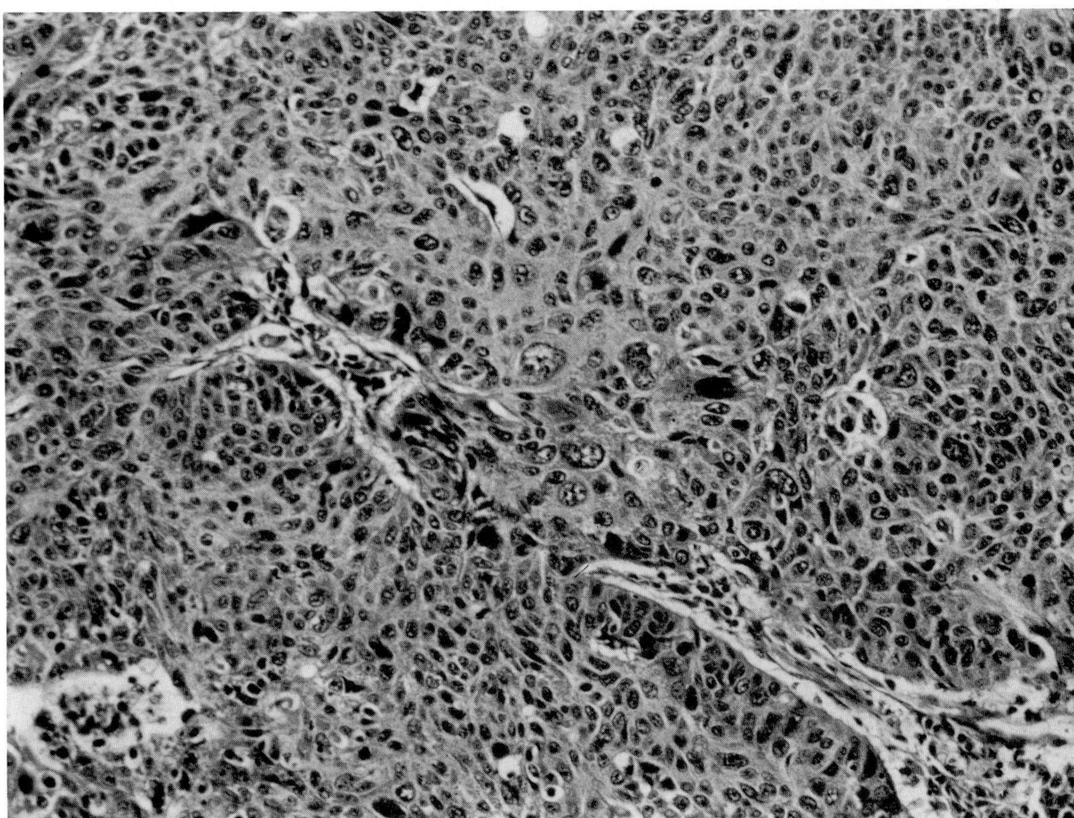

Figure 7–12. With dedifferentiation, variation in nuclear size becomes apparent.

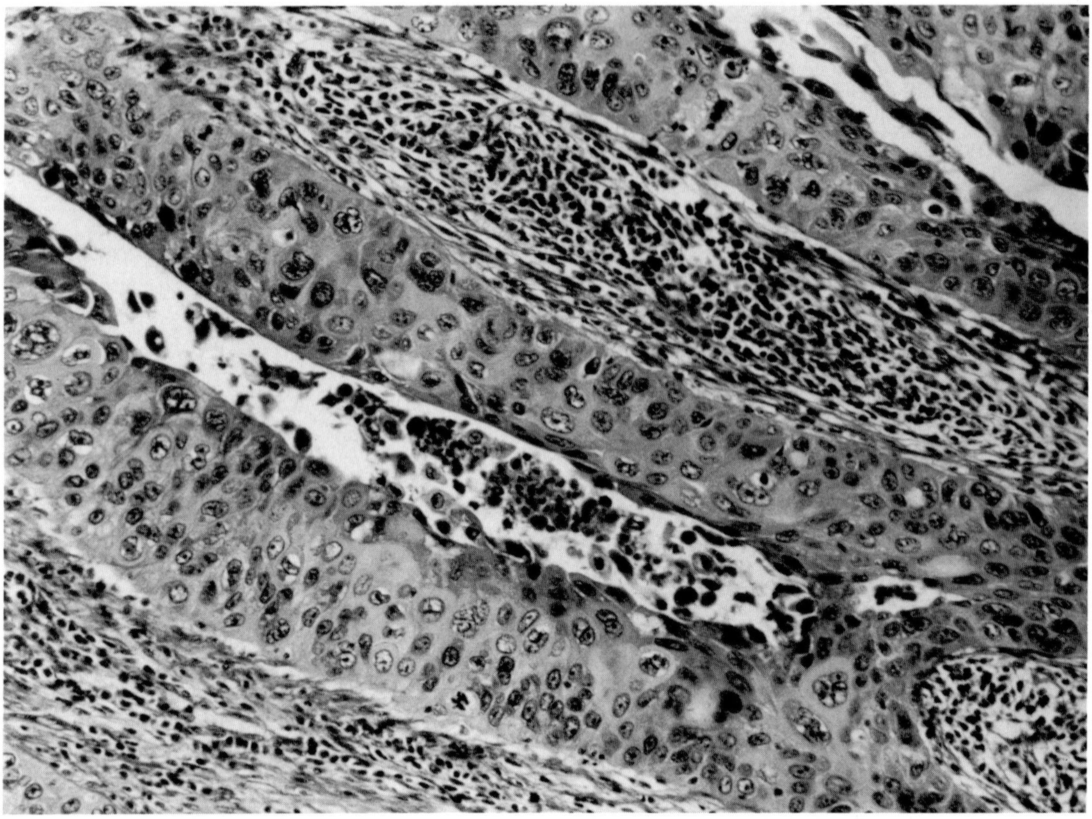

Figure 7–13. Variable nuclear size and shape in a poorly differentiated squamous cell carcinoma.

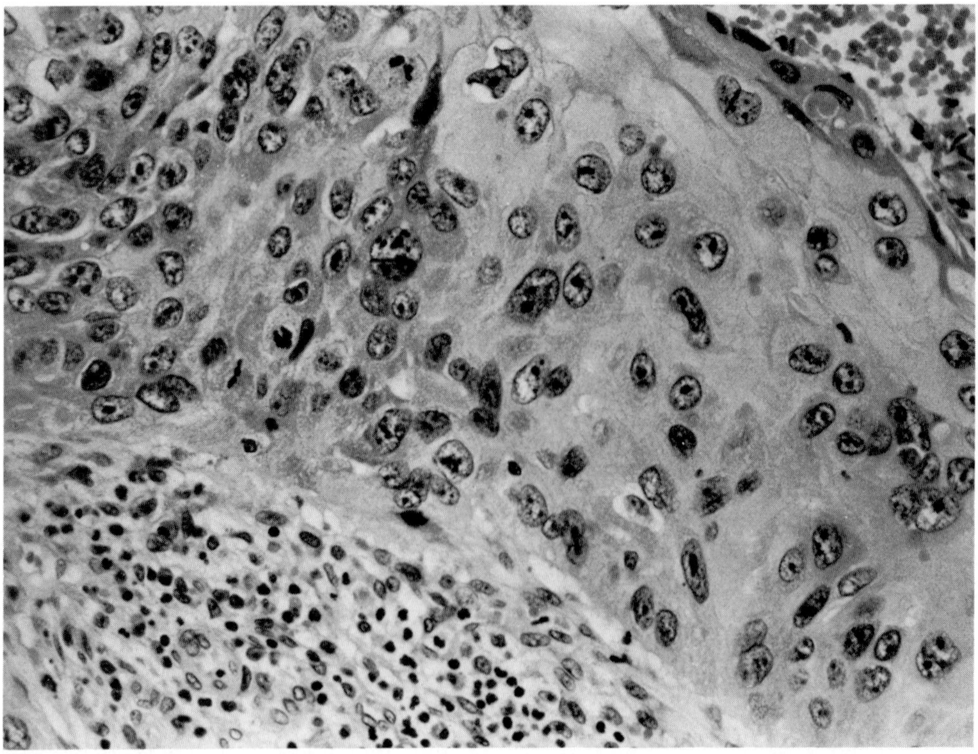

Figure 7–14. The nuclei in this poorly differentiated squamous cell carcinoma vary in size and shape, and many have prominent nucleoli.

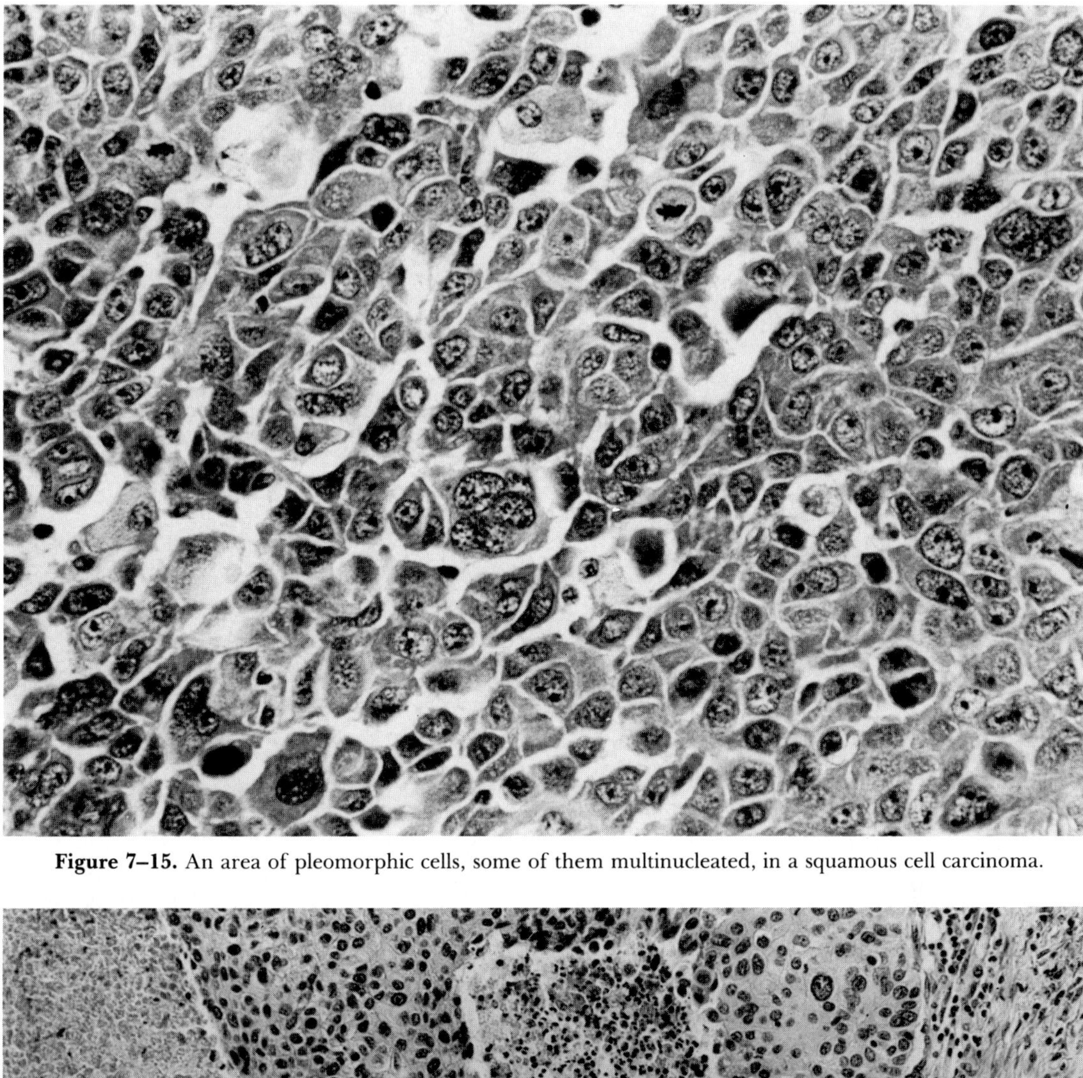

Figure 7–15. An area of pleomorphic cells, some of them multinucleated, in a squamous cell carcinoma.

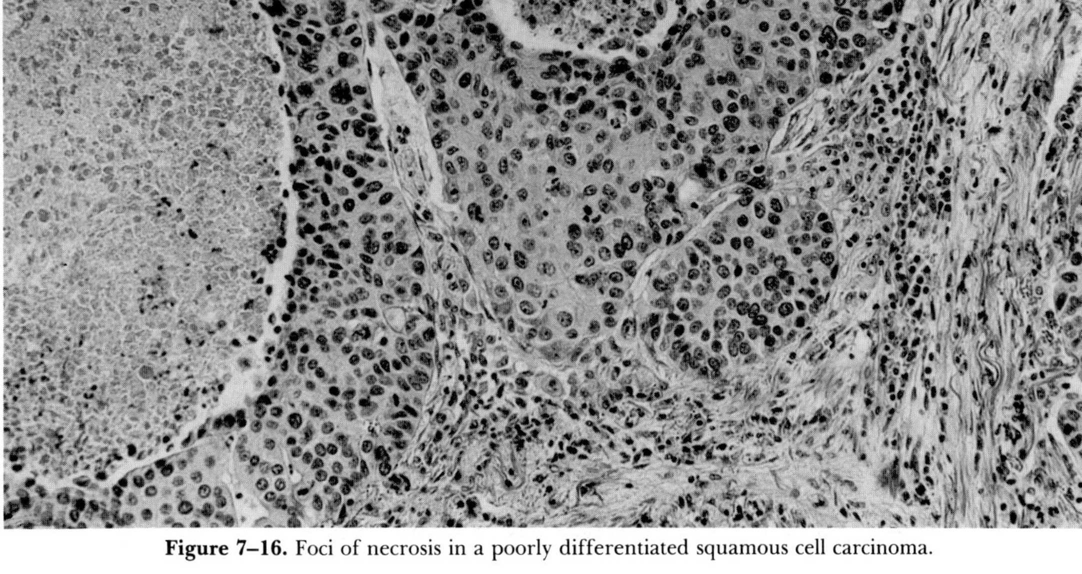

Figure 7–16. Foci of necrosis in a poorly differentiated squamous cell carcinoma.

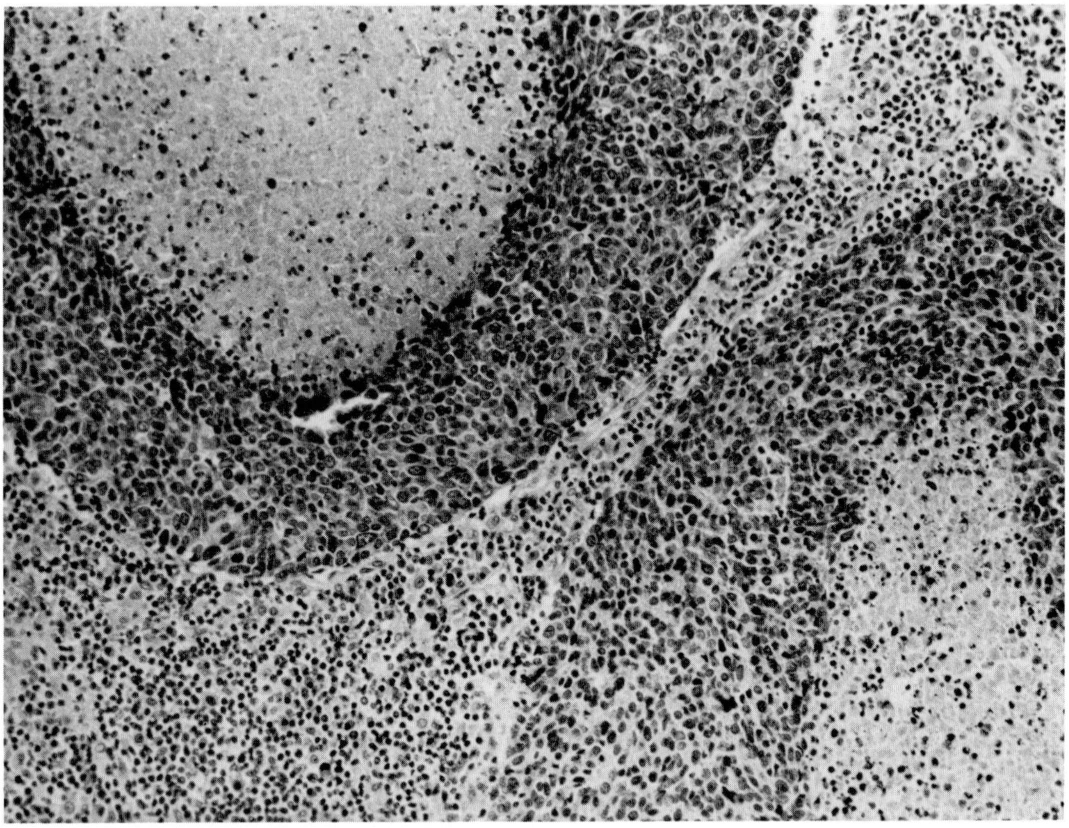

Figure 7–17. The zones of necrosis create an impression of stratification.

HISTOLOGIC GRADE AND SURVIVAL

The prognosis for a patient with squamous cell carcinoma of the lung is better, stage for stage, than for adenocarcinoma. Among the 1,121 resected non–small cell carcinomas reviewed by the Lung Cancer Study Group,[32] patients with squamous cell carcinoma had an outcome superior to those with adenocarcinoma: 65% and 55%, respectively, were expected to survive 5 years. The differences in survival were significant overall and in the T1 N0, T1 N1, and T2 N1 subsets but not in the TNM subsets in stage III disease.

Since the light microscopic appearance of a squamous cell carcinoma of the lung can be quite variable, especially when extensive material is available for evaluation, different pathologists may disagree in their assessment of the histologic grade. Overlap between well- and moderately differentiated tumors and between moderately and poorly differentiated tumors is common. Although assessment of histologic grade is not consistently reproducible among different observers, an attempt was made at the M.D. Anderson Cancer Center to determine the value of grade as a prognostic indicator (Lukeman JM, unpublished study). Two hundred ten surgically resected bronchogenic squamous cell carcinomas from patients admitted to the hospital between 1974 and 1981 were graded using the criteria of presence and extent of keratinization, degree of cellular pleomorphism, and frequency of mitoses. Patients whose tumors were placed in the well- and moderately differentiated categories had similar survival times, while those with poorly differentiated tumors had slightly shorter survivals; the differences were not statistically significant. The single most important factor in assessing prognosis appeared to be the clinical stage of the disease rather than the degree of cellular differentiation. A similar review was carried out by Dr. Mary Matthews (personal communication, 1983), who found that while there was a minimal decrease in survival in patients with poorly differentiated squamous cell carcinomas, the figures were not statistically significant in all three subgroups.

These data are not in agreement with the findings of Katlic and Carter,[26] who reported a 5-year survival of 7% for poorly differentiated squamous cell carcinoma, 20% for moderately differentiated tumors, and 39% for well-differentiated carcinomas. In a more recent review, Carter[7] cites other reported series and notes that the data indicate that squamous cell carcinoma has a better prognosis in all of the staging subsets than that of the other cell types.

Further studies are required to assess the relevance of mitotic activity and nuclear DNA content with regard to survival. Van Bodegom and co-workers[46] studied tumor ploidy in 52 surgically resected stage I (T1 and T2) squamous cell carcinomas with a minimal follow-up of 5 years. Forty-four percent were diploid with a 6-year survival of 53%, while 56% were aneuploid with a 6-year survival of 40%. Diploid tumors tended to recur locally and aneuploid tumors developed distant metastases, but the difference was not significant. However, the percentage of aneuploid tumor cells was a prognostic indicator.

In a flow cytometric study of surgical specimens from 105 untreated patients with squamous cell carcinoma and a minimum follow-up of 5 years, Volm and colleagues[47] concluded that cytometric DNA content did have prognostic importance. Patients with aneuploid tumors died significantly sooner than those with diploid tumors, and patients whose tumors had a high proliferative activity also died significantly sooner.

Nuclear DNA content in 33 squamous cell carcinomas of the lung was analyzed on Feulgen-stained histologic and cytologic preparations with cytophotometry by Yoneyama and co-workers,[49] and 28 had high and scattered DNA values.

CYTOLOGY

In smears, the cells may be in compact clusters (Fig. 7–18) or loosely cohesive aggregates (Fig. 7–19). The cells can have any shape: round, oval, elongated, and tadpole forms are encountered (Figs. 7–20 through 7–23). Nuclei also vary greatly in shape, and they do not always conform to the shape of the whole cell. Indentations and irregularities of the nuclear contour are common but become less conspicuous with loss of differentiation. Occasionally, multinucleated giant forms or clear cells are found. Spindle-shaped squamous carcinoma cells are seldom seen in sputum and are more common in aspirated specimens. The nucleoli increase in size and prominence with loss of differentiation (Fig. 7–24).

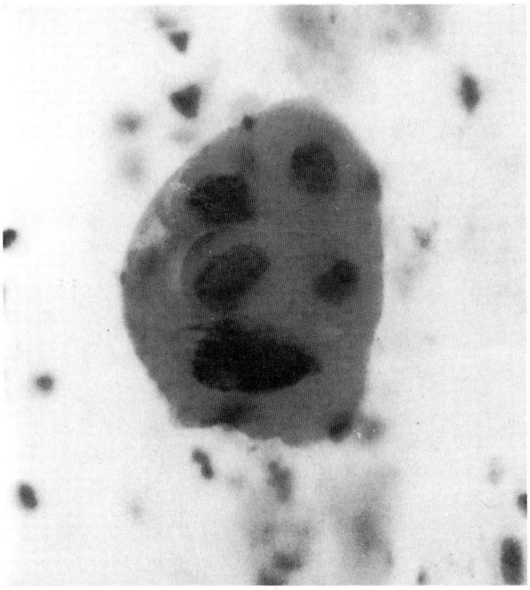

Figure 7–18. A compact cluster of cells in sputum from a squamous cell carcinoma.

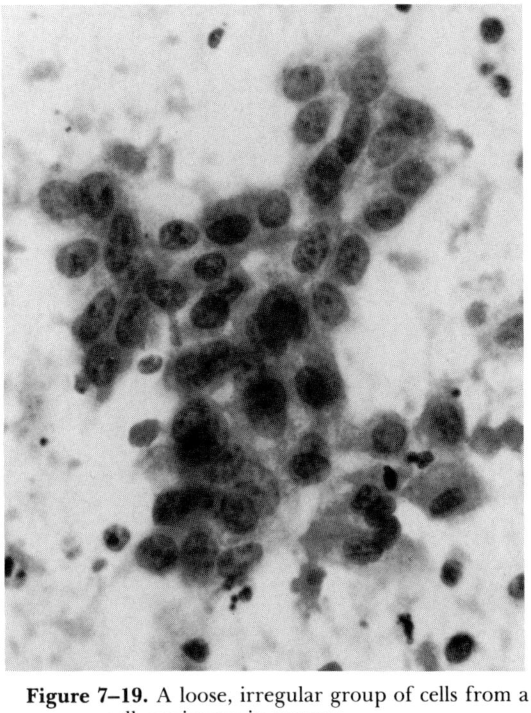

Figure 7–19. A loose, irregular group of cells from a squamous cell carcinoma in sputum.

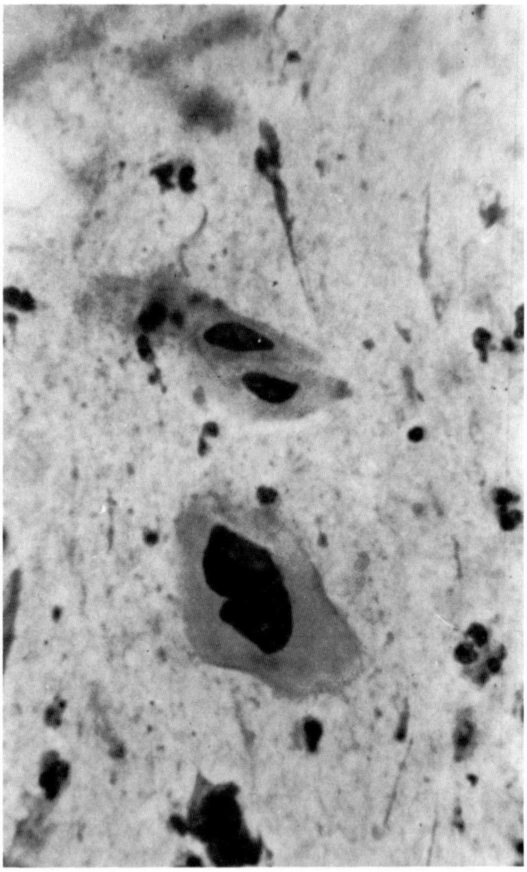

Figure 7–20. Ovoid cells and nuclei from a squamous cell carcinoma.

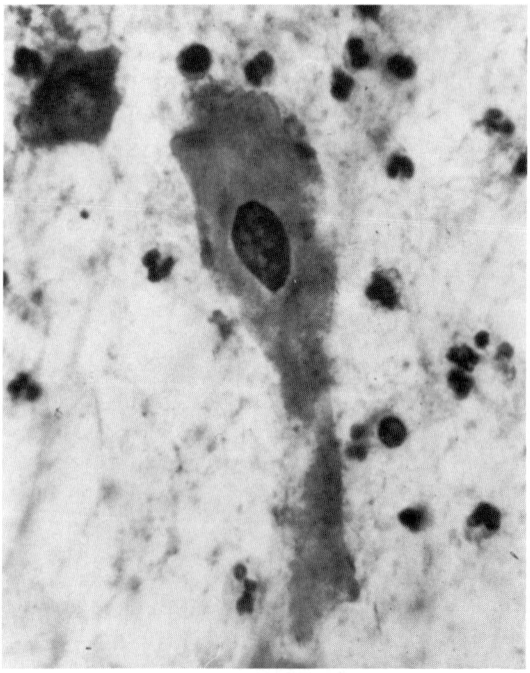

Figure 7–21. A more elongated squamous carcinoma cell.

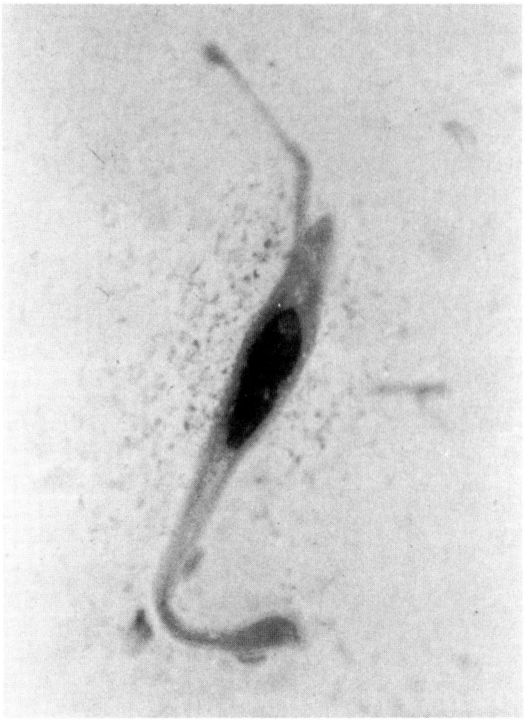

Figure 7–22. Tapering cytoplasm in an elongated squamous carcinoma cell.

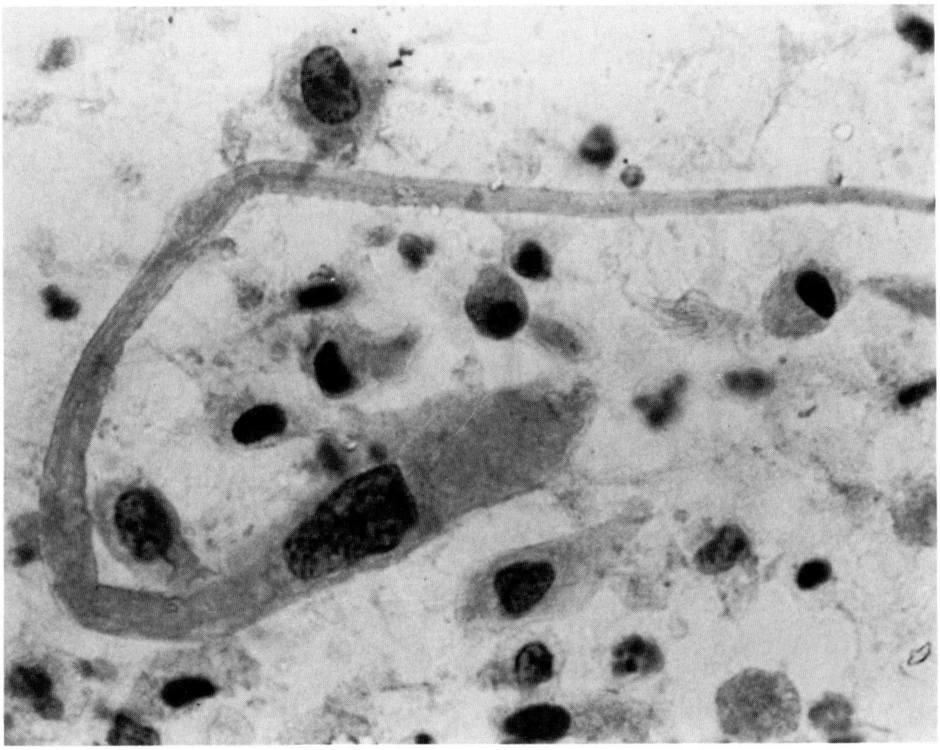

Figure 7–23. A cell from a squamous cell carcinoma has a tadpole shape.

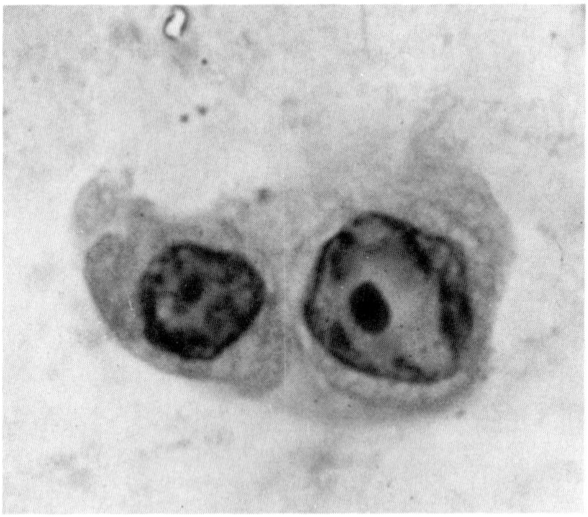

Figure 7–24. A prominent nucleolus is evident in one of the cells from a squamous cell carcinoma.

The cytoplasm is orangeophilic in the well-differentiated cells but basophilic or amphophilic in poorly differentiated cells, depending on the degree to which they are forming keratin. In well-differentiated, keratinizing squamous cell carcinomas, the nuclear/cytoplasmic ratios are relatively low: in moderately differentiated areas, the nuclear diameter is approximately 50% of that of the cell, while in poorly differentiated cells it is of the order of 70%.

IMMUNOHISTOCHEMISTRY

Bronchial basal cells contain cytokeratin proteins similar to those found in squamous epithelial cells (Figs. 7–25 and 7–26).[4] Several investigators[3, 4, 19, 29, 38] have shown that bronchial squamous cell carcinomas have a highly complex cytokeratin pattern, which probably reflects differences in cytokeratin expression between basal, ciliated, and goblet cells.[3, 4] Although the cytokeratin profile of squamous cell carcinomas of the lung is characterized by the presence of stratified (high-molecular-weight) epithelium-type cytokeratins, particularly cytokeratins Nos. 5 and 6, the tumors also contain significant amounts of simple (low-molecular-weight) epithelium-type cytokeratins and minor amounts of cytokeratin No. 13.[3, 4, 19, 29, 38] The mixed stratified and simple epithelium-type pattern is similar to that found in squamous cell carcinomas of the uterine cervix where metaplastic changes are also involved in the development of the tumor.[29, 30] As in bronchial basal cells, reserve cells of the uterine cervix react with certain antibodies considered characteristic of particular forms of stratification.[30]

Maturing cells of human stratified squamous epithelium (epidermis, esophagus, vagina, conjunctiva) synthesize a protein envelope immediately beneath the plasma membrane that is stabilized by cross-linked dipeptide ϵ-(γ-glutamyl) lysine.[36] This envelope or marginal band can be identified by electron microscopy, and it measures approximately 12 nm in thickness.[17] Involucrin (molecular weight, 92 kd), a nonfilamentous protein unrelated to cytokeratins, is a soluble precursor of this protein envelope.[37] Immunohistochemical and biochemical studies of tissue sections and cultured tumor cells have demonstrated that involucrin is absent from basal cells of the normal human epidermis, but as the cells mature it appears in the upper stratum spongiosum and stratum granulosum.[2, 33] Normal bronchial cells do not contain involucrin. When normal tracheal epithelial cells are cultured, typical colonies of keratinocytes with assembled cross-linked envelopes similar to those of epidermal keratinocytes may develop.[2] Further evidence that bronchial epithelium may exhibit a keratinocyte-like pattern of differentiation is provided by the observation of strong immunostaining for involucrin in metaplastic bronchial epithelium.[39] Involucrin in squamous cell carcinomas of the lung thus appears to reflect the presence of a differentiation antigen that is present in larger cells in the center of squamous cell nests and absent in the small basal-oriented cells.

In our experience, immunostaining for involucrin can be useful in the diagnosis of squamous cell carcinomas of the lung, particularly the less differentiated tumors in which evidence of keratinization may be difficult to recognize by routine light microscopic examination. At the present time, a variety of antibodies to involucrin, which can be used on frozen or paraffin sections, are commercially available.

An increasing number of reports have appeared recently describing monoclonal antibodies generated against squamous cell carcinoma–related antigens.[5, 10, 14, 20, 27] Unfortunately, the reactivity of the majority of these antibodies is not restricted to lung cancer or to squamous cell carcinoma, and only a few of them have a potential for application in the classification of lung tumors. Examples of these antibodies are antibody 9.2.2 described by Brenner and co-workers[5] and LuCa3 and LuCa4 developed by Kyoizumi and colleagues,[27] which, when tested against lung tumors, reacted with squamous cell carcinomas but not with adenocarcinomas or small cell carcinomas. Since most monoclonal antibodies react with antigens that are destroyed during tissue fixation and routine embedding procedures, their use in diagnostic surgical pathology is limited.

Epidermal growth factor (EGF) is a small polypeptide (molecular weight, 6 kd) that stimulates the growth and differentiation of a variety of normal and neoplastic epithelial cells.[6] The effect of the EGF on cell proliferation is mediated by its binding to a specific EGF receptor (EGF-R) that is a 170-kd protein located in the cell surface membrane.[1] Studies have demonstrated structural similarities between the sequence of the v-erb-B oncogene of AEV-H (a strain of the avian erythroblastosis virus) and the EGF-R.[12] These observations and the finding of increased EGF-R expression in a variety of epithelial malignant neoplasms suggest that an aberrant expression of EGF-R may be involved in the pathogenesis of certain epithelial tumors.[12, 18, 22, 34] This hypothesis is supported by reports indicating an increase in EGF-R binding in lung carcinoma[8, 22, 24, 41] and a correlation between invasiveness and EGF-R expression in breast carcinoma[15, 40] and bladder carcinoma.[34] Using a murine monoclonal antibody, Hendler and Ozanne[22] found that binding to EGF-R occurred in bronchial squamous cell carcinomas but not in other types of lung carcinoma. In a more recent immunocytochemical study, Sobol and associates[41] found EGF-R expression in all bronchial squamous cell and large cell carcinomas, and in a number of adenocarcinomas, but not in any of the small cell carcinomas examined. The results of these and other studies[8] raise the possibility that immunocytochemical detection of EGF-R expression in lung tumors might find application in the future in distinguishing squamous cell and large cell carcinomas and adenocarcinomas from small cell lung carcinomas. It is also possible that antibodies that are able to pre-

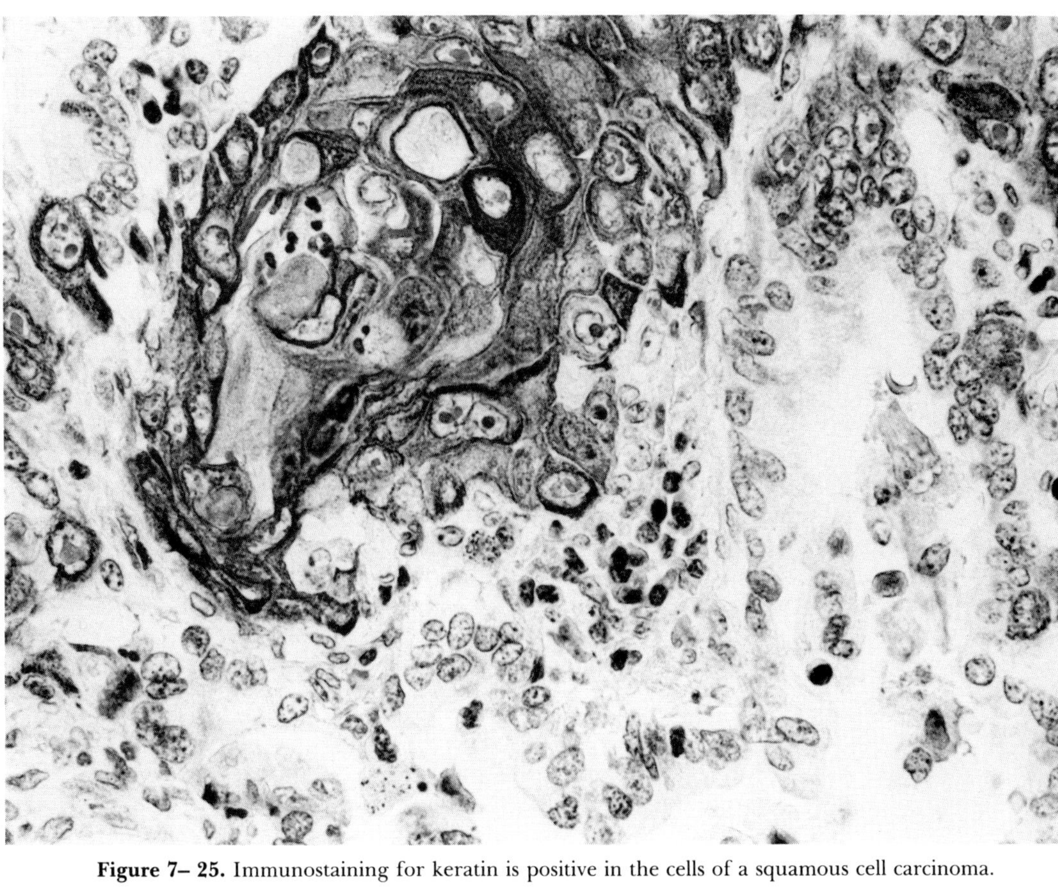

Figure 7–25. Immunostaining for keratin is positive in the cells of a squamous cell carcinoma.

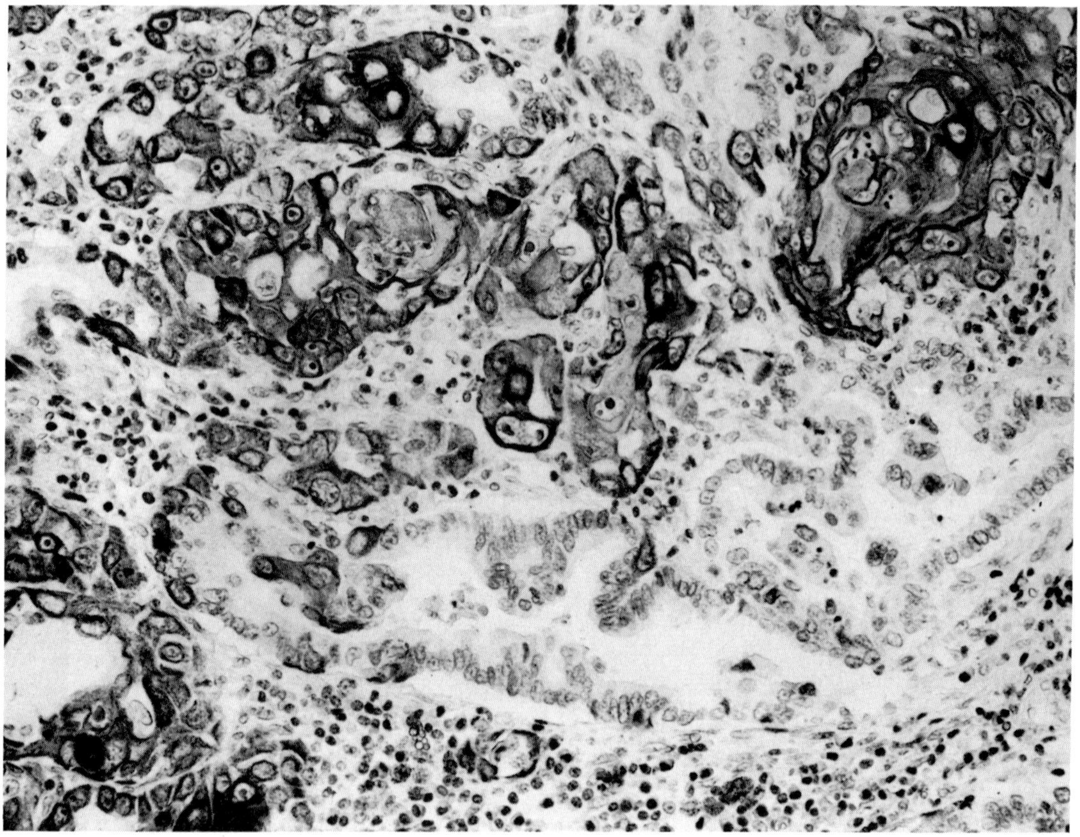

Figure 7–26. Most of the cells lining the small bronchus do not exhibit keratin immunoreactivity.

vent the binding of the EGF to its receptor could interfere with cell replication in pulmonary squamous cell carcinomas since these tumors apparently require a greater amount of EGF for growth. It is thus conceivable that these antibodies might have some therapeutic application.

Recently, a previously unrecognized parathyroid hormone–related protein has been isolated from a lung cancer cell line and its gene cloned.[43] This factor appears to be responsible for the malignant hypercalcemia syndrome that occurs in cancer patients without bony metastases, especially those with bronchogenic squamous cell carcinoma. The diagnostic and biologic potentials of this marker remain to be determined.

ELECTRON MICROSCOPY

Within the nests of a well- to moderately differentiated squamous cell carcinoma there is commonly some separation of adjacent cells, but they remain attached at the sites of desmosomes (Figs. 7–27 and 7–28). This is the ultrastructural basis for the so-called intercellular bridges observed by light microscopy. However, even in the presence of numerous desmosomes, adjacent cell membranes are sometimes apposed (Figs. 7–29 and 7–30). Only a small number of the microvillus-like cytoplasmic protrusions bear desmosomes; many are free-ending filopodia (Fig. 7–31).

The ultrastructural hallmarks of squamous carcinoma cells are the cell junctions and cytokeratin filaments, and in the better differentiated tumors both features are conspicuous. The cell junctions are true desmosomes with intermediate lines, and their prominence is due in part to their length and also to the thickness of their subplasmalemmal densities and the inserting bundles of cytokeratin filaments (Fig. 7–32). The cytokeratin filaments run from the desmosomes into the cytoplasm where they form dense wavy bundles (Fig. 7–32). In some lung tumors diagnosed as squamous cell carcinomas from their light microscopic appearance, the pattern is

Text continued on page 186

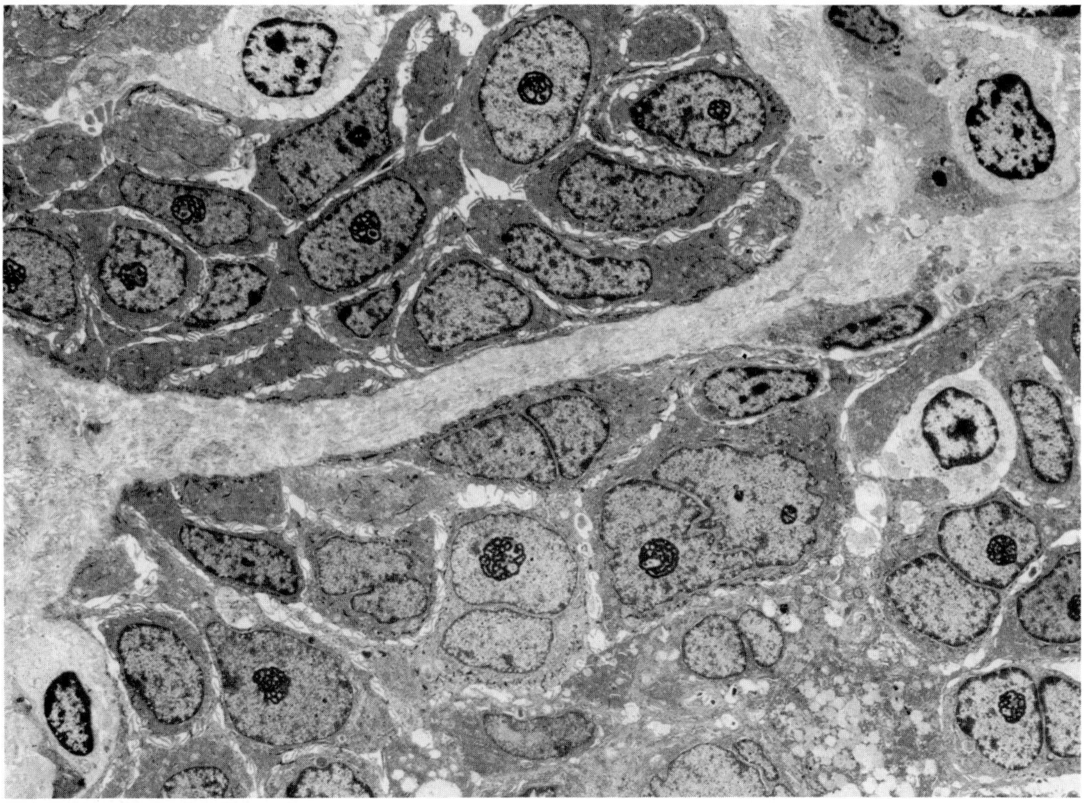

Figure 7–27. The electron micrograph shows nests of cells from a moderately differentiated squamous cell carcinoma within a collagenous stroma. (×2,400)

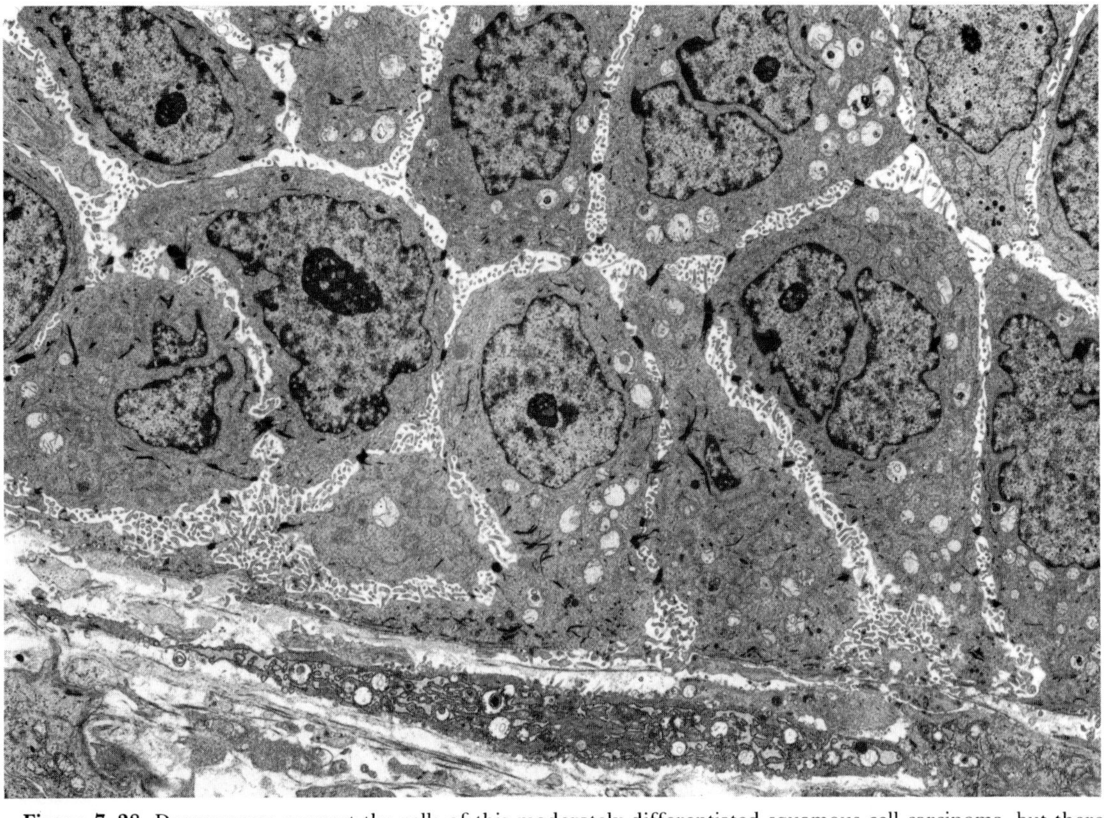

Figure 7–28. Desmosomes connect the cells of this moderately differentiated squamous cell carcinoma, but there are also many filopodia in the clefts between neighboring cells. (×3,300)

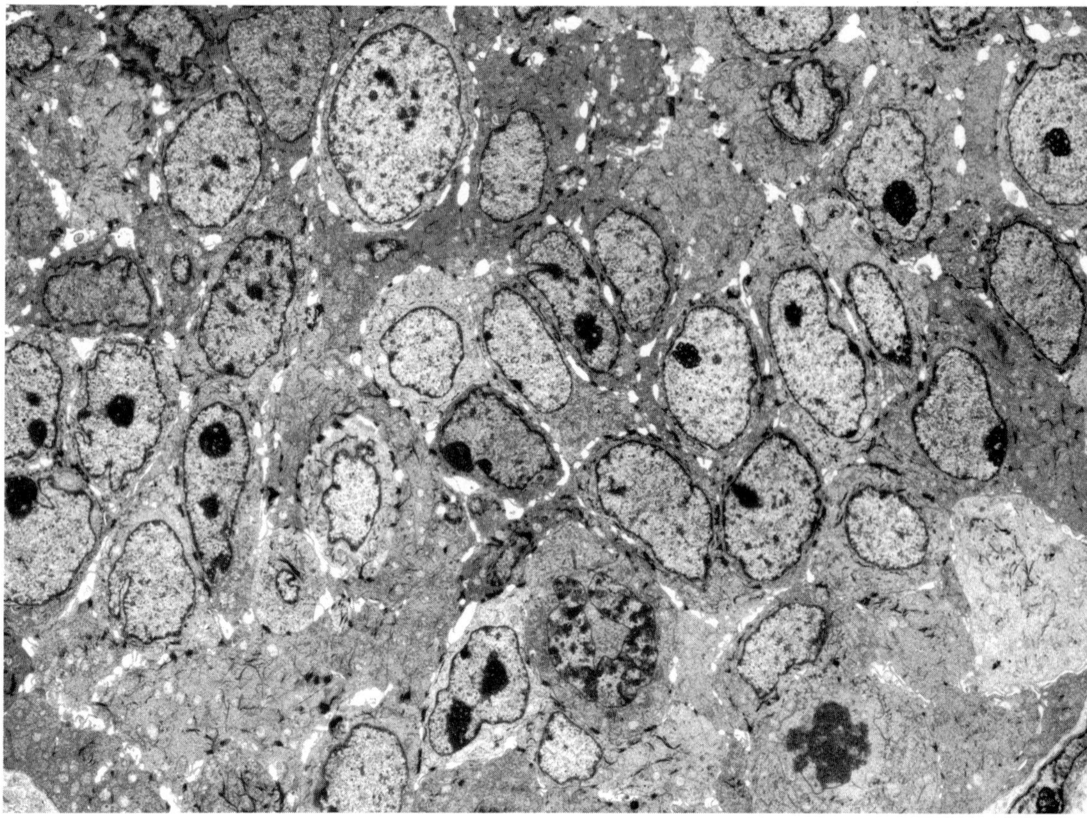

Figure 7–29. Poorly differentiated squamous cell carcinoma. Some cells are apposed while others are separated by slender clefts. (×2,500)

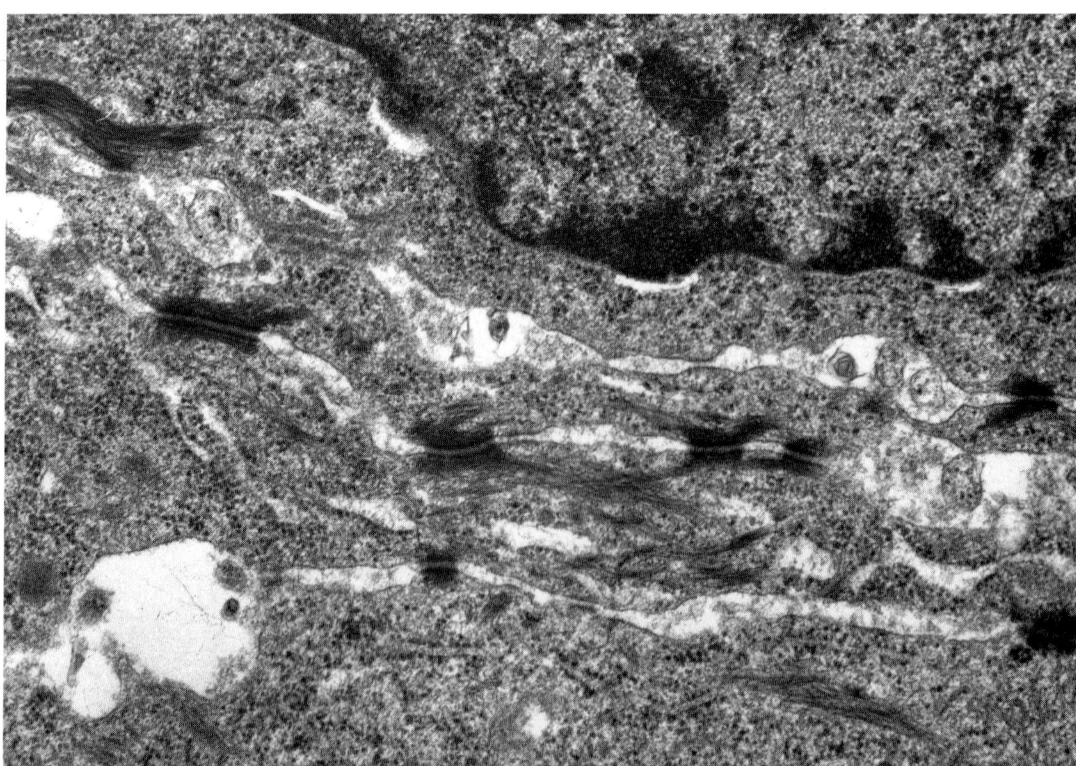

Figure 7–30. There are frequent desmosomes between the cells of this squamous cell carcinoma, but the cells are quite closely apposed. (×24,000)

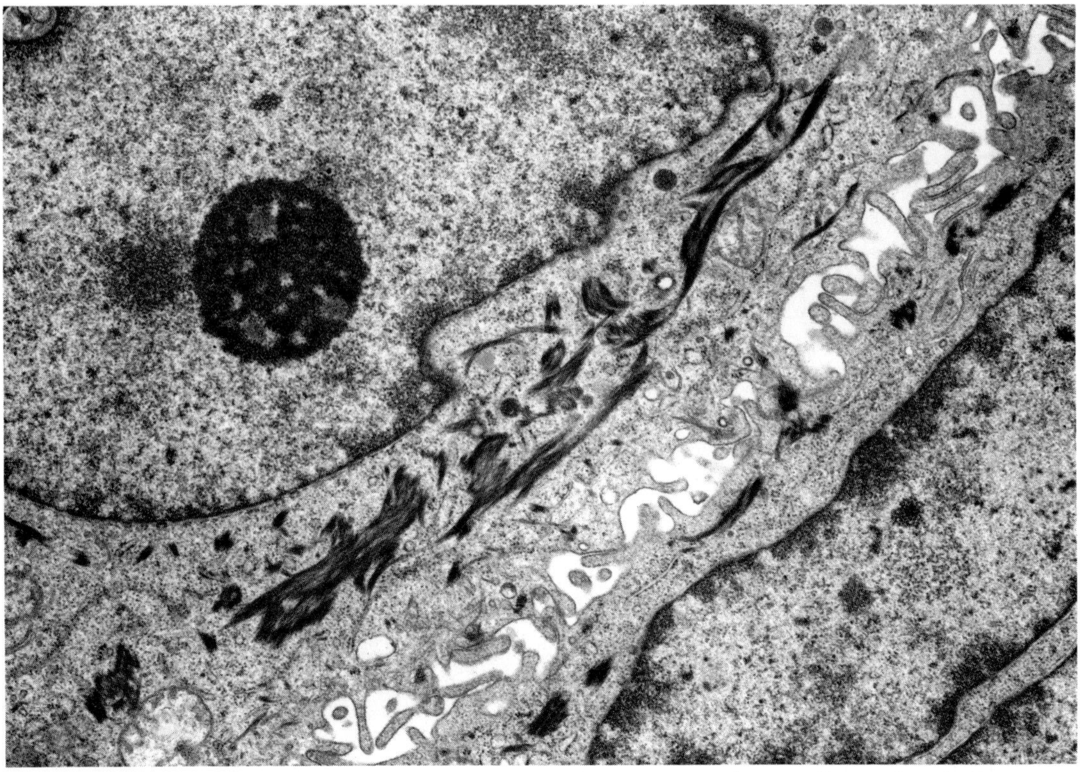

Figure 7–31. Filopodia protrude into the cleft between two squamous carcinoma cells. Cytokeratin filaments are present in the cytoplasm. (×12,500)

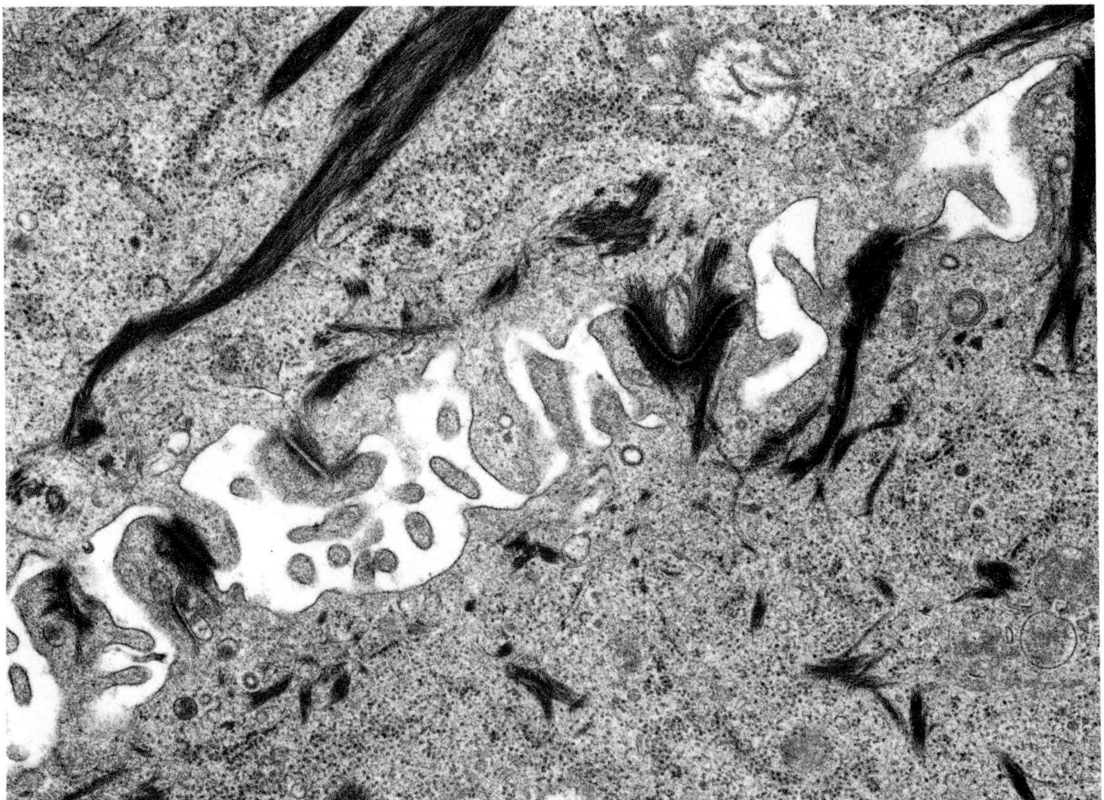

Figure 7–32. Cytokeratin filaments insert into the desmosomes. (×22,000)

orderly and the cells contain plentiful endoplasmic reticulum but cell junctions are small and cytokeratin filament bundles are not apparent (Fig. 7–33). A few small dense-core granules may be detected (Fig. 7–34), but they are probably lysosomes. Linnoila and associates[28] noted that neuroendocrine differentiation is rarely seen in squamous cell carcinoma of the lung.

Dingemans and Mooi[11] examined the interaction of tumor cells and lung parenchyma within the depth of 50 bronchogenic squamous cell carcinomas and found that in most instances a continuous basal lamina surrounded every tumor cell group, even when the groups were isolated by desmoplastic stroma.

With loss of differentiation, there is a progressive diminution in the number and size of the desmosomes, intermediate lines disappear, and the plasmalemmal densities become shorter and thinner. The cell junctions may be merely tiny densities of neighboring cell surfaces. With progressive reduction in the number of desmosomes, cell cohesion is reduced and many cells are detached or separated from their neighbors by broad clefts (Figs. 7–35 and 7–36). The number of cytokeratin filaments also diminishes as the cells dedifferentiate. In the more primitive tumors, only scattered cells contain slender wisps of filaments, and many cells have none. This does not necessarily mean an absence of cytokeratin immunoreactivity. With loss of differentiation, the cells of a bronchogenic squamous cell carcinoma approach a nonspecific morphology in which they are indistinguishable from those of a totally dedifferentiated adenocarcinoma.

The distinctive characteristics of squamous cells may be lost with spindle cell (sarcomatoid) transformation, although this is not always the case. Suster and associates[42] found well-formed intercellular junctions and thick bundles of tonofilaments in one tumor. The two peripheral squamous spindle cell carcinomas reported by Oh and co-workers[35] had a biphasic appearance because of the marked cellular pleomorphism of the spindle cells. Eight sarcomatoid lung carcinomas were

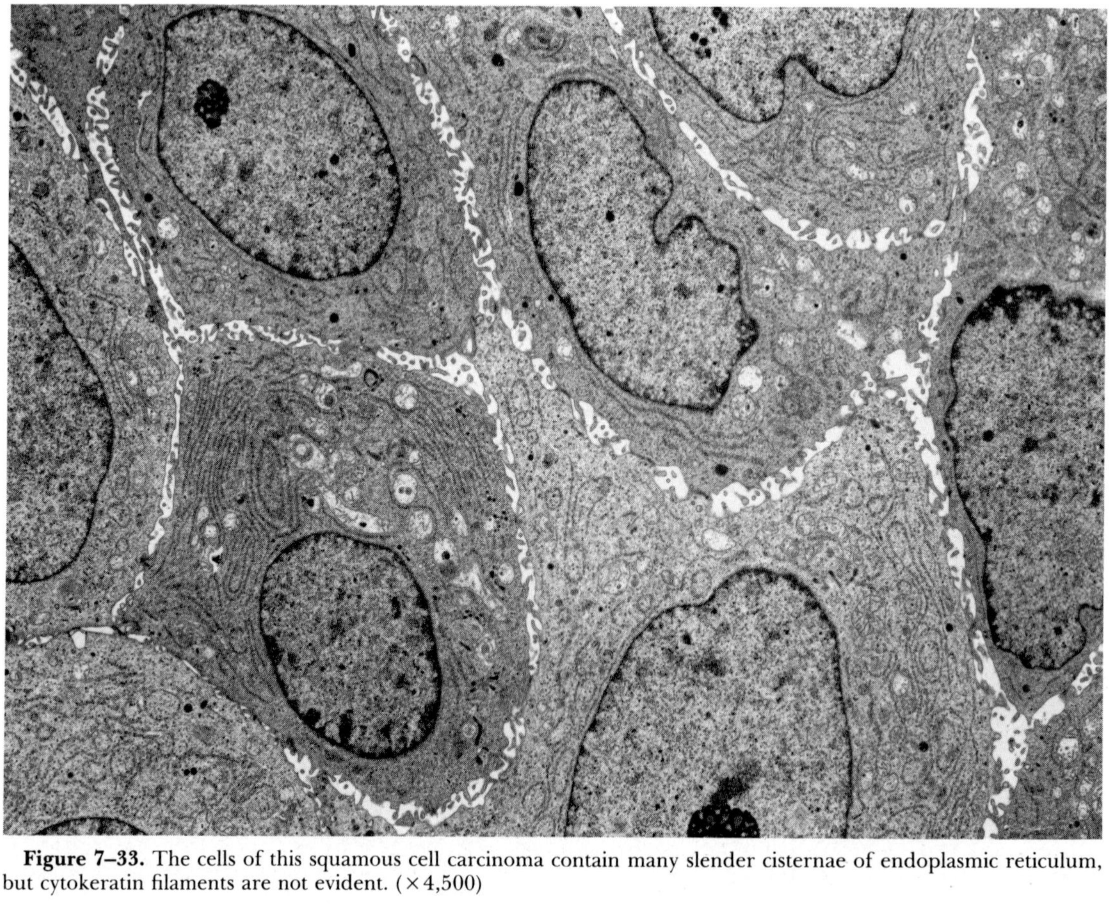

Figure 7–33. The cells of this squamous cell carcinoma contain many slender cisternae of endoplasmic reticulum, but cytokeratin filaments are not evident. (×4,500)

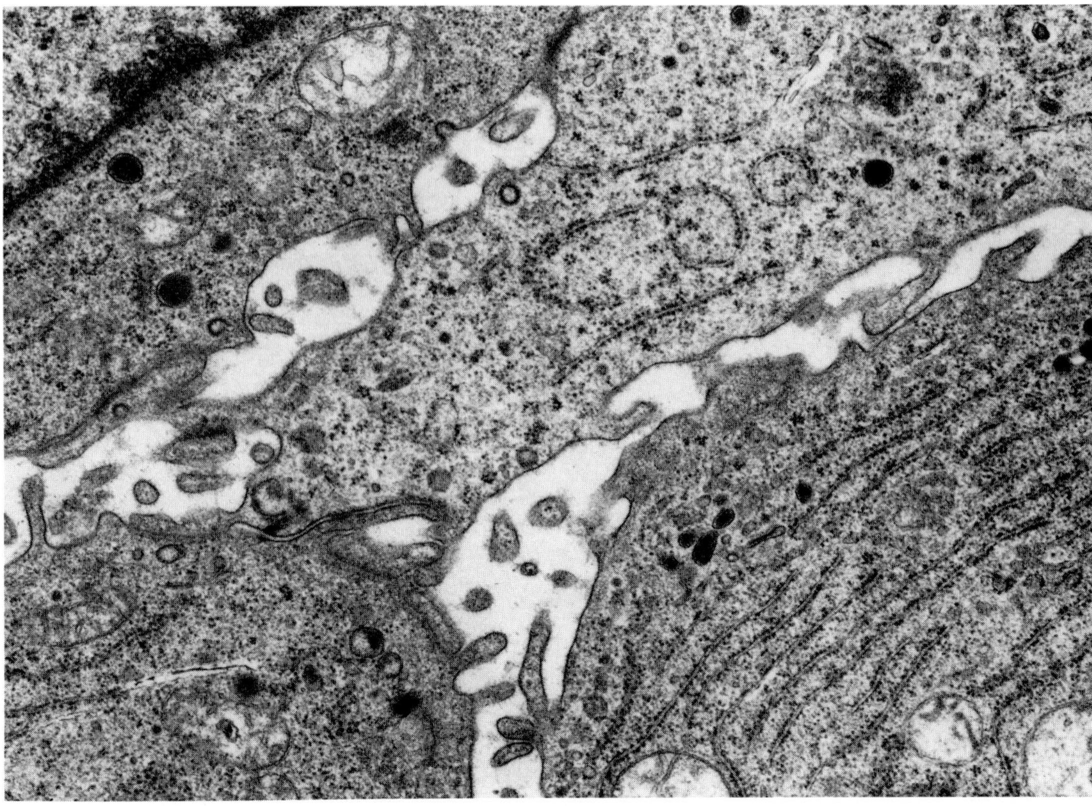

Figure 7–34. Occasional small dense-core granules in a squamous cell carcinoma are probably lysosomes. (×21,000)

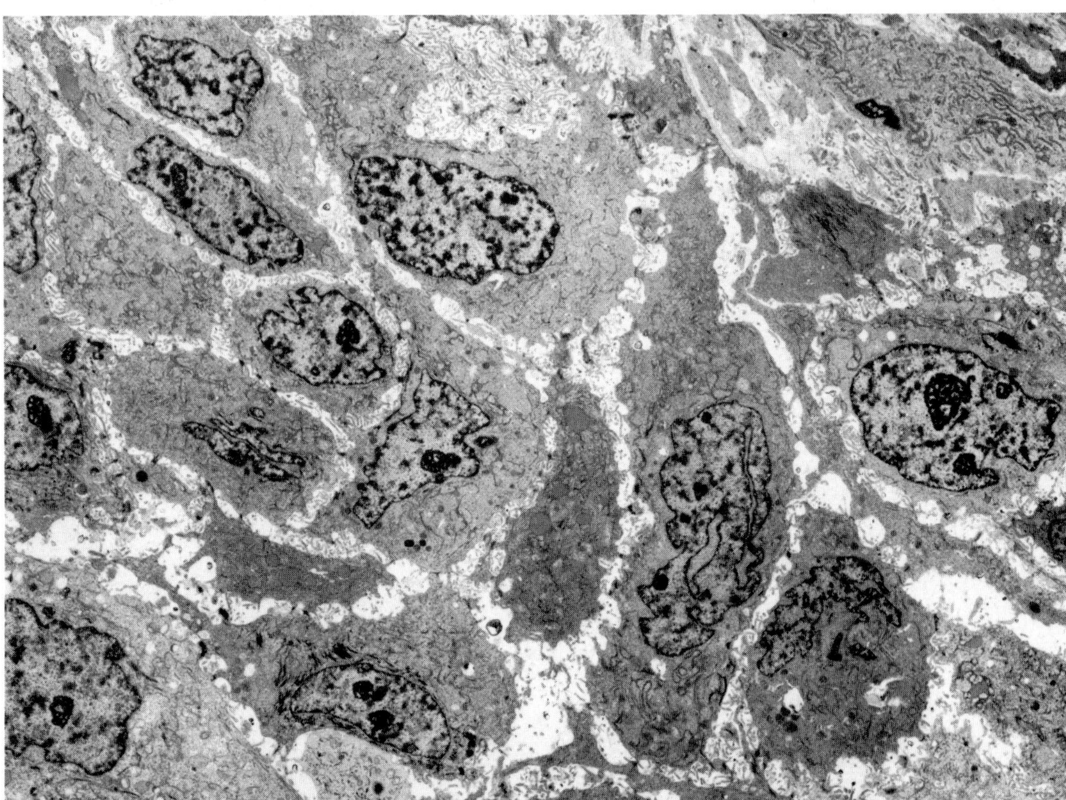

Figure 7–35. Poorly differentiated squamous cell carcinoma. The gaps between the cells are irregular. (×2,600)

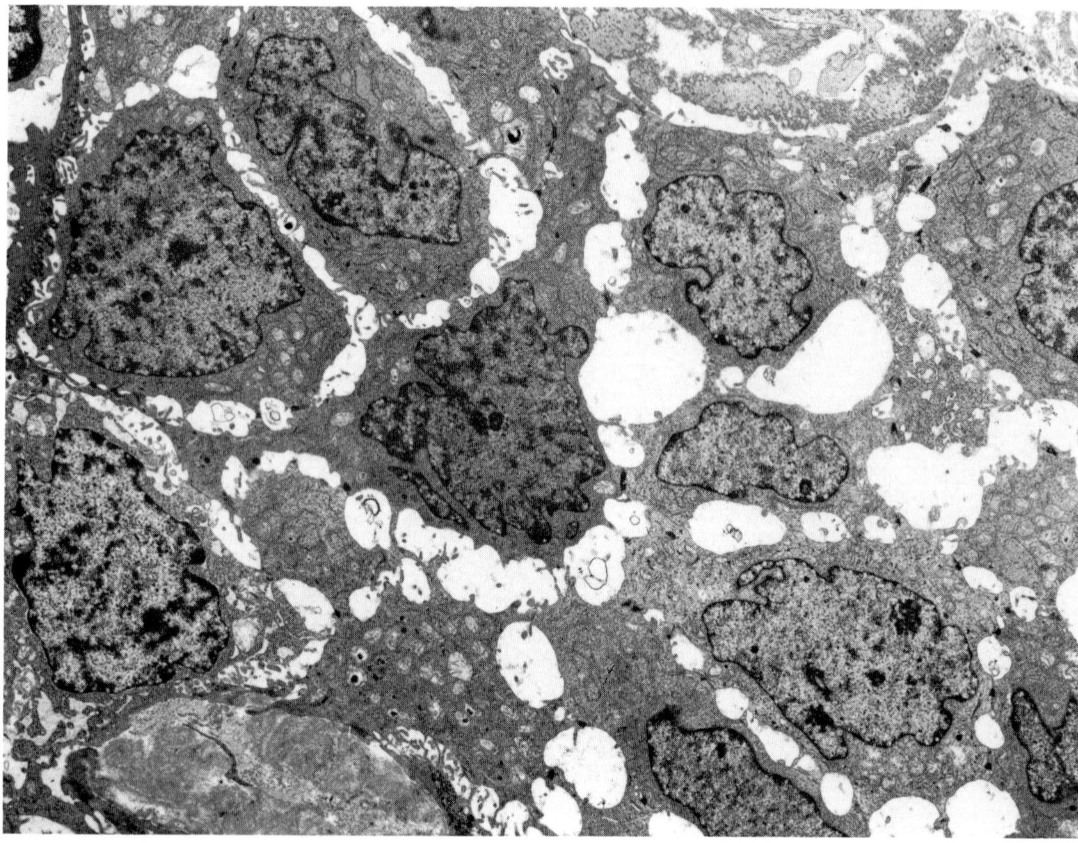

Figure 7–36. Poorly differentiated squamous cell carcinoma. Some large gaps are forming between the cells. (×2,700)

studied with immunocytochemistry and electron microscopy by Humphrey and colleagues.[23] Three of the eight tumors exhibited keratin expression in both the carcinomatous and spindle cell components, but epithelial differentiation was not detected in the sarcomatoid component of five tumors.

REFERENCES

1. Adamson ED, Rees AR: Epidermal growth factor receptors. Mol Cell Biochem 34:129, 1981.
2. Banks-Schlegel S, Green H: Involucrin synthesis and tissue assembly by keratinocytes in normal and cultured human epithelia. J Cell Biol 90:732, 1981.
3. Bejui-Thivolet F, Viac J, Thivolet J et al: Intracellular keratins in normal and pathological bronchial mucosa. Virchows Arch [A] 395:87, 1982.
4. Blobel GA, Moll R, Franke WW et al: Cytokeratins in normal lung and lung carcinomas. Virchows Arch [B] 45:407, 1984.
5. Brenner BG, Jothy S, Shuster J et al: Monoclonal antibodies to human lung from antigens demonstrated by immunofluorescence and immunoprecipitation. Cancer Res 42:3187, 1982.
6. Carpenter G, Cohen S: Epidermal growth factor. Annu Rev Biochem 48:193, 1979.
7. Carter D: Squamous cell carcinoma of the lung: An update. Semin Diagn Pathol 2:226, 1985.
8. Cerny T, Barnes DM, Hasleton P et al: Expression of epidermal growth factor receptor (EGF-R) in human lung tumours. Br J Cancer 54:265, 1986.
9. Collier FC, Enterline TH et al: The prognostic implications of vascular invasion in primary carcinoma of the lung. Arch Pathol 66:594, 1958.
10. Dazord L, Bourel D, Lecorre R et al: A monoclonal antibody (Po66) directed against human lung squamous cell carcinoma immunolocalization of tumour xenografts in nude mice. Cancer Immunol Immunother 24:263, 1987.
11. Dingemans KP, Mooi WJ: Ultrastructure of tumour invasion and desmoplastic response of bronchogenic squamous cell carcinoma. Virchows Arch [A] 411:283, 1987.
12. Downward J, Yarden Y, Mayes E et al: Close similarity of the epidermal growth factor receptor and v-erb-B oncogene protein sequence. Nature 307:521, 1984.
13. Dulmet-Bender E, Jaubert F, Huchon J: Exophytic endobronchial epidermoid carcinoma. Cancer 57:1358, 1986.
14. Fernstein PD, Pekny KW, Reisfeld RA et al: Antigen associated with human squamous cell lung carcinoma defined by murine monoclonal antibodies. Cancer Res 46:2970, 1986.
15. Fitzpatrick SL, Brightwell J, Wittliff JL et al: Epidermal growth factor binding to breast tumor biopsies and relationship to estrogen receptor and

progestin receptor levels. Cancer Res 44:3448, 1984.
16. Fisseler-Eckhoff A, Snyder E, Achatzy R et al: Stromal composition in bronchogenic carcinomas: Morphometric structure analysis. Thorac Cardiovasc Surg 35:160, 1987.
17. Green H: Terminal differentiation of human cultured human epidermal cells. Cell 11:405, 1977.
18. Gullick WJ, Marsden JJ, Whittle N et al: Expression of epidermal growth factor receptors in human cervical, ovarian, and vulvar carcinomas. Cancer Res 46:285, 1986.
19. Gusterson B, Mitchell D, Warburton M et al: Immunohistochemical localization of keratin in human lung tumours. Virchows Arch [A] 394:269, 1982.
20. Hanai N, Shitara K, Yoshida H: Distribution of a squamous cell lung carcinoma–associated antigen, KA-32, in human tissues and some defined by monoclonal antibody KM-32. Cancer Res 46:5206, 1986.
21. Helmuth RA, Strate RW: Squamous carcinoma of the lung in a nonirradiated, nonsmoking patient with juvenile laryngotracheal papillomatosis. Am J Surg Pathol 11:643, 1987.
22. Hendler FJ, Ozanne BW: Human squamous cell lung cancers express increased epidermal growth factor receptors. J Clin Invest 74:647, 1984.
23. Humphrey PA, Scroggs MW, Roggli VL et al: Pulmonary carcinomas with a sarcomatoid element: An immunocytochemical and ultrastructural analysis. Hum Pathol 19:155, 1988.
24. Hunts J, Ueda M, Ozawa S et al: Hyperproduction and gene amplification of the epidermal growth factor receptor in squamous cell carcinomas. Jpn J Cancer Res 76:663, 1985.
25. Johnston WW: Histologic and cytologic patterns of lung cancer in 2,580 men and women over a 15-year period. Acta Cytol 32:163, 1988.
26. Katlic M, Carter D: Prognostic implications of histology: Size and location of primary tumors. In Rosencweig M (ed): Treatment of Lung Cancer, p 143. New York, Raven Press, 1979.
27. Kyoizumi S, Akiyama M, Kouno N et al: Monoclonal antibodies to human squamous cell carcinoma and their application in tumor diagnosis. Cancer Res 45:3274, 1985.
28. Linnoila RI, Mulshine JL, Steinberg SM et al: Neuroendocrine differentiation in endocrine and nonendocrine lung carcinomas. Am J Clin Pathol 90:641, 1988.
29. Moll R: Diversity of cytokeratins in carcinomas. Acta Histochem 34 (suppl):37, 1987.
30. Moll R, Levy R, Czernobilski B et al: Cytokeratins of normal epithelia and some neoplasms of the female genital tract. Lab Invest 49:599, 1983.
31. Morita T, Sugano H: Lung cancer cases reported in the annual of pathological autopsy cases in Japan (1958–1982), with special reference to the characteristics of lung cancer in Japan. Gan No Rinsho 34:416, 1988.
32. Mountain CF, Lukeman JM, Hammar SP et al: Lung cancer classification: The relationship of disease extent and cell type to survival in a clinical trials population. J Surg Oncol 35:147, 1987.
33. Murphy GF, Flynn TC, Rice RH et al: Involucrin expression in normal and neoplastic human skin: A marker for keratinocyte differentiation. J Invest Dermatol 82:453, 1984.
34. Neal AE, Bennett MK, Hall RR et al: Epidermal growth factor receptors in human bladder cancer: Comparison of invasive and superficial tumors. Lancet 1:366, 1985.
35. Oh S, Tsuchiya E, Kitagawa T et al: Spindle cell squamous carcinoma of the lung: Two case reports. Gan No Rinsho 33:293, 1987.
36. Rice RH, Green H: The cornified envelope of terminally differentiated human epidermal keratinocytes consists of cross-linked proteins. Cell 11:417, 1977.
37. Rice RH, Green H: Presence of human epidermal cells of soluble protein precursor in the cross-linked envelope: Activation of cross linking by calcium ions. Cell 18:681, 1979.
38. Said JW, Nash G, Banks-Schlegel S et al: Keratin in human lung tumors: Patterns of localization of different-molecular-weight-keratin proteins. Am J Pathol 113:27, 1983.
39. Said JW, Nash G, Sasoon AF et al: Involucrin in lung tumors: A specific marker for squamous differentiation. Lab Invest 49:563, 1983.
40. Sainsbury JR, Sherbert GV, Fardon JR et al: Epidermal growth factor receptors and estrogen receptors in human breast cancer. Lancet 1:364, 1985.
41. Sobol RE, Astarita RW, Hofeditz C et al: Epidermal growth factor receptor expression in lung carcinomas defined by a monoclonal antibody. JNCI 79:403, 1987.
42. Suster S, Huszar M, Herczeg E: Spindle cell squamous carcinoma of the lung: Immunocytochemical and ultrastructural study of a case. Histopathology 11:871, 1987.
43. Suva LJ, Winslow GA, Wettenhall REA et al: A parathyroid hormone-related protein implicated in malignant hypercalcemia: Cloning and expression. Science 237:893, 1987.
44. Teeter SM, Holmes FF, McFarlane MJ: Lung carcinoma in the elderly population: Influence of histology on the inverse relationship of stage to age. Cancer 60:1331, 1987.
45. Tokudome S, Haratake J, Horie A et al: Histologic types of lung cancers among male Japanese copper smelter workers. Am J Ind Med 14:137, 1988.
46. Van Bodegom PC, Baak JP, Stroet-van-Galen C et al: The percentage of aneuploid cells is significantly correlated with survival in accurately staged patients with stage 1 resected squamous cell lung cancer and long-term follow-up. Cancer 63:143, 1989.
47. Volm M, Mattern J, Muller T et al: Flow cytometry of epidermoid lung carcinomas: Relationship of ploidy and cell cycle phases to survival: A five-year follow-up study. Anticancer Res 8:105, 1988.
48. Watanabe S, Tsugane S, Arimoto H et al: Trend of lung cancers in the National Cancer Center of Japan and comparison with that of Japanese pathological autopsy records. Jpn J Cancer Res 78:460, 1987.
49. Yoneyama K, Erhardt K, Auer G et al: Nuclear DNA content in squamous cell carcinoma, small cell carcinoma, and bronchioloalveolar carcinoma of the lung. Am J Clin Oncol 10:330, 1987.

Chapter

8

UNDIFFERENTIATED LARGE CELL CARCINOMA

Undifferentiated large cell carcinoma is one of the four major lung carcinoma categories in the World Health Organization (WHO) classification.[7, 64] It is sometimes loosely referred to as large cell carcinoma, but this usage is imprecise since squamous cell carcinoma and adenocarcinoma are also large cell carcinomas. An undifferentiated large cell carcinoma is, as its name implies, a non–small cell carcinoma that displays no evidence of either squamous or glandular maturation.[52, 64] Minimal differentiation that is not apparent in conventional light microscopic preparations may be detected in some cases by using immunocytochemical or ultrastructural methods,[9] and greater precision in the diagnosis of undifferentiated large cell carcinoma will consequently be achieved if these procedures are used. For practical purposes, however, the category must be defined as an entity that can be diagnosed by routine light microscopy, and the small degrees of maturation that are identified with more sophisticated techniques may not be clinically relevant. Undifferentiated large cell carcinoma is therefore a non–small cell lung carcinoma that does not show morphologic evidence of differentiation in hematoxylin-eosin–stained sections or secretory activity with mucin stains.

Many pathologists use the term *poorly differentiated carcinoma* when they think they can detect slight differentiation in a non–small cell carcinoma but are uncertain whether it is squamous or glandular. Thresholds for identifying subtle degrees of differentiation in hematoxylin-eosin–stained paraffin sections inevitably vary, and subjective impressions come into play. It is not helpful to a clinician to learn that a tumor is poorly differentiated rather than undifferentiated if the line of maturation is not specified. The unqualified term *poorly differentiated carcinoma* should be avoided whenever possible, even though it serves to inform the clinician that the tumor is a non–small cell carcinoma and for this reason is to be preferred to "unclassified carcinoma." It might be argued that a tumor whose cells are forming cords or nests rather than diffuse sheets is not totally lacking in differentiation, but these primitive patterns are not specific and they are seen in a few small cell "undifferentiated" carcinomas. By definition, therefore, non–small cell carcinomas that lack discernible squamous or glandular features by light microscopy are undifferentiated large cell carcinomas and the poorly differentiated category is a diagnostic wastebasket.

Some undifferentiated large cell carcinomas are composed of diffuse sheets of closely packed uniform cells. In the 1967 WHO classification, four subtypes of large cell carcinoma were described: (1) solid tumors with mucin, (2) solid tumors without mucin, (3) clear cell tumors, and (4) giant cell tumors. In the 1981 revision, the solid tumors with mucin formation were grouped with adenocarcinomas, but the giant cell and clear cell variants were retained.

Pleomorphic carcinomas composed of bizarre and multinucleated giant cells without a squamous or glandular component constitute an anaplastic variant of undifferentiated large cell carcinoma. Hadley and Bullock[18] referred to them as a subtype of anaplastic carcinoma in 1953, and Nash and Stout[40] reported five cases in 1958 and suggested that this form of tumor should be accorded special recognition until more was known about its behavior. Ozello and Stout[43] confirmed its origin by tissue culture. In 1969, Hathaway and co-workers[22] reported 21 cases and analyzed the 118 cases already published.

If some or all of the cells of a large cell lung carcinoma have clear cytoplasm, if the mucin stain is negative, and if there is no evidence of differentiation, the tumor falls within the undifferentiated large cell category. There is probably no merit to recognizing a clear cell subtype of undifferentiated large cell carcinoma. Clear cytoplasm in a lung carcinoma is frequently a sign of degenerative change, particularly in rapidly proliferating tumors. If the cells contain glycogen, metastatic renal cell carcinoma and the rare benign clear cell tumor of the lung enter into the differential diagnosis.[28]

INCIDENCE

Reports based on light microscopy indicate that the frequency of undifferentiated large cell carcinomas is between 10% and 20% of all lung carcinomas.[63] The incidence will be closer to the lower figure when resection specimens are studied and mucin stains are performed and higher if poorly differentiated carcinomas are included.

CLINICAL FEATURES

There are no clinical or radiologic features that will allow a prebiopsy diagnosis of undifferentiated large cell carcinoma.[51] The tumors are often large bulky masses with extensive areas of necrosis or hemorrhage.[60] Glandular differentiation is more common than squamous in resection specimens from patients in whom an initial small biopsy specimen had been reported as undifferentiated large cell carcinoma, an observation that correlates with the common peripheral location and infrequent primary involvement of segmental bronchi. This form of lung cancer is typically aggressive in its behavior and in many instances is rapidly fatal,[12, 13, 23, 24, 36, 52] but patients whose carcinoma has not yet metastasized to regional lymph nodes live longer, and prolonged survival following chemotherapy has been recorded.[58]

LIGHT MICROSCOPY

Some undifferentiated large cell carcinomas are composed of uniform cells in diffuse sheets while others contain larger and often pleomorphic giant cells. Although mixtures of the two patterns are frequently seen, they are described separately for convenience.

Uniform Type

The cells are round to polygonal, and they are compactly grouped without evidence of architectural patterns (Figs. 8–1 and 8–2). A lobular grouping may occur (Fig. 8–3), and occasionally islets of cells are enveloped by a band of fibrous tissue. Some or many cells can have clear cytoplasm that will be mucin negative (Fig. 8–4). The tumor in Figure 8–5 occurred in the lung of a patient from whom a bronchogenic squamous cell carcinoma had been resected: it showed no trace of squamous features and was designated an undifferentiated large cell carcinoma. An impression of stratification can be produced by multilayered sheets of cells surrounding a central focus of necrosis, but this alone is not sufficient evidence for squamous differentiation, although it is so regarded by some pathologists. Zones of necrosis are quite frequently seen, and dropout of individual degenerating cells can create an illusion of glandular lumens. The size of the tumor cells may be the same as that of most adenocarcinomas and squamous carcinomas, but the nuclear/cytoplasmic ratio is higher. Nuclei are round and central, and a large nucleolus is the rule. In rare instances, foci of apparent undifferentiated small cell carcinoma may be found in a predominantly large cell carcinoma, prompting a diagnosis of mixed large cell–small cell carcinoma. Extreme caution must be exercised in making this diagnosis, and support from results of immunostaining and electron microscopy should first be sought.

A mucin stain must always be performed before the diagnosis is made. It will be positive in approximately half of patients suspected of having undifferentiated large cell carcinomas, placing the tumors in the adenocarcinoma category. Solitary mucin-containing cells may be entrapped near the periphery of the groups of tumor cells and can be disregarded. Only intracytoplasmic mucin is significant; surface and stromal staining is

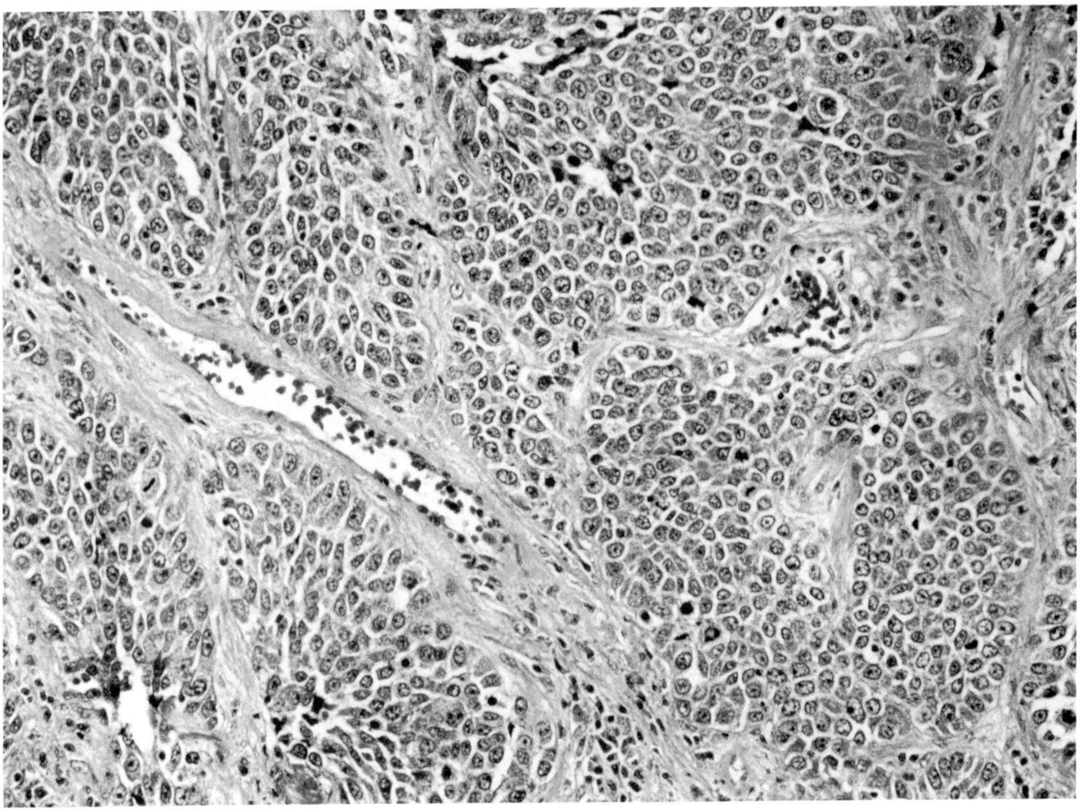

Figure 8–1. Undifferentiated large cell carcinoma, compact type. Solid nests of uniform cells.

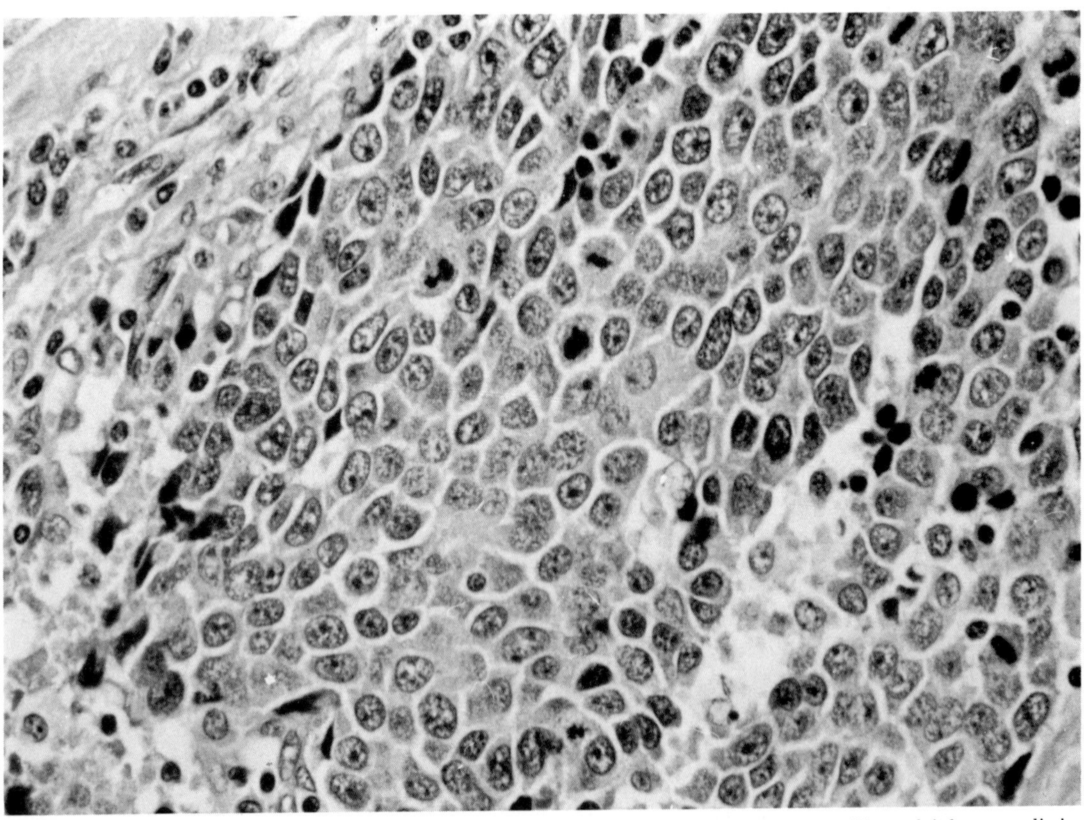

Figure 8–2. Undifferentiated large cell carcinoma, compact type. The round to ovoid nuclei have a distinct chromatin pattern, and a nucleolus is often visible.

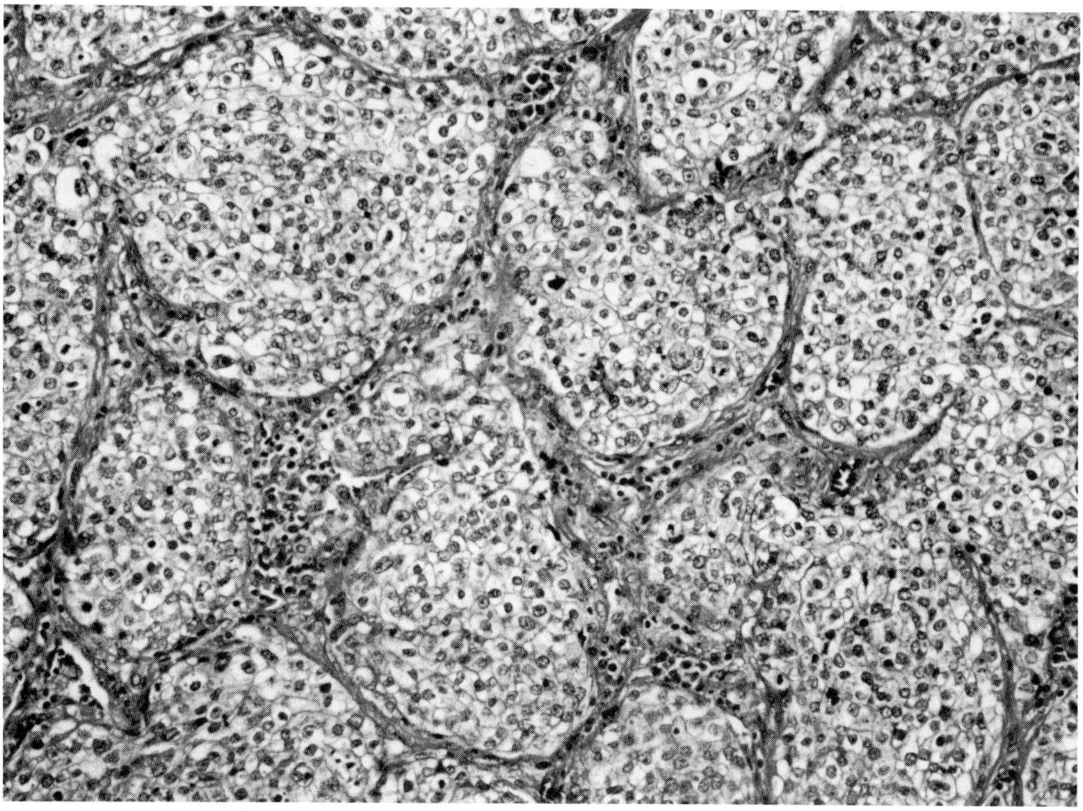

Figure 8–3. Undifferentiated large cell carcinoma. The solid nests of cells are separated by slender bands of stroma.

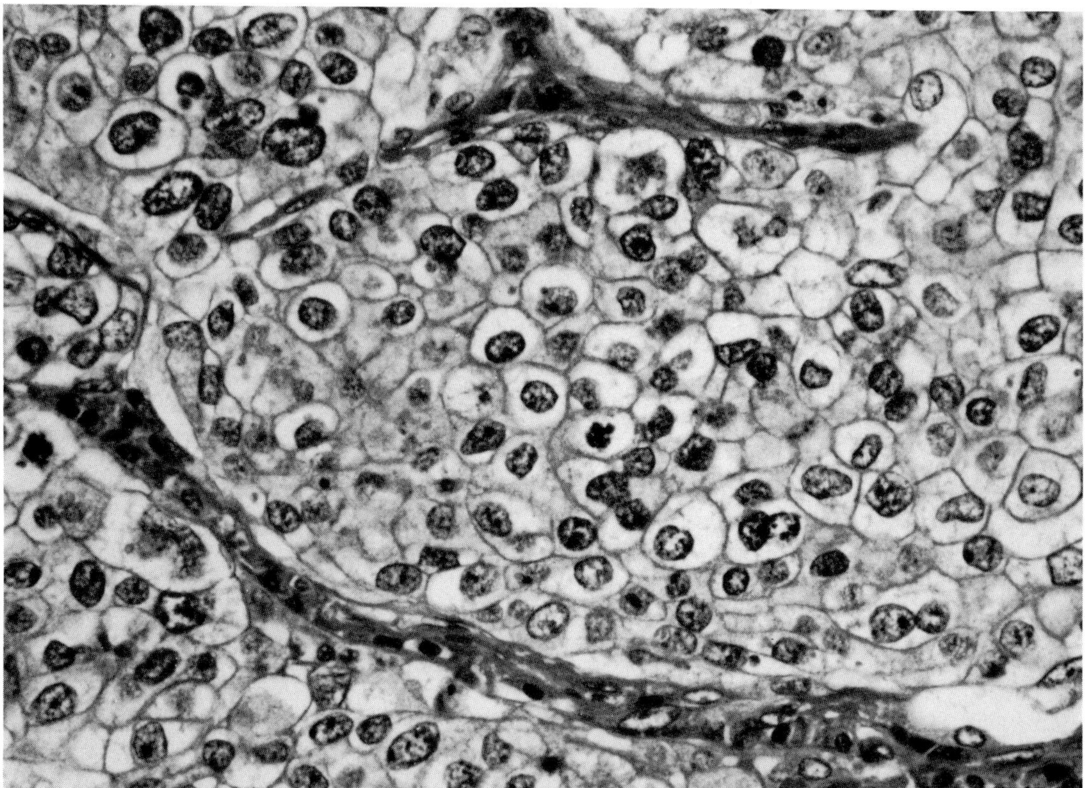

Figure 8–4. Undifferentiated large cell carcinoma. The moderate amount of cytoplasm is evident, and it is clear in some cells. A mucin stain was negative.

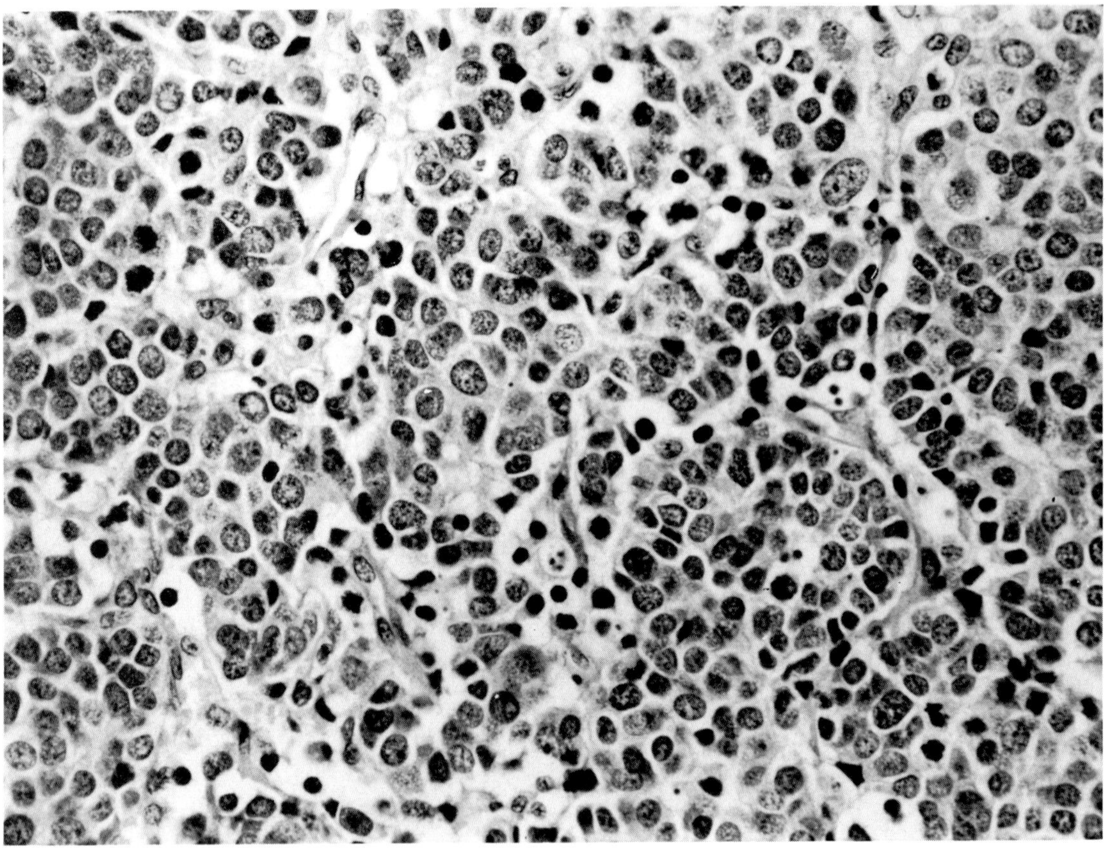

Figure 8–5. Undifferentiated large cell carcinoma. This was a recurrent tumor in a patient who earlier underwent resection of a bronchogenic squamous cell carcinoma.

not relevant. Yesner[63] recommends the alcian blue–periodic acid–Schiff (PAS) procedure, pointing out that it serves to distinguish the pale blue staining of mucopolysaccharides in the stroma from the dark blue to purple acid mucin in the tumor cells. When only glycogen is present, the PAS component is positive. Yesner considers that more than 1% of positive cells are required for a diagnosis of adenocarcinoma. Members of the Lung Cancer Study Group favor Mayer's mucicarmine stain, believing that the bright pink mucin leaves little possibility for misinterpretation, even though it is perhaps a little less sensitive than alcian blue.

Giant Cell Carcinoma

The features of the cells of giant cell carcinoma are extremely variable, but the fundamental property is large size, often accompanied by marked variability in cell and nuclear shape and multinucleation (Figs. 8–6 through 8–8). A significant number of the cells (more than 30% are required by the Lung Cancer Study Group) should display these characteristics before the tumor is designated a giant cell carcinoma. Carter and Eggleston[7] advocate a figure of 40%, and Ferraro and colleagues[12] require 50%. Cell cohesion is often lost (see Fig. 8–6), and the outlines of the cells are then easily perceived. Because of the lack of cohesion, a pleomorphic large cell lymphoma is occasionally considered, and the immunoperoxidase stain for leukocyte common antigen will then be helpful. Necrosis is common, and an extensive infiltration by inflammatory cells is often seen (see Figs. 8–7 and 8–8).[26] In contrast to the high nuclear/cytoplasmic ratio that characterizes the uniform type of undifferentiated large cell carcinoma, much of the cell is made up of cytoplasm. It varies in tinctorial qualities but is often markedly eosinophilic and may be finely vacuolated. Neutrophils or macrophages are sometimes present within degenerating tumor cells.

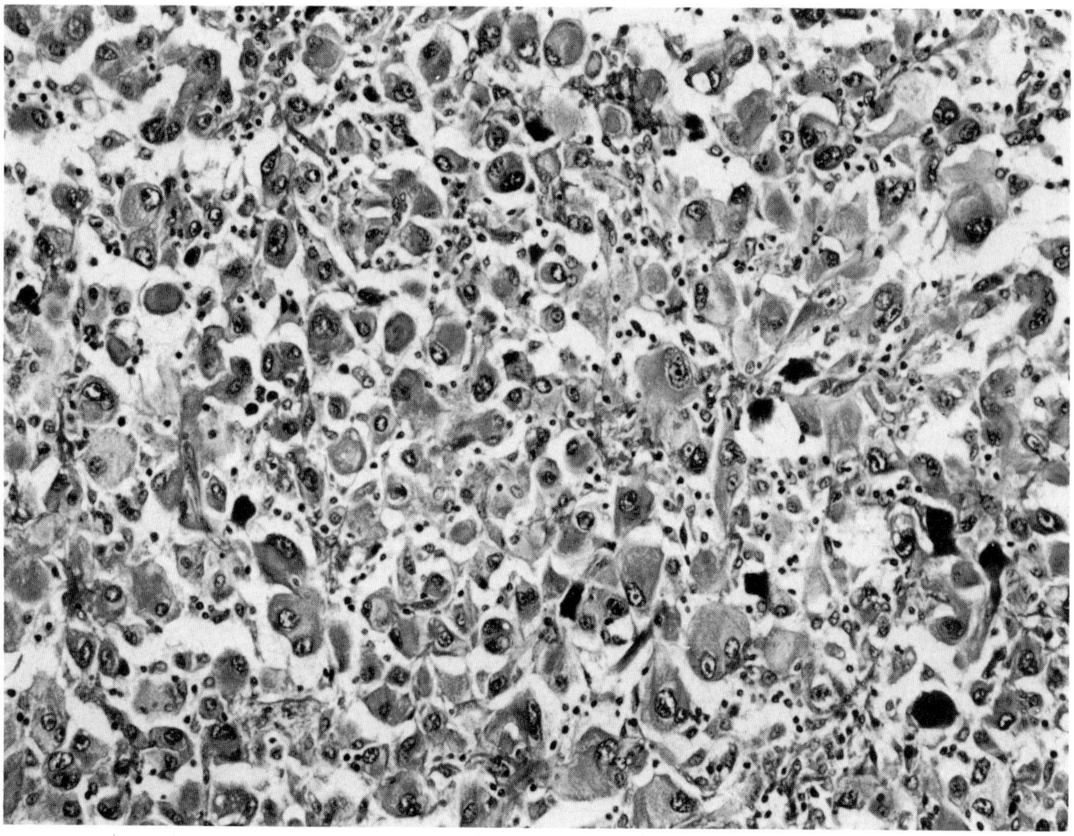

Figure 8–6. Undifferentiated large cell carcinoma composed of loosely cohesive giant cells.

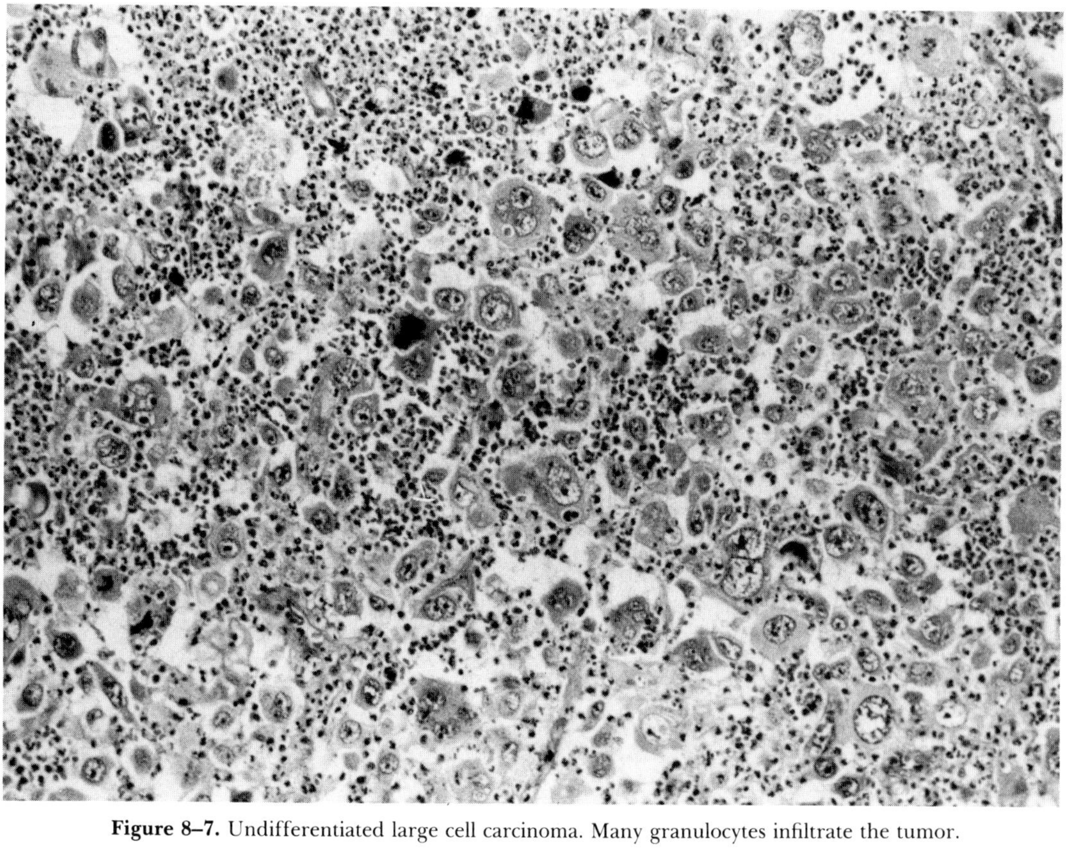

Figure 8–7. Undifferentiated large cell carcinoma. Many granulocytes infiltrate the tumor.

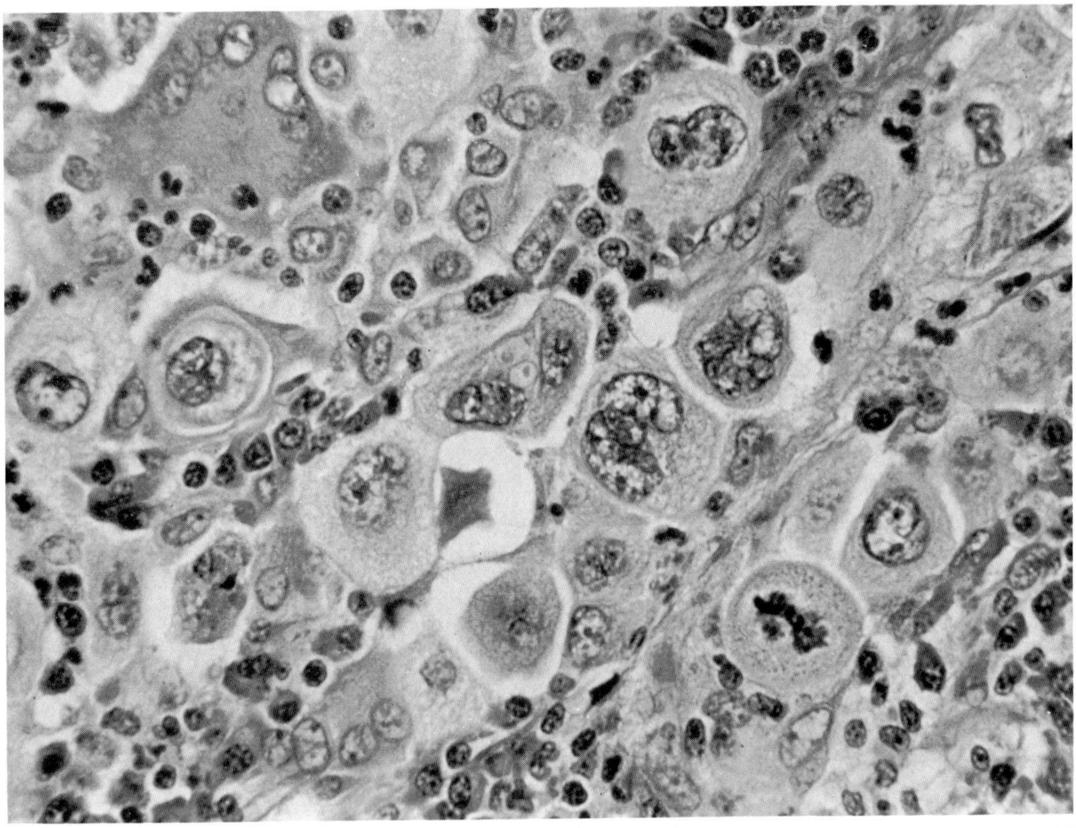

Figure 8–8. Undifferentiated large cell carcinoma. Mononucleate and multinucleate cells coexist with neutrophils and plasma cells.

The single or multiple tumor cell nuclei vary greatly in size and shape. Single nuclei can reach a large size, and they are typically irregular and lobulated in profile with densely clumped chromatin and one or more large nucleoli.[31] Several small nuclei may be present in a single cell.

Giant cell transformation may partially involve an otherwise differentiated carcinoma, and the great majority of these tumors are adenocarcinomas. However, pleomorphic cells also occur in some squamous cell carcinomas (Figs. 8–9 and 8–10). The differentiated component is generally only detected in resection or autopsy material.

CYTOLOGY

Cells of the compact type of undifferentiated large cell carcinoma are oval or polyhedral with finely granular cytoplasm that may appear eosinophilic or basophilic.[6] The nucleus is central and round to ovoid (Fig. 8–11), and it may appear hyperchromatic. One large or several smaller nucleoli are present (Figs. 8–12 and 8–13). In the pleomorphic form, the larger cells often contain several nuclei showing marked irregularity and hyperchromasia (Figs. 8–14 through 8–16),[45] and these cells can occur singly or in clusters among the less pleomorphic cells. In sputum or in aspiration specimens, the cells may lie in loose sheets (Fig. 8–17) or aggregates, which can closely resemble those of poorly differentiated adenocarcinoma; however, they do not form the three-dimensional clusters that are seen in adenocarcinomas and particularly in the bronchioloalveolar subtype.

IMMUNOCYTOCHEMISTRY

Immunocytochemical studies have confirmed that undifferentiated large cell carcinomas constitute a phenotypically heterogeneous group of neoplasms that includes poorly differentiated squamous cell carcinomas and adenocarcinomas[5, 10, 11, 17, 46, 47] and

Text continued on page 201

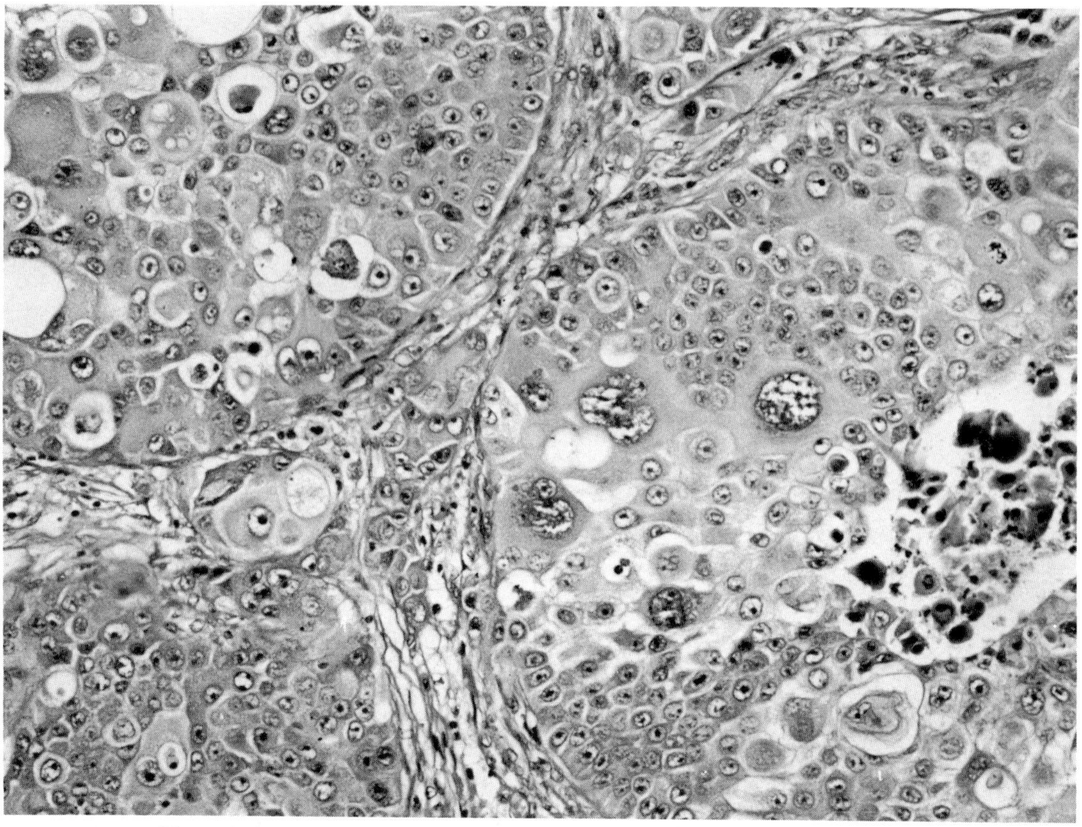

Figure 8–9. Squamous cell carcinoma showing early pleomorphic transformation.

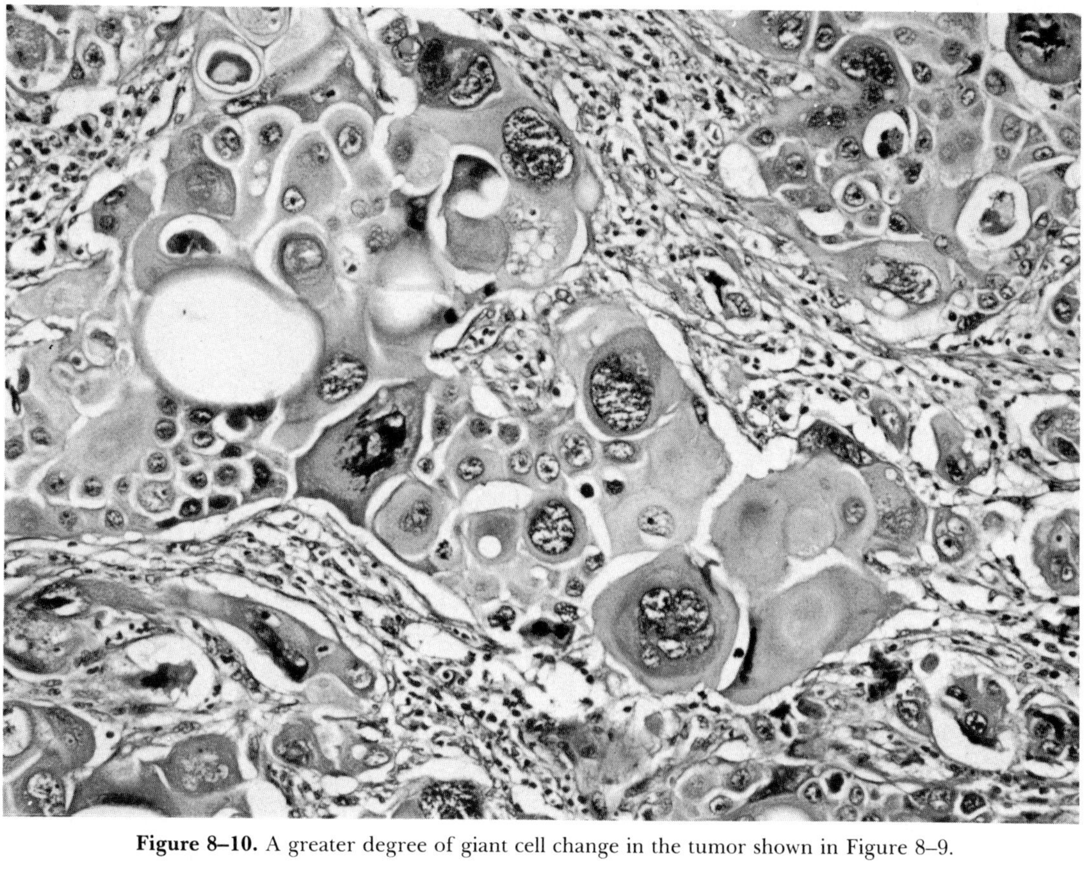

Figure 8–10. A greater degree of giant cell change in the tumor shown in Figure 8–9.

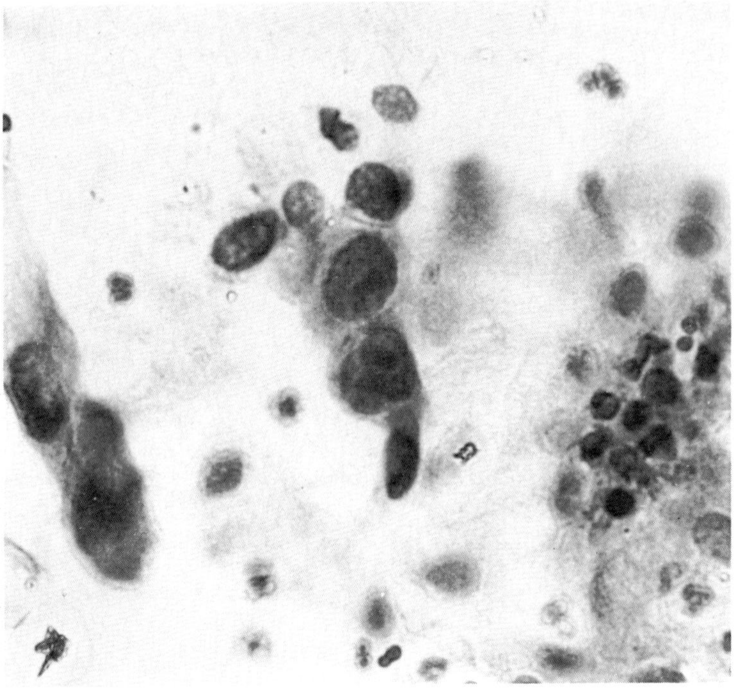

Figure 8–11. Undifferentiated large cell carcinoma. Sputum: the cells are forming irregular small clusters.

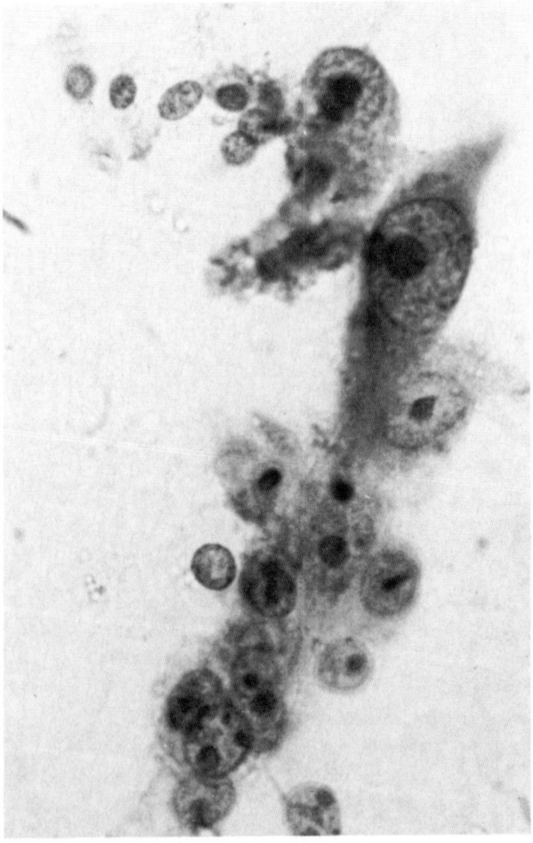

Figure 8–12. Undifferentiated large cell carcinoma. Fine-needle aspiration biopsy: nucleoli are round, dense, and often large.

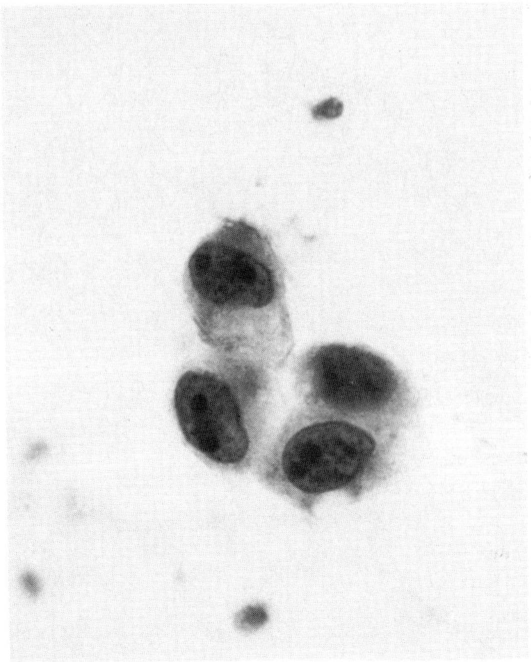

Figure 8–13. Undifferentiated large cell carcinoma. Sputum: two nucleoli are visible in the three focused nuclei.

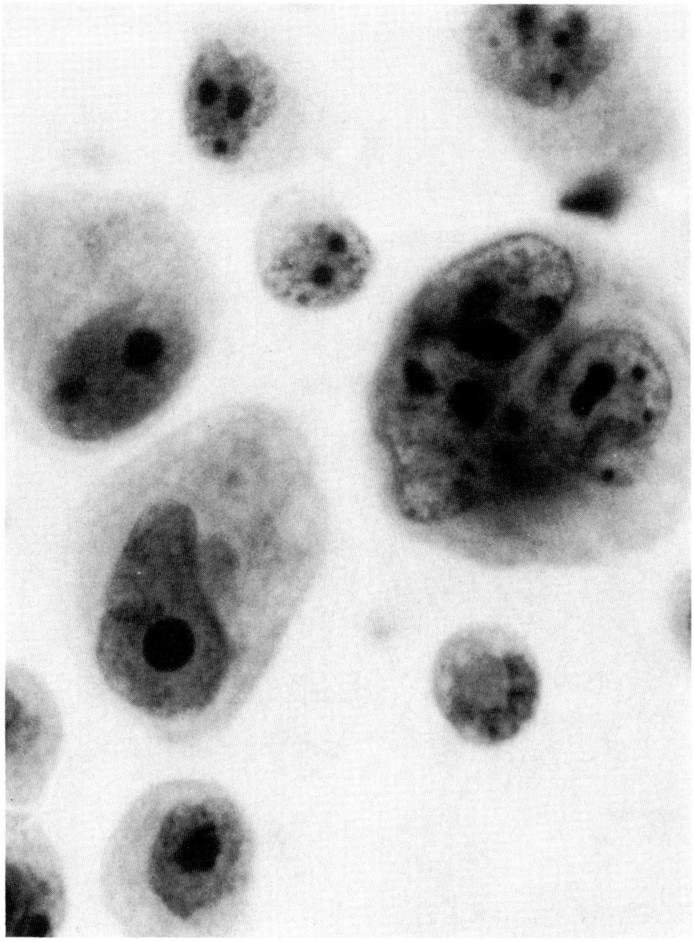

Figure 8–14. Undifferentiated large cell carcinoma. Fine-needle aspiration biopsy: the nuclei contain sharply etched, often multiple nucleoli.

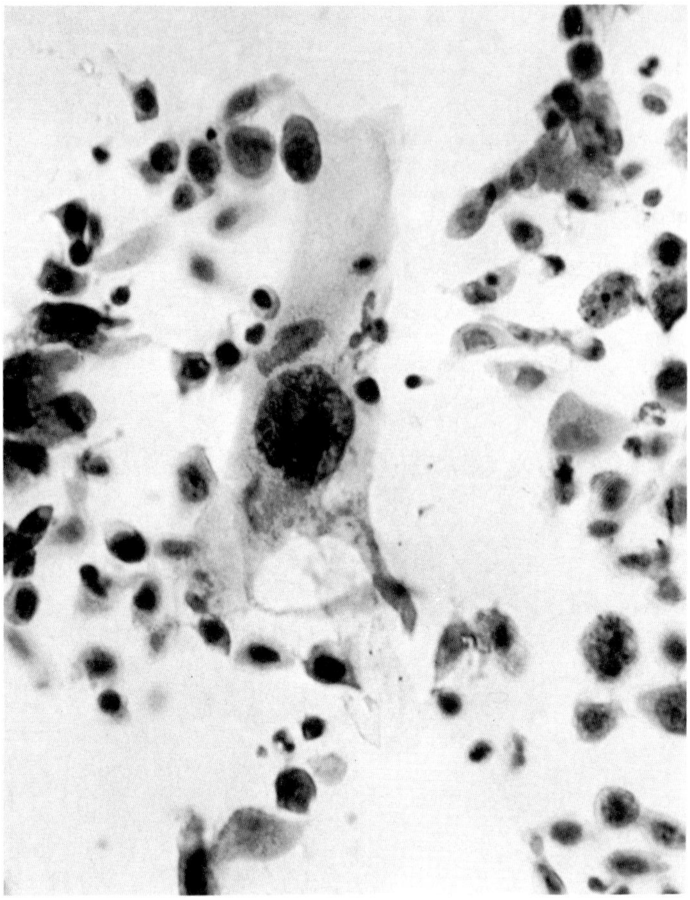

Figure 8–15. Undifferentiated large cell carcinoma. Fine-needle aspiration biopsy: a tumor cell with extensive cytoplasm is surrounded by many inflammatory cells.

Figure 8–16. Undifferentiated large cell carcinoma. Fine-needle aspiration biopsy: there is a mixture of small mononucleate and larger pleomorphic cells with neutrophils and some debris.

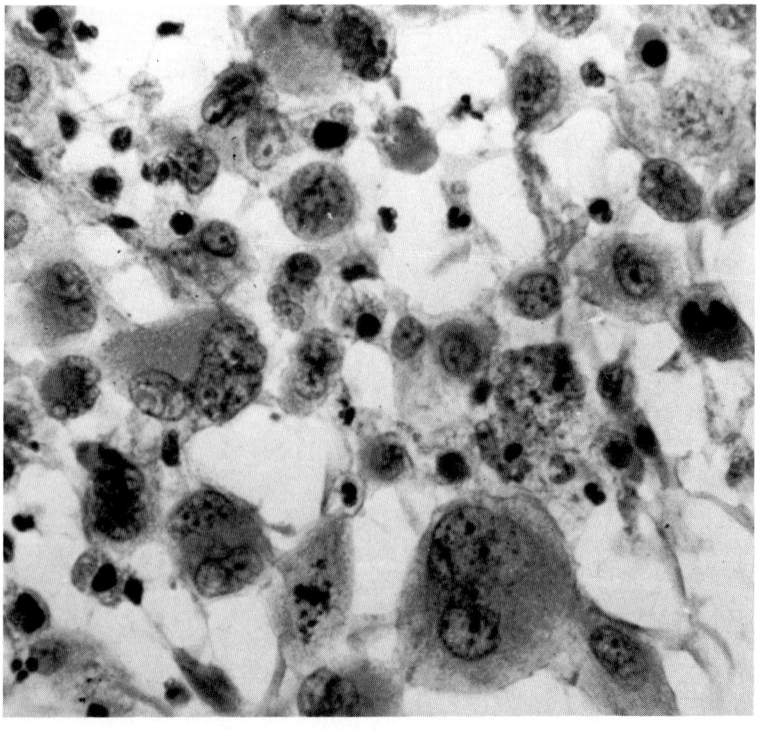

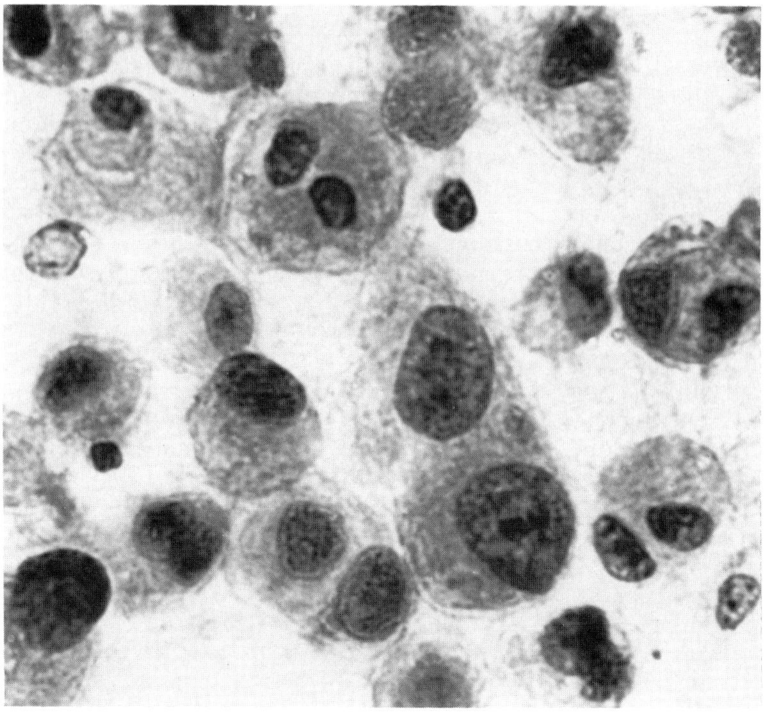

Figure 8–17. Undifferentiated large cell carcinoma. Fine-needle aspiration biopsy: there is considerable variation in cell and nuclear size.

have shown that a few display endocrine differentiation manifested by positive immunostaining for neuron-specific enolase, serotonin, and various neuropeptides.[10, 11, 20, 33, 35, 41] Immunoreactivity for surfactant apoproteins, indicating Clara cell or type II pneumocyte differentiation, has also been reported.[27, 37] Rarely, an undifferentiated large cell carcinoma may produce excessive serum alkaline phosphatase.[44]

Undifferentiated large cell carcinomas can be divided into two groups according to their cytokeratin expression. In one, the cytokeratins are of the type found in simple epithelia, and these tumors can be viewed as poorly differentiated adenocarcinomas. The second type expresses a stratified epithelium–type cytokeratin pattern, indicating that they are poorly differentiated squamous cell carcinomas.[39] The latter group can also be recognized by reactivity with antisera against involucrin, a specific marker for squamous cell differentiation. Six of the 12 tumors studied by Said and co-workers were positive for this protein.[50] In our experience, immunocytochemical studies using antibodies for high- and low-molecular-weight cytokeratins and involucrin will reveal evidence of glandular or squamous differentiation in many undifferentiated large cell carcinomas.

ELECTRON MICROSCOPY

Studies of non–small cell lung carcinomas in which conventional light microscopy has been correlated with electron microscopy have helped to define the nature of undifferentiated large cell carcinoma and elucidate its morphologic features.[1, 3, 8, 15, 19, 25, 31, 32, 55, 61] In Chapters 6 and 7, the changes that take place with loss of differentiation in the cells of adenocarcinomas and squamous cell carcinomas are described and illustrated. In adenocarcinomas, there is a progressive disappearance of lumens and their associated microvilli and tight junctions. In a dedifferentiating squamous cell carcinoma, the number and size of the cell junctions diminish, and the elaborate substructure of the mature desmosomes with their intermediate lines and subplasmalemmal plaques gives way to mere densities of the apposed cell membranes. Cytokeratin filaments become reduced in number and eventually disappear. The progressive loss of specialized characteristics that is seen in both adenocarcinomas and squamous cell carcinomas leads ultimately to a cell type devoid of the specific structural features of the two differentiated categories of non–small cell carcinoma,[53] and this lowest common morphologic denominator constitutes undifferentiated large cell carcinoma. In undifferentiated large cell carcinomas that are ultrastructurally devoid of glandular or squamous features, immunocytochemical studies for epithelial markers such as cytokeratins,[17, 38] desmosomal proteins,[39] or carcinoembryonic antigen[5] may nonetheless be positive.

By electron microscopy, cells of the uniform type of undifferentiated large cell carcinoma are roughly round, but most appear polygonal because of compression from intimate apposition with neighboring cells. Cell surfaces are smooth (a few filopodia may be present), and cell junctions are sparse and poorly developed. Cytokeratin filament bundles are not seen, and organelles are confined to a few mitochondria and short slender cisternae. Nuclei have smooth contours, and in well-fixed tissues the chromatin is fine and evenly dispersed. Nucleoli are round, large, and dense.

From what has been stated about undifferentiated large cell carcinoma, it will be apparent that many tumors that are given this designation by light microscopy are found on ultrastructural examination to have glandular features (Fig. 8–18), or less often they are seen with the electron microscope to possess the mature desmosomes and cytokeratin filaments of a squamous cell carcinoma. There may be only a hint of differentiation, insufficient to clearly indicate the line of maturation. For example, the cell junctions may seem to be more numerous than in a typical undifferentiated large cell carcinoma, or a few bundles of cytokeratin filaments or a small space suggestive of a lumen may be found. These findings indicate that the tumor is not totally lacking in differentiation, but they are not sufficient to justify calling it an adenocarcinoma or squamous cell carcinoma. It is not uncommon to find a suggestion of gland formation as well as prominent cell junctions and cytokeratin in the same tumor.[29] While these features could be viewed as an argument for a diagnosis of poorly differentiated large cell carcinoma,

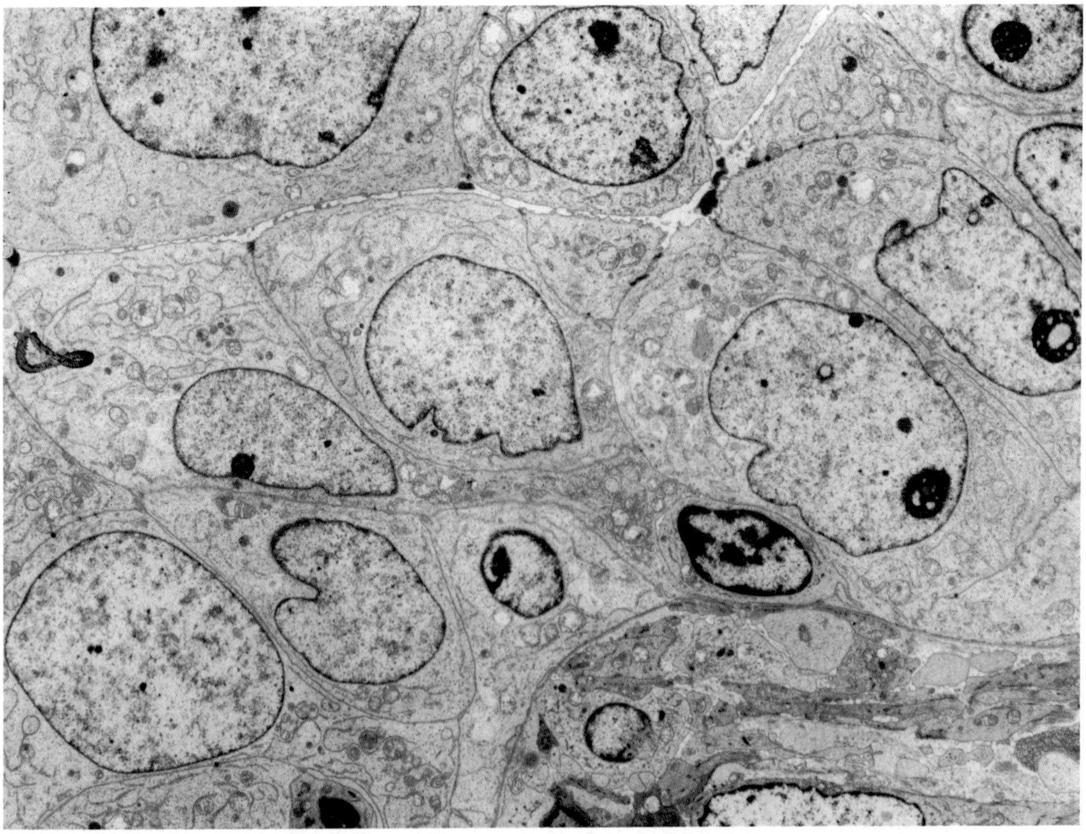

Figure 8–18. Poorly differentiated adenocarcinoma. The tumor was an undifferentiated large cell carcinoma by light microscopy, but electron microscopy showed occasional slender lumens. Note the close apposition of the smooth cell membranes. (×4,500)

use of the term is not encouraged because it lacks clinical value. Cytoplasmic granules comparable in size and appearance to those of Clara cells are occasionally encountered in an otherwise undifferentiated large cell carcinoma. Only rarely, in our experience, does an undifferentiated large cell carcinoma contain cytoplasmic granules of endocrine caliber, and when they are sparse, their nature and significance are uncertain (Fig. 8–19).

A broad range of ultrastructural appearances can be seen in pleomorphic undifferentiated large cell carcinomas (Figs. 8–20 and 8–21). In some tumors, the cells appear epithelial because of their shape and apposition and the presence of well-defined cell junctions and considerable numbers of organelles. The endoplasmic reticulum can be extensive (Fig. 8–20), and lipid droplets and vacuoles of varying sizes are common (Fig. 8–21). The marked nuclear irregularity is shown well in electron micrographs (Fig. 8–21). It can be seen that the cells of the giant cell form of undifferentiated large cell carcinoma generally do not possess specific features, a characteristic they share with pleomorphic carcinomas in other locations.

Electron microscopy is not required in the routine evaluation of a suspected undifferentiated large cell carcinoma because the minor levels of differentiation it may reveal are not known to be of prognostic significance. It is, however, a useful monitoring device to assess the accuracy of diagnoses of undifferentiated large cell carcinoma made by light microscopy and is mandatory if a possibility of small cell carcinoma cannot be ruled out by light microscopy.

Two continuous cancer cell lines were established from patients with large cell undifferentiated lung carcinomas by Anger and co-workers,[3] and the cells showed little evidence of maturation at the ultrastructural level. Some nonspecific cytoplasmic filaments were present in one, and microvilli with rare primitive junctions were found in the second cell line. Both grew as solid tumors in nude mice and failed to show evidence of differentiation. Flow cytometric analysis showed hypertriploid stemlines with high RNA indi-

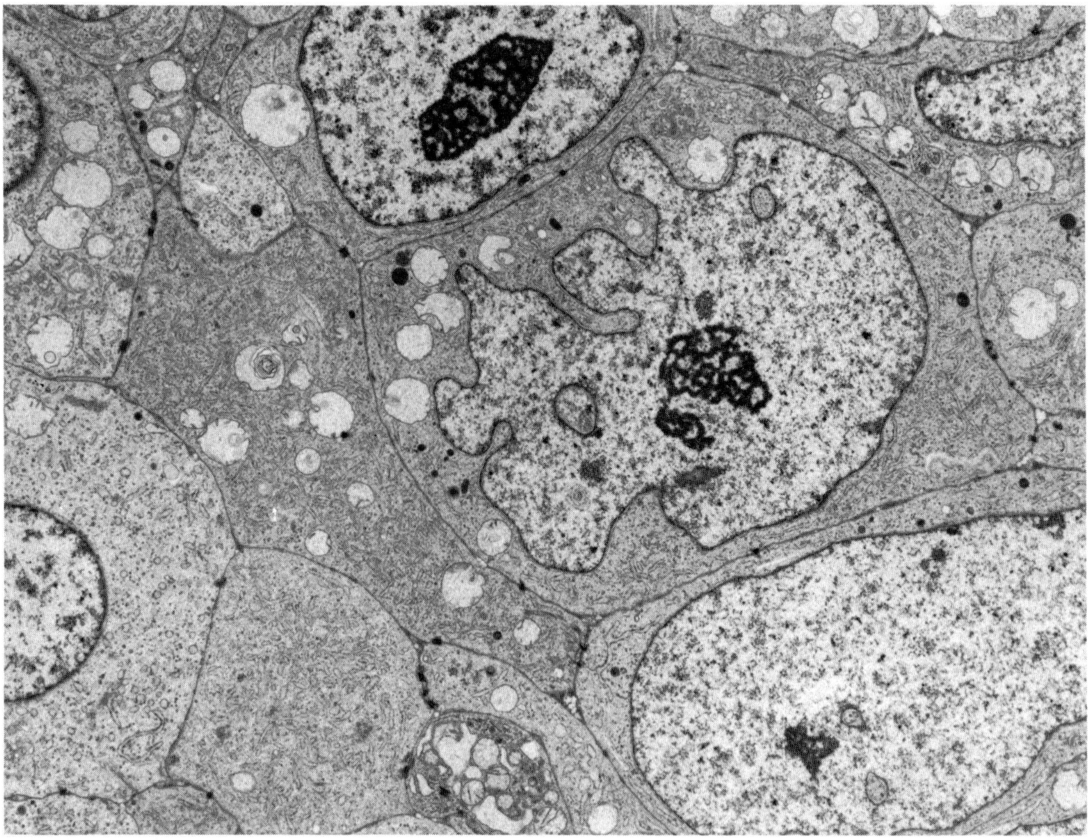

Figure 8–19. Undifferentiated large cell carcinoma composed of cells with closely apposed cell membranes and small cell junctions. A few dense-core granules of endocrine caliber are present. (×5,200)

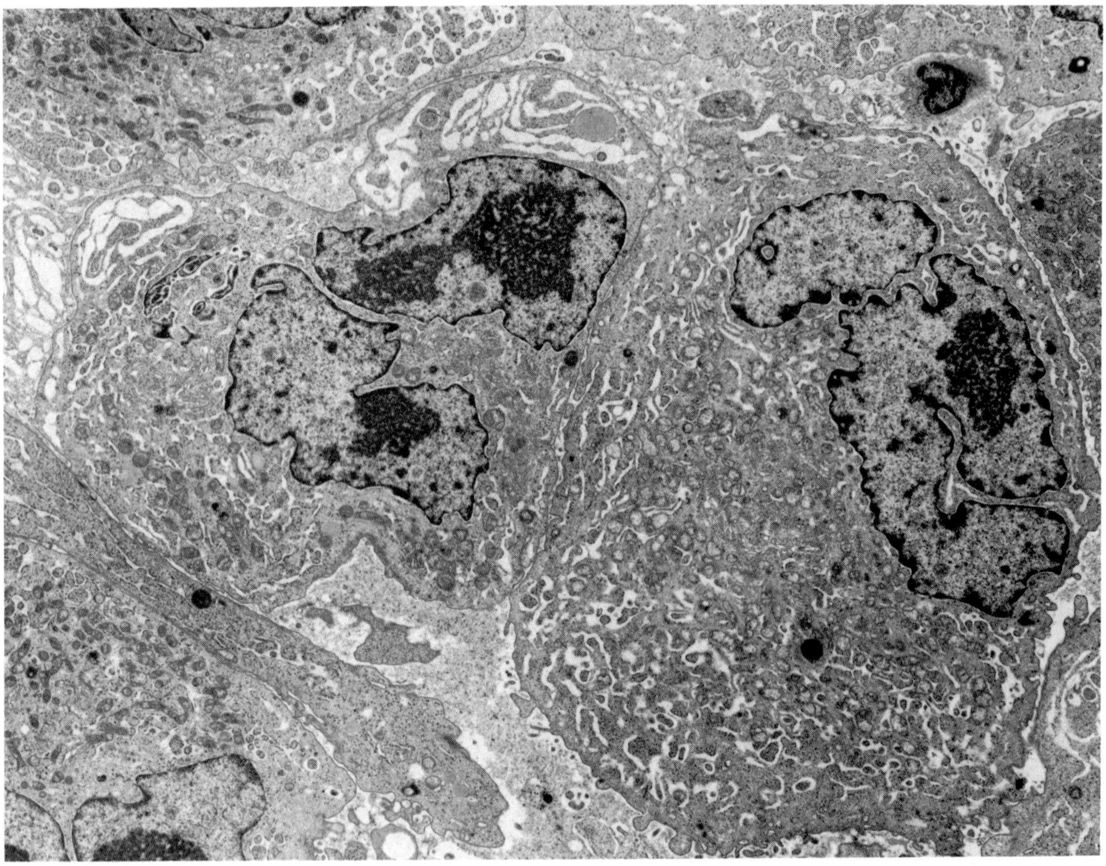

Figure 8–20. Undifferentiated large cell carcinoma. Pleomorphic cells with irregular nuclei, large nucleoli, and abundant organelles. A few short surface protrusions simulate microvilli. Although neighboring cells occasionally contact one another, cell junctions are not evident. (×4,500)

ces, and marker chromosomes were present in both tumor cell lines.

DIFFERENTIAL DIAGNOSIS

Undifferentiated large cell carcinomas are on occasion difficult to distinguish from small cell lung carcinomas, and mixed variants occur.[32] Radice and associates[49] reported that small cell–large cell tumors responded less well to therapy and had shorter survival times than pure small cell carcinomas. Little and co-workers[30] found an amplified c-myc oncogene in cell lines of this type of tumor, but the phenomenon of gene amplification may be unique to *in vitro* cells. The distinction of small cell carcinoma from undifferentiated large cell carcinoma and the occurrence of mixed variants are discussed in Chapter 9. Morphometric studies confirm that there is a spectrum of cell size that encompasses both small and large cell lung cancers.[57] Authentic mixtures of large cell and small cell carcinomas in which both components are undifferentiated must be rare. We have not seen a convincing example at the ultrastructural level. Possible cases have with electron microscopy been found to be made up of cells of a single type varying in the quantity and density of their cytoplasm (see Fig. 9–3).

Rarely an undifferentiated large cell carcinoma can simulate melanoma, large cell lymphoma, or certain sarcomas, and a screening panel of antibodies incorporating those for cytokeratins, S-100 protein or preferably a melanoma-specific antigen, and leukocyte common antigen is extremely useful in narrowing the differential diagnosis. While the clinical data may strongly indicate a primary pulmonary neoplasm, any of these tumors can involve the lung solely or as part of a disseminated disease. If the chest wall is involved, it should be remembered that mesothelioma can mimic both the uniform and the pleomorphic forms of undifferentiated

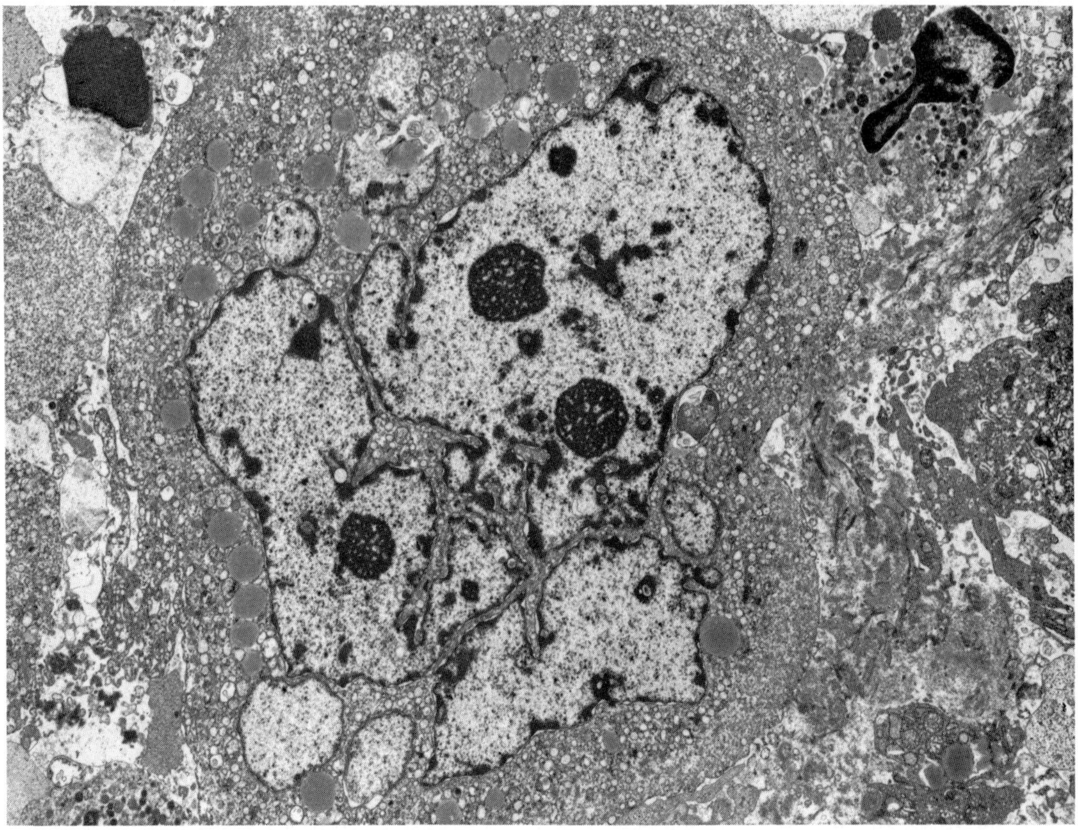

Figure 8–21. Undifferentiated large cell carcinoma. A multilobated tumor cell from an area of necrosis. Nucleoli are large and round. This cell contains many lipid droplets and small vacuoles, and neutrophils lie close to its surface. (×4,500)

large cell carcinoma, and immunostaining for carcinoembryonic antigen may aid in distinguishing between the two tumors (see Chapter 12).

The interpretation of immunostaining for vimentin calls for considerable caution, and this is particularly the case when attempting to distinguish undifferentiated large cell carcinoma from a sarcoma. Although vimentin filaments are typically present in sarcomas and melanomas,[42] co-expression with cytokeratin proteins, and with other types of intermediate filaments, can occur in lung tumors, including undifferentiated large cell carcinoma.[4, 14, 34, 56] In an immunocytochemical study of 285 formalin-fixed lung carcinomas, Upton and co-workers[56] found reactivity for vimentin in 11 (8.5%) of 129 adenocarcinomas and in 15 of 61 (24.6%) anaplastic large cell carcinomas. Although the authors did not observe staining for this marker in any of the 51 squamous cell carcinomas or 35 small cell carcinomas included in their series, vimentin reactivity in these tumors has been reported by others.[34, 56]

Production of β-human chorionic gonadotropin (hCG) has been found to be associated with all histologic types of lung cancer,[16] but especially with undifferentiated large cell carcinoma.[21, 35, 59, 62] In an immunohistochemical study of 127 lung tumors, Wachner and associates[59] were able to demonstrate β-hCG in 12 (9%), and the highest incidence was in the undifferentiated large cell carcinoma group (4 of the 12 cases were positive). It is conceivable that an undifferentiated large cell carcinoma producing β-hCG might be confused with choriocarcinoma, but primary choriocarcinoma of the lung is an extremely rare neoplasm and the presence of trophoblastic elements will establish the diagnosis. The serum hCG titer is also of great value in making this distinction.[48, 54]

It is beyond the scope of this text to detail the ultrastructural features of the various metastatic tumors that can be confused with undifferentiated large cell carcinoma of the lung, but the value of selected immunostaining procedures and/or electron microscopy merits emphasis. The range of ultrastructural appearances that can be encountered among soft tissue sarcomas is extremely broad. Undifferentiated large cell carcinoma may mimic rhabdomyosarcoma, liposarcoma, osteosarcoma, and other sarcomas, but a sarcoma within the lung is almost always metastatic with clinical evidence of a primary tumor elsewhere.

REFERENCES

1. Addis BJ, Dewar A, Thurlow NP: Giant cell carcinoma of the lung: Immunohistochemical and ultrastructural evidence of dedifferentiation. J Pathol 155:231, 1988.
2. Albain KS, True LD, Golomb HM et al: Large cell carcinoma of the lung: Ultrastructural differentiation and clinicopathologic correlations. Cancer 56:1618, 1985.
3. Anger B, Bockman R, Andreeff M et al: Characterization of two newly established human cell lines from patients with large cell anaplastic lung carcinoma. Cancer 50:1518, 1982.
4. Azumi N, Battifora H: Distribution of vimentin and keratin in epithelial and nonepithelial neoplasms: A comparison of the immunohistochemical study on formalin and alcohol-fixed tumors. Am J Clin Pathol 88:286, 1987.
5. Brockmann M, Brockmann I, Herberg U et al: Adenocarcinomas of the lung: Immunohistochemical findings (keratin/CEA). J Cancer Res Clin Oncol 113:379, 1987.
6. Broderick PA, Corvese NL, LaChance T et al: Giant cell carcinoma of lung: A cytologic evaluation. Acta Cytol 19:225, 1975.
7. Carter D, Eggleston JC: Tumors of the Lower Respiratory Tract, 2nd ed. Washington, DC, Armed Forces Institute of Pathology, 1980.
8. Churg A: Fine structure of large cell undifferentiated carcinoma of lung. Hum Pathol 9:143, 1978.
9. Churg A, Warnock ML: The fine structure of large cell undifferentiated carcinoma of the lung: Evidence for its relation to common adeno- and squamous cell carcinomas. Lab Invest 36:334, 1977.
10. Delmonte VC, Alberti O, Saldiva PHN: Large cell carcinoma of the lung: Ultrastructural and immunohistochemical features. Chest 90:524, 1986.
11. Dhillon AP, Rode J, Dhillon DP et al: Neural markers in carcinoma of the lung. Br J Cancer 51:645, 1985.
12. Ferraro J, Lansing LS, Ruckeldeschel JC: Giant cell carcinoma of the lung: A rapidly fatal histologic variant (abstr). Proc Am Assoc Cancer Res 20:465, 1979.
13. Kallenberg F, Jaque J: Giant cell carcinoma of the lung: Clinical and pathological assessment: Comparison with other large cell anaplastic bronchogenic carcinomas. Scand J Thorac Cardiovasc Surg 13:343, 1979.
14. Gatter KC, Dunnil MS, Van Muijen GNP et al: Human lung tumours may coexpress different classes of intermediate filaments. J Clin Pathol 39:950, 1986.
15. Gould VE: Ultrastructural analysis of undifferentiated pulmonary tumors. Hum Pathol 9:77, 1978.
16. Groop C, Havenmann K, Scheuer A: Ectopic hormones in lung cancer patients at diagnosis and during therapy. Cancer 46:347, 1980.
17. Gusterson B, Mitchell B, Warburton et al: Immunohistochemical localization of keratin in human lung tumors. Virchows Arch [A] 394:269, 1982.
18. Hadley GG, Bullock WK: Autopsy reports of pulmonary carcinoma. Calif Med 79:431, 1958.
19. Hammar S: Adenocarcinoma and large cell undifferentiated carcinoma of the lung. Ultrastruct Pathol 11:263, 1987.
20. Hammond ME, Sause WT: Large cell neuroendocrine tumors of the lung: Clinical significance and histopathologic definition. Cancer 56:1624, 1985.
21. Hatch KD, Shingleton HM, Gore H et al: Case report: Human chorionic gonadotropin-secreting large cell carcinoma of the lung detected during follow-up of a patient previously treated for gastrointestinal trophoblastic disease. Gynecol Oncol 10:98, 1980.
22. Hathaway BM, Copeland K, Gurley J: Giant cell adenocarcinoma of the lung. Arch Surg 98:24, 1969.
23. Hellstrom HR, Fisher ER: Giant cell carcinoma of lung. Cancer 16:1080, 1963.
24. Herman DL, Bullock WK, Waken JK: Giant cell adenocarcinoma of the lung. Cancer 19:1337, 1966.
25. Horie A, Ohta M: Ultrastructural features of large cell carcinoma of the lung with reference to the prognosis of patients. Hum Pathol 12:423, 1981.
26. Johnson RL, Donnell RM: Diffuse granulocytic infiltration of giant cell carcinoma of the lung: A distinctive histologic finding with clinical significance. Lab Invest 40:262, 1979.
27. Katinya JN, Sueishi K, Tanaka K et al: Immunoreactivity of surfactant apoprotein in adenocarcinomas, large cell, and small cell carcinoma of the lung. Acta Pathol Jpn 36:1271, 1986.
28. Katzenstein AA, Prioleau PG, Askin FB: The histologic spectrum and significance of clear cell change in lung carcinoma. Cancer 45:943, 1980.
29. Kodama T, Shimosato Y, Koide T et al: Large cell carcinoma of the lung: ultrastructural and immunohistochemical study. Jpn J Clin Oncol 15:431, 1985.
30. Little CD, Nau M, Carney DN et al: Amplification and expression of the c-myc oncogene in human lung cancer cell lines. Nature 306:194, 1983.
31. Lukeman JM, Mackay B: The cytopathology and histopathology of lung cancer. Semin Respir Med 3:140, 1982.
32. Matthews MJ, Mackay B, Lukeman JM: The pathology of non–small cell carcinoma of the lung. Semin Oncol 10:334, 1983.
33. McDowell EM, Wilson TS, Trump BF: Atypical endocrine tumors of the lung. Arch Pathol Lab Med 105:20, 1981.
34. McNutt MA, Bolen JW, Gown AM et al: Coexpression of intermediate filaments in human epithelial neoplasms. Ultrastruct Pathol 9:31, 1985.
35. Metz SA, Weintraub B, Singer J et al: Ectopic secretion of chorionic gonadotropin by a lung carcinoma: Pituitary gonadotropin subunit secretion and prolonged chemotherapeutic remission. Am J Med 65:325, 1978.
36. Mitchell DM, Morgan PGM, Ball JB: Prognostic features of large cell anaplastic carcinoma of the bronchus. Thorax 35:118, 1980.
37. Mizutani Y, Nakajima T, Morinaga S et al: Immunohistochemical localization of pulmonary surfac-

tant apoproteins in various lung tumors: Special reference to nonmucous-producing lung adenocarcinomas. Cancer 61:532, 1988.
38. Moll R: Diversity of cytokeratins in carcinomas. Acta Histochem (Jena) 34:37, 1987.
39. Moll R, Cowin P, Kapprell HP et al: Desmosomal proteins: New markers for identification and classification of tumors. Lab Invest 54:4, 1986.
40. Nash AD, Stout AP: Giant cell carcinoma of the lung. Cancer 11:369, 1958.
41. Neal MH, Kosinski R, Cohen P et al: Atypical endocrine tumors of the lung: A histologic, ultrastructural, and clinical study of 19 cases. Hum Pathol 17:1264, 1986.
42. Osborn M, Weber K: Biology of disease: Tumor diagnosis by intermediate filament typing: A novel tool for surgical pathology. Lab Invest 48:372, 1987.
43. Ozello L, Stout AP: The epithelial origin of giant cell carcinoma of lung confirmed by tissue culture: Report of a case. Cancer 14:1052, 1961.
44. Pfeffer JM, Stovin PGI: Tumor production of alkaline phosphatase in a patient with giant-cell carcinoma of bronchus. Thorax 33:261, 1978.
45. Pfitser P, Knoblich PG: Giant carcinoma cells of bronchogenic origin. Acta Cytol 12:256, 1968.
46. Piehl MR: Subsets of pulmonary large cell undifferentiated carcinomas defined immunohistochemically. Lab Invest 56:35A, 1967.
47. Piehl MR, Gould VE, Warren WH et al: Immunohistochemical identification of exocrine and neuroendocrine subsets of large cell lung carcinoma. Pathol Res Pract 183:675, 1988.
48. Pushchak MJ, Farhi DC: Primary choriocarcinoma of the lung. Arch Pathol Lab Med 11:477, 1987.
49. Radice PA, Matthews MJ, Ihde DC et al: The clinical behavior of "mixed" small cell–large cell bronchogenic carcinoma compared to "pure" small cell subtypes. Cancer 50:2894, 1982.
50. Said JW, Nash G, Sasoon AF et al: Involucrin in lung tumors: A specific marker for squamous differentiation. Lab Invest 49:563, 1983.
51. Shin MS, Jackson LK, Shelton RW et al: Giant cell carcinoma of the lung: Clinical and roentgenographic manifestions. Chest 89:366, 1986.
52. Spencer H: Pathology of the Lung. New York, Pergamon Press, 1985.
53. Stoebner P, Cussac Y, Porte A et al: Ultrastructure of anaplastic bronchial carcinomas. Cancer 20:286, 1967.
54. Tanimura A, Natsyama H, Kawano M et al: Primary choriocarcinoma of the lung. Hum Pathol 16:1281, 1985.
55. Tateishi R, Hattori S: Ultrastructure of large cell and giant cell carcinomas in the lung in relation to histogenesis. In Shimosato Y, Melamed MR, Nettesheim P (eds): Morphogenesis of Lung Cancer, vol 2, p 45. FL, CRC Press, 1982.
56. Upton MP, Hirohashi S, Tome Y et al: Expression of vimentin in surgically resected adenocarcinoma and large cell carcinomas of the lung. Am J Surg Pathol 10:560, 1986.
57. Vollmer RT: The effect of cell size on the pathologic diagnosis of small and large cell carcinomas of the lung. Cancer 50:1380, 1982.
58. Vosika GJ: Large cell bronchogenic carcinoma: Prolonged disease-free survival following chemotherapy. JAMA 241:594, 1979.
59. Wachner R, Wittekind C, Kleitz S: Localization of CEA, β-HCG, SP1, and keratin in the tissue of lung carcinomas: An immunohistochemical study. Virchows Arch [A] 402:415, 1984.
60. Wagner RI: Clinical and morphological characteristics of giant cell cancer of the lung. Grudn Khir 1:80, 1981.
61. Wang NS, Seemayer TA, Ahmed MN et al: Giant cell carcinoma of the lung: A light and electron microscopic study. Hum Pathol 7:3, 1976.
62. Wilson TS, McDowell EM, McIntire KR et al: Elaboration of human chorionic gonadotropin by lung tumors: An immunocytochemical study. Arch Pathol Lab Med 105:169, 1981.
63. Yesner R: Large cell carcinoma of the lung. Semin Diagn Pathol 2:255, 1985.
64. Yesner R, Sobin L: Histologic Typing of Lung Tumors. Geneva, World Health Organization, 1977.

Chapter

9

SMALL CELL CARCINOMA

Many patients with small cell lung carcinoma (SCLC) can achieve a temporary remission with combination chemotherapy, and the separation of SCLC from non-SCLC is the most important subdivision of lung carcinomas from the point of view of the clinician. As a result, there is pressure on the pathologist to establish the diagnosis of SCLC whenever possible. With good preparations of tissue or cytology specimens, recognition of SCLC is often easy, but the morphologic features overlap with those of other lung carcinomas; and in small, artifactually distorted biopsy specimens, distinctions become blurred and uncertainty and misdiagnosis are common. Many pathologists attempt to subclassify SCLC on the basis of the cell and nuclear shape and size into oat cell and intermediate types, but recent studies indicate that this practice is not reproducible or clinically meaningful.[131]

SCLC has been known since the 19th century as one of the tumor types of the *Bergkrankheit,* the mountain disease of the pitchblende and uranium miners of Bohemia and Saxony.[139, 205] It was believed to be a sarcoma until Barnard[16] recognized that it was a carcinoma and not a mediastinal sarcoma.[195] More detailed accounts by Azzopardi[15] and others followed. In recent years, information on SCLC has accrued from a large number of clinicopathologic studies, from investigations into the biology of the tumors using cell lines and xenografts, and from immunocytochemistry and electron microscopy.

The relative frequency of SCLC is variously given as from 10% to 25% of all primary lung tumors. In a study of 2,580 patients treated at Duke University Medical Center between 1973 and 1986, Johnston and colleagues[148] found that during the first 5 years of the study, SCLC made up 11.6% of the histologically confirmed cases. In the final 5 years, the figure was 23.1%. The relative incidence is similar in young persons:[12] 10% of the 89 patients between the ages of 19 and 39 years who were treated for lung carcinoma at Roswell Park Memorial Institute between 1973 and 1983 had SCLC.

The strong male predominance of as high as 10:1 noted in former years is decreasing. Women made up a larger proportion of patients with SCLC entering clinical trials in the latter part of the 15-year study by Johnston and colleagues.[148] While all types of lung cancer increased in women in Los Angeles County during the 10-year period from 1972 to 1981, SCLC showed the largest rate of annual increase.[311] Among 1,745 patients from five separate trials between 1972 and 1986, the percentage of women with SCLC increased from 21% to greater than 35%.[267]

The central location of two thirds of these tumors is consistent with chronic mucosal irritation and increased absorption of carcinogens at points of bifurcation of the bronchial passages, and cigarette smoking is a major etiologic factor.[109] In a study of 383 cases of lung cancer in uranium miners, Saccomanno and associates[250] found that SCLC was the most common type, and a synergistic or additive effect of cigarette smoking and α-radiation from radon gas was suggested.

CLINICAL FEATURES

Most patients who are diagnosed as having SCLC already have symptoms, but they are of brief duration and have often been present for less than 3 months. Cough is common, but because of the customary submucosal spread of the tumor, hemoptysis is not frequent. There are some rare associated symptoms, including the Leser-Trélat syndrome.[127] On radiography, the tumor typically appears as a central mass without cavitation.

The tumors may produce ectopic hormones,[3, 17, 75, 110, 121, 176, 180, 198, 199, 235, 284, 314, 317] but clinical evidence of endocrine hyperfunction is relatively uncommon. Bondy and Gilby[31] assessed the endocrine status of 106 patients with SCLC prior to the initiation of therapy and concluded that the pattern of hormone abnormality observed in this group of patients was relatively specific for SCLC and different from that observed in other pulmonary tumors. Almost one half of the patients had evidence of abnormal control of adrenocortical steroids, two had the ectopic ACTH secretion syndrome, 38% showed evidence of inappropriate antidiuretic hormone secretion, approximately one half had evidence of abnormal glucose tolerance, and many also had a paradoxical rise of plasma growth hormone concentration after glucose administration. Severe hypercalcemia is occasionally encountered:[128] in the case reported by Yoshimoto and co-workers,[319] the plasma immunoreactive parathyroid hormone concentration was markedly elevated and Northern blot analysis revealed parathyroid hormone mRNA in the tumor. Serum levels of hormones and other SCLC products have been used to monitor the progress of patients receiving chemotherapy.[50, 51, 275]

Sculier and associates[259] found that 189 (29.5%) of 641 patients with SCLC had at least one neurologic disorder either at the time of presentation or during progression of the tumor. The most common were metastases involving, in decreasing frequency, the brain, meninges, spinal cord, and epidural tissues. One percent of patients had the Lambert-Eaton syndrome, a myasthenic disorder[63, 83, 151, 157, 221, 306] characterized by proximal muscle weakness that improves with exercise. The cause is an IgG-mediated reduction in the number of presynaptic voltage-gated calcium channels at the neuromuscular junction.[58] Circulating neuronal antinuclear antibodies have been detected in the Lambert-Eaton syndrome,[81, 108] but while Grisold and co-workers[113] found them in 17 of 40 patients with SCLC, only 1 patient displayed a sensory neuropathy. A visual paraneoplastic syndrome has been noticed in some patients with SCLC, and Grunwald and colleagues[114] documented loss of retinal ganglion cells and their processes in a patient who had high levels of cerebrospinal fluid immunoglobulin and immune deposits in the retina.

Metastases

Schultz and associates[257] studied the localization and incidence of metastases in 383 patients with bronchogenic carcinoma and found that SCLC showed the highest metastatic frequency. At the time of diagnosis, as many as two thirds of patients with SCLC have clinically detectable metastases in one or more sites.[85, 142, 172] Approximate figures are bone, 35%; liver, 25%; and 10% each in central nervous system, lymph nodes, subcutaneous tissue, and pleura. An increased number of metastatic sites over a 15-year period has been identified,[267] and this can in part be attributed to improvements in staging and longer survival.

Bone is the most common site of extrapulmonary spread of SCLC, and the detection of bone metastases is an important aspect of the pretreatment evaluation.[46, 62, 130, 142] Monoclonal antibodies have been used for the purpose.[269] Berendsen and colleagues[22] used immunofluorescence for the monoclonal antibody MOC1 associated with a membrane antigen of SCLC on 53 bone marrow aspirates from 30 patients: reactive cells were detected in 19 patients (63%). Simultaneous histopathologic examination of the bone marrow biopsy specimens detected tumor cells in only six cases (20%), indicating that the method is more sensitive than conventional histochemical staining of bone marrow aspirates.

Liver metastases[216] may be detected by peritoneoscopy,[78] but the procedure is not widely practiced now that computed tomographic (CT) scanning is available for the delineation of both intrathoracic and metastatic disease.[303]

Metastases to the brain and spinal cord are common in SCLC, and prophylactic therapy is frequently included in SCLC protocols.[43, 68, 80, 99, 134, 135, 149, 162, 218, 225] The frequency of brain metastases in untreated patients ranges up to 23% in published reports, and as many as 30% of patients develop clinical evidence in the course of therapy. The incidence is reduced by brain irradiation. Improvements in survival have been accompanied by an increase in the incidence of cerebral metastases, and they are present at autopsy in almost half of patients with SCLC. Tumor foci within the central nervous system may be protected by the blood–brain barrier from systemic chemotherapy with the consequence that the tumor survives within the confines of the nervous system after it has been eradicated in other locations. Meningeal carcinomatosis also seems to have increased with longer patient survival.[8, 13, 37, 248] At the time of diagnosis it is present in fewer than 5% of patients, but it is demonstrated in up to 20% more during therapy. Cytologic examination of the cerebrospinal fluid does not always reveal the presence of the tumor, but elevated protein and lowered glucose in the cerebrospinal fluid may be an indication that meningeal carcinomatosis is present.

Extension to the mediastinum almost invariably occurs:[195] among patients who underwent curative resection and then died within 30 days from causes not related to the tumor, 70% had mediastinal node or distal metastatic involvement at autopsy. SCLC is the most common cause of the vena cava syndrome.[185, 258]

Metastases to a wide variety of relatively infrequent sites are also seen at autopsy or detected before death. Recent examples are reports of metastasis of SCLC to small bowel,[203] colon,[298] testis,[271] and pineal gland.[297]

STAGING

With a higher labeling index and shorter doubling time than other lung carcinomas,[111] SCLC is an aggressive tumor that is generally disseminated at the time of diagnosis. The criteria that are used to stage non–SCLC do not have the same applicability for SCLC.[9, 126, 141] The Veterans Administration Lung Cancer Study Group advocated subdivision of inoperable cases into limited disease, confined to one hemithorax including ipsilateral scalene nodes, and extensive disease, being any disease beyond the confines of the definition of limited disease.[9] Among the patients who present with localized disease, roughly half have a complete response to therapy but the majority suffer a recurrence after a short interval.[53]

PROGNOSTIC FACTORS

Since conventional staging is of limited value, attempts have been made to detect useful prognostic indicators in patients with SCLC.[230, 231, 270, 287] Johnston and co-workers[148] found that the disease seemed slightly less aggressive in women, with a median survival of 13 versus 10 months. The size of the tumor is less helpful: Hainsworth and associates[120] reviewed records and chest films of 101 patients with limited-stage SCLC and found that initial tumor volume calculated from tumor measurements on chest radiography was unrelated to survival.

Vincent and colleagues[287] examined 333 consecutive patients with SCLC and detected 15 parameters with individual prognostic significance, the most powerful being serum albumin level, bone marrow aspirate, disease extent, and performance status. They did not find prognostic significance in age, sex, pleural involvement, or the superior vena cava syndrome. Hainsworth and associates[120] found that an elevated serum lactic acid dehydrogenase (LDH) level predicted improved survival.

In the review of 1,745 patients with SCLC by the Cancer and Leukemia Group B between 1972 and 1986,[267] the impact of pretreatment prognostic factors on outcome was assessed. Multivariate analysis showed that female gender was predictive of improved response. A performance status of 0 or 1 was associated with improved response rates in both subsets but was statistically significant only for overall objective response in patients with limited disease. Performance status was, however, a highly significant predictor of survival in both groups. Supraclavicular lymph node involvement, while still within the definition of limited disease, had a borderline unfavorable impact on survival compared with a lesser extent of limited disease. In patients with extensive disease, a decrease in survival rates was associated with an increased number of metastatic sites.

When the overall survival of patients with a neurologic disorder was compared with those who did not have neurologic problems,[259] there was no difference in the survival curves for the first year and a half, but patients without the neurologic complications had a greater probability of long-term survival. There were no statistically significant differences when this comparison was made according to stage of disease. When a neurologic disorder associated with cancer appeared, the survival time was usually short and the neurologic disorder was the primary cause of death in the majority of cases.

SURVIVAL

Prior to the use of chemotherapy, the median survival for patients with SCLC was less than 6 months and the 5-year survival was less than 1%. Now median survival has improved to over 1 year in most reports, and the number of long-term disease-free survivors has increased.[224] Up to 90% of patients will experience an objective response to therapy and at least 10% will survive for 3 years or more clinically free of disease. George and co-workers [97] found that the median survival for a group of 101 patients with SCLC was 51 weeks but noted that there was no evidence of improvement in response or survival during the 6 years covered by their study. One reason for the plateau in therapeutic progress in the past decade[125] is inadequacy of the current staging system, and improved methods to detect micrometastases are needed.

Patients with authentic limited disease can be expected to have longer survival times, particularly if the lesion is detected early and resected.[67] In a group of 33 patients studied by Ishida and associates[143] to evaluate surgical treatment of SCLC, the overall 5-year survival rate was 38%, but for stage I patients it was 57% as against only 11% in those with stage III disease. Hitchins and co-workers[136] assessed the outcome in 280 patients with SCLC 2 to 7 years after treatment with combination chemotherapy, with or without chest or cranial radiation therapy. Fourteen patients (6.7%) survived free of cancer for 30 months or longer, and 9 of them had limited disease at diagnosis while 4 others had extensive disease with only one metastatic site. Eighteen percent of the 101 patients in George and co-workers'[97] study were alive at 130 weeks (2.5 years), and patients who had surgery with adjuvant therapy had better survivals; when they were excluded, only 12% survived for 130 weeks. Gephart and colleagues[98] reviewed 17 tumors varying in size from 1.9 to 3.5 cm, all considered to be resectable and without clinical or radiologic evidence of metastases: seven patients (41%) died of recurrent or metastatic carcinoma with an average survival of 1.7 years.

Long-term survivors make up an extremely small percentage of patients with SCLC.[72, 100, 136, 196, 272, 290, 291] Two of Hitchins and colleagues'[136] 280 patients were alive and disease free more than 5 years after diagnosis (the median survival was 3.2 years), and the authors note that a 30-month survival cannot be considered a cure since late relapses do occur. Twenty-one of 500 (4%) patients in a Charleston series survived 30 months or longer, but 6 eventually had relapses occurring as late as 88 months after diagnosis.[150] Hitchins and colleagues[136] concluded that late toxicity from aggressive therapy does not outweigh the benefits of long-term survival and potential cure. Longer survival does however carry the risk of complications,[88, 89] including the possibility of developing a non–SCLC.[144,166]

GROSS APPEARANCE

The tumor arises in the vicinity of the hilum in over 70% of cases. The cut surface is grayish white, soft, and friable with areas of necrosis. Tumor cells may initially proliferate beneath the mucosa of a major bronchus and impart to it a pipestem appearance, and circumferential extension can stenose the lumen. Only occasionally does SCLC show exophytic growth: Watkin and associates[296] reported an instance of endobronchial involvement in which residual carcinoma could not be found in the lobectomy specimen. Blackman and co-workers[26] described the unusual case of a 42-year-old woman with multiple tracheal and bronchial tumors that suggested benign tracheobronchial papillomatosis.

LIGHT MICROSCOPY

The quality of the material provided for the pathologic evaluation of SCLC is often inadequate for a number of reasons. Biopsy specimens obtained at bronchoscopy[39, 189] are small, and they may be fragmented and are prone to squashing artifact. Drying effect is often superimposed. Caution should be exercised when interpreting a small, distorted biopsy specimen. Non–SCLC is often mistaken for SCLC because of artifactual changes in the specimen. Additional sections may show improved areas, but sometimes there is no alternative to requesting an additional biopsy specimen.

Most tumors lack an architectural pattern and monotonous sheets of uniform cells separated by slender partitions of connective tissue are characteristic (Fig. 9–1). Groups of tumor cells can be sharply demarcated with some palisading at their periphery (Fig. 9–2).

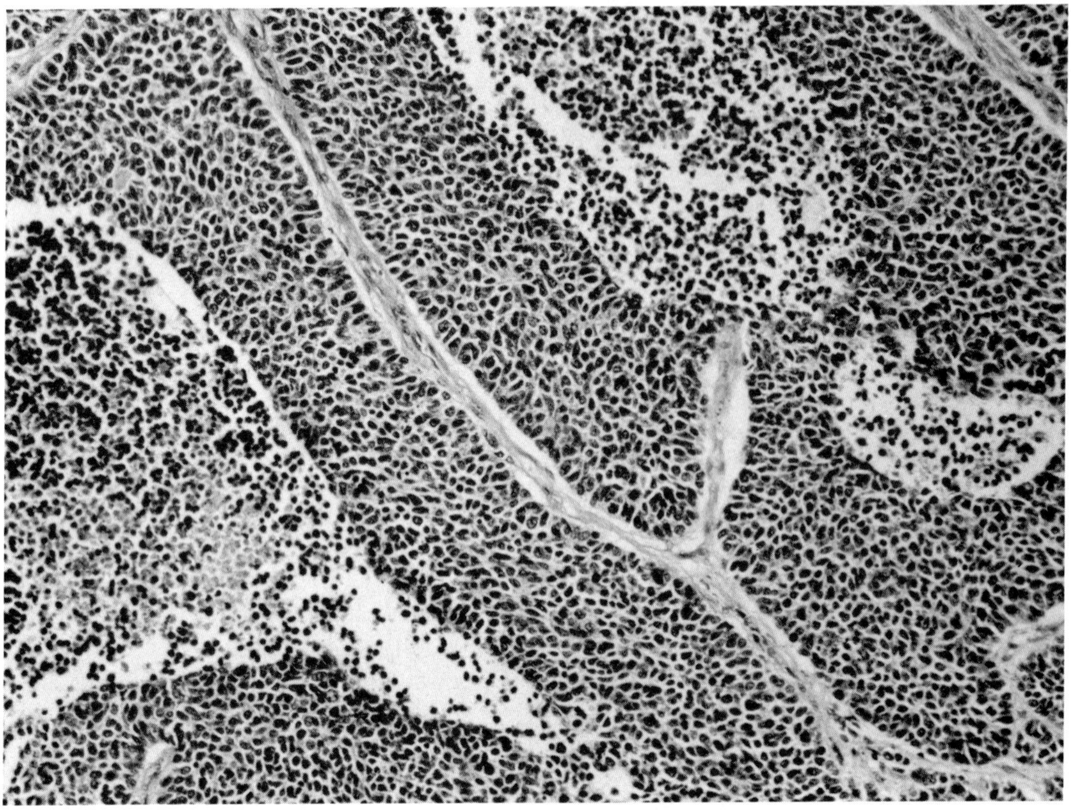

Figure 9–1. Small cell carcinoma. Diffuse sheets of cells surround zones of necrosis.

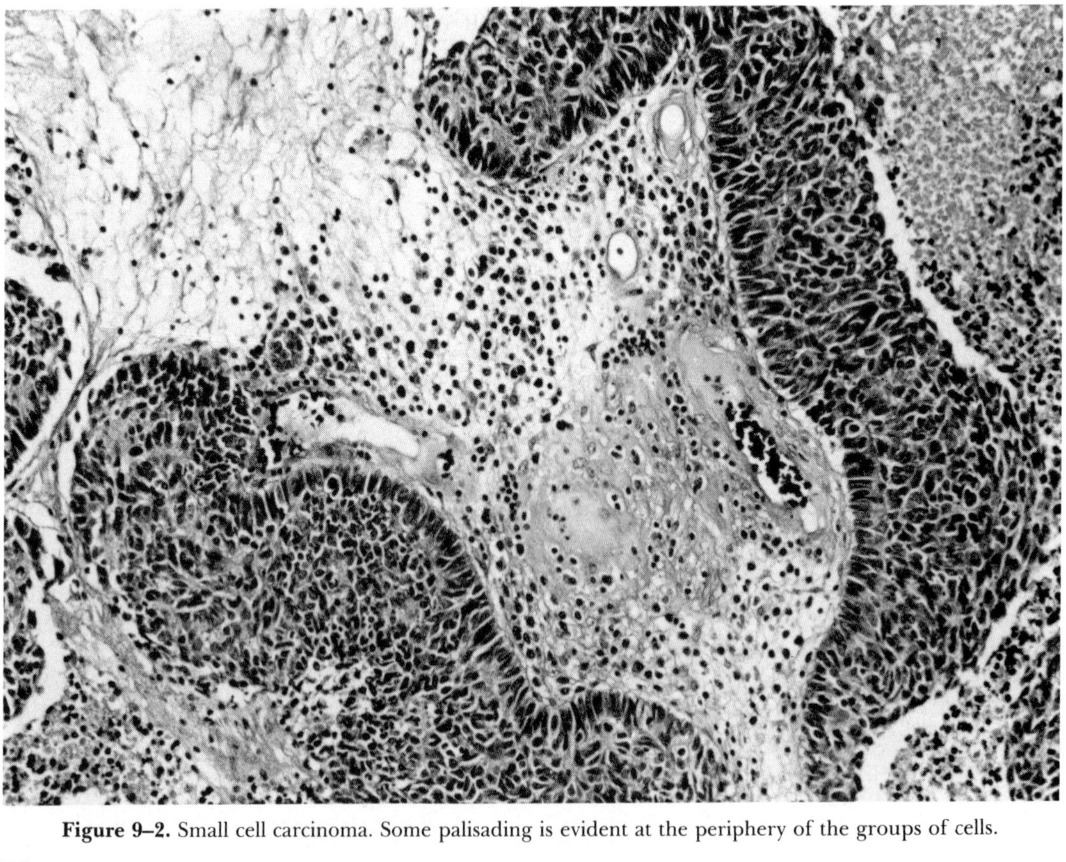

Figure 9–2. Small cell carcinoma. Some palisading is evident at the periphery of the groups of cells.

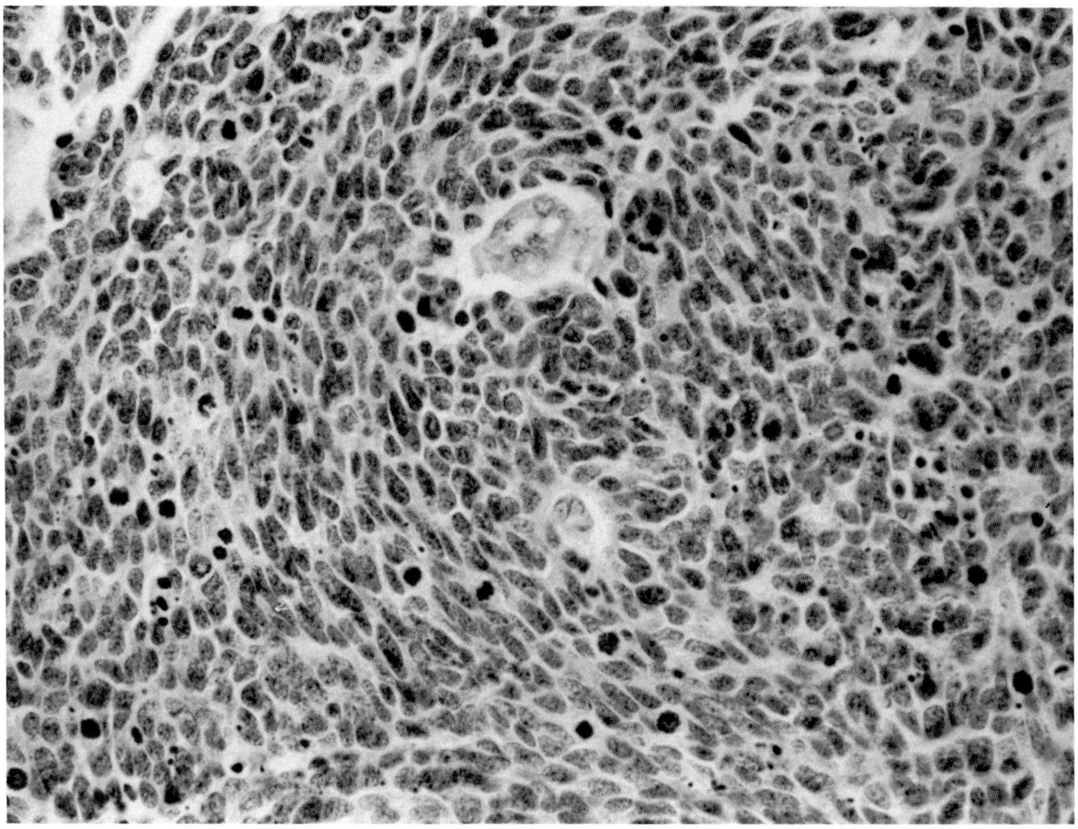

Figure 9–3. Small cell carcinoma. Very little cytoplasm can be seen, and the nuclei appear to be close together. Mitotic figures are present.

Foci of necrosis are almost always present (see Figs. 9–1 and 9–2), ranging from small zones at the center of sheets of cells to extensive areas of the tumor. The individual tumor cells are small (Fig. 9–3), and although they may appear round in some areas (Fig. 9–4) they are generally ovoid and can be elongated (Fig. 9–5) or even fusiform (Fig. 9–6). Cells that look round may be elongated cells in cross section. The nucleus mirrors the shape of the cell. The hyperchromatic appearance of the tumor at low magnification is striking and results from the close packing of the cells and their small amounts of cytoplasm. Nuclear chromatin is finely but evenly clumped in well-preserved tissue (see Figs. 9–4 and 9–5), and the small nucleoli are rendered less conspicuous by the diffuse density of the nucleoplasm. The nuclear/cytoplasmic ratio is typically high, and the thin rims of cytoplasm are barely visible in tissue sections (Figs. 9–3 through 9–7).

While sheets of cells devoid of organization are typical, rosettes may be present within the diffuse areas (see Fig. 9–7) or rarely they occupy an extensive area of the tumor (Fig. 9–8). The cells can form broad cords (Fig. 9–9). DNA from broken-down cells may accumulate within vessel walls, imparting to them an appearance that has been referred to as hematoxyphil vascular change[7] or basophilic encrustation (Fig. 9–10). SCLC cells are vulnerable to squashing, and crushing effect is a frequent finding, particularly in small biopsy specimens: it should not be used as a diagnostic criterion, since an identical appearance can be produced in non–SCLC or in chronic bronchitis. The bronchial epithelium overlying the tumor may show pagetoid invasion, but usually the surface of the tumor is separated from the epithelium by a layer of submucosa.

If an architectural pattern is present, it can aid in distinguishing SCLC from lymphoma, but provided the material available for study is well preserved and free of crushing artifact, it is the size, shape, and cytologic features of the nuclei that serve to distinguish the tumor cells from lymphocytes or lymphoma cells within the lung and in metastatic

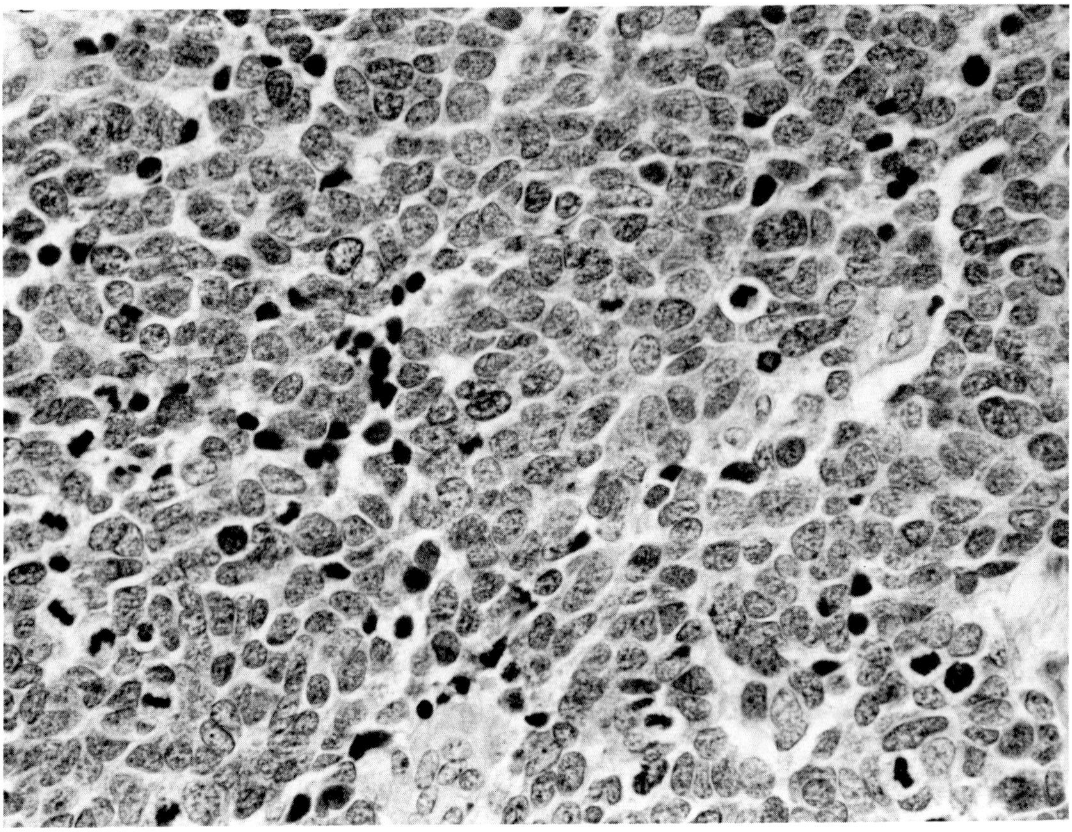

Figure 9–4. Small cell carcinoma. The nuclei have finely clumped chromatin and inconspicuous nucleoli.

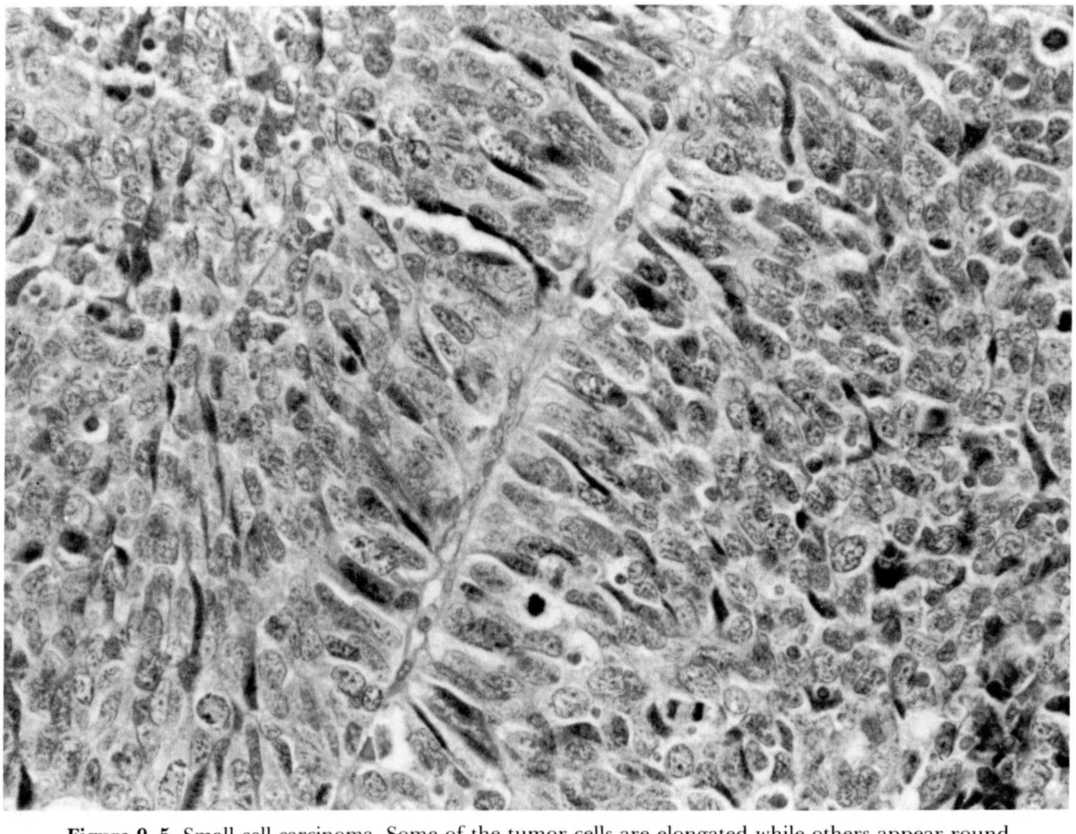

Figure 9–5. Small cell carcinoma. Some of the tumor cells are elongated while others appear round.

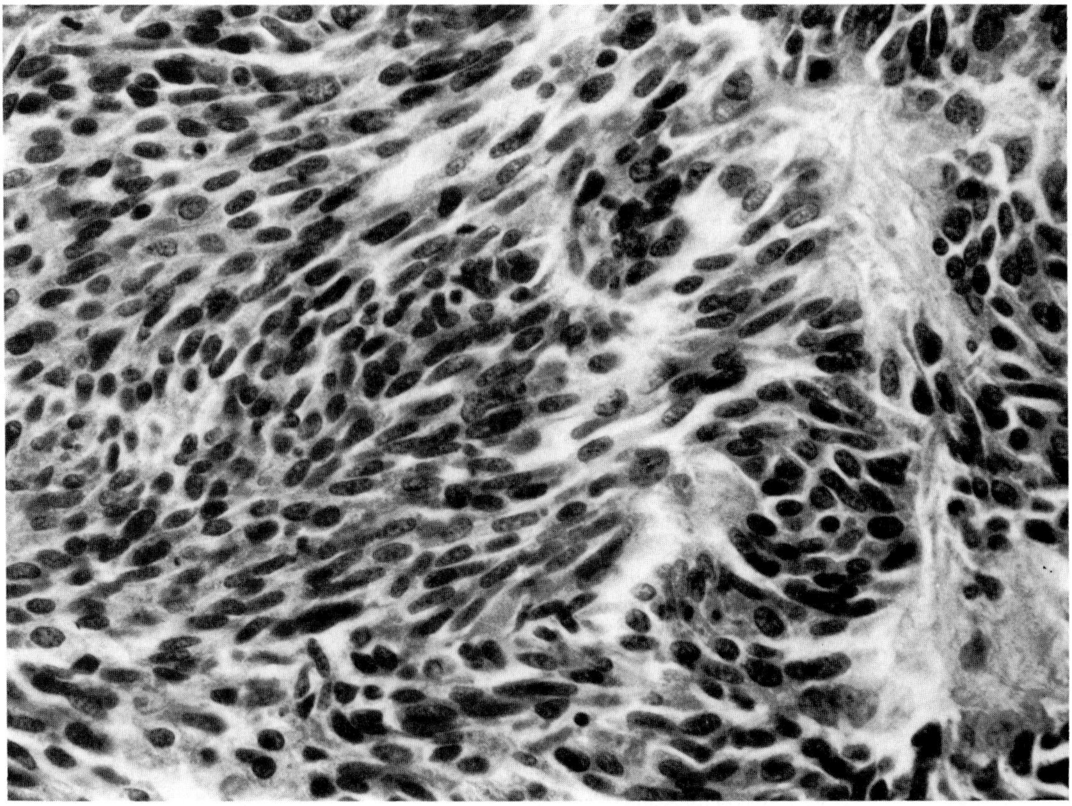

Figure 9–6. Small cell carcinoma with a predominance of fusiform cells.

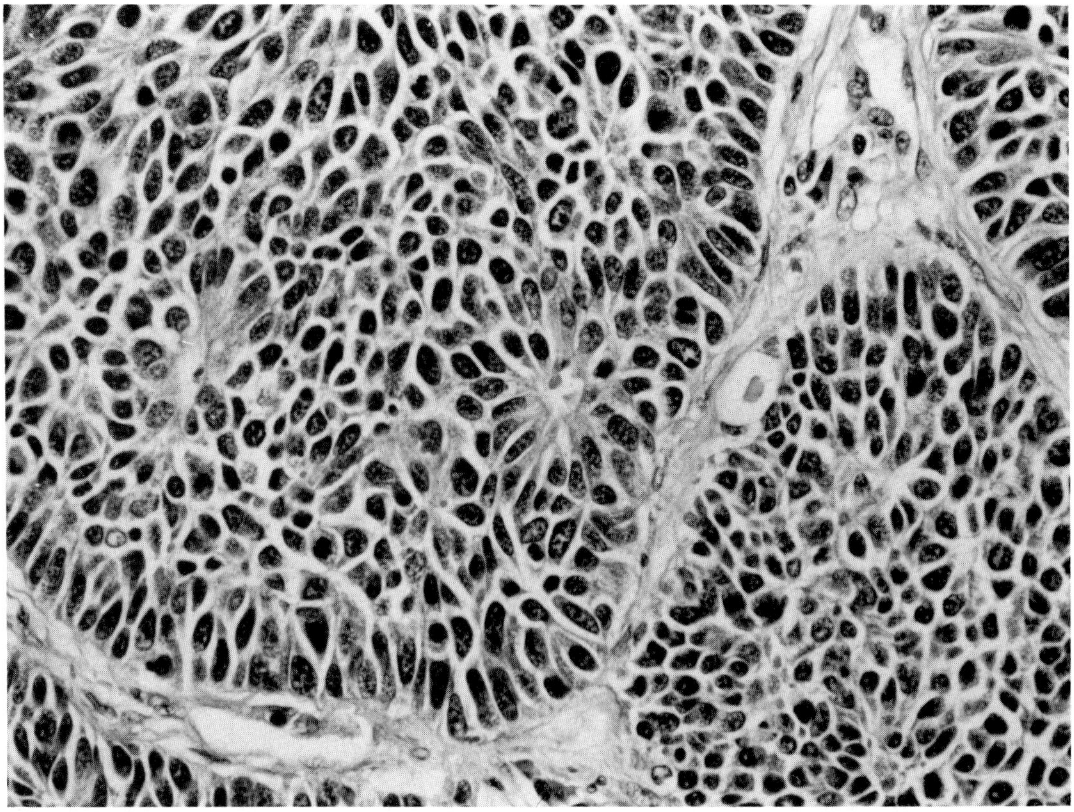

Figure 9–7. Small cell carcinoma. An occasional small rosette is visible.

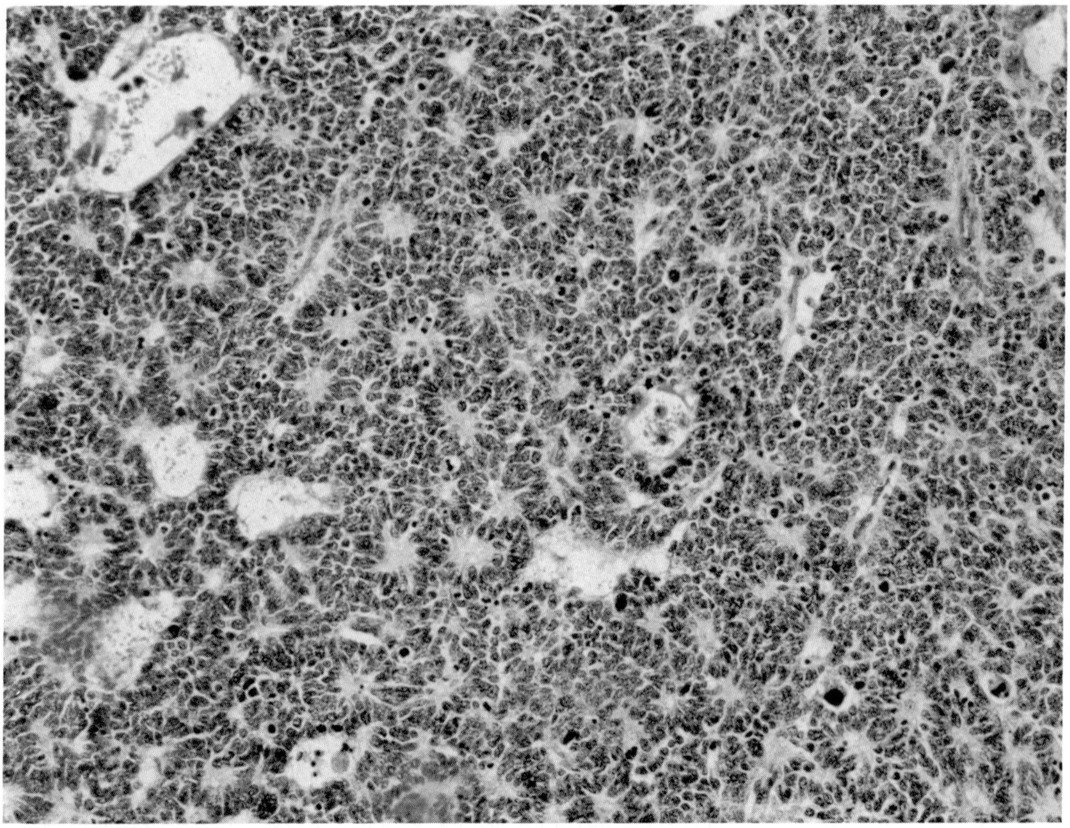

Figure 9–8. Small cell carcinoma. Prominent rosette formation was present in an area of this tumor.

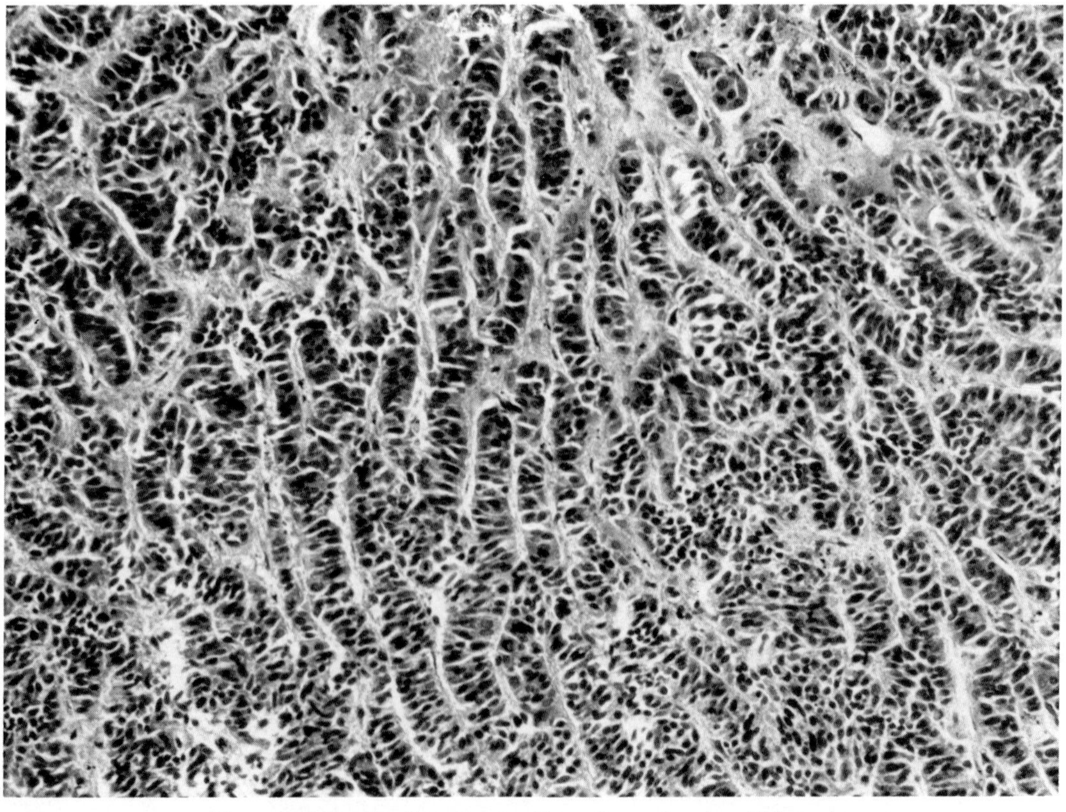

Figure 9–9. Small cell carcinoma. The cells are forming thick cords.

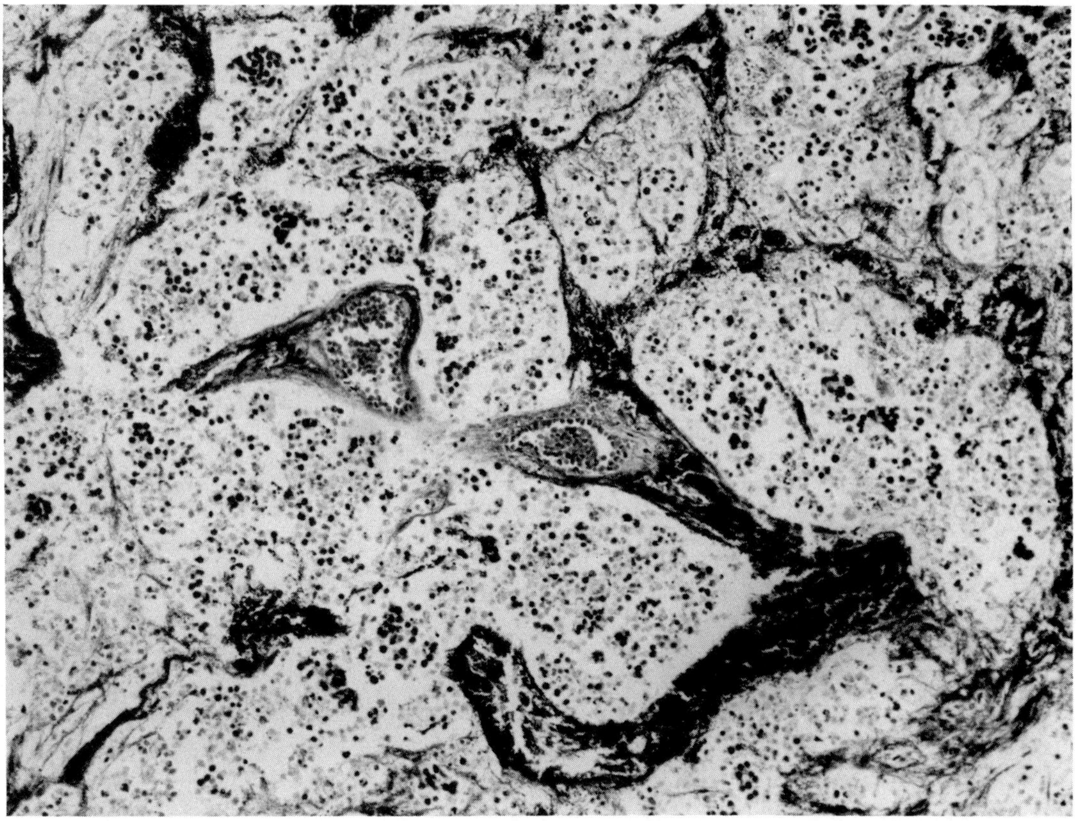

Figure 9–10. Small cell carcinoma. Hematoxyphil encrustation of vessels in an area of necrosis.

sites (Figs. 9–11 and 9–12). Following therapy, and particularly in metastases, SCLC cells will sometimes undergo morphologic changes.[2] There may be a transition to a larger cell type that resembles undifferentiated large cell carcinoma[194] or displays squamous or glandular features, or scattered cells can show varying degrees of pleomorphism with bizarre, giant, and multinucleated forms.[19] The latter is a common finding in necrotic areas. Phagocytic activity has been observed in the tumor cells.[76]

Two variants of SCLC can cause difficulty in diagnosis when material is scanty or distorted. One consists of a mixture of small cells with larger cells, and it may be termed a small cell–large cell carcinoma.[6] Coexistence of SCLC and differentiated non–SCLC[36] is more common and has been designated the combined variant of SCLC[131, 186] (see the section on subtyping later in this chapter and the accompanying figures). In their study of heterogeneity in lung cancer, Roggli and co-workers[246] found that seven cases of SCLC were homogeneous while eight showed mixtures with other cell types.

CYTOLOGY

The diagnosis of SCLC can be made from cytologic preparations in a high percentage of cases.[14, 147, 206, 282, 299] Cells in sputum, aspiration biopsy specimens, and bronchial washings and brushings are essentially similar in appearance to those seen in tissue sections, although the character of the nuclear chromatin and the size of nucleoli are seen better in carefully prepared cytologic slides.[181, 182] The tumor cells tend to be loosely cohesive, but they are often found in small clusters or in chains, and the tendency to aggregate may help distinguish SCLC from a lymphoma in which clumping and molding are not characteristic.

In cytologic smears, the moderately hyperchromatic nuclei with their smooth surfaces and ovoid or elongated profiles may have a naked appearance because of the thinness of the investing cytoplasm or from it becoming frayed or lost during preparation (Fig. 9–13). The cytoplasm is more visible in fine-needle aspiration biopsy specimens (Figs. 9–14 and 9–15) than in sputum or washing or brushing

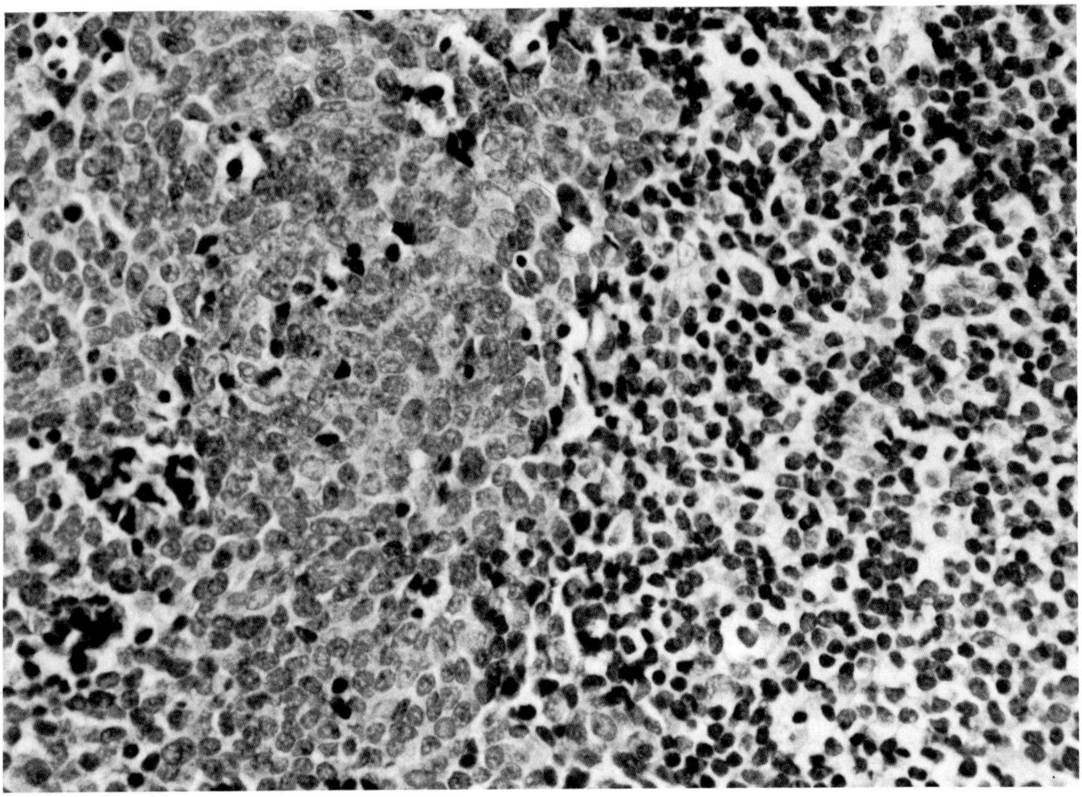

Figure 9–11. Small cell carcinoma, metastatic in a lymph node. The contrast in size and nuclear chromatin between the tumor cells and the lymphocytes can be appreciated.

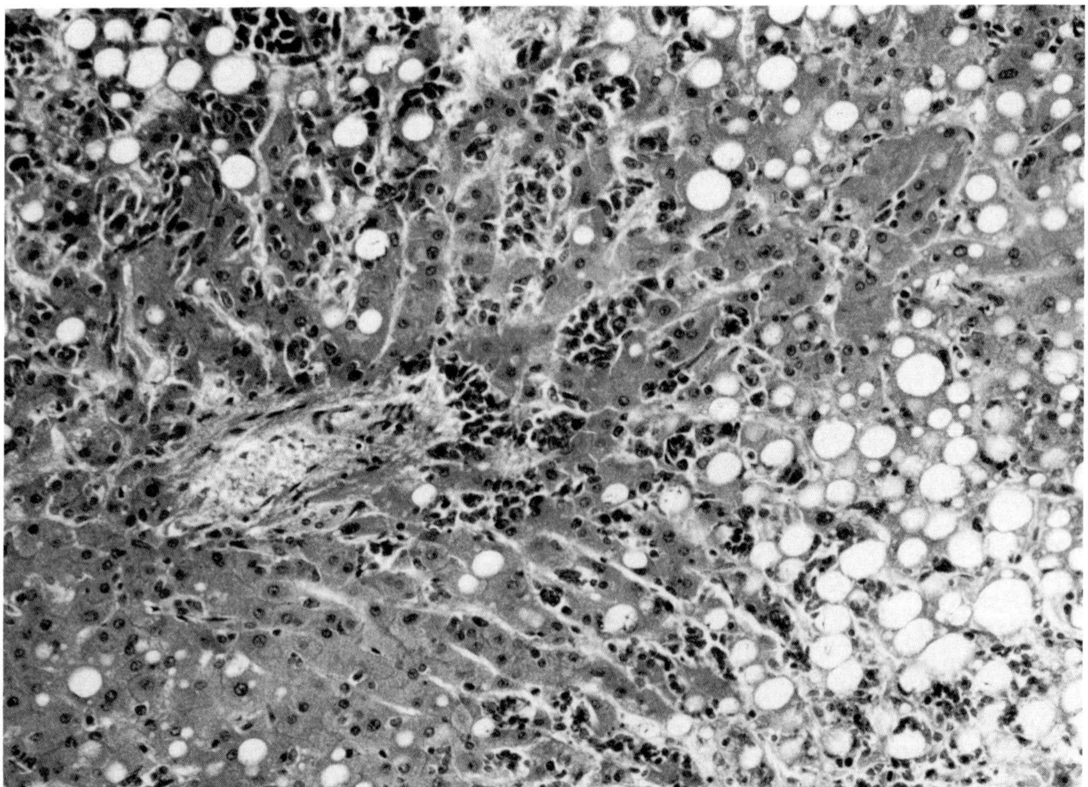

Figure 9–12. Small cell carcinoma, metastatic in liver. The cells resemble lymphocytes at low magnification, but their larger size, ovoid nuclei, and finely clumped nuclear chromatin were evident on closer inspection.

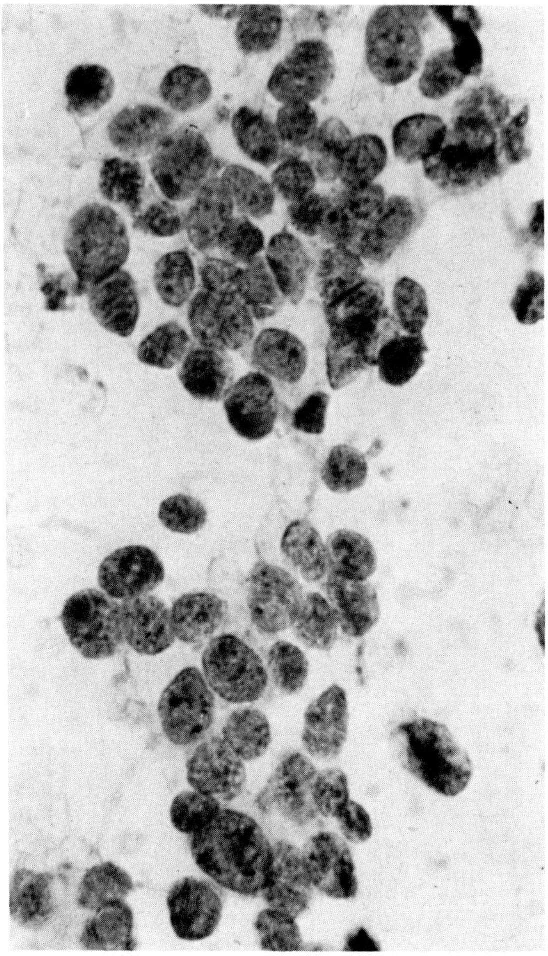

Figure 9–13. Small cell carcinoma. In this preparation from sputum, nuclei appear bare but an occasional trace of cytoplasm is visible.

specimens, but the nuclei still seem to be close together. Fine-needle aspiration biopsy specimens are effective preparations from which to establish a diagnosis of SCLC.[82]

IMMUNOCYTOCHEMISTRY

The histologic diagnosis of SCLC can be facilitated by employing general (broad spectrum) immunocytochemical markers that will recognize neuroendocrine features in neoplastic cells and certain markers for the detection of specific neuroendocrine cell products (specific regulatory substances). Markers included in the former category are expressed independent of the production of regulatory peptides by the tumor, and they therefore have more practical application in surgical pathology. Included in this group are some cytoskeletal filaments, particularly cytokeratins, and neurofilament proteins; cytosolic proteins, such as neuron-specific enolase and protein gene product 9.5; intragranular matrix proteins including chromogranins and Leu-7; and the membrane glycoprotein synaptophysin. Among the regulatory polypeptides, bombesin (gastrin releasing peptide), ACTH, and calcitonin are most frequently detected in SCLC and are therefore potentially of value in the diagnosis. Because of their variable sensitivity and specificity for endocrine differentiation, the two groups of markers can be used singly or in combination.

Broad-Spectrum Neuroendocrine Markers

The cytoskeletal composition of neuroendocrine tumors of the bronchopulmonary tract has been a source of controversy and confusion for years. Early reports stated that carcinoids and SCLC were negative for cytokeratins but positive for neurofilament pro-

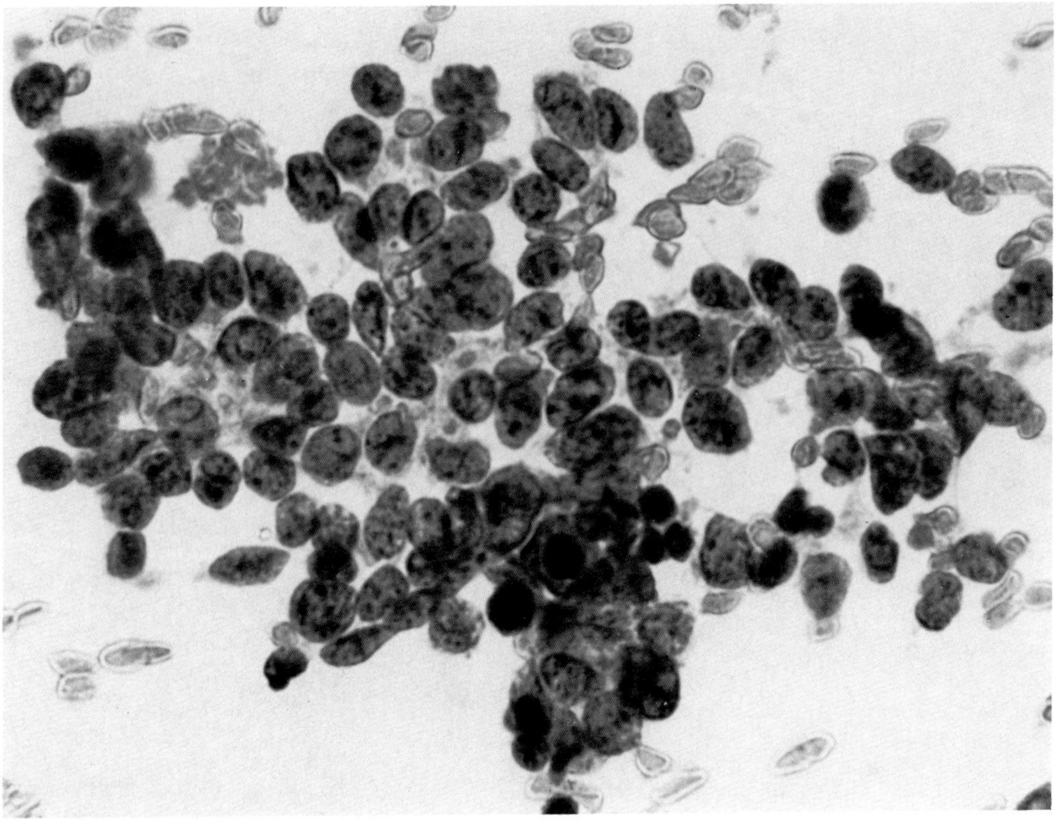

Figure 9–14. Small cell carcinoma in a fine-needle aspiration biopsy. Some of the cells are loosely cohesive. A few nucleoli can be seen.

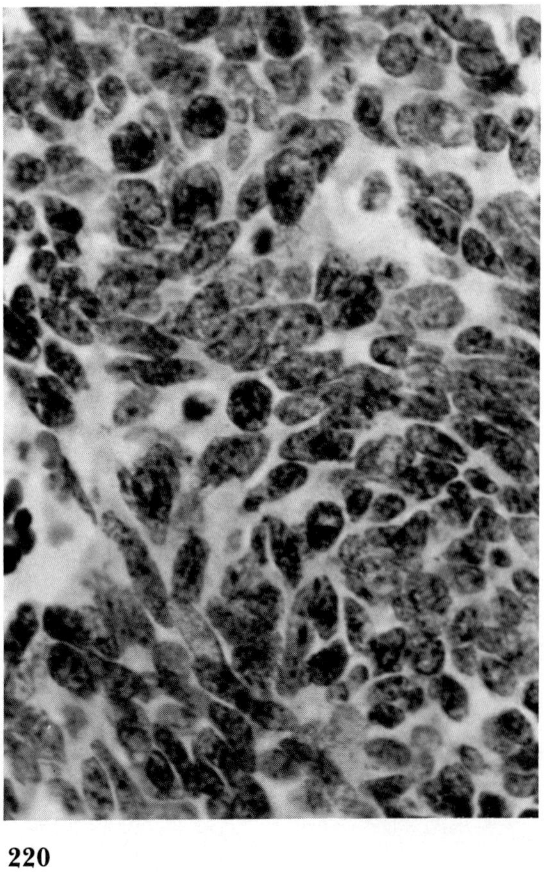

Figure 9–15. Small cell carcinoma in a fine-needle aspiration biopsy. Fusiform cells predominate. Marked anisokaryosis is present.

teins.[10, 168–170, 240] Recent studies have demonstrated cytokeratins, specifically polypeptides Nos. 8, 18, and small amounts of 19, in SCLC,[28, 105, 171, 207, 238] but some investigators have been unable to confirm the presence of neurofilament proteins.[60, 105, 171, 285] It is probable that the inability of early studies to demonstrate cytokeratin in these tumors may have been due to the use of antibodies with restricted reactivity for different members of the keratin family.

Neurofilaments are protein triplets composed of three distinct subunits with respective molecular weights of 68, 150, and 200 kd that can be found in all classes of nerves.[229] Immunocytochemical studies have shown neurofilament proteins in various tumors with neural features, including ganglioneuroma, ganglioneuroblastoma, neuroblastoma, esthesioneuroblastoma, medulloblastoma, and pinealoma.[32, 159, 167, 213, 236] In addition, neurofilament reactivity has been found in cutaneous neuroendocrine (Merkel cell) carcinomas, pancreatic islet cell tumors, carcinoid tumors, and SCLC.[169, 170, 240] While the expression of neurofilament proteins in bronchial carcinoids is widely accepted, although by no means frequent, this finding in SCLC remains controversial.[105, 171] If coexpression of neurofilament protein and cytokeratin does occur in SCLC, it is evidently a rare phenomenon.

The glycolytic enzyme enolase is ubiquitous in its distribution and has three distinct subunits, which have been designated α, β, and γ.[91, 187, 244] Five forms of the enzyme have been identified: three homodimers (αα, ββ, and γγ) and two hybrids (αβ and αγ). The β-enolase form is found predominantly in muscle. The α-isoenzyme, also designated non-neural enolase, is the most common form and is found in most tissues. The term neuron-specific enolase was initially used to designate the γγ-isoenzyme enolase, which is the main isoenzyme form of enolase in the brain, where it corresponds to the 14.3.2 neuron-specific protein.[30] When this designation is used for locations other than brain, it refers to the concentration of the subunits that can occur as γγ or αγ-isoenzymes. In addition to its presence in the brain, neuron-specific enolase has been recognized in a variety of normal and neoplastic neuroendocrine cells.[233, 254, 261, 274] It has been reported to be useful as a tumor marker for SCLC in both serum[50, 87, 93, 94, 286] and tissue specimens[5, 23, 223, 251, 268] (Fig. 9–16). Using immunocytochemical procedures, neuron-specific enolase reactivity has been found in 60% to 100% of SCLC.[23, 93, 156, 242, 268] Recent studies have shown that neuron-specific enolase is also expressed in a variety of normal nonendocrine cells, such as smooth muscle cells,[155] blood platelets and lymphocytes,[154] and epithelial cells of the loop of Henle and macula densa of the kidney,[118] and in nonendocrine tumors, including carcinomas of the kidney, breast, and ovary and seminomas, chordomas, some sarcomas (leiomyosarcoma, rhabdomyosarcoma, alveolar soft part sarcoma), and lymphomas.[119, 159, 165, 220, 228, 289] Because neuron-specific enolase can be found in a non–SCLC that does not possess evidence of neuroendocrine differentiation,[77, 94, 242, 251] immunostaining for this substance is not a reliable criterion with which to differentiate SCLC from non–SCLC. In our experience, neuron-specific enolase is a useful marker in this context only when it is used to support observations based on conventional morphology.

Protein gene product 9.5 (PGP 9.5) is a 27-kd cytosolic protein of unknown function that, like neuron-specific enolase, was isolated from the brain.[277] This protein is widely distributed in neurons and is found in neuroendocrine tumors.[245] PGP 9.5 immunostaining was reported in 4 of 14 cases of SCLC and in 8 of 18 cases of non–SCLC studied by Rode and co-workers.[245] The results of this study, as well as those obtained by others,[5, 77] indicate that this marker is less sensitive or specific than neuron-specific enolase for the detection of neuroendocrine differentiation and the recognition of SCLC.

Chromogranin comprises a group of acidic polypeptides known as chromogranin A, B, and C that form a major part of the soluble proteins in secretory granules where they are believed to stabilize the intragranular matrix.[11, 308] These proteins were originally extracted from the adrenal medulla where they are stored in and released from catecholaminergic granules.[27, 226, 255] The three chromogranins correspond to previously described proteins: chromogranin A is equivalent to (parathyroid) secretory protein I[163]; chromogranin B has also been called secretogranin I[247]; and chromogranin C corresponds to pituitary tyrosin sulfated protein (TSP) or secretogranin II.[247] Chromogranin has been found to be widely distributed by virtue of its presence in endocrine cells that contain secretory granules. Chromogranin A is the

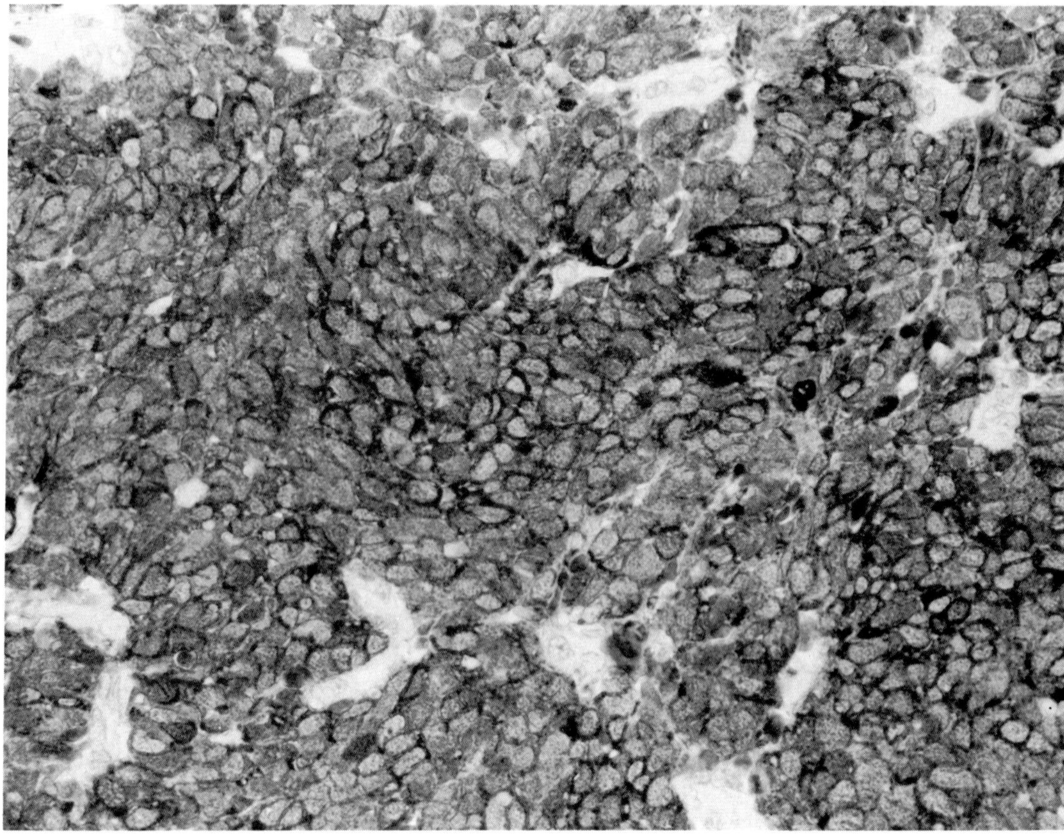

Figure 9–16. Small cell carcinoma showing strong reactivity for neuron-specific enolase.

most abundant and has a molecular weight of 75 kd.[117] Several studies have indicated that chromogranin A can be used as a marker for endocrine tumors.[179, 251, 256, 307] Using a recently developed mouse monoclonal antibody to chromogranin A (LK2H10), a strong correlation has been found between chromogranin reactivity and the results of Grimelius staining in pancreatic endocrine neoplasms, suggesting that the basis of the Grimelius reaction may involve binding to chromogranin.[178] Demonstration of chromogranin A immunoreactivity in SCLC using the monoclonal antibody LK2H10 has been inconsistent.[174, 179, 251, 295] While one group of investigators was able to find focal immunoreactivity in 19 of 32 (59%) cases,[174] others have been unable to demonstrate any immunostaining with this marker.[251] Deftos and associates[73] demonstrated reactivity for chromogranin in 11 of 18 classic SCLC cell lines by immunostaining. Also, chromogranin mRNA was found in all five cases of SCLC studied.[129] Since the positive immunocytochemical reaction relates to the number of secretory granules, it is possible that the discrepancies among the reported immunocytochemical results may be due, at least in part, to the diagnostic criteria used in the selection of the cases. Non–SCLC with neuroendocrine differentiation can be confused with SCLC when only a light microscopic assessment of the tumor is made. In spite of the high specificity of chromogranin for endocrine differentiation, SCLC that contains small and sparse endocrine granules tends to react weakly or not at all, and as many as one third of these tumors do not contain granules. Consequently, immunostaining for this endocrine marker is of limited value in the diagnosis of SCLC, particularly when only small amounts of tissue are examined, as in bronchial biopsies.

The monoclonal antibody HNK-1 reacts with Leu-7, a human differentiation antigen initially described in a subpopulation of lymphocytes that have a natural killer cell function.[4] It also binds to an antigenic constituent of myelin-associated glycoprotein found in adult central and peripheral myelin sheaths.[202, 265] Leu-7 reactivity has been found in various neuroendocrine cells and tumors, including enterochromaffin cells,[263] pancreatic islet cells and islet cell tumors,[263] carcinoid tumors of the intestine, lungs, and small intestine,[174, 192, 281] pheochromocytomas,[42, 79, 281] and SCLC.[42, 64, 256, 273, 281, 283] Immunocytochemical and immunoblot analyses have shown that the HNK-1 antibody apparently reacts with the carbohydrate moiety of a protein (molecular weight, 75 kd) localized in the matrix of the chromaffin granule.[281] Several studies have indicated that Leu-7 could be a useful marker in the diagnosis of SCLC,[42, 64, 252, 273, 283] especially since it can be detected in formalin-fixed, paraffin-embedded specimens. Linnoila and co-workers[174] reported Leu-7 reactivity in 56% (18 of 32 tumors) of cases of SCLC and in 22% of cases of non-SCLC. Since monoclonal antibodies detect only one determinant on a macromolecule, there is the possibility of cross reactivity with antigenic sites present on unrelated molecules. This problem is well illustrated by demonstration of Leu-7 immunoreactivity in hypertrophic and neoplastic prostatic epithelium.[249] Therefore, positive immunostaining for Leu-7 in non–SCLC should be interpreted with caution and should not be viewed as unequivocal evidence of endocrine differentiation in these tumors. Because of its inconsistent expression in SCLC and its expression in about one fifth of the cases of non–SCLC, we believe that the value of Leu-7 in the diagnosis of SCLC is limited.

Synaptophysin (or P38) is a major integral membrane glycoprotein originally isolated from presynaptic vesicles of bovine brain. By using a monoclonal antibody (SY38), synaptophysin was demonstrated in the small (30 to 80 nm in diameter) vesicles that, ultrastructurally, have clear contents, and occur in human neuroendocrine cells and related tumors.[40, 56, 107, 276, 304] Several studies have indicated that synaptophysin can be used as a broad-spectrum neuroendocrine marker for establishing the histopathologic diagnosis of SCLC.[40, 156, 305] Kayser and co-workers[156] found reactivity for synaptophysin in 49 of 68 (79%) cases of SCLC and 6 of 74 (8%) cases of non–SCLC. Since the same non–SCLC cases that reacted for synaptophysin also stained for other neuroendocrine markers, it is possible that these cases may have had a neuroendocrine cell component that was responsible for the synaptophysin expression in these particular tumors.

Synaptophysin has the advantage over other panendocrine markers, such as neuron-specific enolase and PGP 9.5, of being more specific for neuroendocrine differentiation. It also has a superiority over chromogranin in being more widely expressed in endocrine tumors, reacting in those that do not present argyrophilia or a positive reaction for chromogranin A, such as β-cell islet cell tumor of the pancreas, as well as the great majority of SCLC cases. In spite of these clear benefits of synaptophysin over other broad-spectrum markers, it has the drawback that the immunostaining usually is weak and often negative when it is performed on routinely fixed, paraffin-embedded tissue specimens. In order to obtain optimal results, the immunoreaction procedure should be performed on frozen sections or in ethanol-fixed, paraffin-embedded tissue sections. Good results have been reported with specimens that have been briefly fixed (2–4 hours) in formalin or in Bouin's solution.[138]

Specific Neuroendocrine Cell Products

A variety of peptides and biogenic amines that can be used as endocrine markers are produced by SCLC. In an immunocytochemical study of 22 tumors, 6 were reactive for bombesin, 3 for ACTH, and 1 each for calcitonin, somatostatin, Leu-enkephalin, and serotonin.[106] Based on these results, as well as on the findings from other studies,[33, 86, 103, 106, 251] it has been stated that the diagnosis of SCLC can be facilitated by the immunocytochemical detection of bombesin or of the C-terminal flanking peptide of probombesin.[5, 122, 268] These peptides are not only highly specific endocrine markers but also are often expressed in SCLC.

Bombesin is a tetradecapeptide originally isolated from amphibian skin and found to be closely related to the gastrin releasing peptide (GRP) present in the human nervous system and in the neuroendocrine cells from the bronchopulmonary and gastrointestinal tracts.[237] Bombesin reactivity has been reported in SCLC cell lines but not in cell lines from other types of lung cancer.[208, 209] It has also been postulated to have an autocrine function in SCLC, causing a stimulation of growth.[69] Bombesin/GRP reactivity has been reported in 20% to 69% of SCLC cases by immunocytochemical procedures.[5, 122, 156, 219, 233, 251] In contrast to chromogranin, the reactivity for this marker does not correlate with the density of neurosecretory granules in the tumor cells.[251] Bombesin has also been found in a few cases of non–SCLC[156, 251]; however, evidence of endocrine differentiation in up to 10% of the non–SCLC cases has been reported.[5]

It is not uncommon to encounter negative immunostaining of a neuroendocrine tumor when antibodies to a single bioactive form of a peptide are used. This could result from the tumor containing little peptide stored in a particular form, or the cells could be inappropriately producing an abnormal molecular form of the hormone.[25] Under these circumstances, by using immunostaining for probombesin derivatives, some authors have found a larger number of tumors reacting for C-flanking peptide of human probombesin than for bombesin, a finding that could facilitate the diagnosis.[268] The probombesin molecule consists of a signal peptide, the bioactive bombesin molecule, and a large C-terminal flanking peptide.[5] In a study of 361 endocrine tumors of the lung, Hamid and co-workers[122] found immunostaining for the C-terminal peptide of human probombesin in 70% of cases of SCLC and 63% of cases of atypical (aggressive) carcinoids, but in only 16% of cases of benign carcinoids. Based on these results, as well as on the finding of a higher concentration of C-flanking peptide of human probombesin than bombesin in the more malignant endocrine tumors, these authors postulated that immunostaining for C-flanking peptide of human probombesin is not only useful as a histopathologic marker but also may have a biologic value predicting the course of the disease. Other regulatory peptides, such as ACTH or calcitonin, can be helpful in the diagnosis of some cases, but since they are infrequently expressed in SCLC, their diagnostic value for this tumor is limited.

ELECTRON MICROSCOPY

Good material is essential for the proper evaluation of the fine structure of any tumor, and it is vital in SCLC since the tumors are prone to crushing artifact. There has been speculation on why this should be, including the unlikely suggestion that it might be due to the action of myofibroblasts within the tumor.[52] Myofibroblasts are often seen in tumors in which crushing artifact is not a characteristic finding, and other properties of the neoplastic small cells, and in particular their puny cytoskeleton, are more likely to be responsible. Figure 9–17 shows the consequences on the fine structure of SCLC cells of a moderate amount of crushing. The nuclei are quite dense with coarse aggregates of chromatin, and some have irregular profiles. It is difficult to make out details of the cytoplasm or to tell where one cell ends and the next begins. The scanty cytoplasm and organelles are consistent with this tumor being a SCLC, but it would be unwise to make the diagnosis from the electron microscopy alone.

The usual appearances of SCLC at the ultrastructural level[47, 65, 84, 123, 152, 181–184, 199, 204, 210–212] are shown in Figures 9–18 through 9–21. At low magnification (see Fig. 9–18), the nuclei seem very close together, an appearance that correlates with the cellularity in light microscopic sections. More detail can be appreciated in Figure 9–19. The cells are predominantly ovoid to elongated, and with so little cytoplasm the shape of the nucleus tends to parallel that of the cell. Some nuclei have angular or slightly irregular profiles, but for the most part their contours are fairly smooth; marked nuclear irregularity in well-preserved material is unusual. There are slender gaps between some of the cells in this illustration, possibly an indication of slight shrinkage artifact. Usually adjacent cells are closely apposed (Figs. 9–20 and 9–21).

The high nuclear/cytoplasmic ratio is shown well by electron microscopy, although it is not evident in every cell. Since many of the cells are ovoid, they have more cytoplasm at the poles of the nuclei, so the plane of section can make a difference in the appearance in thin sections. The periphery of the cells is smooth and filopodia are a rare finding. The cell membranes of neighboring cells are intimately apposed without infoldings, but the number and appearance of the cell junctions are quite variable. In some SCLC there are frequent desmosomes that are small but mature, with thin bundles of tonofilaments that quickly disappear as they extend off into the cytoplasm. More often, the junctions are intermediate and they can be mere tiny densities of the cell membranes that require some searching for their detection.

Organelles are sparse in SCLC cells, a feature that contrasts the tumors to differentiated non–SCLC, but undifferentiated large cell carcinomas of the compact type may have comparably small numbers of organelles. In SCLC cells, the organelles are typically con-

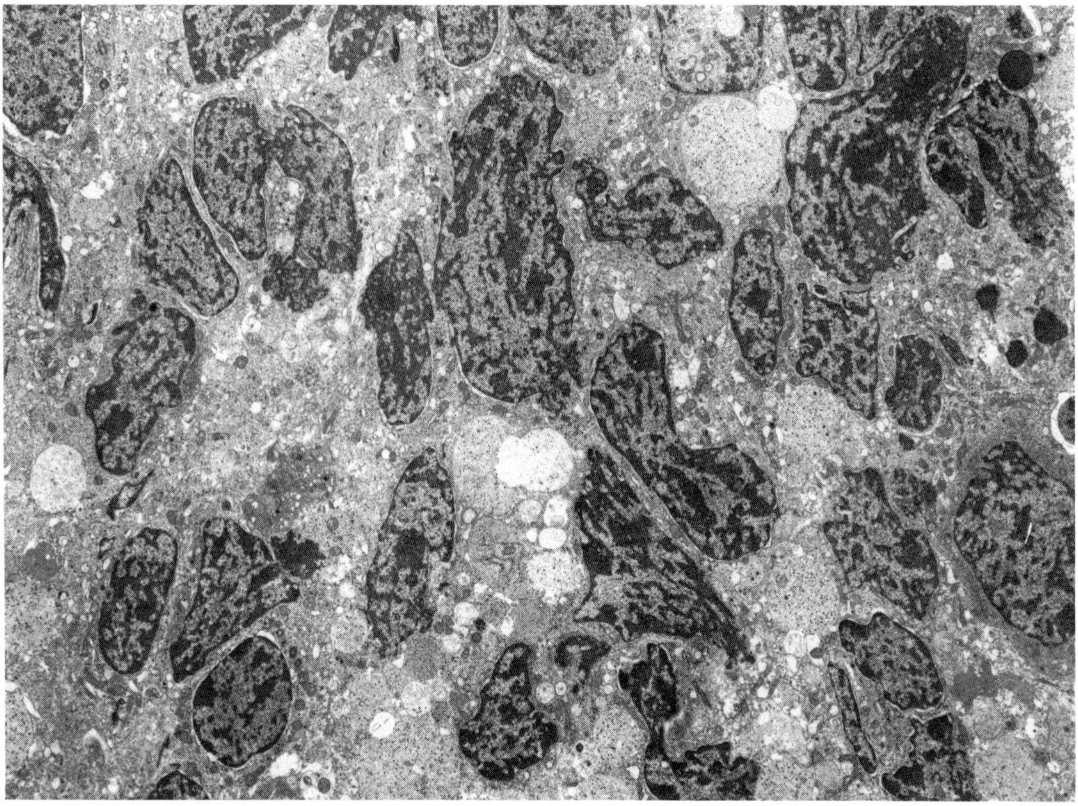

Figure 9–17. Small cell carcinoma. The electron micrograph shows marked distortion in an area of moderate crushing artifact. (×2,900)

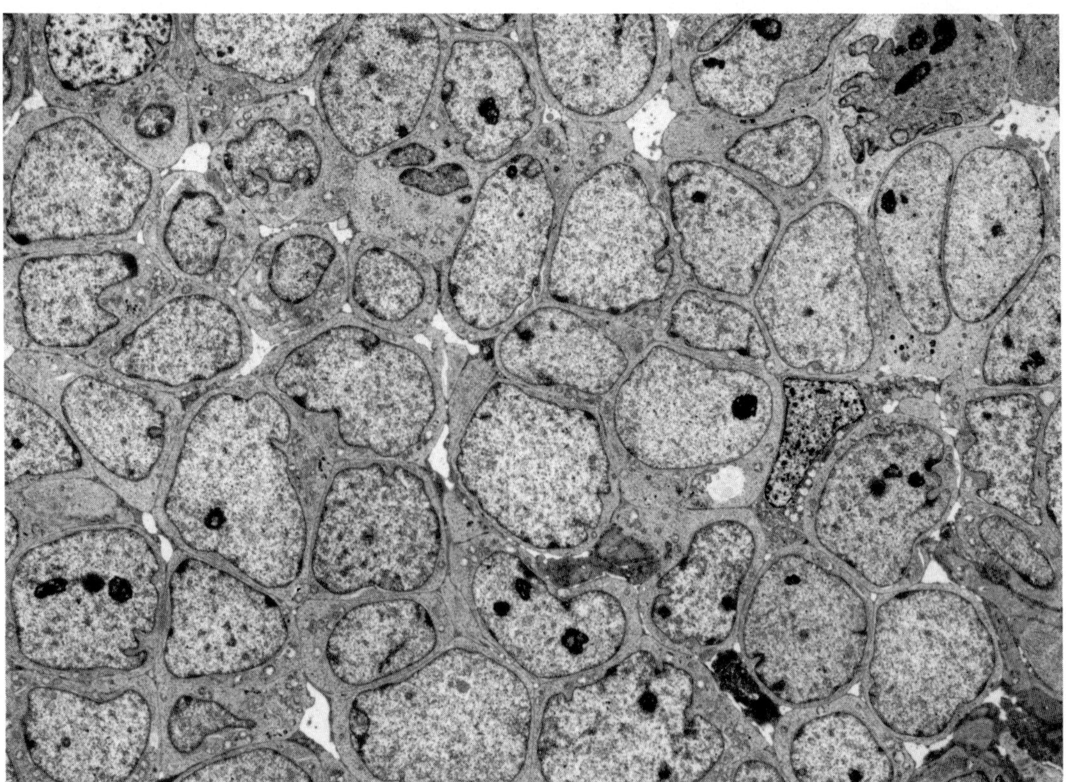

Figure 9–18. Small cell carcinoma. The typical appearance of the tumor as seen in a low-magnification electron micrograph. The high nuclear/cytoplasmic ratio can be appreciated. (×2,100)

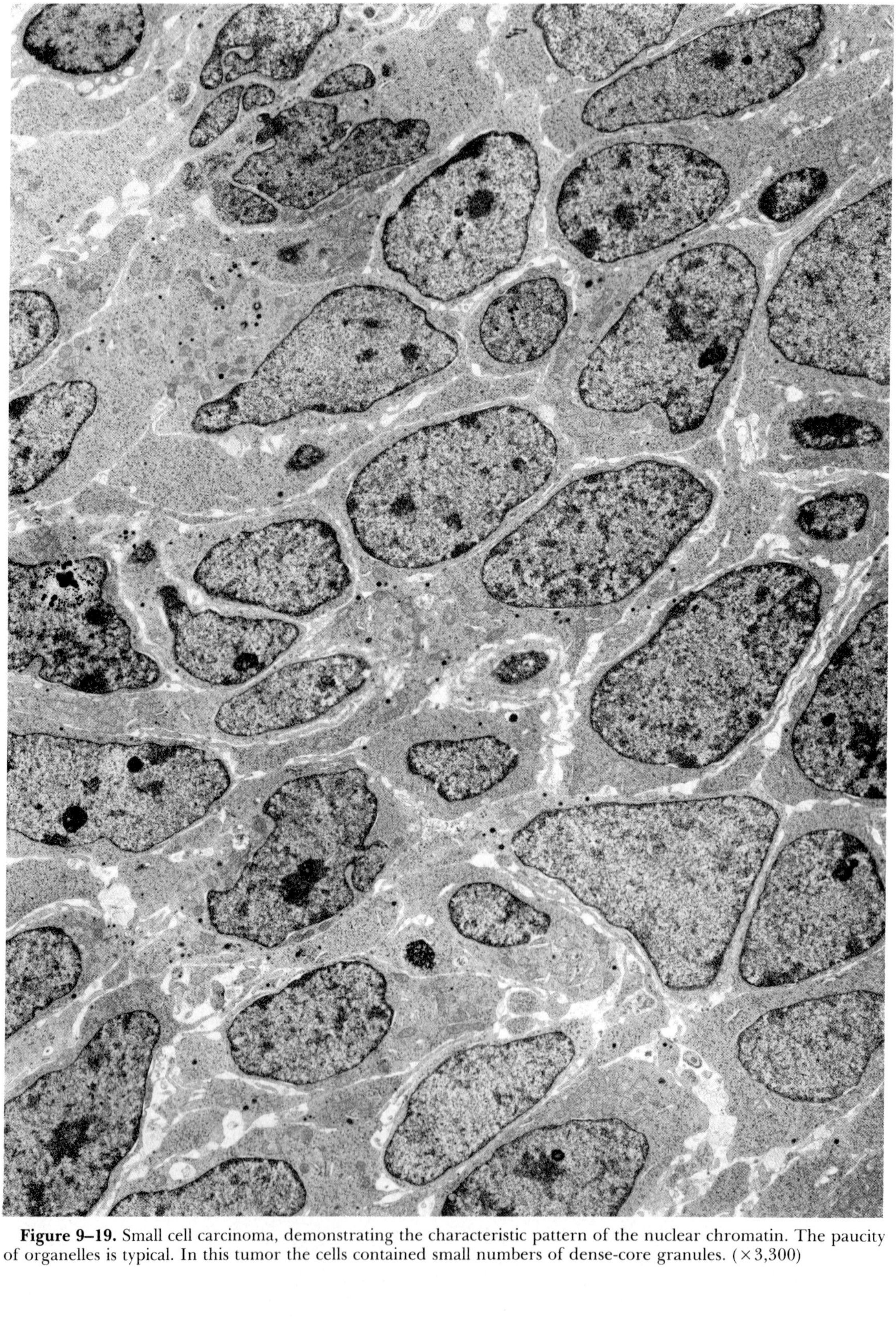

Figure 9–19. Small cell carcinoma, demonstrating the characteristic pattern of the nuclear chromatin. The paucity of organelles is typical. In this tumor the cells contained small numbers of dense-core granules. (×3,300)

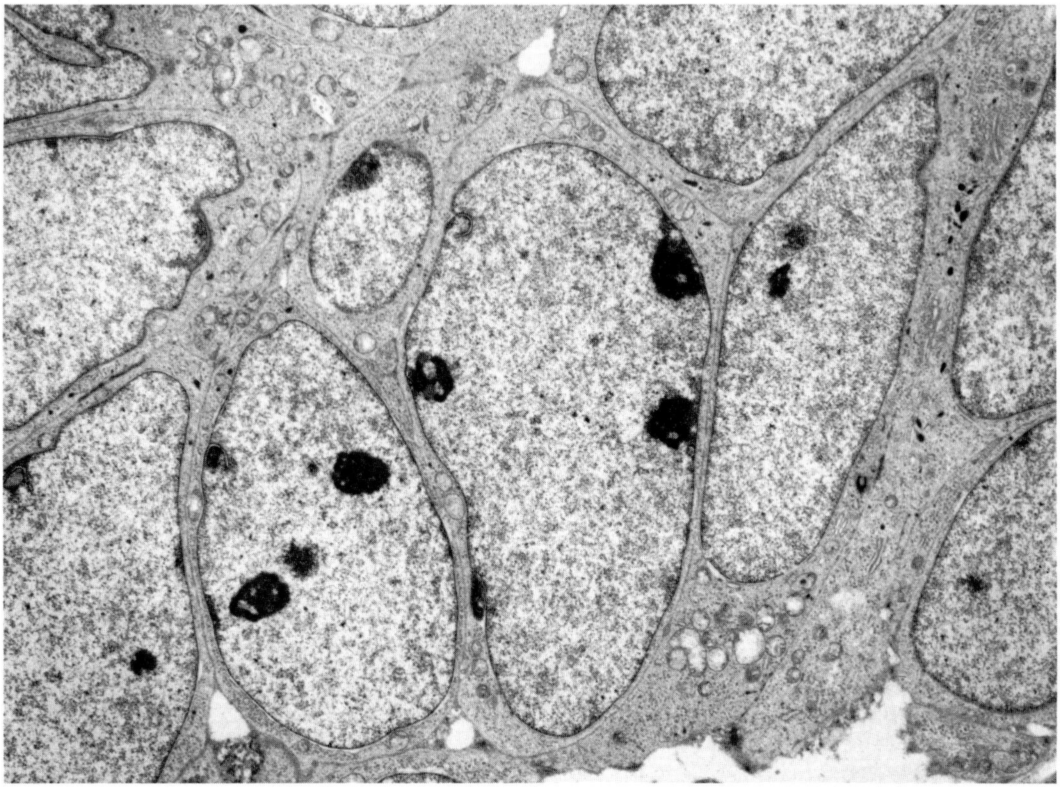

Figure 9–20. Small cell carcinoma. An occasional mitochondrion can be seen within the thin rim of cytoplasm. Nucleoli are more prominent than usual. The small dense bodies in the cytoplasm are irregular, and they are probably lysosomes. (×4,000)

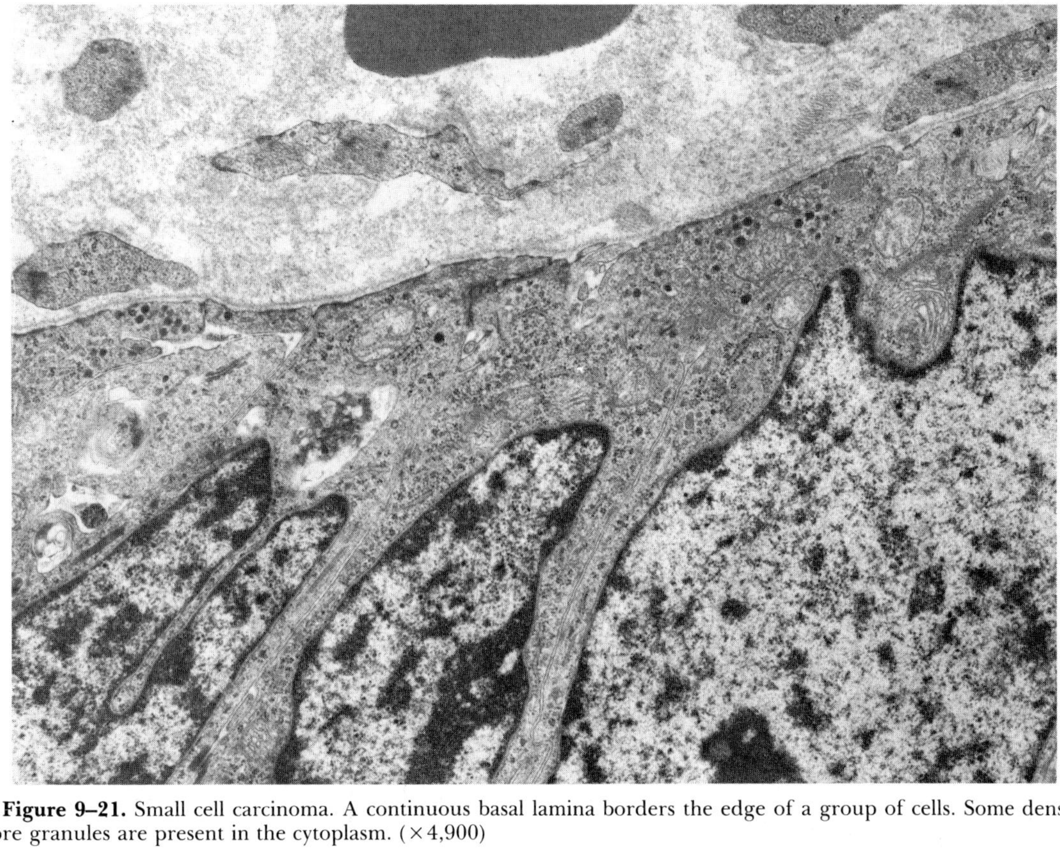

Figure 9–21. Small cell carcinoma. A continuous basal lamina borders the edge of a group of cells. Some dense-core granules are present in the cytoplasm. (×4,900)

fined to a few mitochondria and short slender cisternae. A small Golgi complex may be seen. The presence of even moderate numbers of organelles in many of the cells should raise the possibility that the tumor is not SCLC. The paucity of cytoplasm and organelles is evident in Figure 9–19.

Tiny dots within the cytoplasm in Figure 9–19 are dense-core secretory granules; at higher magnification they were round and uniform. The few irregular dense bodies in Figure 9–20 are probably lysosomes. Dense-core granules are widely considered to be a characteristic finding in SCLC. They are often present, but in our material they are sparse in about one third of the cases and in at least 10% of the tumors they cannot be found. In contrast, carcinoids always contain granules and usually they are present in considerable numbers. Hammar and coworkers[124] found that about 10% of 100 SCLC studied did not have neuroendocrine features. Granules were absent in 11.5% of a group of 52 tumors.[294] The granules are more consistently detected in cell lines.

SCLC granules are consistently small and uniform, spherical, and approximately 120 nm in diameter, and the limiting membrane is separated by a narrow halo from the dense core.[183] The granules are similar in size to those of extrapulmonary neuroendocrine carcinomas and neuroblastomas. The SCLC granules may be present throughout the cytoplasm, but they tend to cluster; and if dendritic processes are present, the granules accumulate within them. Exocytosis of the granules has been described.[214] A basal lamina is found in a small number of these tumors at the edge of sharply demarcated groups of cells. Secretory granules are present in Figure 9–21 near the basal lamina and in a dendritic process of a tumor cell in Figure 9–22. The process is more visible because neighboring cells are fragmented. It also contains a few microtubules: they are common in the dendrites of neuroblastoma cells but are not often seen in SCLC.

The typical appearances have been described, but there is some variation at the ultrastructural level among SCLC, even

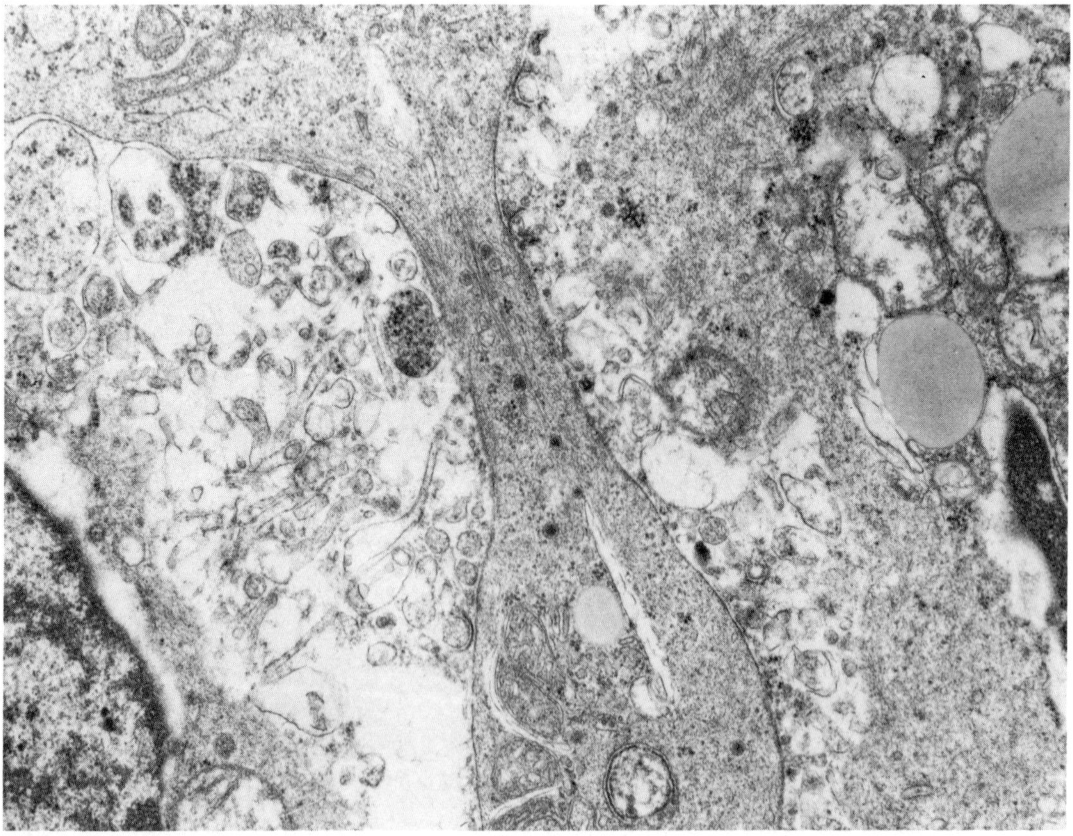

Figure 9–22. Small cell carcinoma. A slender process of a tumor cell contains a few small granules and an occasional microtubule. (×23,000)

within a single tumor, and because of this, several areas of a tumor should be examined if the diagnosis is in question. A small sampling can give a misleading impression. The size of the cells and their nuclei overlap those of carcinoid tumors and undifferentiated large cell carcinomas, and some cells have a fair amount of cytoplasm and moderate numbers of organelles. It is not unusual to find that some or even all the nuclei in a particular tumor have fine, evenly dispersed chromatin and multiple prominent nucleoli, as shown in Figure 9–20. Electron microscopy is highly precise in defining the morphologic features of a tumor, provided well-preserved and undistorted tissue is available for study, and it is the most reliable method with which to establish the diagnosis of SCLC. However, since variations do occur, and overlap with other tumor types is recognized, caution must be exercised when evaluating the ultrastructural findings if they do not conform to the typical features of SCLC. It must further be remembered that the samples of tissue provided for electron microscopy are meager and do not display the range of variation that is often seen by light microscopy in lung tumors. It is good practice to routinely correlate the appearance of the thick sections of the plastic-embedded tissue with the paraffin sections and/or cytologic preparations.

Vollmer and co-workers[294] studied 52 SCLC by electron microscopy, correlating the findings with tumor stage and survival. Thirty-nine of the specimens were glutaraldehyde-fixed and 13 were from paraffin. Dense-core granules were absent in 11.5%. Cell junctions were identified in 90%, and tonofilaments were seen in 17%. Glandular and squamous differentiation were found in 2 tumors, glandular differentiation and SCLC in 1, and a combination of SCLC with non–SCLC in 11. When the ultrastructural findings were compared with the clinical stage, most tumors from patients with stage I disease had desmosomes while most of the tumors from patients with stage III disease did not, and this was a statistically significant association. Neither the presence nor the number of granules bore a relation to stage or survival. The study raises the possibility that an absence of junctions in SCLC may be a poor prognostic sign and a contraindication to surgery. Only the type of cell junction was of prognostic importance with respect to survival; patients whose tumors had intermediate junctions and especially desmosomes had a significantly greater chance to have more localized disease and a resectable tumor and consequently a longer survival. The median survival periods for patients without identifiable junctions, with intermediate junctions, and having desmosomes were 6.4, 8.2, and 11.3 months, respectively.

SUBTYPING

The four histologic groups of lung cancer proposed by Marchesani in 1924[188] (basal cell carcinoma, polymorphocellular carcinoma, keratinizing squamous cell carcinoma, cylindrical cell adenocarcinoma) were expanded by the World Health Organization (WHO) in 1962, and two subtypes of SCLC, oat cell and polygonal forms, were recognized.[160] The classification was adapted and tested by the Veterans Administration Oncology Group[315] and was further modified in the first WHO classification of 1967.[161] Four categories were recommended: lymphocyte-like or oat cell, fusiform, polygonal, and "others."

In 1973, pathologists of the Working Party for the Therapy of Lung Cancer reduced the four groups to two, lymphocyte-like (oat cell) and intermediate, the latter merging the fusiform and polygonal types in the first WHO classification.[193] The revision of the WHO classification published in 1981 adopted these two categories but added a combined subtype for SCLC with a component of squamous cell or adenocarcinoma.[310]

Oat cell carcinoma was defined in the 1981 WHO classification as "a malignant tumour composed of uniform small cells, generally larger than lymphocytes, having dense round or oval nuclei, diffuse nucleoli, and very sparse cytoplasm," while SCLC of the intermediate cell type was "a malignant tumour composed of small cells, with nuclear characteristics similar to the oat cell but with more abundant cytoplasm. The cells may be polygonal or fusiform and are less regular in appearance than those of oat cell carcinoma."[310] The descriptions are sufficiently similar to indicate that separation of the two subtypes might not be easy, and many pathologists experienced difficulty in practice.

A number of groups have addressed the problem of subdividing SCLC on the basis of its histologic appearance and attempted to assess the possible prognostic relevance of such subtyping; the published reports have to some degree been conflicting.[44, 59, 70, 71, 90,

[116, 132, 133, 153, 164, 175, 222, 260, 292, 293] The variations in the findings can in part be attributed to the fact that not all observers used the same criteria to separate the subtypes. Roggli and co-workers[246] found that agreement for the diagnosis of SCLC was 98% among a group of observers, but it was only 72% for subtyping. Ultrastructural studies do not provide support for SCLC subtyping.[183]

Members of the pathology panel of the International Association for the Study of Lung Cancer concluded that there were no clinical, biologic, or ultrastructural differences between SCLC of the oat cell and intermediate types. They proposed that the terms *oat cell* and *intermediate* be deleted but recommended that two variants be recognized: mixed small cell–large cell carcinoma composed of small cells with a significant population of large cells arranged in nests diffusely throughout the tumor, and combined SCLC composed of a combination of SCLC with neoplastic squamous cell carcinoma or adenocarcinoma.[131] The evolution of the nomenclature for SCLC is shown in Table 9–1.

Mixed histology small cell–large cell carcinoma[239] has been recognized as an uncommon but distinct pathologic variant of SCLC associated with lower response rates and shorter survival than tumors composed exclusively of small cells. We have not seen a convincing example in an untreated patient, but the appearance that has been described can be simulated by an undifferentiated large cell carcinoma with a component of smaller cells; the ultrastructural appearance of such a tumor is shown in Figure 9–23. The diagnosis certainly should not be made from poorly preserved or distorted material, and it is probably only valid in pretherapy specimens since a consequence of therapy is that some of the small cells enlarge.

Combined SCLC is rare; the tumors are more readily diagnosed in resection or autopsy specimens where there is sufficient tissue for adequate histologic study. However, 9 of 429 patients with SCLC seen at Vanderbilt University between 1977 and 1983 had a combined subtype at the time of diagnosis that was established by bronchoscopy in 6 patients, fine-needle aspiration in 1, lymph node biopsy in 1, and thoracotomy in 1.[186] There were no differences in median age, sex, performance status, and stage of disease with other subtypes of SCLC, but patients with combined subtype histology had a higher incidence of peripheral lesions on chest radiography (56% versus 14%) and a lower median lactic acid dehydrogenase value at diagnosis. The overall response to chemotherapy and median survival of 8 versus 10 months were similar to those of the other subtypes. Two of the patients with combined histology, both of whom underwent surgical resection and received chemotherapy, survived for at least 5 years.

Figures 9–24 through 9–27 show an example of the combined variant of SCLC in which small nests of squamous cells are present within the SCLC (see Fig. 9–24). Their presence can be highlighted by cytokeratin immunostaining (see Fig. 9–25). Electron microscopy revealed close apposition between the small cell component and the squamous nests (Fig. 9–26), although the two cell types were clearly distinct and transitional forms were not identified. The squamous cells were united by prominent desmosomes that contrasted to the small desmosomes between the small cells, and some of the larger desmosomes were also present within the cytoplasm of the squamous cells (Fig. 9–27). Entrapped gland-like structures within an SCLC (Fig. 9–28) should not be misinterpreted as evidence of a second neoplastic component. The

Text continued on page 235

Table 9–1. Evolution of Nomenclature for Small Cell Lung Cancer Subtyping

<table>
<tr><th>Kreyberg (1962)</th><th>WHO (1967)</th><th>WP-L (1973)
WHO (1981)</th><th>IASLC (1988)</th></tr>
<tr><td>Oat cell</td><td>Lymphocyte-like</td><td>Oat cell</td><td>Small cell carcinoma</td></tr>
<tr><td rowspan="3">Polygonal</td><td>Polygonal</td><td rowspan="2">Intermediate</td><td rowspan="2">Mixed small cell/large cell</td></tr>
<tr><td>Fusiform</td></tr>
<tr><td>Other</td><td>Combined oat cell carcinoma</td><td>Combined small cell carcinoma</td></tr>
</table>

WHO, World Health Organization; WP-L, Working Party for Therapy of Lung Cancer; IASLC, International Association for the Study of Lung Cancer.

From Hirsch FR, Matthews DJ, Aisner S et al: Histopathologic classification of small cell lung cancer: Changing concepts and terminology. Cancer 62(5):974, 1988.

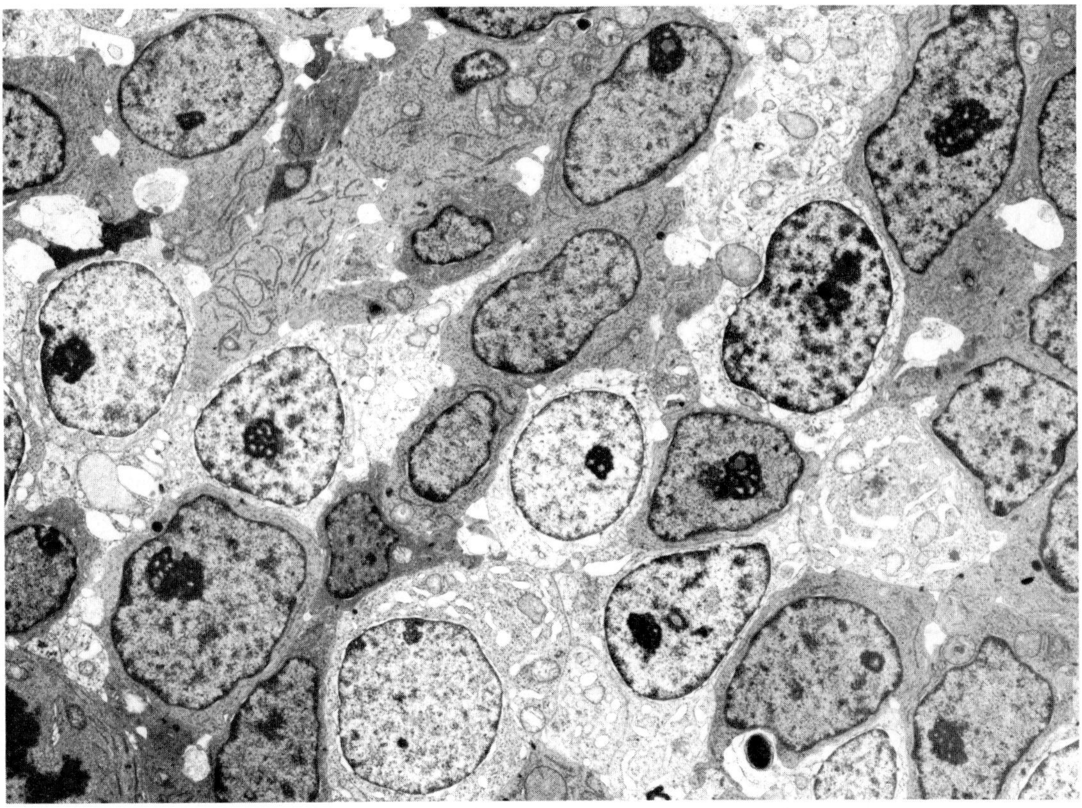

Figure 9–23. Undifferentiated large cell carcinoma with a component of smaller, darker cells simulating a small cell–large cell variant of small cell carcinoma. (×4,700)

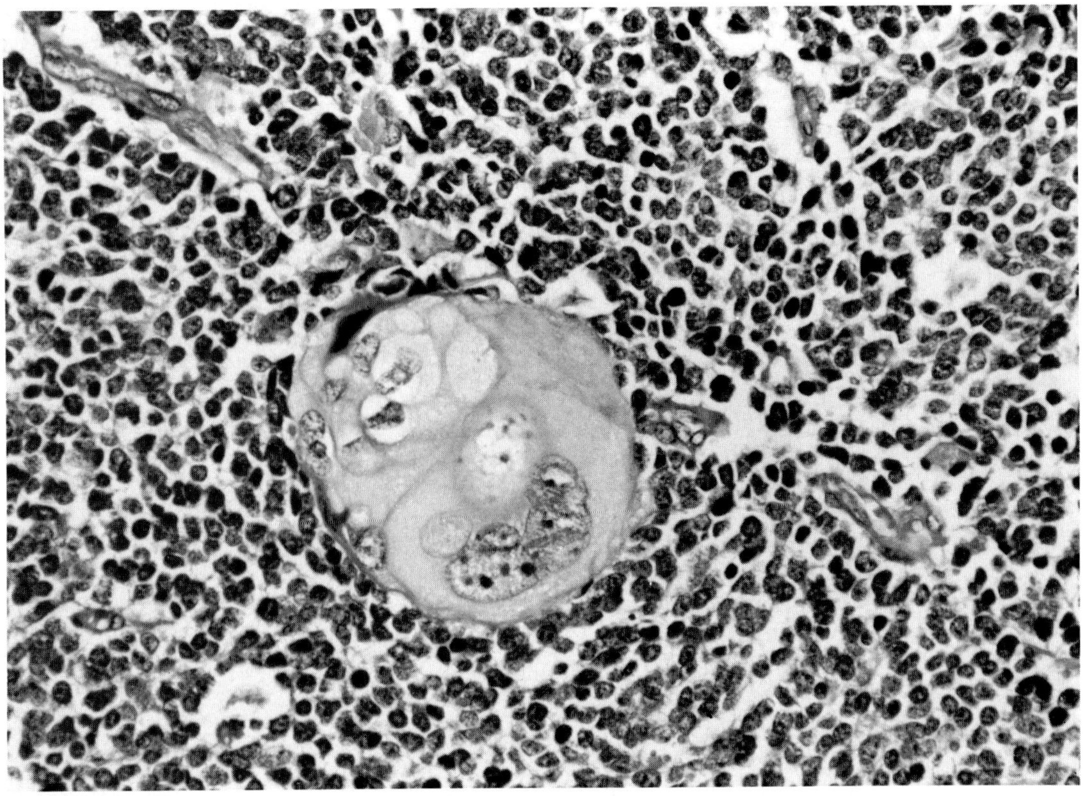

Figure 9–24. Small cell carcinoma, combined variant. Numerous small islands of squamous differentiation were present among the small cells.

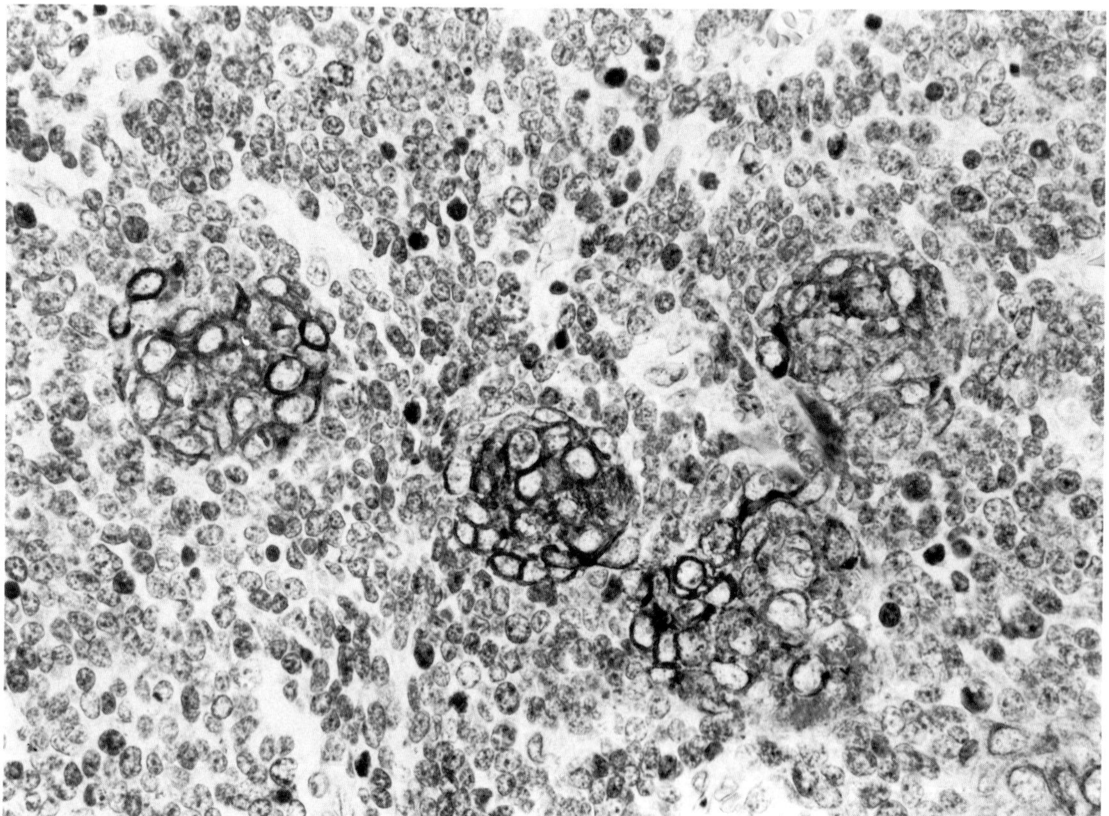

Figure 9–25. The same tumor stained for keratin 903, highlighting the squamous cells.

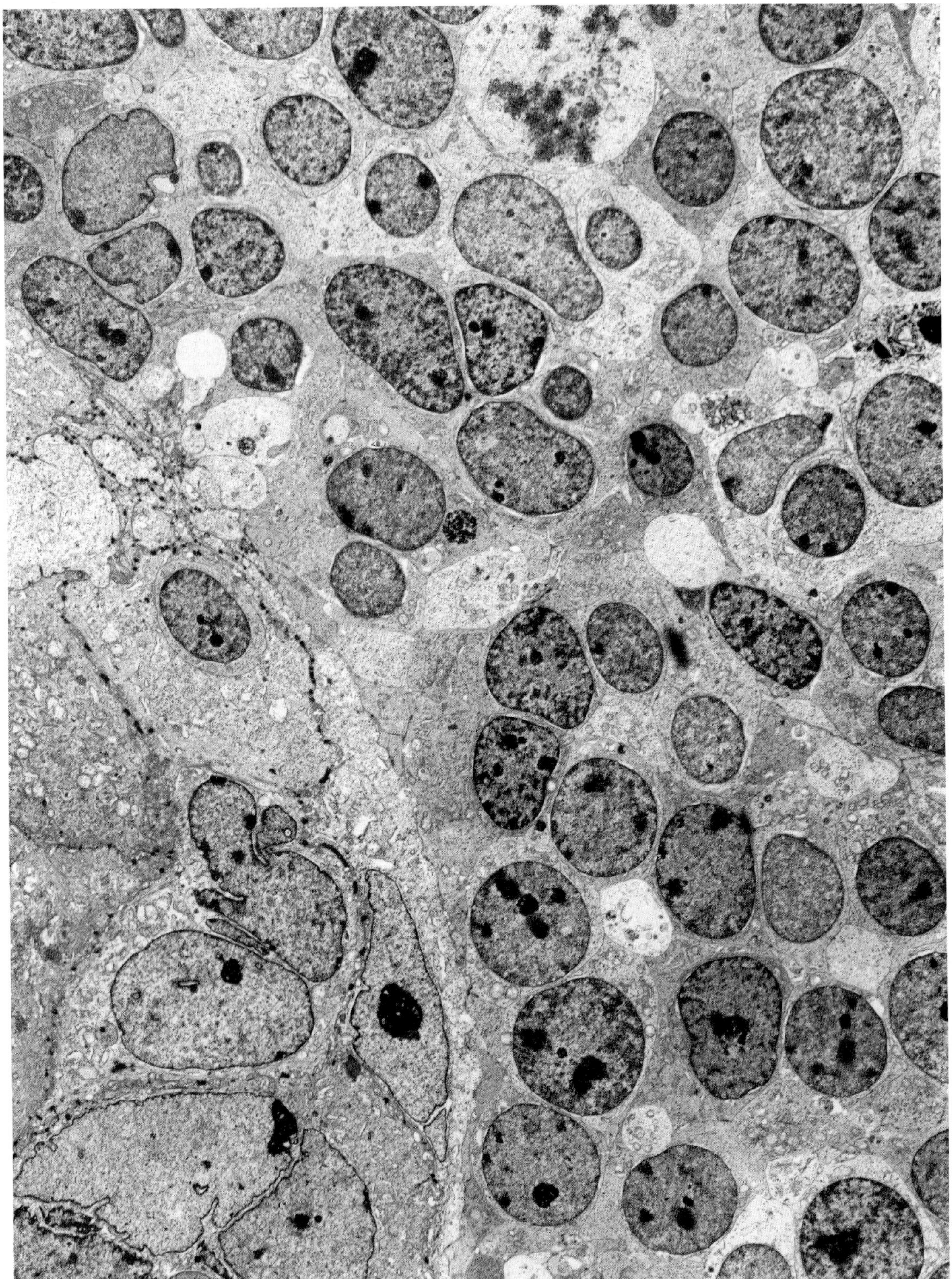

Figure 9–26. The same tumor in a low-power electron micrograph that shows the close apposition of the small cells and squamous cells. (×4,500)

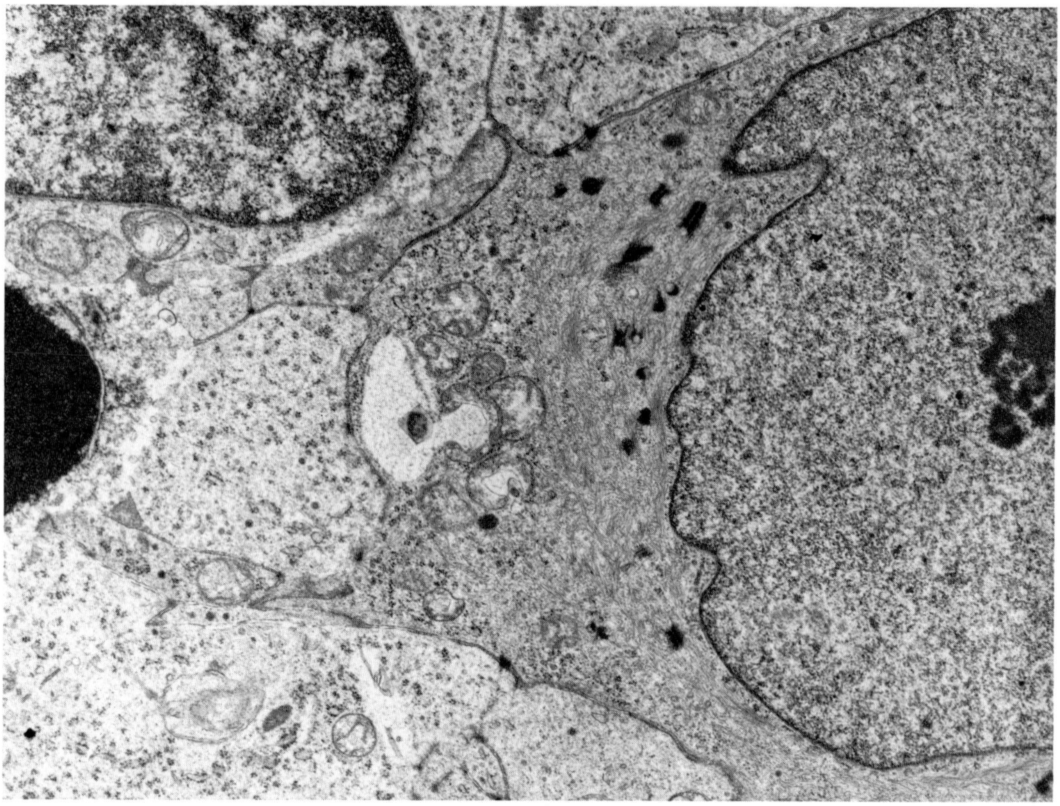

Figure 9–27. Same tumor as in Figures 9–24 through 9–26. Intracytoplasmic desmosomes can be seen within the cytoplasm of the squamous cell in company with intermediate filaments. (×11,500)

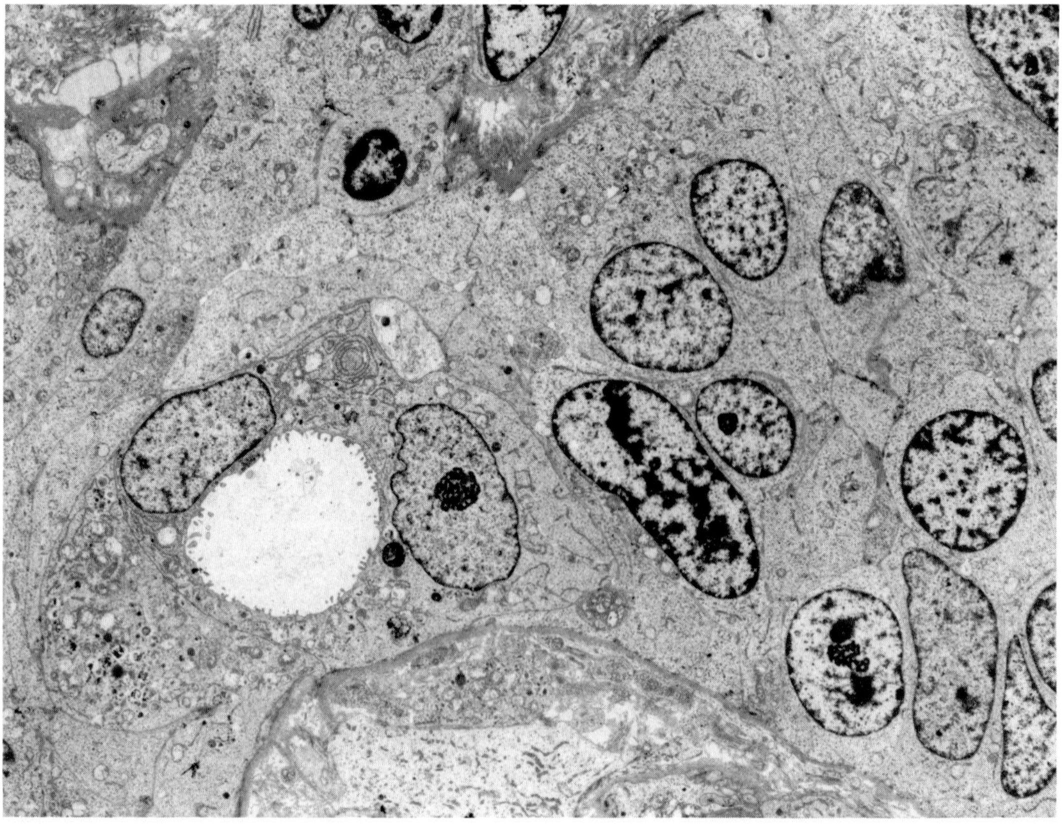

Figure 9–28. Small cell carcinoma. A small acinus is present, but it represents an entrapped structure. (×2,650)

non–SCLC portion of a combined variant may also be an adenocarcinoma or an undifferentiated large cell carcinoma. The two components of a combined variant of SCLC are usually distinct, and they may not be in contact; when they are contiguous, intimate intermingling of the cells is not seen and the appearance is rather that of a collision tumor.

DIFFERENTIAL DIAGNOSIS

The importance of good material from which to make the diagnosis of SCLC has already been stressed. When it is available, the diagnosis can usually be reached with confidence from tissue sections or cytologic smears. An occasional squamous cell carcinoma with smaller cells than usual[61] can cause confusion with SCLC, especially in a small biopsy specimen, and while the distinction should be possible in a resection specimen, it is always reassuring to have material for electron microscopy available for study.

Small cell carcinomas histologically identical to primary SCLC can occur in the trachea,[20, 54, 241, 278] larynx,[20, 101, 173, 215, 300, 309] and esophagus.[55, 137, 146, 243] Extrapulmonary SCLC[104, 140] have been reported in many locations,[300] and some tumors show neuroendocrine differentiation, manifested by positive staining with neuron-specific enolase or chromogranin and variably with other immunocytochemical procedures, and at the ultrastructural level by the presence of dendritic processes and small dense-core granules. Since many cases of SCLC are diagnosed from metastatic sites, the possibility of an extrapulmonary primary condition must always be considered, and the pathology findings should always be interpreted in the context of the clinical data.

ANALYTICAL CYTOLOGY

Highly precise measurements of cell and nuclear dimensions can be obtained by performing morphometric analysis on low-magnification electron micrographs.[184] Table 9–2 shows the mean values and standard deviations for statistically derived descriptors obtained in this manner for a group of lung tumors and illustrates the degree of overlap that occurs among histologic types. The findings underscore the difficulty of subtyping SCLC in paraffin sections. Nomori and coworkers[223] used morphometry together with immunocytochemistry and electron microscopy to study surgically resected tumors and identified four subtypes: oat cell, intermediate cell, and combined and undifferentiated SCLC, the latter presumed to be nonneuroendocrine. However, the morphometric analysis, performed under oil immersion, showed considerable overlap among the first three types with respect to cell and nuclear area and nuclear/cytoplasmic ratio.

Separation of SCLC from non–SCLC is nevertheless possible with morphometric techniques. Marchevsky and colleagues[190] examined 42 cytologic specimens from bronchial brushings, 15 of which contained SCLC cells. Nuclear and cytoplasmic diameters were determined and nuclear/cytoplasmic ratios calculated, and the data enabled the classification of the tumors when they were treated as unknowns. Maubon and associates[197] also used material from bronchial brushings to study by image analysis

Table 9–2. Mean Values and Standard Deviations for Statistically Derived Tumor Descriptors for Lung Tumor Groups

	Maximum cell diameter		Minimum cell diameter		Maximum nuclear diameter		Minimum nuclear diameter		Cytoplasmic area		Nuclear area		N:C ratio*	
Tumor type	*Mean*	*SD*	*Mean*	*SD*	*Mean*	*SD*	*Mean*	*SD*	*Mean*	*SD*	*Mean*	*SD*	*Mean*	*SD*
Adenocarcinoma	16.6	2.8	10.4	1.7	9.3	1.0	6.5	0.79	116	37	45	11.0	0.42	0.09
Squamous cell carcinoma	15.0	3.1	9.6	2.2	9.0	0.94	6.2	0.88	98	47	41	11.0	0.47	0.09
Undifferentiated large cell carcinoma	14.8	1.8	9.9	1.3	9.1	9.1	6.3	0.64	98	22	43	9.0	0.46	0.06
Small cell carcinoma	11.0	1.6	7.3	0.8	7.8	1.0	5.4	0.60	55	12	30	6.0	0.58	0.17
Carcinoid	12.0	1.6	7.7	1.2	7.2	7.0	5.0	0.56	63	18	26	6.0	0.44	0.05

*Ratio of nuclear to cytoplasmic area.

From Mackay B, Ordóñez NG, Bennington JL et al: Ultrastructural and morphometric features of poorly differentiated and undifferentiated lung tumors. Ultrastruct Pathol 13:569, 1989.

eight specimens of poorly differentiated squamous cell carcinomas and 10 specimens of SCLC. The technique permitted differentiation between the two types of tumors, with heterogeneity of the malignant nuclei indicating an epidermoid carcinoma and homogeneity indicating an SCLC. Thunnissen and Diegenbach[279] used histologic sections to examine examples of adenocarcinoma, squamous cell carcinoma, and SCLC by digital nuclear image analysis and found that for each group of digital nuclear image features, the nuclei of SCLC were correctly classified in a higher percentage (80% to 100%) than were the nuclei of adenocarcinoma (46% to 74%) and squamous cell carcinoma (29% to 68%).

Nuclear DNA may be an effective prognostic indicator for SCLC.[29, 41, 280, 288] Abe and associates[1] reported that patients with tumor cells having hyperdiploid patterns had significantly shorter survival times than those with near diploid patterns. However, attempts to assess the nuclear DNA pattern from the cytomorphology were unreliable. Oud and colleagues[232] found a good correlation between DNA analyses by flow and image cytometry, but recommended that care be taken when interpreting DNA histograms of SCLC metastases. Vindelov and co-workers[288] concluded from their flow cytometric studies that SCLC is heterogeneous and that different subpopulations can be demonstrated, separated *in vitro,* and grown as heterotransplants in nude mice or in tissue culture. *In vivo* evidence indicated that treatment failure results from selection and overgrowth of resistant subpopulations.

BIOLOGY

Cytogenetic studies have revealed chromosomal abnormalities in patients with SCLC.[45, 312, 316] A deletion of part of the short arm of chromosome 3 has been reported,[30, 35, 145, 301] but some laboratories have found SCLC cell lines without this defect.[262] Similar alterations can occur in some patients with non–SCLC[18] and in those with other tumors.[302] De Fusco and associates[74] point out that most of the previous studies were performed on long-term cultures of cell lines, and they used primary SCLC specimens grown in short-term cultures. A chromosomally abnormal clone was observed in each of the 11 cases, and an abnormality of chromosome 3 was found in six of the tumors.

Many cell lines have been established from SCLC.[48, 49, 95, 96, 227, 266] By using serum-free HITES medium,[217] a success rate of as high as 75% can be achieved, and on the basis of its behavior in culture, SCLC has been separated into classic and variant subtypes. Image analysis has confirmed the morphologic differences.[38] Scarpa and colleagues[253] compared the ability of the two types of SCLC cell lines to synthesize the extracellular glycoproteins, fibronectin and laminin, and found that the cell lines of the pure type did not produce either whereas those of the variant type synthesized laminin. They postulate that the variant form may be derived from a primitive neuroectodermal cell with both neural and epithelial features, whereas the classic type is derived from a more mature cell with predominantly neuronal features.

Oncogenes have received considerable attention in connection with the behavior of SCLC.[24, 112, 115, 177, 318] The myc oncogenes c-myc, n-myc, and l-myc are primarily activated in SCLC.[34] Kiefer and co-workers[158] reported amplification and expression of 16 proto-oncogenes examined in 12 established SCLC cell lines. Seven of the 12 showed a 20- to 35-fold amplification of the c-myc oncogene, 3 cell lines showed an 80- to 130-fold amplification of n-myc oncogene, and 1 cell line had a simultaneous amplification of c-myc and n-myc oncogenes.

It is possible that *in vitro* findings using material from treated patients and metastases may not parallel those obtained from primary tumors prior to the institution of therapy. Observations of radioresistance and amplification of the c-myc oncogene may therefore not be directly applicable to clinical practice.[262] Berendsen and colleagues[21] reported studies on three classic-type SCLC cell lines established from one patient during follow-up: in the course of this period, the tumor changed from sensitive to completely resistant to chemotherapy. No major changes were seen between the biopsy and cell line obtained before the start of therapy and later specimens.

HISTOGENESIS

The common assumption that SCLC is an endocrine neoplasm is the basis of classification schemes that place SCLC at the undifferentiated end of a spectrum that includes carcinoid and atypical carcinoid.[92, 103, 105, 234, 313] There are, however, distinct differences between a typical SCLC and a typical carcinoid in morphology, epidemiology,[102] and behavior (see Chapter 10). That some SCLC have endocrine features cannot be questioned. The paraneoplastic syndromes, immunostaining properties, and dense-core granules provide incontrovertible evidence. Nevertheless, a minority of the tumors do not possess dense-core granules, and an even smaller number have as a component a differentiated carcinoma, either squamous cell or adenocarcinoma. Transition of SCLC to a form with larger cells or even frank non–SCLC occurs *in vitro* and *in vivo* following therapy.

Searching in normal respiratory epithelium for a progenitor cell for bronchial carcinoids, the endocrine (Kulchitsky) cell is the obvious choice, but the reserve cells of the bronchial mucosa more closely resemble the cells of SCLC. It is reasonable therefore to speculate that at least some SCLC are derived from the reserve cells. If one accepts the hypothesis of a common cell of origin for all the cell types in the respiratory mucosa, as evidently occurs in the gut[57, 66, 264] the existence of SCLC possessing or devoid of endocrine features,[124] the occurrence of atypical endocrine tumors morphologically intermediate between carcinoid and SCLC,[191, 201, 212] the occasional non–SCLC with neuroendocrine features,[174, 210] and the combination of SCLC with differentiated non–SCLC[200] can be more readily explained.

REFERENCES

1. Abe S, Makimura S, Itabashi K et al: Nuclear DNA content, cytomorphologic features and clinical characteristics of small cell carcinoma of the lung. Anal Quant Cytol Histol 9:495, 1987.
2. Abeloff MD, Eggleston JC: Morphologic changes following therapy. In Greco FA, Oldham RK, Bunn PA (eds): Small Cell Lung Cancer, p 235. New York, Grune & Stratton, 1981.
3. Abeloff MD, Trump DL, Baylin SB: Ectopic adrenocorticotrophic (ACTH) syndrome and small cell carcinoma of the lung: Assessment of clinical implications in patients on combination chemotherapy. Cancer 48:1082, 1981.
4. Abo T, Balch CM: A differentiation antigen of human NK and K cells identified by a monoclonal antibody (HNK-1). J Immunol 127:1024, 1981.
5. Addis BJ, Hamid Q, Ibrahim NB et al: Immunohistochemical markers of small cell carcinoma and related neuroendocrine tumours of the lung. J Pathol 153:137, 1987.
6. Adelstein DJ, Tomashefski JF, Snow NJ et al: Mixed small cell and non–small cell lung cancer. Chest 89:699, 1986.
7. Ahmed A: Some ultrastructural observations of haematoxyphil vascular change in oat-cell carcinoma. J Pathol 112:1, 1974.
8. Aisner J, Aisner SC, Ostrow S et al: Meningeal carcinomatosis from small cell carcinoma of the lung: Consequences of improved survival. Acta Cytol 23:292, 1979.
9. Aisner J, Whitley NYO: Current staging of lung cancer: An overview of current and newer approaches. In Hansen HH (ed): Basic and Clinical Concepts of Lung Cancer, p 183. Boston, Kluwer Academic Publishers, 1989.
10. Altmannsberger M, Osborn M, Droese M et al: Diagnostic value of intermediate filament antibodies in clinical cytology. Klin Wochenschr 62:114, 1984.
11. Angeletti RH: Chromogranin and neuroendocrine secretion. Lab Invest 55:387, 1986.
12. Antkowiak JG, Regal AM, Takita H: Bronchogenic carcinoma in patients under age forty. Ann Thorac Surg 47:391, 1989.
13. Aroney RS, Dalley DN, Chan WK et al: Meningeal carcinomatosis in small cell carcinoma of the lung. Am J Med 71:26, 1981.
14. Atay Z: Possibilities and limitations of cytological diagnoses of small cell bronchogenic carcinoma. Recent Results Cancer Res 98:25, 1985.
15. Azzopardi JG: Oat cell carcinoma of the bronchus. J Pathol Bacteriol 78:513, 1959.
16. Barnard WG: The nature of the "oat-celled sarcoma" of the mediastinum. J Pathol Bacteriol 29:241, 1926.
17. Baylin SB, Mendelson G: Ectopic (inappropriate) hormone production by tumors: Mechanisms involved and the biological and clinical implications. Endocrinol Rev 1:45, 1980.
18. Becker D, Sahin AA: Loss of heterozygosity at chromosomal regions 3p and 13q in non–small cell carcinoma of the lung represents low-frequency events. Genome 4:97, 1989.
19. Bègin P, Sahai S, Wang NS: Giant cell formation in small cell carcinoma of the lung. Cancer 52:1875, 1983.
20. Benisch BM, Tawfik B, Breitenbach EE: Primary oat cell carcinoma of the larynx: An ultrastructural study. Cancer 36:145, 1975.
21. Berendsen HH, de Leij L, de Vries EG et al: Characterization of three small cell lung cancer cell lines established from one patient during longitudinal follow-up. Cancer Res 48:6891, 1988.
22. Berendsen HH, de Leij L, Postmus PE et al: Detection of small cell lung cancer metastases in bone marrow aspirates using monoclonal antibody directed against neuroendocrine differentiation antigen. J Clin Pathol 41:273, 1988.
23. Bergh J, Esscher T, Steinholtz L et al: Immunocytochemical demonstration of neuron-specific enolase (NSE) in human lung cancers. Am J Clin Pathol 84:1, 1985.
24. Birrer MJ, Minna JD: Molecular genetics of lung cancer. Semin Oncol 15:226, 1988.
25. Bishop AE, Power RF, Polak JM: Markers for neuroendocrine differentiation. Pathol Res Pract 183:119, 1988.
26. Blackman F, Chung HR, McDonald RJ et al: Oat cell carcinoma with multiple tracheobronchial papillomatous tumors. Chest 83:817, 1983.
27. Blaschko H, Comlin RS, Schnieder FH et al: Secretion of a chromaffin granule protein, chrom-

ogranin, from adrenal glands after splanchnic stimulation. Nature 215:56, 1967.

28. Blobel GA, Gould VE, Moll R et al: Coexpression of neuroendocrine markers and epithelial cytoskeletal proteins in bronchopulmonary neuroendocrine neoplasms. Lab Invest 52:39, 1985.
29. Blöndal T, Pontèn J: DNA ploidy in small cell carcinoma of the lung. Anticancer Res 3:47, 1983.
30. Bock E, Dissing J: Demonstration of enolase activity connected to brain specific protein 14-3-2. Scand J Immunol 4:31, 1975.
31. Bondy PK, Gilby ED: Endocrine function in small cell undifferentiated carcinoma of the lung. Cancer 50:2147, 1982.
32. Borit A, Ordonez NG, Brooks TE et al: Central neural antigens: Detection and diagnostic applications. CRC Lab Sci 23:219, 1986.
33. Bostwick DG, Roth KA, Evans CJ et al: Gastrin-releasing peptide, a mammalian analog of bombesin, is present in human neuroendocrine lung tumors. Am J Pathol 117:195, 1984.
34. Brambilla E, Wuyam B, Brambilla C: Oncogenes and bronchial cancer. Rev Mal Respir 5:535, 1988.
35. Brauch H, Johnson B, Hovis J et al: Molecular analysis of the short arm of chromosome 3 in small cell and non–small cell carcinoma of the lung. N Engl J Med 317:1109, 1987.
36. Brereton HD, Matthews MD, Costa J et al: Mixed anaplastic small cell and squamous cell carcinoma of the lung. Ann Intern Med 88:805, 1978.
37. Brereton HD, O'Donnell JF, Kent CH et al: Spinal meningeal carcinomatosis in small cell carcinoma of lung. Ann Intern Med 88:517, 1978.
38. Broers JL, Pahlplatz MM, Katzko MW et al: Quantitative description of classic and variant small cell lung cancer cell lines by nuclear image cytometry. Cytometry 9:426, 1988.
39. Bruya TE, Morris JF, Barker AF: Bronchoscopy and bone marrow examinations: An efficient strategy to establish the diagnosis of small cell carcinoma of the lung. Chest 79:423, 1981.
40. Buffa R, Rindi G, Sessa F et al: Synaptophysin immunoreactivity and small clear vesicles in neuroendocrine cells and related tumours. Mol Cell Probes 2:367, 1988.
41. Bunn PA, Carney DN, Gazdar AF et al: Diagnostic and biological implications of flow cytometric DNA content analysis in lung cancer. Cancer Res 43:5032, 1983.
42. Bunn PA, Linnoila J, Minna JD et al: Small cell lung cancer, endocrine cells of fetal bronchus, and other neuroendocrine cells express the Leu-7 antigenic determinant present in natural killer cells. Blood 65:764, 1985.
43. Bunn PA, Nugent JL, Matthews MJ: Central nervous system metastases in small cell bronchogenic carcinoma. Semin Oncol 5:314, 1978.
44. Burdon JG, Sinclair RA, Henderson MM: Small cell carcinoma of the lung: Prognosis in relation to histologic subtype. Chest 76:302, 1979.
45. Campbell L, Brown J, Garson OM et al: Cytogenetic abnormalities in lung cancer. In Hansen HH (ed): Basic and Clinical Concepts of Lung Cancer, p 123. Boston, Kluwer Academic Publishers, 1989.
46. Campling B, Quirt I, DeBoer G et al: Is bone marrow examination in small cell lung cancer really necessary?. Ann Intern Med 105:508, 1986.
47. Carlson G, Sibley RK: Ultrastructural features of pulmonary neoplasms. In Russo J, Sommers SC (eds): Tumor Diagnosis by Electron Microscopy, vol 3, Philadelphia, Field and Wood, 1989, p 93.
48. Carney DN, de Leij L: Lung cancer biology. Semin Oncol 15:199, 1988.
49. Carney DN, Gazdar AF, Bepler G et al: Establishment and identification of small cell lung cancer cell lines having classic and variant features. Cancer Res 45:2913, 1985.
50. Carney DN, Marangos PJ, Ihde DC et al: Serum neuron-specific enolase: A marker for disease extent and response to therapy of small cell lung cancer. Lancet 1:583, 1982.
51. Carney DN, Zweig MH, Ihde DC et al: Elevated serum creatine kinase BB levels in patients with small cell lung cancer. Cancer Res 44:5399, 1984.
52. Carstens PHB: Electron microscopy of small cell carcinoma of the lung with special reference to the crush phenomenon. Ultrastruct Pathol 4:253, 1983.
53. Carter D: Small cell carcinoma of the lung. Am J Surg Pathol 7:787, 1983.
54. Chaffin JG, Herrera GA, Roberts C: Oat cell carcinoma of the trachea: A case report with electron microscopy. Ultrastruct Pathol 4:61, 1983.
55. Chaudhry AP, Setchidanand S, Prezyna A et al: Oat cell carcinoma (apudoma) of esophagus. NY State J Med 81:1212, 1981.
56. Cheifec G, Falkmer S, Grimelius L et al: Synaptophysin: A new marker for pancreatic neuroendocrine tumors. Am J Surg Pathol 11:241, 1987.
57. Cheng H, Leblond CP: Origin, differentiation and renewal of the four main epithelial cell types in the mouse small intestine: V. Unitarian theory of the origin of the four epithelial cell types. Am J Anat 141:537, 1974.
58. Chester KA, Lang B, Gill J et al: Lambert-Eaton syndrome antibodies: Reaction with membranes from a small cell lung cancer xenograft. J Neuroimmunol 18:97, 1988.
59. Choi H, Byhardt RW, Clowry LJ et al: The prognostic significance of histologic subtyping in small cell carcinoma of the lung. Am J Clin Oncol 7:389, 1984.
60. Christen B, Trojanowski JQ, Pietra GG: Immunohistochemical demonstration of phosphorylated and nonphosphorylated forms of human neurofilament subunits in human pulmonary carcinoids. Hum Pathol 18:997, 1987.
61. Churg A, Johnston WH, Stulbarg M: Small cell squamous and mixed small cell squamous–small cell anaplastic carcinomas of the lung. Am J Surg Pathol 4:255, 1980.
62. Clamon GH, Edwards WR, Hamous JE et al: Patterns of bone marrow involvement with small cell lung cancer. Cancer 54:100, 1984.
63. Clamon GH, Evans WK, Shepherd FA: Myasthenic syndrome and small cell cancer of the lung. Arch Intern Med 144:999, 1984.
64. Cole SPC, Mirski S, McGarry RC et al: Differential expression of the Leu-7 antigen on human lung tumor cells. Cancer Res 45:4285, 1985.
65. Copple B, Wright SE, Moatamed F et al: Electron microscopy in small cell lung carcinoma: Clinical correlation. J Clin Oncol 2:910, 1984.
66. Cox WF, Pierce GB: The endodermal origin of the

endocrine cells of an adenocarcinoma of the colon of the rat. Cancer 50:1530, 1982.
67. Crisci C, Nutini S, Righi R et al: Role of surgery in undifferentiated small cell carcinoma of the lung: Preliminary results of an international multicenter study. Minerva Chir 44:589, 1989.
68. Cruz JM, Jackson DV, Muss HB et al: Detection of brain metastasis at diagnosis of small cell carcinoma of the lung. J Neurooncol 2:67, 1984.
69. Cuttitta F, Carney DN, Mulshine J et al: Bombesin-like peptides can function as autocrine growth factors in human small cell lung cancer. Nature 316:823, 1985.
70. Davis S, Sobel H: Histologic subtypes of small cell carcinoma of the lung: response to therapy. Eur J Cancer 17:351, 1981.
71. Davis S, Stanley KE, Yesner R et al: Small cell carcinoma of the lung: Survival according to histologic subtype: A Veterans Administration Lung Group Study. Cancer 47:1863, 1981.
72. Davis S, Wright PW, Schulman SF et al: Long-term survival in small cell carcinoma of the lung: A population experience. J Clin Oncol 3:80, 1985.
73. Deftos LJ, Linnoila RI, Carney DN: Demonstration of chromogranin A in human neuroendocrine cell lines by immunohistology and immunoassay. Cancer 62:92, 1988.
74. De Fusco PA, Frytak S, Dahl RJ et al: Cytogenetic studies in 11 patients with small cell carcinoma of the lung. Mayo Clin Proc 64:168, 1989.
75. De la Monte SM, Hutchins GM, Moore GW: Paraneoplastic syndromes and constitutional symptoms in prediction of metastatic behavior of small cell carcinoma of the lung. Am J Med 77:851, 1984.
76. Desimone PA, East R, Powell RD: Phagocytic tumor cell activity in oat cell carcinoma of the lung. Hum Pathol 11:535, 1980.
77. Dhillon AP, Rode J, Dhillon DP et al: Neural markers in carcinoma of the lung. Br J Cancer 51:645, 1985.
78. Dombernowsky P, Hirsh F, Hansen HH et al: Peritoneoscopy in the staging of 190 patients with small cell anaplastic carcinoma of the lung with special reference to subtyping. Cancer 41:2008, 1978.
79. Doria M, Franklin WA: Leucocyte antigens in small cell lung carcinoma. Lung Invest 54:17, 1986.
80. Doyle TJ: Brain metastases in the natural history of small cell lung cancer 1972–1979. Cancer 50:752, 1982.
81. Dropcho EJ, Stanton C, Oh SJ: Neuronal antinuclear antibodies in a patient with Lambert-Eaton myasthenic syndrome and small cell lung carcinoma. Neurology 39:249, 1989.
82. Duggan CJ, Delohery JF, Philips JN: Aspiration biopsy of palpable lymph nodes and the diagnosis of lung carcinoma. Aust NZ J Med 19:241, 1989.
83. Eckman MH, Robert NJ, Parkinson DR et al: Eaton-Lambert syndrome and small cell lung cancer: Side effects and certainty. Med Decis Making 6:174, 1986.
84. Elema JD, Kemming HM: The ultrastructure of small cell lung carcinoma in bronchial biopsy specimens. Hum Pathol 16:1133, 1985.
85. Elliott JA, Osterlind K, Hirsch FR et al: Metastatic patterns in small cell lung cancer: Correlation of autopsy findings with clinical parameters in 537 patients. J Clin Oncol 5:246, 1987.
86. Erisman MD, Linnoila RI, Hernandez O et al: Human lung small cell carcinoma contains bombesin. Proc Natl Acad Sci USA 79:2379, 1982.
87. Esscher T, Steinholtz L, Bergh J et al: Neurone-specific enolase: A useful diagnostic serum marker for small cell carcinoma of the lung. Thorax 40:85, 1985.
88. Feld R: Late complications associated with the treatment of small cell lung cancer. In Hansen HH (ed): Basic and Clinical Concepts of Lung Cancer, p 301. Boston, Kluwer Academic Publishers, 1989.
89. Feld R, Payne D, Hodson I et al: Complications of treatment of small cell carcinoma of the lung: Experience from a recent Canadian trial. Antibiot Chemother 41:204, 1988.
90. Fer MF, Rodgers LW, Richardson RL et al: The intermediate subtype of small cell lung cancer: A frequently unrecognized neoplasm. Clin Res 27:384, 1979.
91. Fletcher L, Rider CC, Taylor CB: Enolase isoenzymes: III. Chromatographic and immunological characteristics of rat brain enolase. Biochim Biophys Acta 452:245, 1976.
92. Forster BB, Muller NL, Miller RR et al: Neuroendocrine carcinomas of the lung: Clinical, radiologic, and pathologic correlation. Radiology 170:441, 1989.
93. Fujita K, Haimoto H, Imaizumi M et al: Evaluation of T-enolase as a tumor marker for lung cancer. Cancer 60:362, 1987.
94. Gasser RW, Herold M, Müller-Holzner E et al: Neuronspezifische Enolase als Tumormarker beim kleinzelligen Bronchuskarzinom. Dtsch Med Wochenschr 113:1708, 1988.
95. Gazdar AF, Minna JD: Cell lines as an investigational tool for the study of biology of small cell lung cancer. Eur J Cancer Clin Oncol 22:909, 1986.
96. Gazdar AF, Oie HK: Cell culture methods for human lung cancer. Cancer Genet Cytogenet 19:5, 1986.
97. George TK, Fitzgerald D, Brown BS et al: Long-term survival in limited-stage small cell lung carcinoma: Experience in Rochester, New York from 1975 to 1981. Cancer 58:1193, 1986.
98. Gephardt GN, Grady KJ, Ahmad M et al: Peripheral small cell undifferentiated carcinoma of the lung: Clinicopathologic features of 17 cases. Cancer 61:1002, 1988.
99. Gianonne L, Johnson DH, Hande KR et al: Favorable prognosis of brain metastases in small cell lung cancer. Ann Intern Med 106:386, 1987.
100. Ginsberg SJ, Comis RL, Gottlieb AJ et al: Long-term survivorship in small cell anaplastic lung carcinoma. Cancer Treat Rep 63:1347, 1979.
101. Gnepp DR, Ferlito A, Hyams V et al: Primary anaplastic small cell (oat cell) carcinoma of the larynx: Review of the literature and report of 18 cases. Cancer 51:1731, 1983.
102. Godwin JD, Brown CC: Comparative epidemiology of carcinoid and oat cell tumors of the lung. Cancer 40:1671, 1977.
103. Gould VE: Neuroendocrinomas and neuroendocrine carcinomas: APUD-cell system neoplasms and their aberrant secretory activities. Pathol Annu 12:33, 1977.
104. Gould VE: Neuroendocrine tumors in "miscellaneous" primary sites: Clinical, pathologic and histogenetic implications. In Fenoglio CM, Wolff

M (eds): Progress in Surgical Pathology, vol IV, p 181. New York, Masson, 1982.
105. Gould VE, Lee I, Warren WH: Immunohistochemical evaluation of neuroendocrine cells and neoplasms of the lung. Pathol Res Pract 183:200, 1988.
106. Gould VE, Linnoila RI, Memoli VA et al: Neuroendocrine cells and neuroendocrine neoplasms of the lung. Pathol Annu 18:287, 1983.
107. Gould VE, Wiedenmann B, Lee I et al: Synaptophysin expression in neuroendocrine neoplasms as determined by immunocytochemistry. Am J Pathol 126:243, 1987.
108. Graus F, Elkon KB, Cordon-Cardo C et al: Sensory neuropathy and small cell lung cancer: Antineuronal antibody that also reacts with the tumor. Am J Med 80:45, 1986.
109. Greco FA, Einhorn LH, Richardson RL et al: Small cell lung cancer: Progress and perspectives. Semin Oncol 5:323, 1978.
110. Greco FA, Hainsworth J, Sismani A et al: Hormone production and paraneoplastic syndromes. In Greco FA, Oldham RK, Bunn PA (eds): Small Cell Lung Cancer, p 177. New York, Grune & Stratton, 1981.
111. Greengard O, Head JF, Goldberg SL et al: Biochemical measure of the volume doubling time of human pulmonary neoplasms. Cancer 55:1530, 1985.
112. Griffin CA, Baylin SE: Oncogene expression in human small cell lung carcinoma. Recent Results Cancer Res 99:237, 1985.
113. Grisold W, Drlicek M, Popp W et al: Antineuronal antibodies in small cell lung carcinoma: Significance for paraneoplastic syndromes. Acta Neuropathol 75:199, 1987.
114. Grunwald GB, Kornguth SE, Towfighi J et al: Autoimmune basis for visual paraneoplastic syndrome in patients with small cell lung carcinoma: Retinal immune deposits and ablation of retinal ganglion cells. Cancer 60:780, 1987.
115. Gu J, Linnoila RI, Seibel NL et al: A study of myc-related gene expression in small cell lung cancer by *in situ* hybridization. Am J Pathol 132:13, 1988.
116. Hage E, Hansen M, Hirsch FR: Electron microscopic subclassification of small cell carcinoma of the lung. Acta Pathol Jpn 33:671, 1983.
117. Hagn C, Schmid W, Fisher-Colbrie R et al: Chromogranin A, B, and C in human adrenal medulla and endocrine tissues. Lab Invest 55:405, 1986.
118. Haimoto H, Takahashi Y, Koshikawa T et al: Immunohistochemical localization of γ-enolase in normal human tissues other than nervous and neuroendocrine tissues. Lab Invest 52:257, 1985.
119. Haimoto H, Takashi M, Koshikawa T et al: Enolase isozymes in renal tubules and renal cell carcinoma. Am J Pathol 124:488, 1986.
120. Hainsworth JD, Johnson DH, Farese RV et al: Limited stage small cell lung cancer: Analysis of clinical prognostic factors. South Med J 80:1518, 1987.
121. Hainsworth JD, Workman R, Greco FA: Management of the syndrome of inappropriate antidiuretic hormone secretion in small cell lung cancer. Cancer 51:161, 1983.
122. Hamid QA, Addis BJ, Springall DR et al: Expression of the C-terminal peptide of human probombesin in 361 lung endocrine tumors, a reliable marker and possible prognostic indicator for small cell carcinoma. Virchows Arch [A] 411:185, 1987.
123. Hammar SP: Common neoplasms. In Dail D, Hammar SP (eds): Pulmonary Pathology, p 727. New York, Springer-Verlag, 1988.
124. Hammar SP, Bockus D, Remington F et al: Small cell undifferentiated carcinomas of the lung with nonneuroendocrine features. Ultrastruct Pathol 9:319, 1988.
125. Hansen HH, Rorth M: Therapy of lung cancer—any progress? An overview of the last decade. In Hansen H (ed): Lung Cancer: Basic and Clinical Aspects, p 249. Boston, Martinus Nijhoff, 1989.
126. Harper PG: Staging of small cell lung cancer. Clin Oncol 4:85, 1985.
127. Hattori A, Umegae Y, Kataki S et al: Small cell carcinoma of the lung with Leser-Trélat sign. Arch Dermatol 118:1017, 1982.
128. Hayward ML, Howell DA, O'Donnell JF et al: Hypercalcemia complicating small cell carcinoma. Cancer 48:1643, 1981.
129. Helman LJ, Gazdar A, Ahn TG: Patterns of gene expression: A novel approach to tumor classification. Proc Am Soc Clin Oncol 6:9, 1987.
130. Hirsch FR, Hansen HH: Bone marrow involvement in small cell anaplastic carcinoma of the lung: Prognostic and therapeutic aspects. Cancer 46:206, 1980.
131. Hirsch FR, Matthews MJ, Aisner S et al: Histopathologic classification of small cell lung cancer: Changing concepts and terminology. Cancer 62(5):973, 1988.
132. Hirsch FR, Matthews MJ, Yesner R: Histopathologic classification of small cell carcinoma of the lung: Comments based on an interobserver examination. Cancer 50:1360, 1982.
133. Hirsch FR, Osterlind K, Hansen HH: The prognostic significance of histopathologic subtyping of small cell carcinoma of the lung according to the classification of the World Health Organization: A study of 375 consecutive patients. Cancer 52:2144, 1983.
134. Hirsch FR, Paulson OB, Hansen HH et al: Intracranial metastases in small cell carcinoma of the lung: Correlation of clinical and autopsy findings. Cancer 50:2433, 1982.
135. Hirsch FR, Paulson OB, Hansen HH et al: Intracranial metastases in small cell carcinoma of the lung: Prognostic aspects. Cancer 51:529, 1983.
136. Hitchins RN, Phillips J, Woods RL: Long term survival in small cell lung carcinoma. Aust NZ J Med 18:3, 1988.
137. Ho K-J, Herrera GA, Jones JM et al: Small cell carcinoma of the esophagus: Evidence for a unified histogenesis. Hum Pathol 15:460, 1984.
138. Hoog A, Gould VE, Grimelius L et al: Tissue fixation methods alter the immunohistochemical demonstrability of synaptophysin. Ultrastruct Pathol 12:673, 1988.
139. Horacek J: Der Joachimsthaler Lungenkrebs nach dem zweiten Weltkrieg. Z Krebforsch 72:52, 1969.
140. Ibrahim NB, Briggs JC, Corbishley CM et al: Extrapulmonary oat cell carcinoma. Cancer 54:1645, 1984.
141. Ihde DC, Hansen HH: Staging procedures and prognostic factors in small cell carcinoma of the lung. In Greco FA, Oldham RK, Bunn PA (eds):

Small Cell Lung Cancer, p 261. New York, Grune & Stratton, 1981.
142. Ihde DC, Simms EB, Matthews MJ et al: Bone marrow metastases in small cell carcinoma of the lung: Frequency, description, and influence on chemotherapeutic toxicity and prognosis. Blood 53:677, 1979.
143. Ishida T, Nishino T, Oka T et al: Surgical treatment of patients with small cell carcinoma of the lung: A histochemical and immunohistochemical study. J Surg Oncol 40:188, 1989.
144. Johnson BE, Ihde DC, Matthews MJ et al: Non–small cell lung cancer: A major cause of late mortality in patients with small cell lung cancer. Am J Med 80:1103, 1986.
145. Johnson BE, Sakaguchi AY, Gazdar AF et al: Restriction fragment length polymorphism studies show consistent loss of chromosome 3p alleles in small cell lung cancer patients' tumors. J Clin Invest 82:502, 1988.
146. Johnson FE, Clawson MC, Bashiti HM et al: Small cell undifferentiated carcinoma of the esophagus: Case report with hormonal studies. Cancer 53:1746, 1984.
147. Johnston WW: Cytology and lung cancer. In McVie JG, Bakker W, Wagenaar SS (eds): Clinical and Experimental Pathology of Lung Cancer, p 65. Boston, Martinus Nijhoff, 1986.
148. Johnston WW: Histologic and cytologic patterns of lung cancer in 2,580 men and women over a 15-year period. Acta Cytol 32:163, 1988.
149. Joss R, Goldhirsch A, Sonntag R et al: Metastasen im Beriech des zentralen Nervensystems beim anaplastischen kleinzelligen Bronchuskarzinom. Schweiz Med Wochenschr 111:48, 1981.
150. Jubelirer SJ: Long-term survivors of small cell carcinoma of the lung. W Va Med J 85:183, 1989.
151. Kalter S, Dhingra HM, Farha P: Primary therapy for small cell lung cancer reversing the Eaton-Lambert syndrome. South Med J 78:197, 1985.
152. Kameya T, Kodama T, Shimosato Y: Ultrastructure of small cell carcinoma of the lung in relation to histogenesis and to carcinoid tumor. In Shimosato Y, Melamed MR, Nettesheim P (eds): Morphogenesis of Lung Cancer, vol II, p 15. Boca Raton, FL, CRC Press, 1982.
153. Kasimis BS, Wuerker RB, Hunt JD et al: Relationship between changes in the histologic subtype of small cell carcinoma of the lung and the response to chemotherapy. Am J Clin Oncol 9:318, 1986.
154. Kato K, Asia R, Shimuzu A et al: Immunoassay of three enolase enzymes in human serum and blood cells. Clin Chem Acta 127:353, 1983.
155. Kato K, Ishiguro Y, Suzuki F et al: Distribution of nervous system-specific forms of enolase in peripheral tissues. Brain Res 237:441, 1982.
156. Kayser K, Schmid W, Elbert W et al: Expression of neuroendocrine markers (neuron specific enolase, synaptophysin and bombesin) in carcinoma of the lung. Pathol Res Pract 183:412, 1988.
157. Khurana RK, Koski CL, Mayer RF et al: Autonomic dysfunction in Lambert-Eaton myasthenic syndrome. J Neurol Sci 85:77, 1988.
158. Kiefer PE, Bepler G, Kubasch M et al: Amplification and expression of protooncogenes in human small cell lung cancer cell lines. Cancer Res 47:6236, 1987.
159. Kizmits R, Schernthaner G, Krisch K: Serum neuron specific enolase: A marker for response to therapy in seminoma. Cancer 60:1017, 1987.
160. Kreyberg L: Histological lung cancer types. Acta Pathol Microbiol Scand [Suppl] 157:1, 1962.
161. Kreyberg L: Histologic Typing of Lung Tumors. In: International Classification of Tumors. Geneva, World Health Organization, 1967.
162. Kristjansen PEG, Pedersen AG: CNS therapy in small cell lung cancer. In Hansen HH (ed): Basic and Clinical Concepts of Lung Cancer, p 275. Boston, Kluwer Academic Publishers, 1989.
163. Kruggel W, O'Connor DT, Lewis RV: The amino terminal sequences of bovine and human chromogranin A and secretory protein 1 are identical. Biochem Biophys Res Commun 127:380, 1985.
164. Lamb D: Histological classification of lung cancer. Thorax 39:161, 1984.
165. Leader M, Collins M, Patel J et al: Antineuron specific enolase staining reactions in sarcomas and carcinomas: Its lack of neuroendocrine specificity. J Clin Pathol 39:1186, 1986.
166. Lee JS, McMurtrey MJ, Ro SY et al: Second primary lung cancer: A remediable treatment failure for small cell lung cancer. Cancer Bull 39:228, 1987.
167. Lee V, Wu HL, Schlaepfer WW: Monoclonal antibodies recognize individual neurofilament triplet proteins. Pro Natl Acad Sci USA 79:6089, 1982.
168. Lehto V-P, Miettinen M, Dahl D et al: Bronchial carcinoid cells contain neural-type intermediate filaments. Cancer 54:624, 1984.
169. Lehto V-P, Miettinen M, Virtanen I: A dual expression of cytokeratin and neurofilaments in bronchial carcinoid cells. Int J Cancer 35:421, 1985.
170. Lehto V-P, Stenman S, Miettinen M et al: Expression of a neural type of intermediate filament as a distinguishing feature between oat cell carcinoma and other lung cancers. Am J Pathol 110:113, 1983.
171. Leube RE, Wiedenmann B, Franke WW: Differentiation markers as an aid in the histological diagnosis of small cell carcinoma of the lung: Synopsis of intermediate filament protein and synaptophysin expression. Klin Wochenschr 66(suppl XI):80, 1988.
172. Levenson RM, Ihde DC, Matthews MJ et al: Small cell carcinoma presenting as an extrapulmonary neoplasm: Sites of origin and response to chemotherapy. JNCI 67:607, 1981.
173. Lindell MM, Jin B-S, Mackay B: Primary oat cell carcinoma of the larynx. AJR 137:555, 1981.
174. Linnoila RI, Mulshine JL, Steinberg SM et al: Neuroendocrine differentiation in endocrine and nonendocrine lung carcinomas. Am J Clin Pathol 90:641, 1988.
175. Linssen GC, Bosman FT, Ten-Velde GP: Histopathological subclassification of small cell carcinoma of the lung: Evaluation of its prognostic significance. Neth J Med 29:313, 1986.
176. List AF, Hainsworth JD, Davis BW et al: The syndrome of inappropriate secretion of antidiuretic hormone (SIADH) in small cell lung cancer. J Clin Oncol 4:1191, 1986.
177. Little CD, Nau MH, Carney DN et al: Amplification and expression of the c-myc oncogene in human lung cancer cell lines. Nature 306:194, 1983.

178. Lloyd RV, Mervak T, Schmidt K et al: Immunohistochemical detection of chromogranin and neuron specific enolase in pancreatic endocrine neoplasms. Am J Surg Pathol 8:607, 1984.
179. Lloyd RV, Wilson BJ: Specific endocrine tissue marker defined by a monoclonal antibody. Science 222:628, 1983.
180. Lokich JJ: The frequency and clinical biology of the ectopic hormone syndromes of small cell carcinoma. Cancer 50:2111, 1982.
181. Lukeman JM, Mackay B: The cytopathology and histopathology of lung cancer. Semin Respir Med 3:140, 1982.
182. Lukeman JM, Mackay B: Diagnosis of poorly differentiated carcinoma of the lung. In Greco FE (ed): Biology and Management of Lung Cancer, p 87. Boston, Martinus Nijhoff, 1983.
183. Mackay B: Ultrastructure of lung neoplasms. In Straus MJ (ed): Lung Cancer: Clinical Diagnosis and Treatment, 2nd ed, p 85. New York, Grune & Stratton, 1983.
184. Mackay B, Ordonez NG, Bennington JL et al: Ultrastructural and morphometric studies on lung carcinomas. Ultrastruct Pathol 13:561, 1989.
185. Maddox A-M, Valdivieso M, Lukeman JM et al: Superior vena cava obstruction in small cell bronchogenic carcinoma: Clinical parameters and survival. Cancer 52: 2165, 1983.
186. Mangum MD, Greco FA, Hainsworth JD et al: Combined small cell and non–small cell lung cancer. J Clin Oncol 7:607, 1989.
187. Marangos PJ, Zis AP, Clark RL et al: Neuronal, non-neuronal and hybrid forms of enolase in brain: Structural, immunological and functional comparisons. Brain Res 150:117, 1978.
188. Marchesani W: Über den primären Bronchialkrebs. Frankfurt Z Pathol 30: 158, 1924.
189. Marchevsky AM, Chuang MT, Teirstein AS et al: Problems in the diagnosis of small cell carcinoma of the lungs by fiberoptic bronchoscopy. Cancer Detect Prev 7:253, 1984.
190. Marchevsky AM, Hauptman E, Shepard C: Computerized interactive morphometry of brushing cytology specimens. Acta Cytol 32:341, 1988.
191. Mark EJ, Ramirez JF: Peripheral small cell carcinoma of the lung resembling carcinoid tumor: A clinical and pathologic study of 14 cases. Arch Pathol Lab Med 109:263, 1985.
192. Martin JME, Maung RM: Differential staining characteristics of carcinoid tumors with S-100 and Leu-7. Lab Invest 54:40, 1986.
193. Matthews MJ: Morphologic classification of bronchogenic carcinoma. Cancer Chemother Rep 4:299, 1973.
194. Matthews MJ: Effects of therapy on the morphology and behavior of small cell carcinoma of the lung: A clinicopathologic study. In Muggia M, Rozencweig M (eds): Lung Cancer: Progress in Therapeutic Research, p 155. New York, Raven Press, 1979.
195. Matthews MJ: Pathology of small cell carcinoma of the lung: Changing concepts. In McVie JG, Bakker W, Wagenaar SS: Clinical and Experimental Pathology of Lung Cancer, p 34. Boston, Martinus Nijhoff, 1986.
196. Matthews MJ, Rozencweig M, Staquet MJ et al: Long term survivors with small cell carcinoma of the lung. Eur J Cancer 16:527, 1980.
197. Maubon I, Cottier M, Pasteur X et al: Bronchial carcinoma and image analysis: Differentiation between poorly differentiated epidermoid carcinoma and small cell carcinoma. Anal Quant Cytol Histol 9:499, 1987.
198. Maurer LH: Ectopic hormone syndromes in small cell carcinoma of the lung. Clin Oncol 4:67, 1985.
199. McDowell EM, Keenan KP, Trump BF: The pathogenesis of hormone-producing tumors of the lung. Recent Results Cancer Res 99:94, 1985.
200. McDowell EM, Trump BF: Pulmonary small cell carcinoma showing tripartite differentiation in individual cells. Hum Pathol 12:286, 1981.
201. McDowell EM, Wilson TS, Trump BF: Atypical endocrine tumors of the lung. Arch Pathol Lab Med 105:20, 1981.
202. McGarry RC, Helfand SL, Quarles RH et al: Recognition of myelin-associated glycoprotein by the monoclonal antibody HNK-1. Nature 306:376, 1983.
203. McNeill PM, Wagman LD, Neifeld JP: Small bowel metastases from primary carcinoma of the lung. Cancer 59:1486, 1987.
204. Mendelsohn G, Suarez M, Hassan MO et al: Histopathologic, immunohistochemical, and ultrastructural studies of lung carcinoma. Prog Surg Pathol 6:127, 1986.
205. Meyer JA, Parker FB: Small cell carcinoma of the lung. Ann Thorac Surg 30:602, 1980.
206. Miyamoto H, Inoue S, Abe S et al: Relationship between cytomorphologic features and prognosis in small cell carcinoma of the lung. Acta Cytol 26:429, 1982.
207. Moll R, Franke WW: Cytochemical cell typing of metastatic tumors according to their cytoskeletal proteins. In Lapis K, Liotta LA, Rabson AS (eds): Biochemistry and Molecular Genetics of Cancer Metastasis, p 101. Boston, Martinus Nijhoff, 1986.
208. Moody TW, Pert CB, Gazdar AR et al: High levels of intracellular bombesin characterize human small cell lung carcinoma. Science 214:1246, 1981.
209. Moody TW, Bertness V, Carney DN: Bombesin-like peptides and receptors in human tumor cell lines. Peptides 4:683, 1983.
210. Mooi WJ, Dewar A, Springall D et al: Non–small cell lung carcinomas with neuroendocrine features: A light microscopic, immunohistochemical and ultrastructural study of 11 cases. Histopathology 13:329, 1988.
211. Mooi WJ, Dingemans KP, van Zandwijk N: Prevalence of neuroendocrine granules in small cell lung carcinoma: Usefulness of electron microscopy in lung cancer classification. J Pathol 149:41, 1986.
212. Mooi WJ, van Zandwijk N, Dingemans KP et al: The "grey area" between small cell and non–small cell lung carcinomas: Light and electron microscopy versus clinical data in 14 cases. J Pathol 149:49, 1986.
213. Mukai M, Torikata C, Iri H et al: Expression of neurofilament triplet proteins in human neural tumors: An immunohistochemical study of paraganglioma, ganglioneuroma, ganglioneuroblastoma, and neuroblastoma. Am J Pathol 122:28, 1986.
214. Mukherjee TM, Swift JG, Smith K et al: Exocytosis of neurosecretory granules in small cell undifferentiated carcinoma. Ultrastruct Pathol 4:187, 1983.

215. Mullins JD, Newman RK, Coltman CA: Primary oat cell carcinoma of the larynx: A case report and review of the literature. Cancer 43:711, 1979.
216. Mulshine JL, Makuch RW, Johnson-Early A et al: Diagnosis and significance of liver metastases in small cell carcinoma of the lung. J Clin Oncol 2:733, 1984.
217. Mulshine JL, Natale RB, Avis I et al: Autocrine growth factors and lung cancer. In Hansen HH (ed): Basic and Clinical Concepts of Lung Cancer, p 107. Boston, Kluwer Academic Publishers, 1989.
218. Murphy KC, Feld R, Evans WK et al: Intramedullary spinal cord metastases from small cell carcinoma of the lung. J Clin Oncol 1:99, 1983.
219. Nakajima T, Shimosato Y, Morinaga S et al: Immunohistochemical study of small cell lung carcinoma with special reference to the neuroendocrine markers aromatic L-amino acid decarboxylase and gastrin-releasing peptide. Jpn J Clin Oncol 16:223, 1986.
220. Nemeth J, Galian A, Mikol J et al: Neuron-specific enolase and malignant lymphomas (23 cases). Virchows Arch [A] 412:89, 1987.
221. Nesom-Davis J: Lambert-Eaton myasthenic syndrome. Semin Immunopathol 8:129, 1985.
222. Nixon DW, Murphy GF, Sewell CW et al: Relationship between survival and histologic type in small cell anaplastic carcinoma of the lung. Cancer 44:1045, 1979.
223. Nomori H, Shimosato Y, Kodama T et al: Subtypes of small cell carcinoma of the lung: Morphometric, ultrastructural, and immunohistochemical analysis. Hum Pathol 17:604, 1986.
224. Nou E: The natural five-year course in bronchial carcinoma: Epidemiologic results. Cancer 53:2211, 1984.
225. Nugent JL, Bunn PA, Matthews MJ et al: CNS metastases in small cell bronchogenic carcinoma: Increasing frequency and changing pattern with lengthening survival. Cancer 44:1885, 1979.
226. O'Connor DT, Frigon RP: Chromogranin A, the major catecholamine vesicle soluble protein. J Biol Chem 259:3237, 1984.
227. Olson L, Sorensen HR, Behnke O: Intratumoral phenotypic diversity of cloned human lung tumor cell lines and consequences for analysis with monoclonal antibodies. Cancer 54:1757, 1984.
228. Ordóñez NG, Ro JY, Mackay B: Alveolar soft part sarcoma: An ultrastructural and immunoyctochemical investigation of its histogenesis. Cancer 63:1721, 1989.
229. Osborn M, Weber K: Biology of disease: Tumor diagnosis of intermediate filament typing: A novel tool for surgical pathology. Lab Invest 48:372, 1983.
230. Osterlind K: Prognostic factors in small cell lung cancer: An analysis of 874 consecutive patients. In Hansen HH (ed): Lung Cancer: Basic and Clinical Aspects, p 129. Boston, Martinus Nijhoff, 1986.
231. Osterlind K, Anderson PK: Prognostic factors in small cell lung cancer: Multivariate model based on 778 patients treated with chemotherapy with or without irradiation. Cancer Res 46:4189, 1986.
232. Oud PS, Pahlplatz MM, Beck JL et al: Image and flow DNA cytometry of small cell carcinoma of the lung. Cancer 64:1304, 1989.
233. Pahlman S, Esscher T, Bergh J et al: Neuron specific enolase as a marker for neuroblastoma and small cell carcinoma of the lung. Tumor Biol 5:119, 1984.
234. Paladugu RR, Benfield JR, Pak HY et al: Bronchopulmonary Kulchitzky cell carcinomas: A new classification scheme for typical and atypical carcinoids. Cancer 55:1303, 1985.
235. Passamonte PM: Hypouricemia, inappropriate secretion of antidiuretic hormone, and small cell carcinoma of the lung. Arch Intern Med 144:1569, 1984.
236. Perentes E, Rubinstein LJ: Recent applications of immunoperoxidase histochemistry in human neuro-oncology. Arch Pathol Lab Med 111:796, 1987.
237. Polak JM, Hobbs R, Bloom SR et al: Distribution of bombesin-like peptide in human gastrointestinal tract. Lancet 1:1109, 1976.
238. Quinlan RA, Schiller DL, Hatzfeld M et al: Patterns of expression of organization of cytokeratin intermediate filaments. Ann NY Acad Sci 455:282, 1985.
239. Radice PA, Matthews MJ, Ihde DC et al: The clinical behavior of "mixed" small cell-large cell bronchogenic carcinoma compared to "pure" small cell subtypes. Cancer 50:2894, 1982.
240. Ramaekers FCS, Puts JJG, Moesker O et al: Antibodies to intermediate filament proteins in the immunohistochemical identification of human tumours: An overview. Histochem J 15:691, 1983.
241. Rashid RK, Mackay B, Silva EG et al: Small cell (oat cell) carcinoma of the trachea with endocrine features: Report of a case and results of ultrastructural and immunohistochemical study. Arch Pathol Lab Med 108:149, 1984.
242. Reeve JG, Stewart J, Watson JV et al: Neuron-specific enolase expression in carcinoma of the lung. Br J Cancer 53:519, 1986.
243. Reyes CV, Chejfec G, Jao W et al: Neuroendocrine carcinomas of the esophagus. Ultrastruct Pathol 1:367, 1980.
244. Rider CC, Taylor CB: Enolase isoenzymes in rat tissues. Electrophoretic, chromatographic, immunological and kinetic properties. Biochim Biophys Acta 365:285, 1974.
245. Rode J, Dhillon AP, Doran JF et al: PGP 9.5, a new marker for human neuroendocrine tumors. Histopathology 9:147, 1985.
246. Roggli VL, Vollmer RT, Greenberg SD et al: Lung cancer heterogeneity: A blinded and randomized study of 100 consecutive cases. Hum Pathol 16:569, 1985.
247. Rosa P, Hille A, Lee RW et al: Secretogranins I and II: Two tyrosine-sulfated secretory proteins common to a variety of cells secreting polypeptides by the regulated pathway. J Cell Biol 101:1999, 1985.
248. Rosen ST, Aisner J, Makuch RW et al: Carcinomatous leptomeningitis in small cell lung cancer: A clinicopathologic review of the National Cancer Institute experience. Medicine 61:45, 1982.
249. Rusthoven JJ, Robinson JB, Kolin A et al: The natural killer cell–associated HNK-1 (Leu-7) antibody reacts with hypertrophic and malignant prostatic epithelium. Cancer 56:289, 1985.
250. Saccomanno G, Huth GC, Auerbach O et al: Relationship of radioactive radon daughters and

cigarette smoking in the genesis of lung cancer in uranium miners. Cancer 62:1402, 1988.

251. Said JW, Vinadalal S, Nash G et al: Immunoreactive neuron-specific enolase, bombesin, and chromogranin as markers for neuroendocrine lung tumors. Hum Pathol 16:236, 1985.

252. Sato Y, Watanabe S, Kodama T et al: Stainability of lung cancer cells with Leu-7 and OKT-9 monoclonal antibodies. Jpn J Clin Oncol 15:357, 1985.

253. Scarpa S, Morstyn G, Carney DH et al: Small cell lung cancer cell lines: Pure and variant types can be distinguished by their extracellular matrix synthesis. Eur Respir J 1:639, 1988.

254. Schmechel D, Marangos PJ, Brightman MW: Neuron specific enolase is a marker for peripheral and central neuroendocrine cells. Nature 276:834, 1978.

255. Schmeider FH, Smith AD, Winkler H: Secretion from the adrenal medulla: Biochemical evidence for exocytosis. Br J Pharmacol Chemother 31:94, 1967.

256. Schuller-Petrovic S, Gebhart W, Lassmann H et al: A shared antigenic determinant between natural killer cells and nervous tissue. Nature 306:179, 1983.

257. Schultz G: The frequency and localization of hematogenic distant metastases of bronchial carcinoma. Z Erkr Atmunsorgane 172:99, 1989.

258. Sculier JP, Evans WK, Feld R et al: Superior vena caval obstruction syndrome in small cell lung cancer. Cancer 57:847, 1986.

259. Sculier JP, Feld R, Evans WK et al: Neurologic disorders in patients with small cell lung cancer. Cancer 60:2275, 1987.

260. Sehested M, Hirsch FR, Osterlind K et al: Morphologic variations of small cell lung cancer: A histopathologic study of pretreatment and post-treatment specimens in 104 patients. Cancer 57:804, 1986.

261. Sheppard MN, Corrin B, Bennett MH et al: Immunocytochemical localization of neuron-specific enolase in small cell carcinomas and carcinoid tumours of the lung. Histopathology 8:171, 1984.

262. Shimosato Y, Nakajima T, Hirohashi S et al: Biological, pathological and clinical features of small cell lung cancer. Cancer 33:241, 1986.

263. Shioda Y, Nagura H, Tsutsumi Y et al: Distribution of Leu-7 (HNK-1) antigen in human digestive organs: An immunohistochemical study with nonoclonal antibody. Histochemical J 16:843, 1986.

264. Sidhu GS: The endodermal origin of digestive and respiratory tract APUD cells: Histopathologic evidence and a review of the literature. Am J Pathol 96:5, 1979.

265. Smolle J, Walter GF, Kerl H: Myelin-associated glycoprotein in neurogenic tumours of the skin: An immunohistochemical study using Leu-7 monoclonal antibody. Arch Dermatol Res 277:141, 1985.

266. Sorenson GD, Pettingill OS, Brinck-Johnsen T et al: Hormone production by cultures of small cell carcinoma of the lung. Cancer 47:1289, 1981.

267. Spiegelman D, Maurer LH, Ware JH et al: Prognostic factors in small cell carcinoma of the lung: An analysis of 1,521 patients. J Clin Oncol 7:344, 1989.

268. Springall DR, Ibrahim NBN, Rode J et al: Endocrine differentiation of extrapulmonary small cell carcinoma demonstrated by immunohistochemistry using antibodies to PGP 9.5, neuron specific enolase and the C-flanking peptide of human pro-bombesin. J Pathol 150:151, 1986.

269. Stahel RA, Mabry M, Skarin AT et al: Detection of bone marrow metastases in small cell lung cancer by monoclonal antibodies. J Clin Oncol 3:455, 1985.

270. Stanley KE: Prognostic factors for survival in patients with inoperable lung cancer. JNCI 65:25, 1980.

271. Stein A, Sova Y, Lurie M et al: Bilateral testicular metastases of pulmonary small cell carcinoma: A rare incidental finding following orchiectomy for prostatic carcinoma. Br J Urol 63:552, 1989.

272. Suga J, Saijo N, Shinkai T et al: Long-term survival in patients with small cell lung cancer. Jpn J Clin Oncol 16:309, 1986.

273. Tabatowski K, Vollmer RT, Tello JW et al: The use of a panel of monoclonal antibodies in ultrastructurally characterized small cell carcinomas of the lung. Acta Cytol 32:667, 1988.

274. Tapia FJ, Polak JM, Barbosa AJA et al: Neuron-specific enolase is produced by neuroendocrine tumours. Lancet 1:808, 1981.

275. Teeling M, McGing P, Johnston P et al: Clinical correlation of tumor endocrine markers in lung cancer. In Hansen HH (ed): Basic and Clinical Concepts of Lung Cancer, p 137. Boston, Kluwer Academic Publishers, 1989.

276. Thomas L, Hartung K, Langosch D et al: Identification of synaptophysin as a hexameric channel protein of the synaptic vesicle membrane. Science 242:1050, 1988.

277. Thompson RJ, Doran JF, Jackson P et al: PGP 9.5: A new marker for vertebrate neurones and neuronendocrine cells. Brain Res 278:224, 1983.

278. Thornley PE, Howatson SR: Primary carcinoma of the trachea: Mixed squamous and oat cell type. Thorax 35:72, 1980.

279. Thunnissen EB, Diegenbach PC: Classification of lung carcinoma by means of digital nuclear image analysis. Anal Quant Cytol Histol 8:301, 1986.

280. Tirindelli-Danesi D, Teodoria L, Mauro F et al: Prognostic significance of flow cytometry in lung cancer: A 5-year study. Cancer 60:844, 1987.

281. Tischler AS, Mobtaker H, Mann K et al: Anti-lymphocyte monoclonal antibody Leu-7 (HNK-1) recognizes a constituent of neuroendocrine granule matrix. Lab Invest 54:64, 1986.

282. Truong LD, Underwood RD, Greenberg SD et al: Diagnosis and typing of lung carcinomas by cytopathologic methods: A review of 108 cases. Acta Cytol 29:379, 1985.

283. Tsutsumi Y: Leu-7 immunoreactivity as histochemical marker for paraffin-embedded neuroendocrine tumors. Acta Histochem Cytochem 17:15, 1984.

284. Umsawasdi T, Valdivieso M: Paraneoplastic syndromes in lung cancer. Semin Respir Med 3:200, 1982.

285. Van Muijen GNP, Ruiter DJ, van Leeumwen C et al: Cytokeratin and neurofilament in lung carcinomas. Am J Pathol 116:363, 1984.

286. Villard JL, Caillaud DC, Kantelip B et al: Enzymatic determination of serum neuron-specific

enolase in small cell lung cancers. Chest 93:1255, 1988.

287. Vincent MD, Ashley SE, Smith IE: Prognostic factors in small cell lung cancer: A simple prognostic index is better than conventional staging. Eur J Cancer Clin Oncol 23:1589, 1987.
288. Vindelov LL, Engelholm SA, Spang-Thomsen M: Flow cytometric DNA analysis in the study of small cell carcinomas of the lung. In McVie JG, Bakker W, Wagenaar SS (eds): Clinical and Experimental Pathology of Lung Cancer, p 105. Boston, Martinus Nijhoff, 1989.
289. Vinores SA, Bonnin JM, Rubinstein LJ et al: Immunohistochemical demonstration of neuron-specific enolase in neoplasms of the CNS and other tissues. Arch Pathol Lab Med 108:536, 1984.
290. Vogelsang GB, Abeloff MD, Ettinger DS et al: Long-term survivors of small cell carcinoma of the lung. Am J Med 79:49, 1985.
291. Volk SA, Mansour RF, Gandara DR et al: Morbidity in long-term survivors of small cell carcinoma of the lung. Cancer 54:25, 1984.
292. Vollmer RT, Birch R, Ogden L et al: Subclassification of small cell cancer of the lung: The Southeastern Cancer Study Group experience. Hum Pathol 16:247, 1985.
293. Vollmer RT, Ogden L, Crissman JD: Separation of small cell from non–small cell lung cancer: The Southeastern Study Group pathologists' experience. Arch Pathol Lab Med 108:792, 1984.
294. Vollmer RT, Shelburne JD, Iglehart JD: Intercellular junctions and tumor stage in small cell carcinoma of the lung. Hum Pathol 18:22, 1987.
295. Walts AE, Said JW, Shintaku IP et al: Chromogranin as a marker of neuroendocrine cells in cytologic material: An immunocytochemical study. Am J Clin Pathol 84:273, 1985.
296. Watkin SW, Soorae AJ, Green JA: Bronchoscopic "resection" of small cell carcinoma. Endoscopy 21:186, 1989.
297. Weber P, Shepard KV, Vijayakumar S: Metastases to pineal gland. Cancer 63:164, 1989.
298. Wegener M, Borsch G, Reitemeyer E et al: Metastasis to the colon from primary bronchogenic carcinoma presenting as occult gastrointestinal bleeding: Report of a case. Z Gastroenterol 26:358, 1988.
299. Weisbrod GL, Cunningham I, Tao LC et al: Small cell anaplastic carcinoma: Cytological histological correlations from percutaneous fine-needle aspiration biopsy. J Can Assoc Radiol 38:204, 1987.
300. Wenig BM, Gnepp DR: The spectrum of neuroendocrine carcinomas of the larynx. Semin Diagn Pathol 6:329, 1989.
301. Whang-Peng J: 3p deletion and small cell lung carcinoma. Mayo Clin Proc 64:256, 1989.
302. Whang-Peng J, Lee EC, Minna JD et al: Deletion of 3(p14p23) in secondary erythroleukemia arising in long-term survivors of small cell lung cancer. JNCI 80:1253, 1988.
303. Whitley NO, Mirvis SE: Abdominal CT in the staging of small cell carcinoma of the lung. CRC Crit Rev Diagn Imaging 29:103, 1989.
304. Wiedemann B, Franke WW, Kuhn C et al: Synaptophysin: A marker protein for neuroendocrine cells and neoplasms. Proc Natl Acad Sci USA 83:3500, 1986.
305. Wiedenmann B, Kuhn C, Schwecheimer K et al: Synaptophysin identified in metastases of neuroendocrine tumors by immunocytochemistry and immunoblotting. Am J Clin Pathol 88:560, 1987.
306. Willcox N, Demaine AG, Newsom-Davis J et al: Increased frequency of IgG heavy chain marker GLM(2) and of HLA-B8 in Lambert-Eaton myasthenic syndrome with and without associated lung cancer. Hum Immunol 14:29, 1985.
307. Wilson BS, Lloyd RV: Detection of chromogranin in neuroendocrine cells with a monoclonal antibody. Am J Pathol 115:458, 1984.
308. Winkler H: The composition of adrenal chromaffin granules: An assessment of controversial results. Neuroscience 1:65, 1976.
309. Woodruff JM, Huvos AG, Erlandson RE et al: Neuroendocrine carcinomas of the larynx: A study of two types, one of which mimics thyroid medullary carcinoma. Am J Surg Pathol 9:771, 1985.
310. World Health Organization Histological Typing of Lung Tumours, 2nd ed. Am J Clin Pathol 77:123, 1982.
311. Wu AH, Henderson BE, Thomas DC et al: Secular trends in histologic types of lung cancer. JNCI 77:53, 1986.
312. Wurster-Hill DH, Cannizzaro LA, Pettengill OS et al: Cytogenetics of small cell carcinoma of the lung. Cancer Genet Cytogenet 13:303, 1984.
313. Yellin A, Benfield JR: The pulmonary Kulchitsky cell (neuroendocrine) cancers: From carcinoid to small cell carcinomas. Curr Probl Cancer 9:1, 1985.
314. Yesner R: Spectrum of lung cancer and ectopic hormones. Pathol Annu 13:207, 1978.
315. Yesner R. Gerstl B, Auerbach O: Application of the World Health Organization classification of lung carcinoma to biopsy material. Ann Thorac Surg 1:33, 1965.
316. Yokota J, Wada M, Shimosato Y et al: Loss of heterozygosity on chromosomes 3, 13, and 17 in small cell carcinoma and on chromosome 3 in adenocarcinoma of the lung. Proc Natl Acad Sci USA 84:9252, 1987.
317. Yoshida Y, Mori M, Sonoda T et al: Ultrastructural-immunohistochemical and biochemical studies on amylase and ACTH producing lung cancer. Virchows Arch [A] 408:163, 1985.
318. Yoshimoto K, Hirohashi S, Sekiya T: Increased expression of the C-myc gene without gene amplification in human lung cancer and colon cancer cell lines. Jpn J Cancer Res 77:540, 1986.
319. Yoshimoto K, Yamasaki R, Sakai H et al: Ectopic production of parathyroid hormone by small cell lung cancer in a patient with hypercalcemia. J Clin Endocrinol Metab 68:976, 1989.

Chapter

10

CARCINOID TUMORS

The application of ultrastructural and immunohistochemical methods to the study of endocrine cells and the tumors derived from them has greatly expanded our knowledge of the morphology and secretory activity of endocrine neoplasms. There is much variation and considerable overlap in the light microscopic appearances and immunocytochemical reactions of these tumors. Because the tumors are functionally heterogeneous, the relevance of the term *carcinoid* has come under scrutiny,[51] but it is hallowed by long usage and connotes an entity to clinicians. In recent studies on bronchial carcinoids, atypical forms and the relationship of carcinoids to small cell lung carcinoma have received particular attention.

The pathology of carcinoid tumors was described by Lubarsch[111] in 1888, and Obendorfer[130] introduced the term *carcinoid* in 1907 when he noticed that the small bowel neoplasms were less aggressive than adenocarcinomas of the intestine. Bronchial carcinoids were recognized by Laennec[100] in 1831 and described in an autopsy report by Mueller[124] in 1882, but they did not become widely known until the reviews by Kramer (1930)[97] and Hamperl (1937).[77] In the past 2 decades, a considerable number of cases have been reported.[10, 11, 14, 18, 23, 27, 30, 42, 54, 65, 75, 88, 101, 118, 132, 138, 148, 152, 169, 171, 172, 190]

Carcinoids make up approximately 2% of primary lung tumors. Godwin[66] gives age-adjusted incidence rates for small cell lung carcinoma and carcinoid of 4.60 and 0.21, respectively, per 100,000 of population. The average age at the time of diagnosis is 50, which is younger than for carcinoma, and there is no predilection for either sex. In the 203 cases reviewed by Okike,[132] the average age was 48 years and the sex distribution was almost equal. The mean age of the 52 patients in the series of Abdi and colleagues[1] was 60.2 years, and 9 were female. Lung carcinoids also occur in children[20, 50, 95, 186]: in a review of 230 primary lung tumors in children, Hartman and Shochet[79] observed that the largest group were bronchial adenomas, among which carcinoids were the most common, and that 8% of the carcinoids were malignant. There is no evidence to indicate that bronchial carcinoids are related to smoking, occupation, or other environmental factors.

CLINICAL FEATURES

A patient with a carcinoid tumor in the lung is often asymptomatic, particularly when the lesion is small and located in the lung periphery. Although all carcinoid tumors contain dense-core granules, and most can be shown by immunostaining to elaborate several hormonal polypeptides or other substances, endocrine symptoms are not manifested in the majority of patients. The reason might be that the products are biologically inactive or are being rapidly degraded, or they may be released only intermittently. However, some patients do present with endocrine symptoms,[115] and it is possible that others have mild effects from the tumor secretions that simply are not noticed. Unlike enterochromaffin tumors, lung carcinoids do not have to produce liver metastases in order for symptoms to become clinically apparent, but it is unusual for a lung carcinoid to elicit the fully developed carcinoid syndrome[84, 140, 160] (flushing of the skin, diarrhea, bronchoconstriction, and valvular lesions involving the right side of the heart with elevation of the serotonin metabolite 5-hydroxyindoleacetic acid in the urine[129]). Endocrine manifestions of bronchial carcinoids include antidiuretic hormone, ACTH, and growth hormone hypersecretion.[52, 85, 90, 116, 133, 145, 151, 188] The endocrine symptoms can disappear with removal of the tumor: we have seen a patient with marked hypercalcemia whose serum calcium level returned to normal after a 1.5-cm peripheral lung carcinoid was resected. Farhangi and colleagues[57] reported a patient who, along with two family members, had multiple endocrine neoplasia type 1 with carcinoid.

An abnormality on the plain chest film was present in 69 of the 72 patients with bronchial adenomas reviewed by Lawson and coworkers.[101] Of the 72 tumors, 67 were carcinoids. The common findings were effects of bronchial obstruction with collapse and/or consolidation, which were seen in 53 patients, all of whom were asymptomatic. Bronchiectasis was present distal to the tumor in 25 patients. A well-defined opacity was seen in 13 asymptomatic patients. Choplin and coworkers[37] described the radiographic features of 32 atypical carcinoids. The most frequent finding was a round or ovoid lobulated peripheral mass, but other appearances included poorly defined infiltrates, thin-walled cavities, and mediastinal masses. Computed tomography of the chest may provide discriminating information in the preoperative assessment.[59, 112]

Since the tumor is usually covered by normal mucosa, the diagnosis is rarely made from sputum cytology, and bronchial washings and brushings are frequently negative. A fine-needle aspiration biopsy specimen may indicate the tumor type,[109] but cytology preparations are often unrewarding.[59] Most of the tumors can be reached with the bronchoscope, but a deep biopsy is needed, and because carcinoids are vascular, brisk bleeding may be produced. Nishikawa and associates[128] diagnosed an atypical carcinoid in sputum, but the cells had exfoliated immediately after fiberoptic bronchoscopy and the tissue specimens did not contain tumor. Transbronchial needle aspiration may be successful.[64] Leonhardt and Gosse[106] reviewed 14 central and 16 peripheral tumors. For the central tumors, cytology of imprints or smears of tissue were judged superior to the tissue specimens themselves, from which 5 of 11 were misdiagnosed on biopsy as small cell carcinomas. Among the 16 peripheral tumors, 5 were diagnosed by cytology, 3 by catheter aspiration, and 2 by transthoracic needle biopsy.

BEHAVIOR

Greengard and co-workers[73] presented quantitative evidence for the long doubling time of carcinoid *in vivo*. However, invasiveness and large size are associated with a relatively high incidence of metastases.[168] Direct spread through the lung parenchyma can give rise to extensive tumor. Suzuki and co-workers[161] reported a case with evidence of intrapulmonary dissemination by aerogenous spread in which multiple implanted foci were present in the periphery of the lung without destruction of alveolar structure. Skinner and Ewen[156] described "carcinoid lung" due to diffuse infiltration by a multifocal bronchial carcinoid.

When there is severe atypia, metastases are present in roughly two thirds of patients, and the 5-year survival is approximately 50%. Abdi and colleagues[1] found three cases (27%) of peripheral carcinoids with regional lymph node metastases but no systemic metastases. Altschuler and associates[5] reported resection of mediastinal metastasis of a malignant bronchial carcinoid 32 years after a pneumonectomy had been performed. Beyond the regional lymph nodes, metastases have been recorded in a wide range of locations, including liver,[42, 132] spleen,[42] brain,[42] ovary,[32] bone,[13, 41] choroid,[61] skin,[94] and breast.[78, 176]

A more conservative resection is feasible for the typical carcinoids than for atypical tumors, in which the possibility of nodal spread must be considered. Even with the attempt to be conservative, pneumonectomy is sometimes necessary. Of 46 patients reviewed by Brandt[30] and co-workers, 21 underwent pneumonectomy, but the series extended over a 37-year period and the authors point out that some of the earlier patients may have been candidates for conservative resection by today's criteria. Abdi and colleagues[1] found that 4 patients required wedge resection and 6 needed lobectomy for peripheral tumors. Wilkins and associates[184] have reviewed changes in the surgical management.

Okike and co-workers[132] reported that 94% of patients survive for 5 years and gave a 10-year figure of 87% and a 25-year survival rate of 66%. Greenberg and colleagues[72] evaluated 151 bronchopulmonary carcinoids, and the overall 5-year survival rate was 87.6%; lack of surgical treatment and advanced stage were independently associated with unfavorable prognosis.

GROSS APPEARANCE

Central and peripheral carcinoids occur in a ratio of approximately 4:1. The tumor is most frequent in the lobar bronchi where endocrine cells are at their greatest concentration, and the incidence diminishes distally and proximally; tracheal carcinoids are uncommon.[31, 136] Abdi and colleagues[1] studied a series of 52 bronchial carcinoids, and only 11 (21.1%) were peripheral. The sizes ranged from 1 to 5 cm with a mean of 2.4 cm. Multiple bronchial carcinoids are unusual.[98]

LIGHT MICROSCOPY

Criteria for the histopathologic identification of carcinoid tumors cannot be easily summarized because of the range of structural variations that occur, even within the same tumor.[185] In the basic pattern, small groups of cells are separated from their neighbors by slender partitions of connective tissue containing thin-walled vessels (Fig. 10–1). In a common variation on this theme, artifactual separation of the groups of tumor cells from the delicate fibrous sheets creates many narrow clefts (Fig. 10–2). Broad cords of cells may branch and combine (Fig. 10–3), or slender columns of tumor cells will simulate an Indian file arrangement (Fig. 10–4). The cords of cells can vary in width (Fig. 10–5) and can curve and form concentric configurations (Fig. 10–6). Some tumors have small glandular lumens or even papillary projections and an adenocarcinoma may be simulated, but a papillary pattern in which a thin layer of tumor cells clothes fibrous cores (Fig. 10–7) is uncommon.[113]

Areas of the tumor may contain zones of fibrous tissue that separate and surround clusters of cells (Fig. 10–8), and an amorphous amyloid-like or true amyloid stroma is occasionally present (Fig. 10–9).[4] The so-

Text continued on page 253

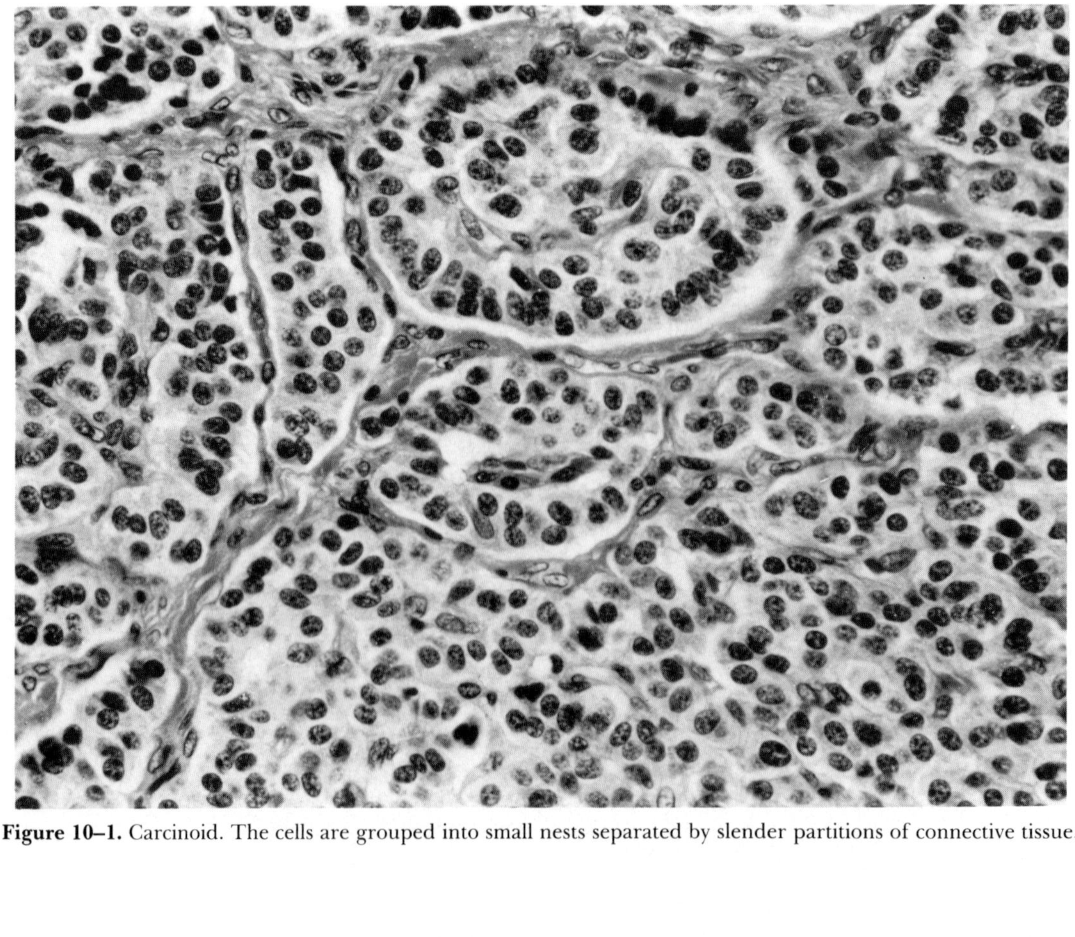

Figure 10–1. Carcinoid. The cells are grouped into small nests separated by slender partitions of connective tissue.

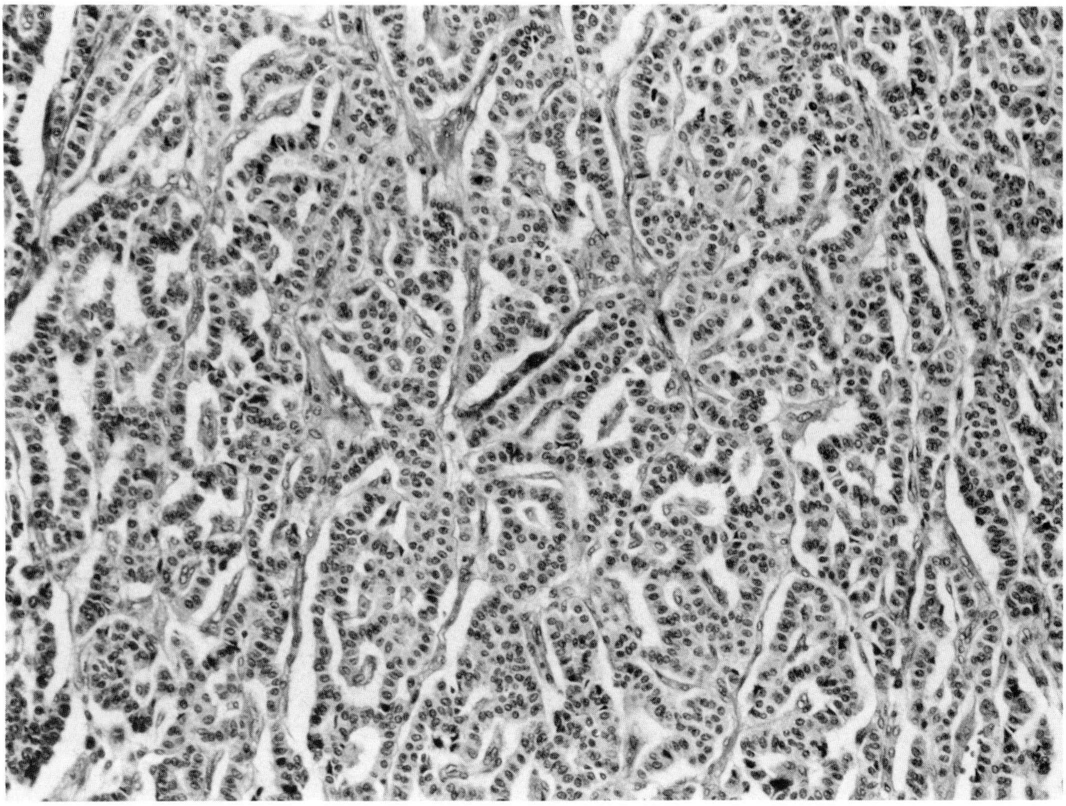

Figure 10–2. Carcinoid. Artifactual clefts have separated some of the nests of cells from the connective tissue framework, producing a pseudoglandular pattern.

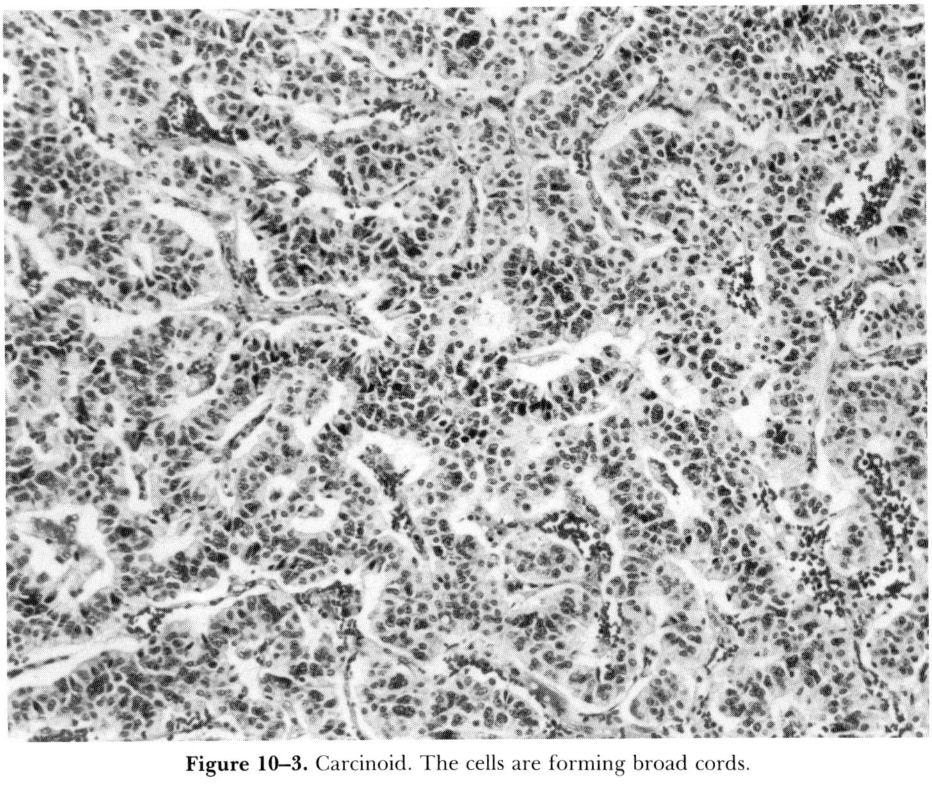

Figure 10–3. Carcinoid. The cells are forming broad cords.

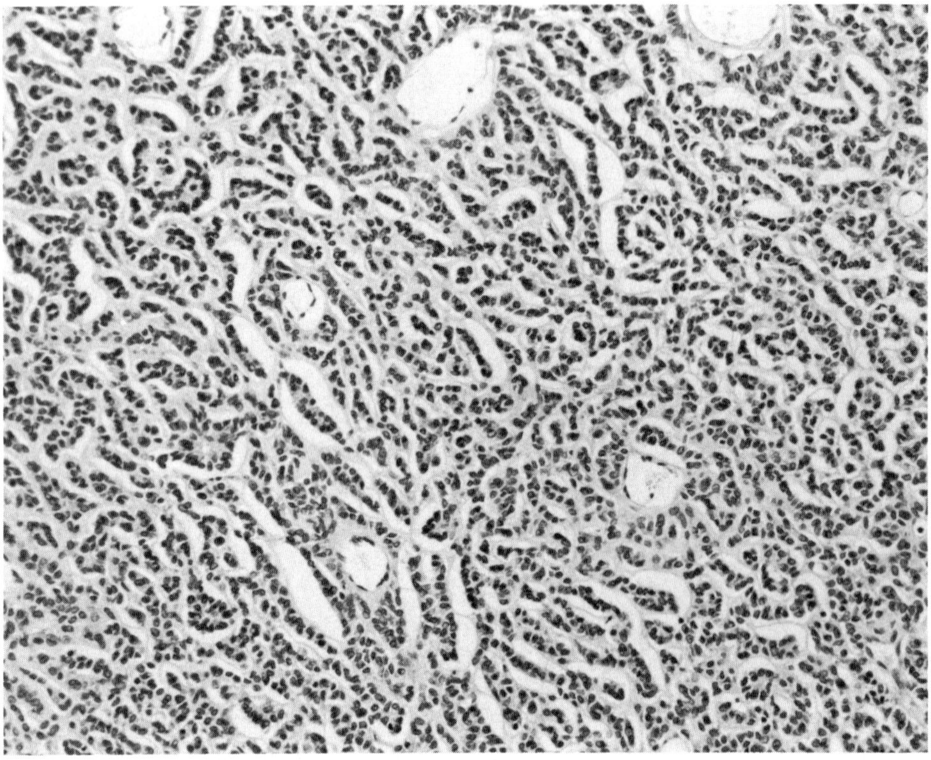

Figure 10–4. Carcinoid. Thin cords one or two cells thick create an Indian file appearance.

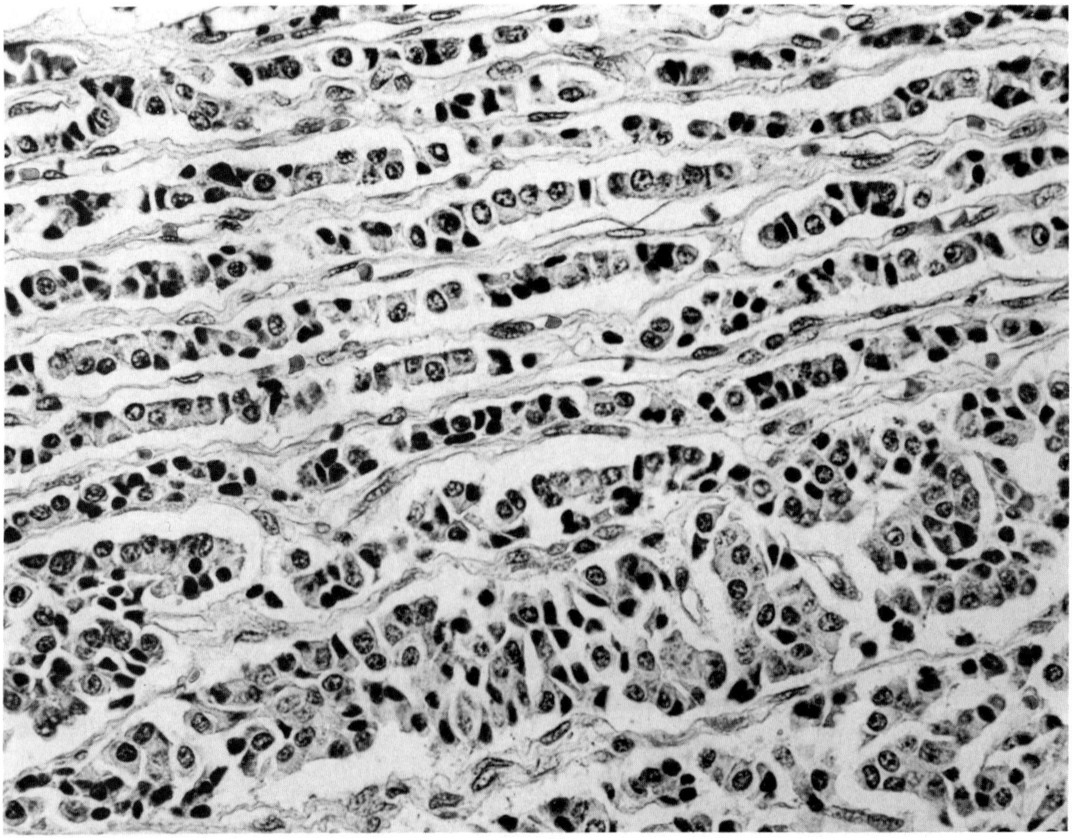

Figure 10–5. Carcinoid. In this area, columns of cells vary in thickness.

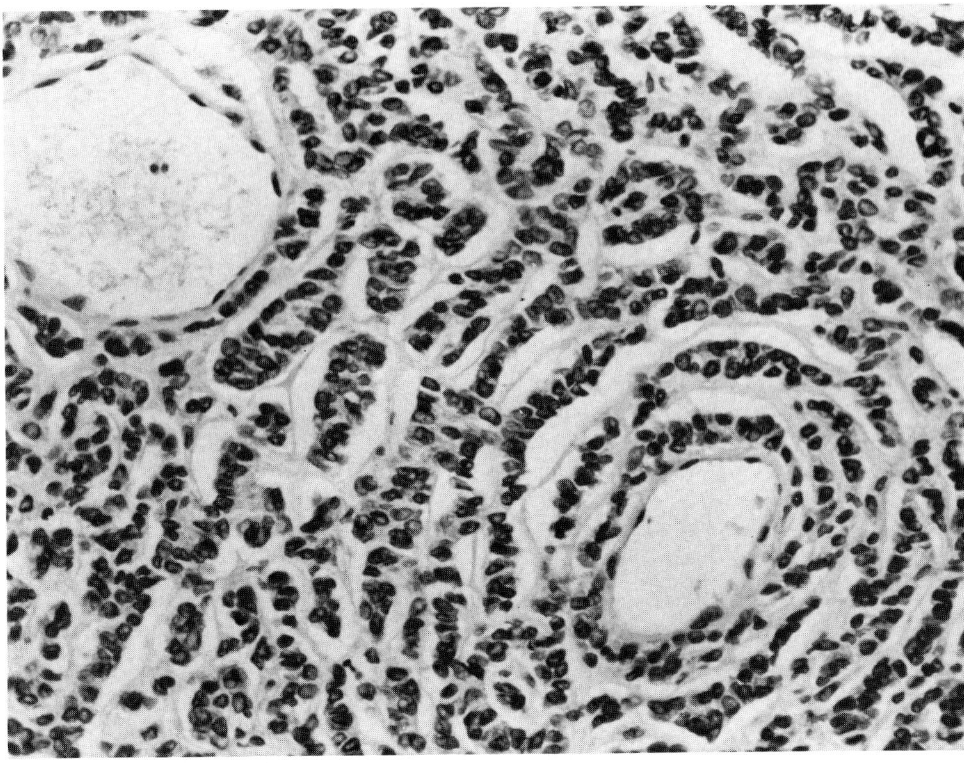

Figure 10–6. Carcinoid. Cords of cells are forming a concentric pattern.

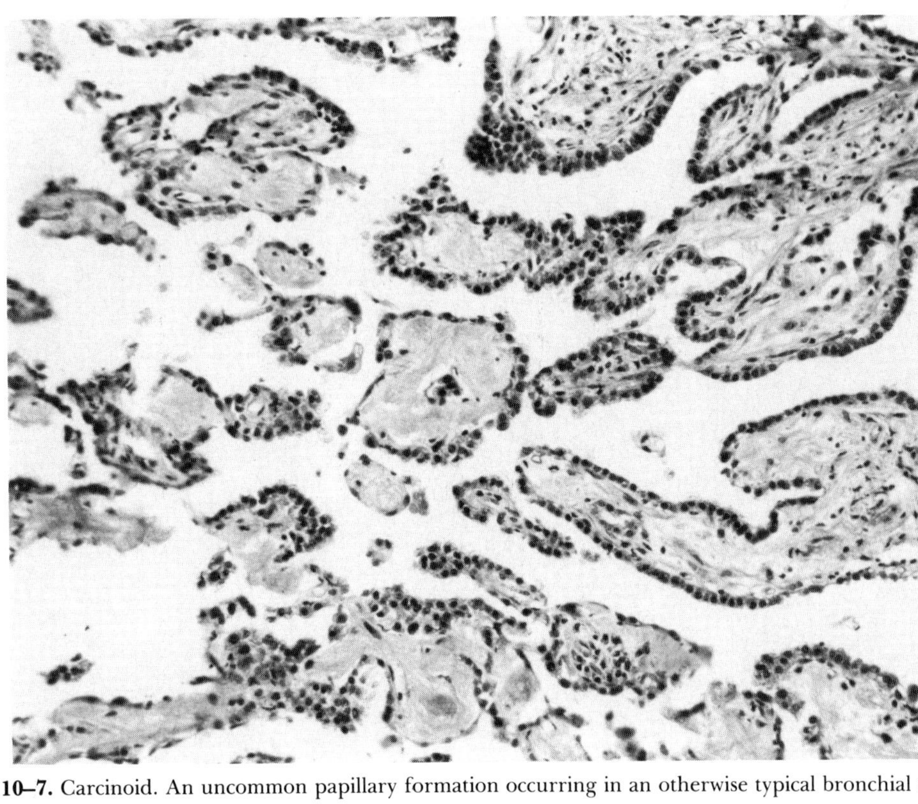

Figure 10–7. Carcinoid. An uncommon papillary formation occurring in an otherwise typical bronchial carcinoid.

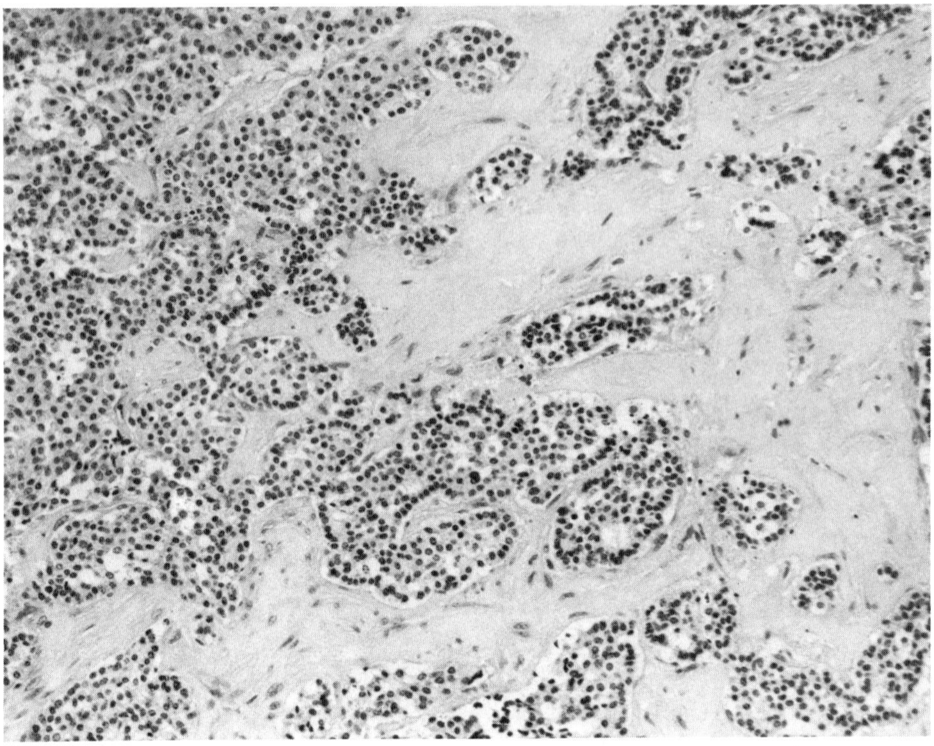

Figure 10–8. Carcinoid. Broad zones of fibrous tissue intervene between groups of tumor cells.

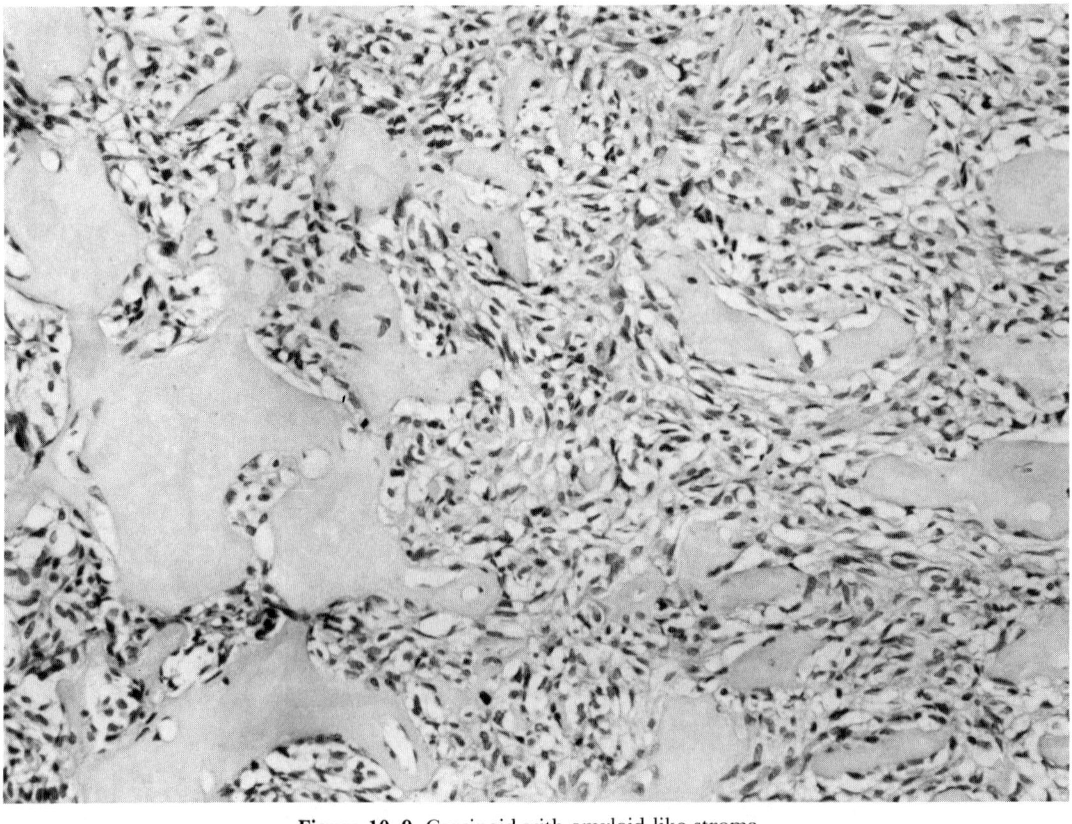

Figure 10–9. Carcinoid with amyloid-like stroma.

called Azzopardi effect, seen frequently in areas of necrosis in small cell lung carcinoma, in which nuclear DNA from disrupted cells becomes encrusted in vessel walls, is not a feature of carcinoids. Mucin can be produced by bronchial carcinoid tumors,[162] but adenocarcinoids are more common in the appendix[43, 143] and stomach[158, 188] than in the lung. Carcinoid cells may stain with the Grimelius method, but other components of the cell including even mucin and glycogen can exhibit some argyrophilia and be confused with endocrine granules. Melanin is an occasional finding, and premelanosomes have been identified by electron microscopy.[36, 69, 71] Psammoma bodies have been reported in metastases.[35] The periphery of a typical carcinoid is sharply delineated at low magnification, but there is no capsule and small aggregates of tumor cells may be found within the alveoli some distance beyond the apparent tumor margin (Figs. 10–10 and 10–11).

A spindle cell pattern is common, particularly in peripheral tumors.[39, 138] The spindle cells may show some attempt at organization into bundles (Fig 10–12), and they can be mixed with groups of polygonal cells. The spindle cell pattern bears some resemblance to a small cell carcinoma composed of fusiform cells, but the more abundant cytoplasm of the carcinoid cells separates the nuclei and creates an appearance that is less cellular or hyperchromatic than that of a small cell carcinoma (Fig. 10–13). Ranchod and Levine[138] studied 35 spindle cell carcinoids. The tumors were peripheral and most often subpleural, and 80% were less than 2 cm in diameter. They were made up principally or entirely of spindle cells that were fairly uniform in length in any one case. The shorter spindle cells often showed an organoid grouping, whereas the longer cells tended to form intersecting fascicles. Microscopic foci of tumor were found in two of the six patients in whom hilar lymph nodes were removed, and one patient had a single microscopic bony metastasis.

Oncocytic transformation is sometimes seen in a bronchial carcinoid (Fig. 10–14),

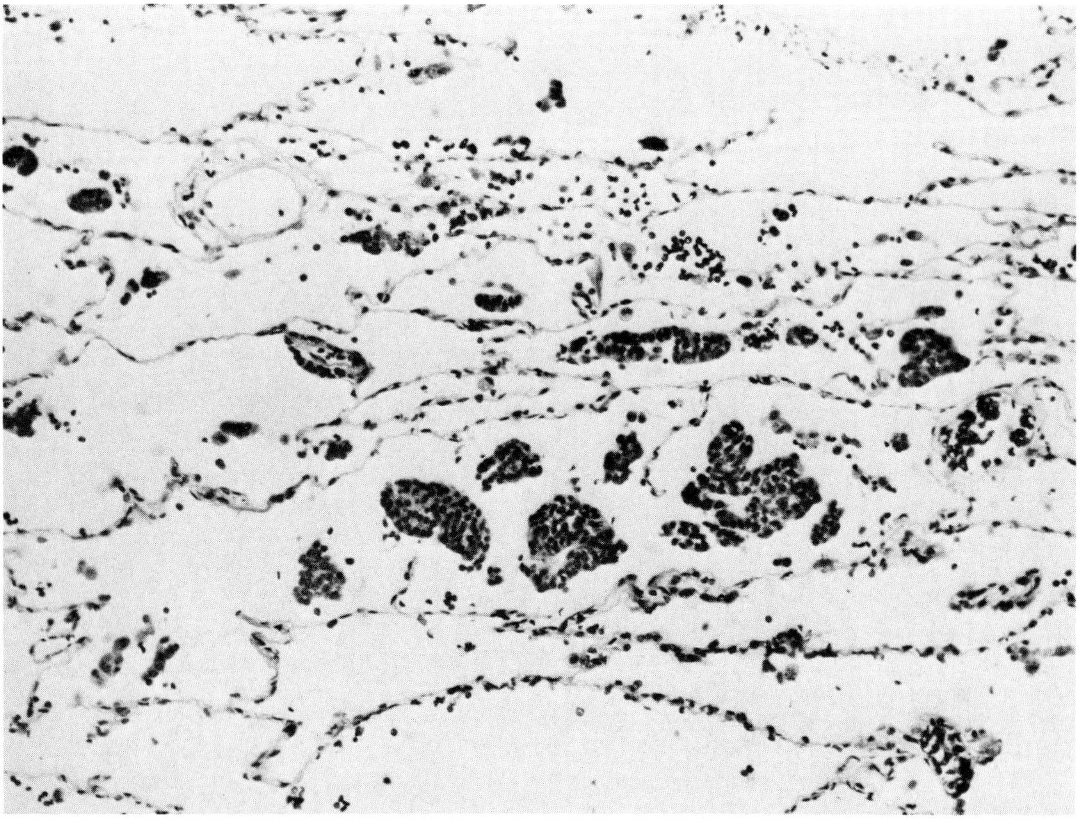

Figure 10–10. Carcinoid. At the periphery of the tumor, small clusters of cells are floating off within the alveolar spaces.

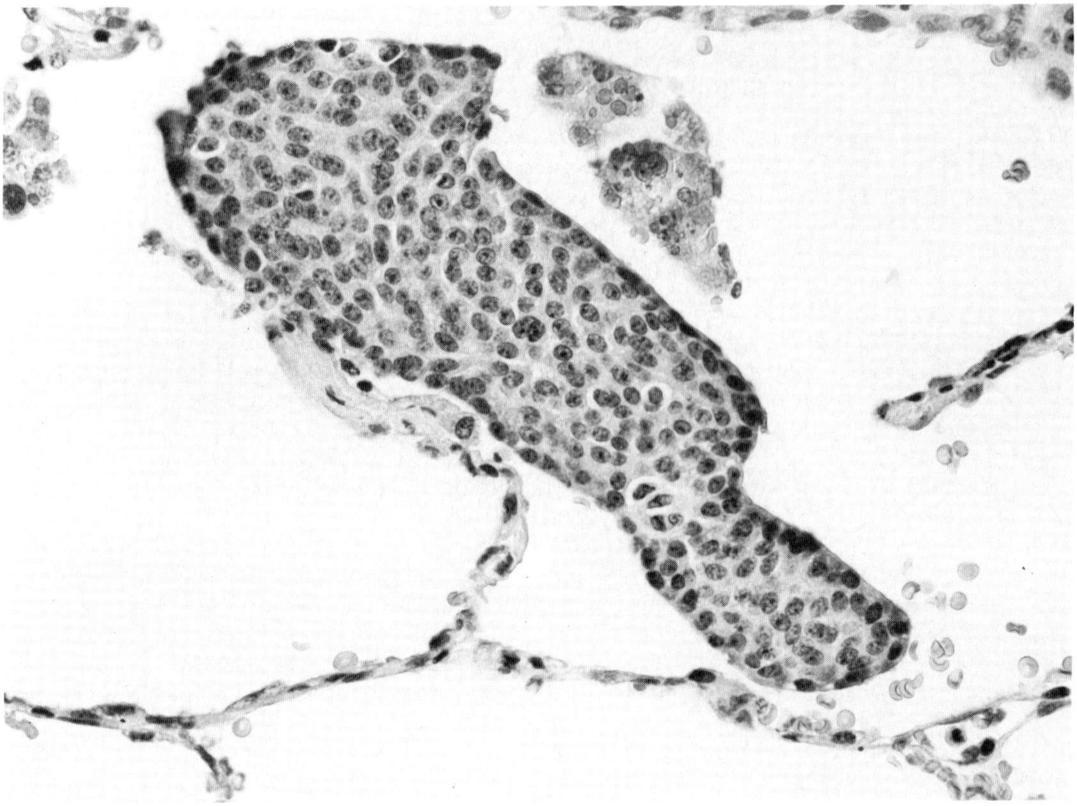

Figure 10–11. Carcinoid. A solid clump of cells some distance from the edge of a cytologically typical carcinoid tumor.

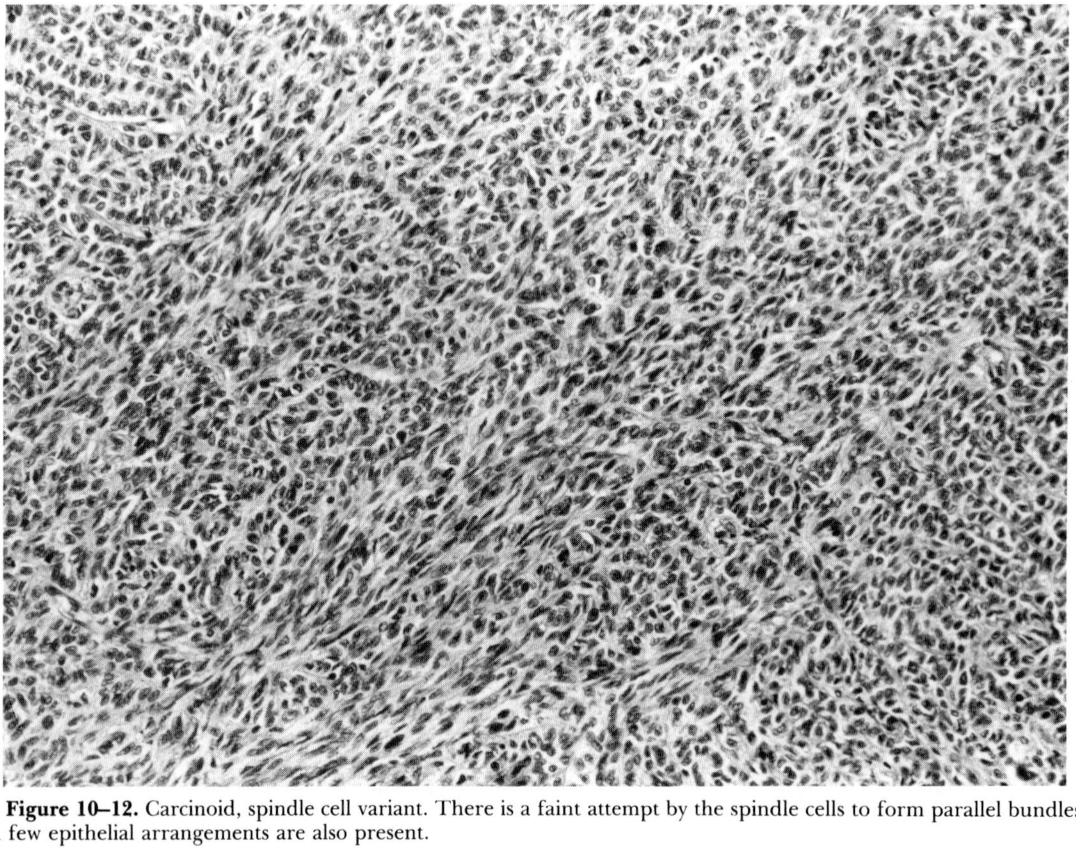

Figure 10–12. Carcinoid, spindle cell variant. There is a faint attempt by the spindle cells to form parallel bundles. A few epithelial arrangements are also present.

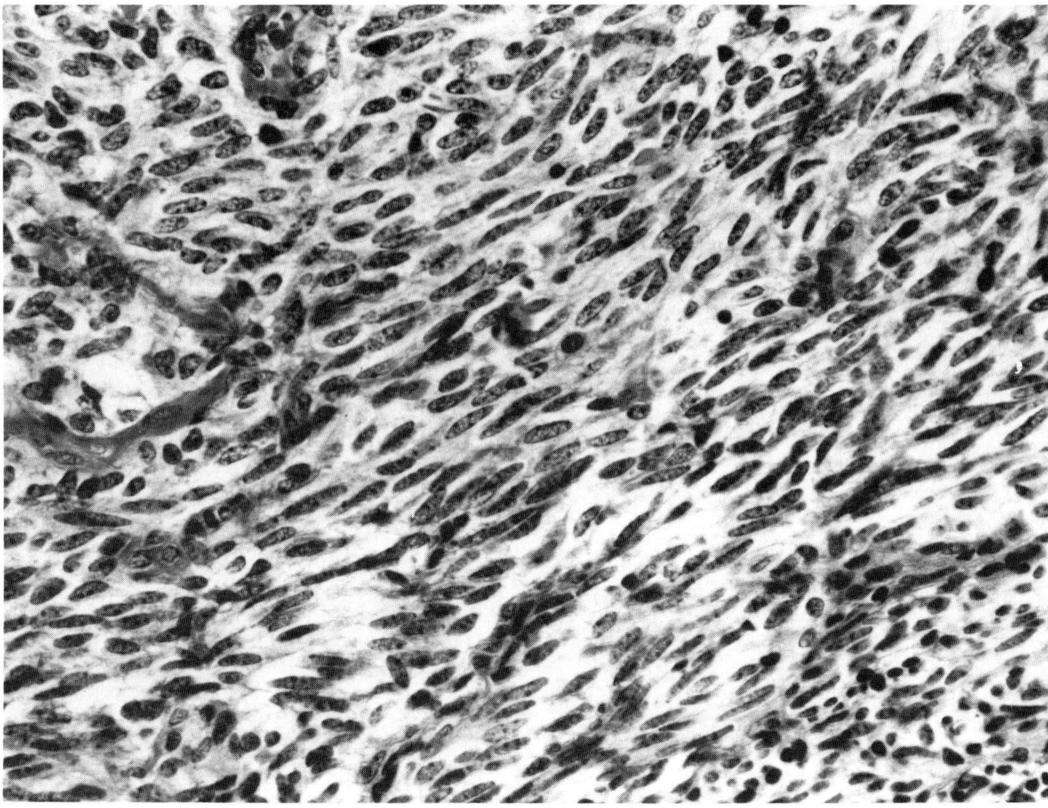

Figure 10–13. Carcinoid, spindle cell variant. The cells are elongated, but they have more cytoplasm than would be seen in a small cell carcinoma with fusiform cells.

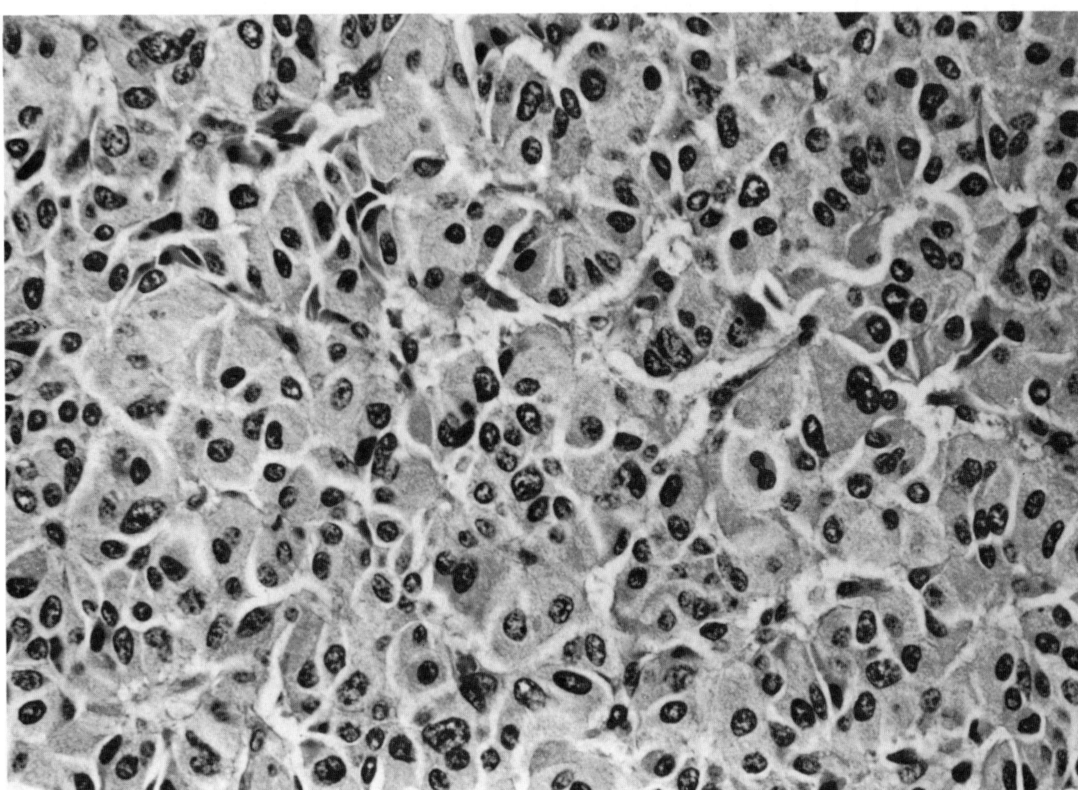

Figure 10–14. Carcinoid, oncocytic variant. The cells have plentiful, finely granular cytoplasm.

and the entire tumor can have this appearance or it may coexist with the more typical forms,[149, 157, 167] in which event transitional zones may be identified.[147] Siwersson and Kindblom[155] described the case of a 13-year-old girl who had an oncocytic carcinoid of the nasal cavity and a bronchial carcinoid that appeared 1 year later. Not all oncocytic tumors show endocrine features,[58] but all should be considered potentially malignant.[127]

Tumorlets

Tumorlets are small groups of endocrine cells adjacent to or encircling bronchi.[28, 40, 137, 191] They have been known since 1926,[134] but Whitwell[182] coined the term in 1955. They are sometimes associated with interstitial fibrosis and obstructive pulmonary disease, and they have been found in irradiated lungs.[164] The endocrine nature of the cells can be demonstrated by immunostaining or electron microscopy,[93] and an association with endocrine hyperfunction (Cushing's syndrome) has been recorded.[142] Watanabe and associates[180] reported an autopsy on a patient with diffuse panbronchiolitis and multiple tumorlets. They studied the number and distribution of the pulmonary endocrine cells singly and in clusters and found that they tended to occur more frequently in the pulmonary segments in which the tumorlets were found. They believed there was transition of the clusters into tumorlets and showed comparable immunostaining in the clusters of endocrine cells and the tumorlets. Although tumorlets are regarded as nonneoplastic proliferations of endocrine cells, distinction from minute carcinoid tumors is not possible on morphologic grounds, and metastases from tumorlets to bronchial lymph nodes have been recorded.[47, 81] Tumorlets must be distinguished from metastatic carcinoid tumor.

Atypical Carcinoids

Atypical cytologic features in a bronchial carcinoid[34, 49] have been shown to have prognostic significance,[10] although the histology does not always accurately predict the subsequent behavior. Minor degrees of atypia may be indicated merely by slight distortion in the histologic pattern, which then appears less orderly in some areas (Fig. 10–15), and the nuclei in these foci are enlarged and show prominent chromatin clumping (Fig. 10–16). Foci of necrosis (Figs. 10–17 and 10–18) are an ominous sign and are often accompanied by cytologic atypia. Increased mitotic activity is seen as the nuclear pleomorphism and architectural disorder increase (Figs. 10–19 through 10–21).

Arrigoni and associates[10] give the history of the development of the concept of carcinoid tumors with cytologically atypical features. The first description of an atypical carcinoid was in 1944 by Engelbreth-Holm,[55] who reported two cases, both without metastases. Arrigoni and associates[10] selected 23 atypical tumors from among 215 patients with lung carcinoids and compared the behavior with 178 classic cases. The atypical tumors showed one or more of the following: increased mitotic activity, nuclear pleomorphism, enlarged nucleoli, hyperchromatic nuclei, abnormal nuclear/cytoplasmic ratio, increased cellularity, disorganized architecture, and tumor necrosis. Of the 23 patients, 16 (70%) developed metastases, whereas only 5.6% of the typical tumors metastasized. Thirty percent of the atypical carcinoid patients were dead at the time of follow-up, the average length of survival being 27 months.

Eleven atypical carcinoids were studied by Grote and co-workers[74] and compared with published cases of typical carcinoids. The only clinical feature to distinguish the atypical from the typical tumors was age at diagnosis (59 versus 49 years). The distinction of an atypical carcinoid from a small cell carcinoma of the lung is usually possible in nodal metastases since the small cell carcinomas are more likely to exhibit perinodal extension.

An aggressive carcinoid tumor spreads through the lungs by extension at its periphery through the alveolar spaces. In addition, lymphatic permeation may be detected (Fig. 10–22), vascular invasion should be searched for (Fig. 10–23), and perineural extension is occasionally encountered (Fig. 10–24).

CYTOLOGY

The cells of typical carcinoids are seldom identified in sputum or bronchial washings or brushings since most of the tumors are covered by an overlying layer of uninvolved mucosa; but if mucosal ulceration occurs, the cells may then appear in cytologic prepara-

Text continued on page 262

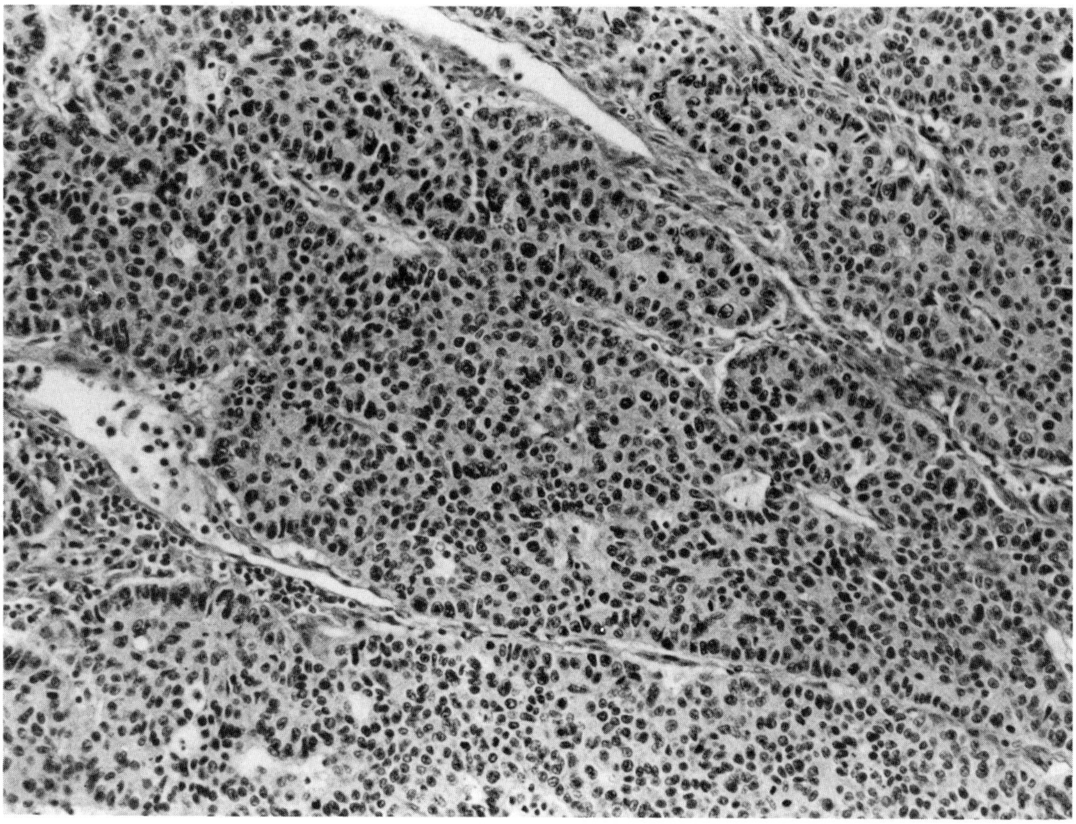

Figure 10–15. Carcinoid, with slight cytologic atypia, occasional mitoses, and early loss of the architectural pattern.

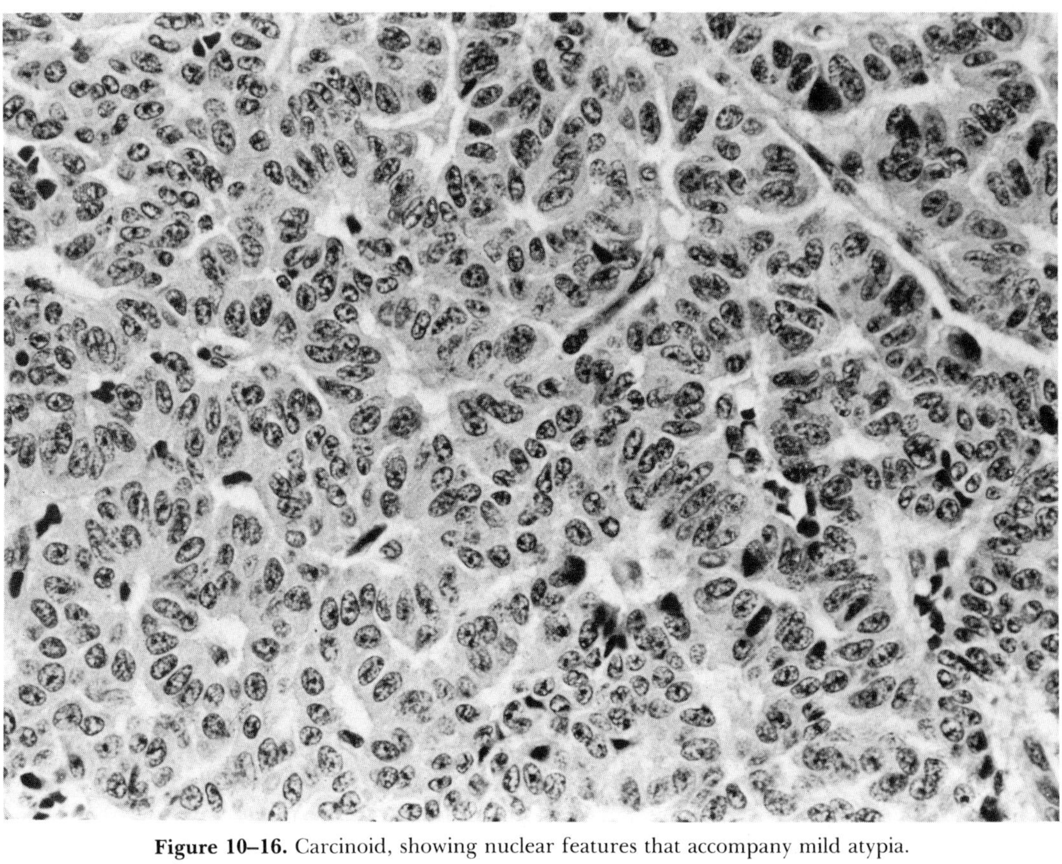

Figure 10–16. Carcinoid, showing nuclear features that accompany mild atypia.

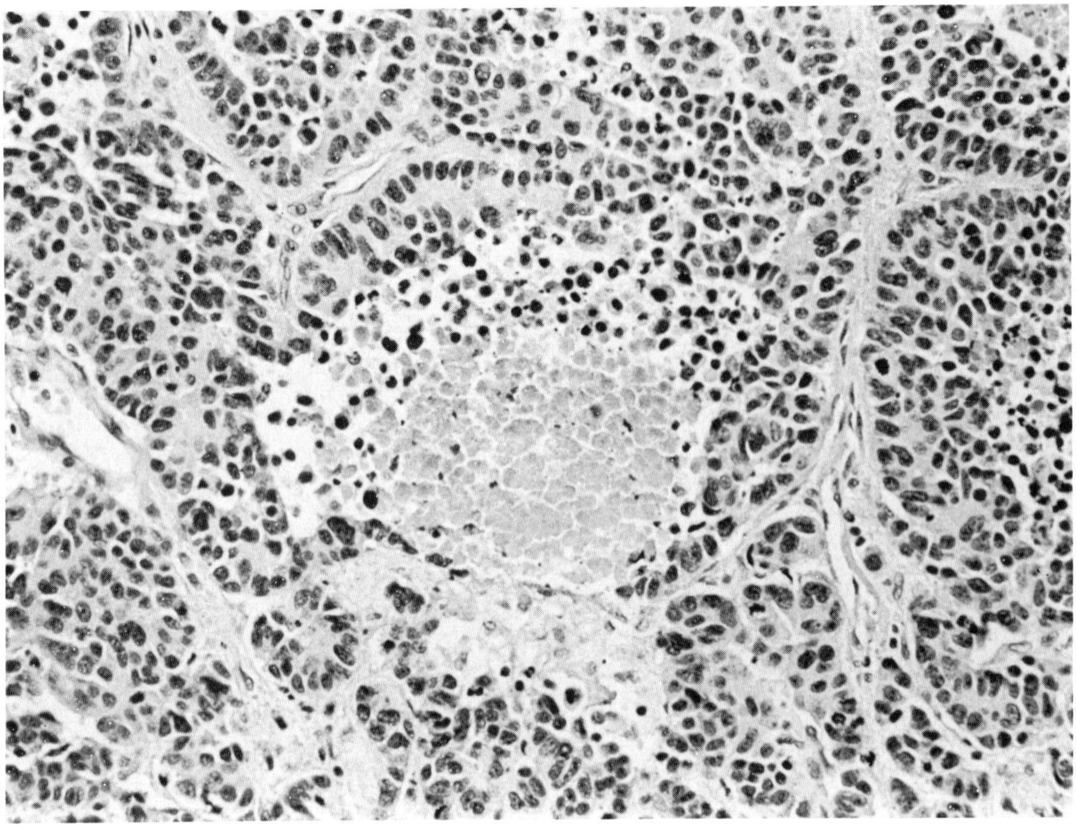

Figure 10–17. Carcinoid. Small foci of necrosis are present in an atypical tumor.

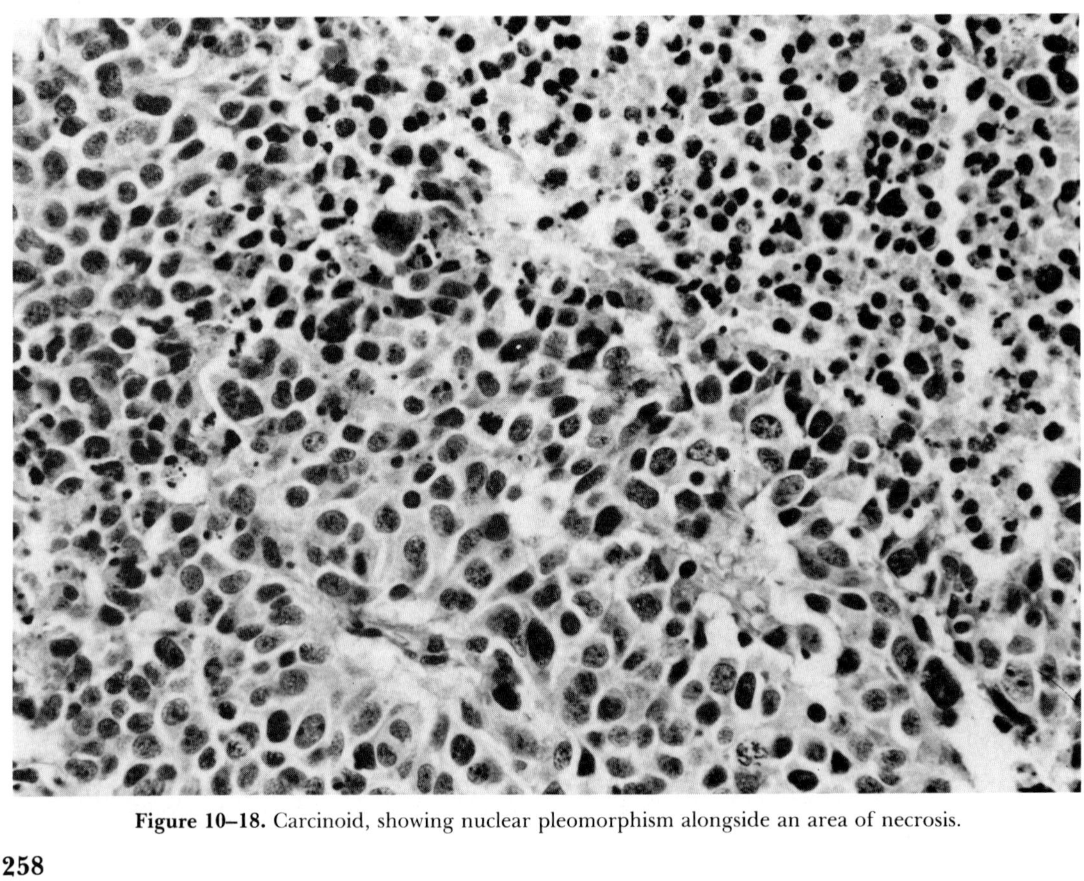

Figure 10–18. Carcinoid, showing nuclear pleomorphism alongside an area of necrosis.

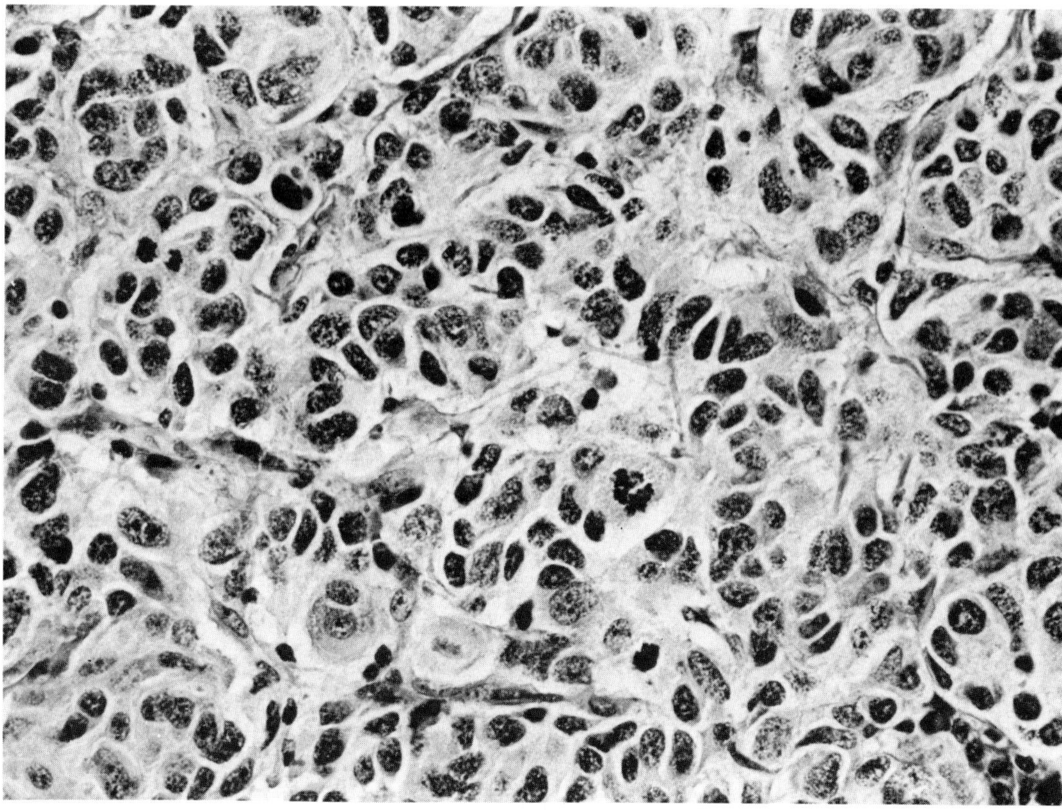

Figure 10–19. Carcinoid. Although the zellballen arrangement is maintained, atypical nuclear features and mitotic activity are evident.

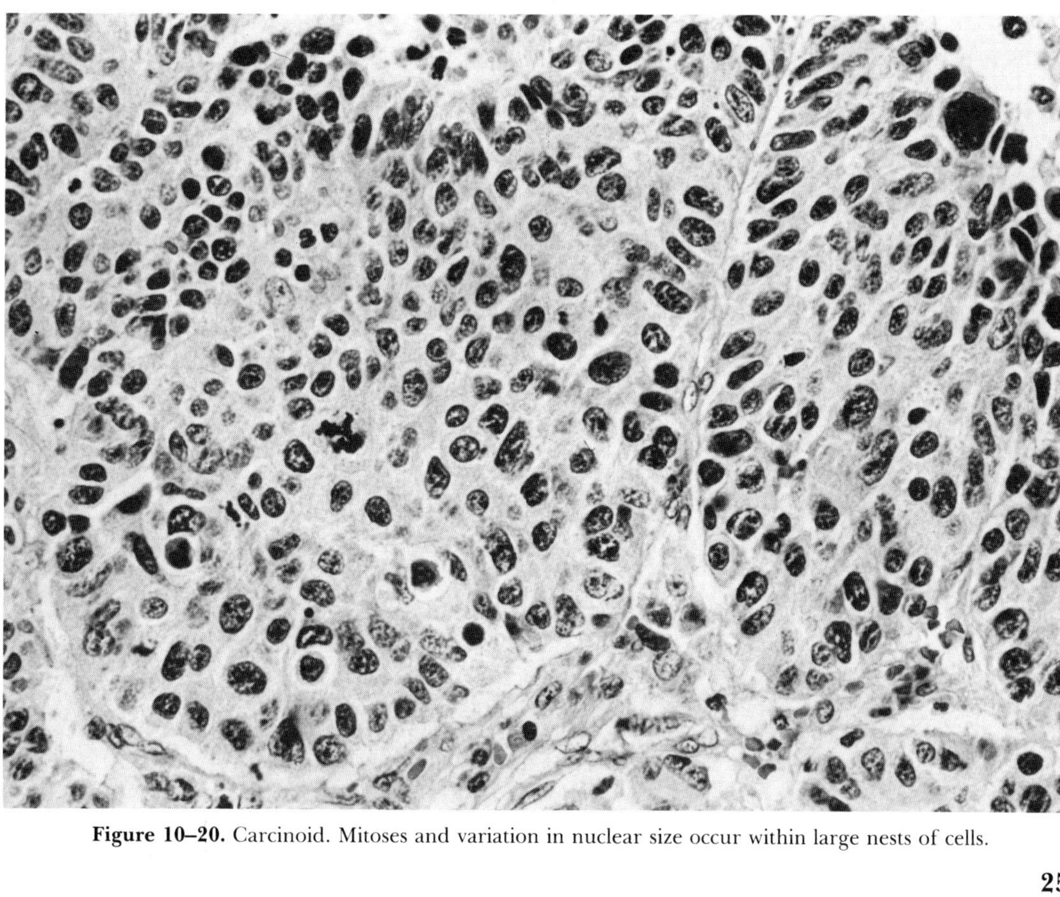

Figure 10–20. Carcinoid. Mitoses and variation in nuclear size occur within large nests of cells.

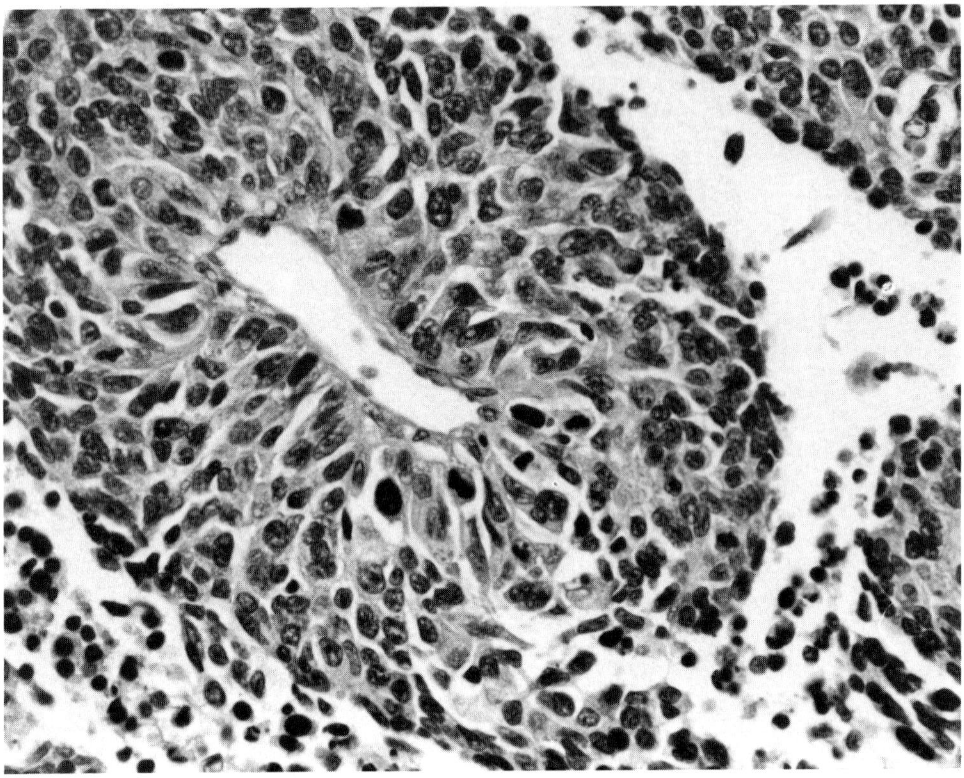

Figure 10–21. Carcinoid. A small group of cells without a nesting pattern surrounds a small vessel within an area of necrosis.

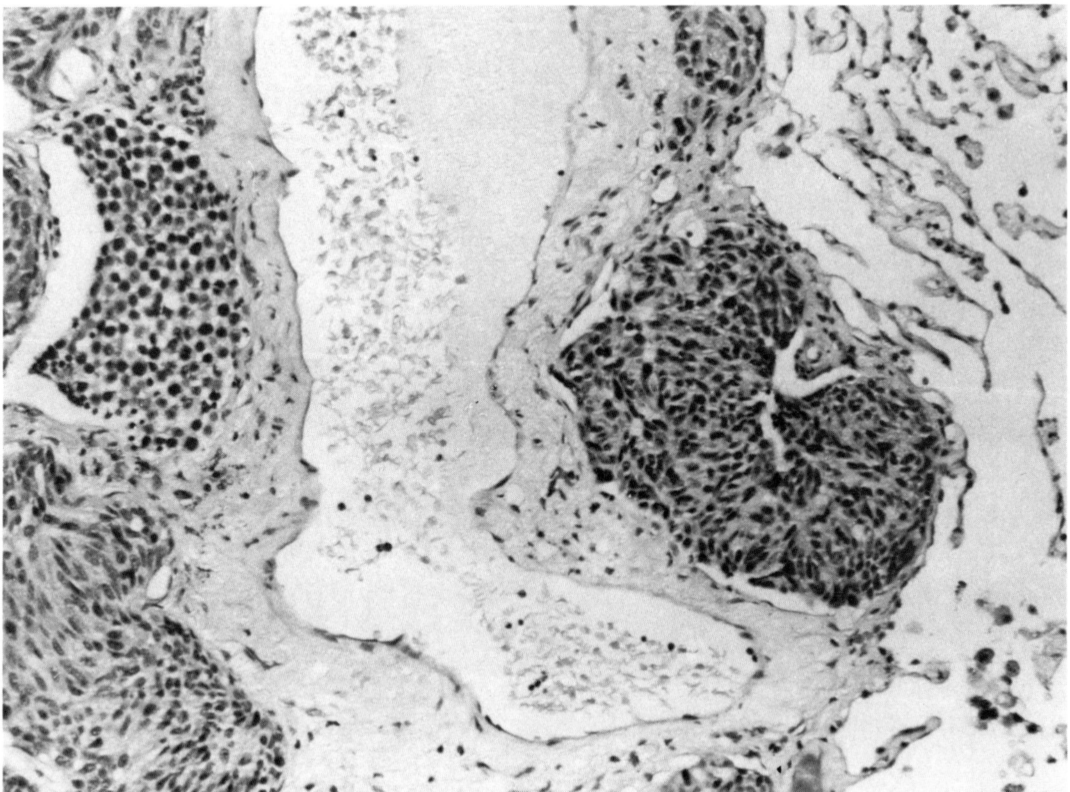

Figure 10–22. Carcinoid. The tumor is permeating lymphatics.

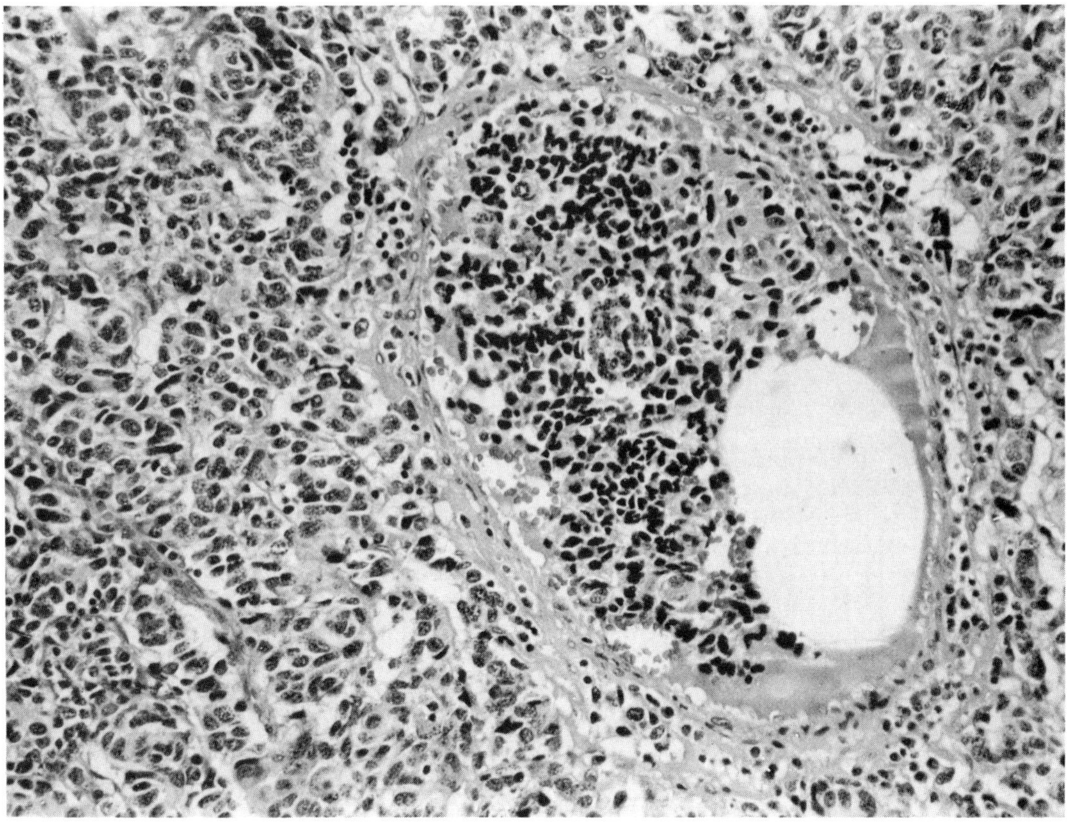

Figure 10–23. Carcinoid. Vascular invasion is occurring in a clearly atypical tumor.

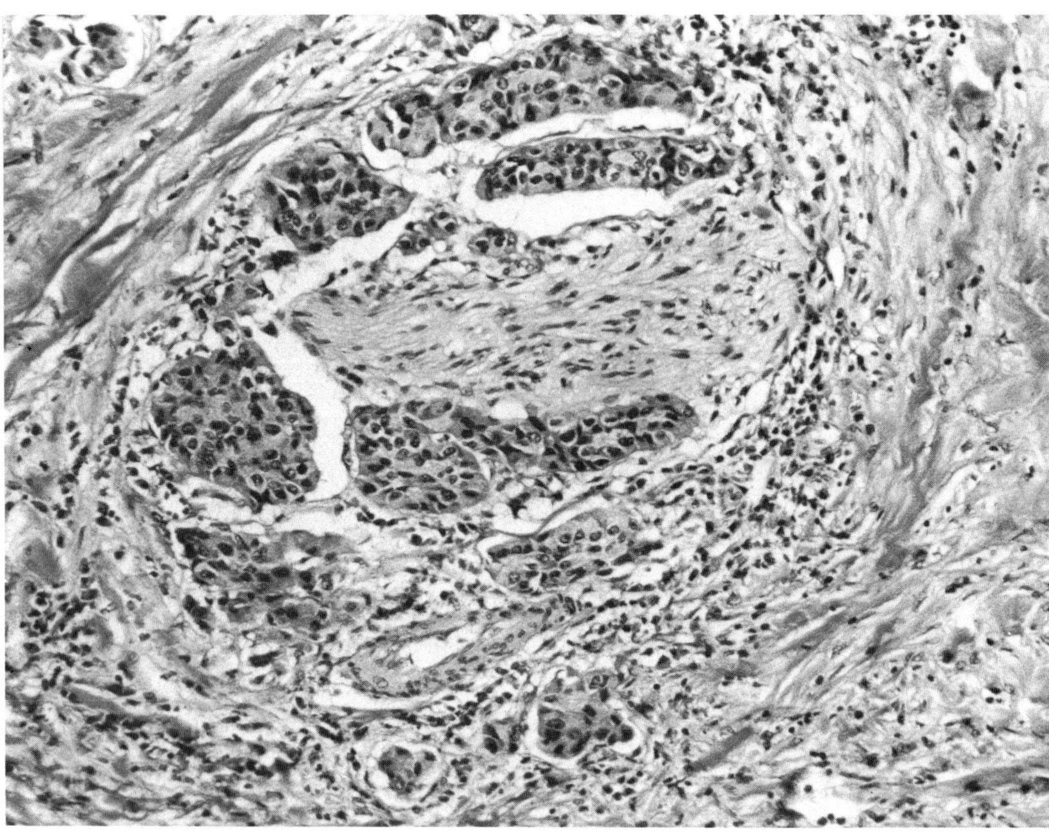

Figure 10–24. Carcinoid. Perineural extension is evident.

tions. Single cells resemble metaplastic cells and are difficult to recognize as tumor. They attract attention when they form small aggregates, and even their innocent appearance should not interfere with a proper diagnosis. The cells in Papanicolaou preparations are typically cuboidal to low columnar, with basophilic cytoplasm and monotonously regular, round central nuclei.[87, 96, 110] The nuclear/cytoplasmic ratio is only minimally higher than in metaplastic cells (Fig. 10–25). A Grimelius stain may be helpful. The nuclear chromatin is more coarsely clumped than that of small cell carcinomas, a useful criterion for spindle cell carcinoids: it can be shown well in touch preparations (Figs. 10–26 and 10–27). Sometimes the chromatin pattern resembles that of a well-differentiated myeloma cell. Nucleoli can be identified, but they are not particularly large.

The presence of atypical features can generally be recognized when adequate material is available for cytologic evaluation,[128] particularly in fine-needle aspiration biopsies.[60] Szyfelbein and co-workers[163] studied 46 fine-needle aspiration biopsy specimens and found that 13 were typical and 3 were atypical carcinoids and the remainder were small cell carcinomas. In atypical carcinoids, the cell and nuclear size and shape are variable. The nuclear/cytoplasmic ratio is high, and the enlarged nuclei contain prominent nucleoli and heavy granular chromatin. Mitoses are frequent, and a background of necrosis may be evident. Two touch preparations (see Figs. 10–26 and 10–27) contrast the cytologic features of a typical and an atypical carcinoid.

IMMUNOCYTOCHEMISTRY

Immunocytochemically, most carcinoid tumors of the lung coexpress epithelial markers such as cytokeratin[22, 25] and desmoplakins,[25] together with one or more general endocrine markers such as neurofilament proteins,[25, 38, 104, 105] neuron-specific enolase,[68, 108, 146, 178] Leu-7,[108] chromogranins,[108, 146] and some specific endocrine cell products.[25, 67, 170, 178, 189] The latter include eutopic substances that are normally present in the lung, including serotonin,[3, 48] bombesin,[46, 48, 107, 179] calcitonin,[21, 46] Leu-enkephalin, and somatostatin,[179] as well as many ectopic substances that are not iden-

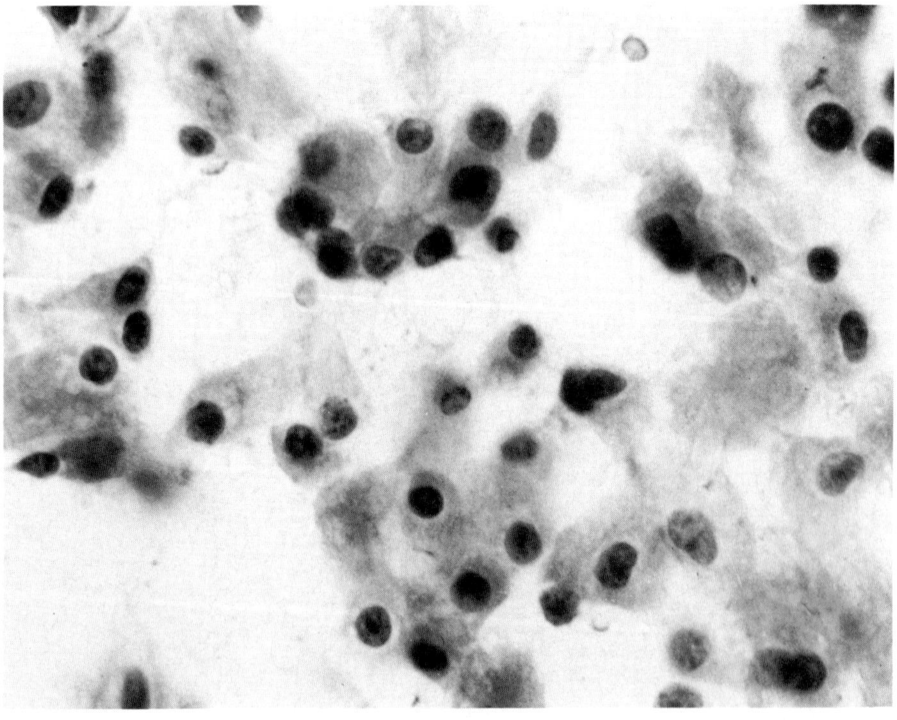

Figure 10–25. Fine-needle aspiration biopsy specimen. The cells contain oval nuclei within ample cytoplasm and recapitulate an acinar-like structure. Nuclei show minimal size variation.

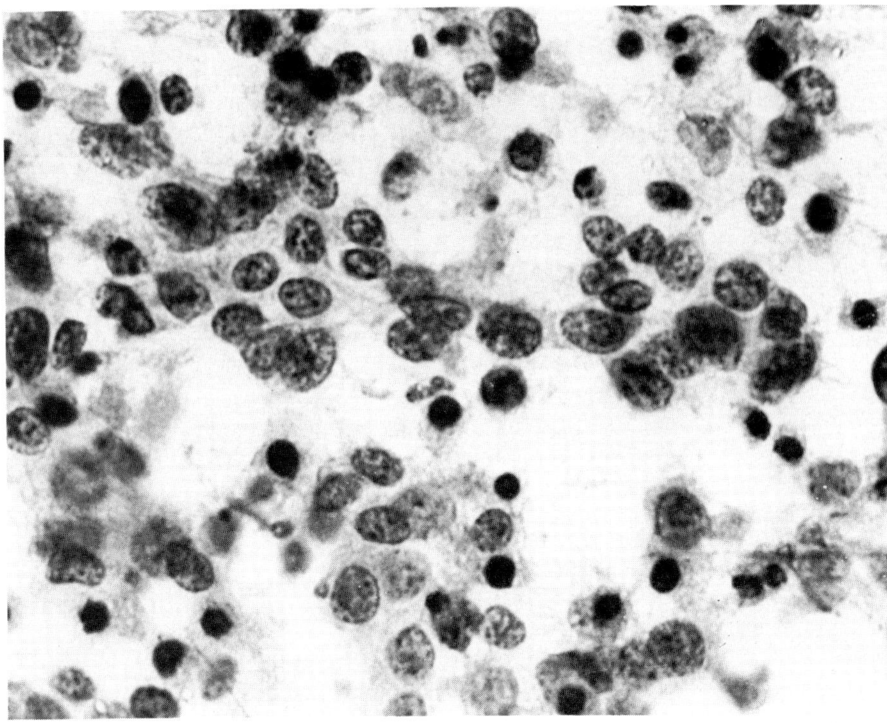

Figure 10–26. Cells of the same tumor in a touch preparation. They have lost their cytoplasm, but nuclear detail is shown.

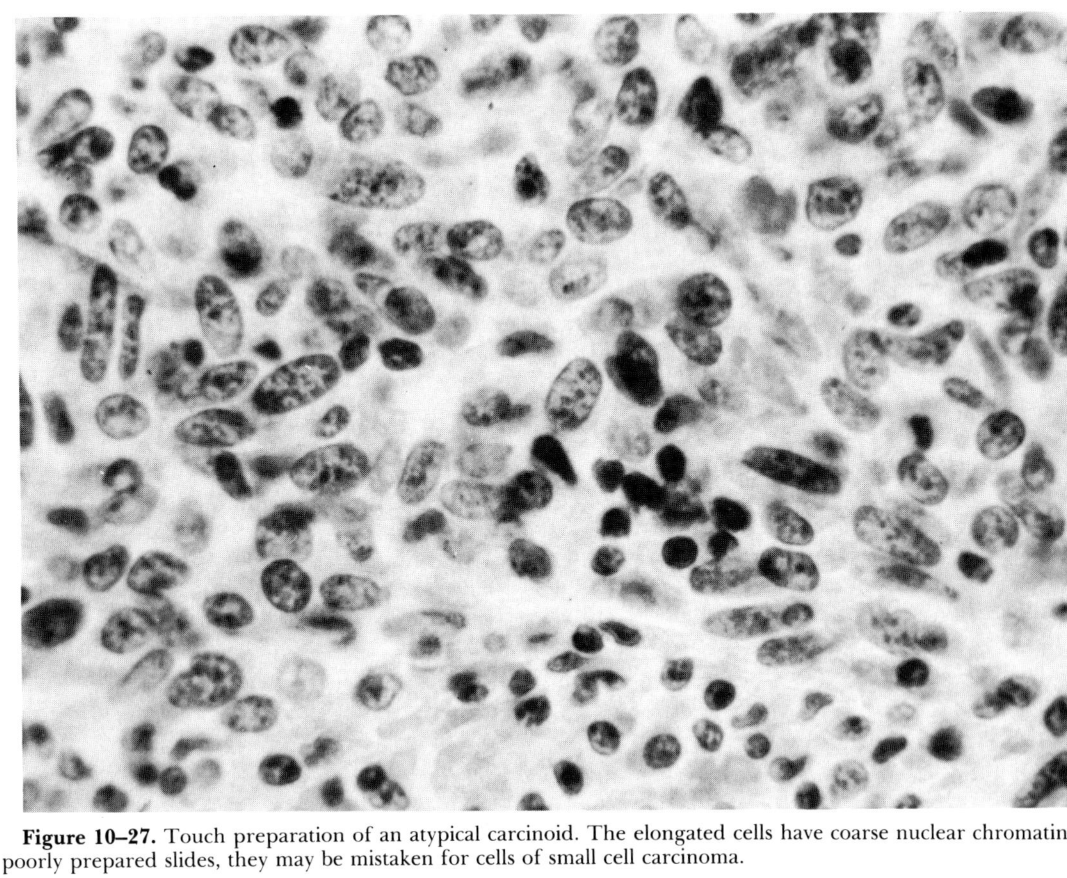

Figure 10–27. Touch preparation of an atypical carcinoid. The elongated cells have coarse nuclear chromatin. In poorly prepared slides, they may be mistaken for cells of small cell carcinoma.

tified in the normal human lung, such as ACTH, vasoactive intestinal polypeptide, antidiuretic hormone, and neurotensin.[67, 108, 170]

Cytokeratins, specifically polypeptides Nos. 8, 9, and 19, constitute the most common intermediate filaments expressed in lung carcinoids.[108] The cytokeratin immunostaining pattern is usually diffuse throughout the cytoplasm, but in some cases the reaction may appear as paranuclear globoid inclusions, which are confirmed by electron microscopy to be aggregates of intermediate filaments[16, 22] (Fig. 10–28). Similar inclusions have been reported in extrapulmonary neuroendocrine tumors,[19, 22, 83, 153] and some authors have attributed a diagnostic value to them, especially in endocrine carcinomas of the skin (Merkel cell tumors).[19, 153] We have not found the inclusions to be common in lung carcinoids or exclusive to endocrine tumors: we were able to find only two tumors with this type of inclusion among 50 lung carcinoids. In one of the two cases, we were able to detect vimentin in the inclusions in addition to cytokeratin. Similar inclusions containing neurofilament proteins have been reported in other endocrine tumors.[153]

Neurofilament proteins are another type of intermediate filament that can be found in lung carcinoids.[25, 38, 104, 105] The expression of these filaments is not as common as that of other neuroendocrine markers, so immunocytochemical studies for neurofilaments have limited value in the routine diagnosis of the tumors. Furthermore, most of the antibodies to neurofilaments that are currently available react poorly or not at all in formalin-fixed, routinely processed tissues.

Neuron-specific enolase is a general endocrine marker that is commonly expressed in lung carcinoids.[68, 108, 146, 159, 178] Unfortunately, this marker has also been detected in a wide variety of nonendocrine tumors,[102, 173] and its diagnostic value is consequently very limited. We found reactivity in 56 of 64 (88%) lung carcinoids, and others have reported similar results.[108, 146]

Because of its frequent expression, its high specificity for endocrine differentiation, and good preservation of antigenicity in formalin-fixed tissue specimens, chromogranin is the most useful general endocrine marker currently available for the immunocytochemical diagnosis of lung carcinoids.[108, 146] Studies have demonstrated that all three types (A, B, and C) are expressed in these tumors.[181] Using a monoclonal antibody (LK2H10) to chromogranin A, we were able to demonstrate immunostaining for this marker in 49 of the 57 (86%) lung carcinoids studied (Fig. 10–29). Although there was a wide variation in the intensity of the reaction from case to case, the intensity of the reaction often correlated with the number of secretory granules seen by electron microscopy. Comparable results were obtained with the recently developed monoclonal antibody PHE-5 (Fig. 10–30).[141] Immunoblot analysis has demonstrated that this antibody reacts with a 90-kd neuroendocrine granule protein that is distinct from chromogranin A.

Leu-7 and synaptophysin are two other general endocrine markers that are often expressed in lung carcinoids.[70, 108] Unfortunately, Leu-7 expression is not exclusive to endocrine cells, as is indicated by its frequent demonstration in prostatic hyperplasia and prostatic carcinomas,[117, 144, 174] while synaptophysin, although highly specific for endocrine differentiation, has the drawback of requiring frozen sections or special fixation in order to obtain reliable results in routinely processed specimens.[86] Despite these limitations, both markers are useful in the diagnosis of lung carcinoids since the tumors do not always display chromogranin reactivity, and Leu-7 and synaptophysin can then serve as complementary markers.

Immunocytochemical studies have demonstrated that the large majority of lung carcinoids react for a variety of eutopic and ectopic hormones and neuropeptides.[25, 67, 170, 178, 189] Bombesin and serotonin, which are present in the normal lung, appear to be the ones most commonly expressed in the lung carcinoids.

Gastrin-releasing peptide (GRP), a peptide of 27 amino acid residues,[119] is considered to be the mammalian form of bombesin.[9, 122, 139] Several studies have reported bombesin and GRP-like immunoreactivity in neuroendocrine tumors of the lung and have indicated that the finding can be helpful in diagnosis.[2, 29, 108, 146, 165, 178] Bombesin/GRP reactivity has been reported in 33 to 75% of lung carcinoids, and we observed it in 26 of 33 cases (67%). We have found it to be the most commonly expressed neuropeptide in lung carcinoids. Immunoreactivity for the C-terminal flanking peptide of human bombesin (CTP) has also been reported in lung carcinoids, but its expression in these tumors is significantly lower than that of bombesin (12% of the cases in one series[2]), and it

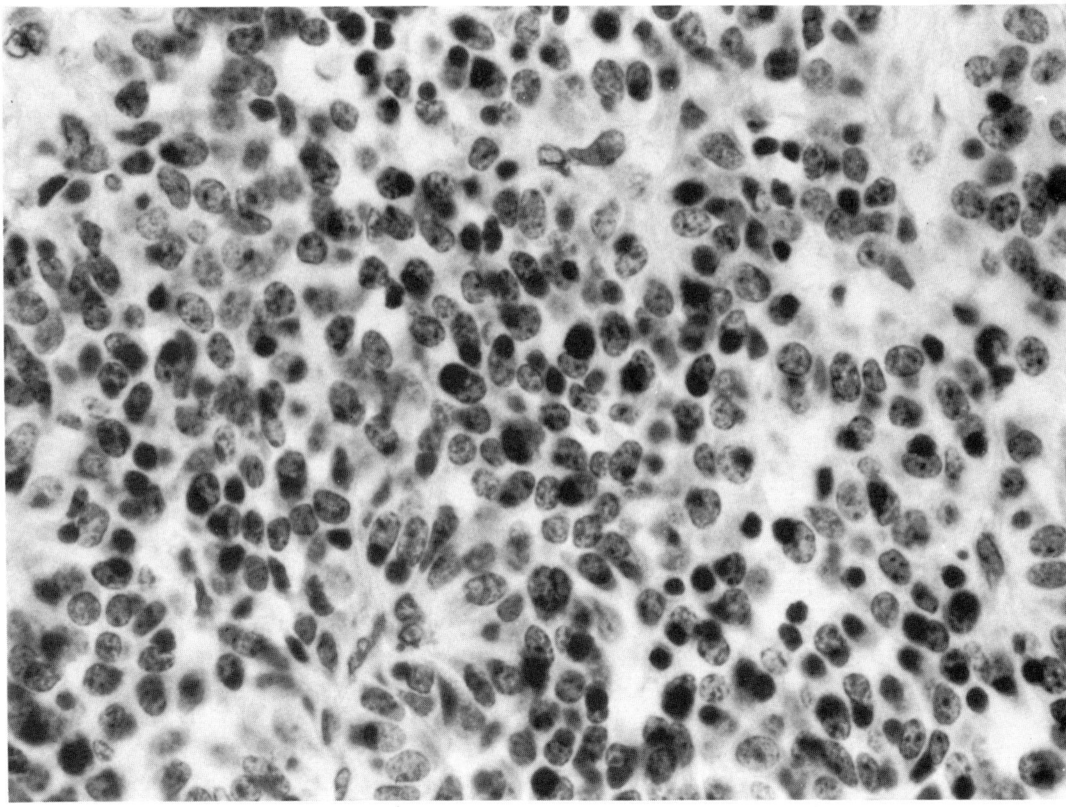

Figure 10–28. Carcinoid. Immunocytochemical preparation demonstrates cytoplasmic globoid inclusions reacting to cytokeratin.

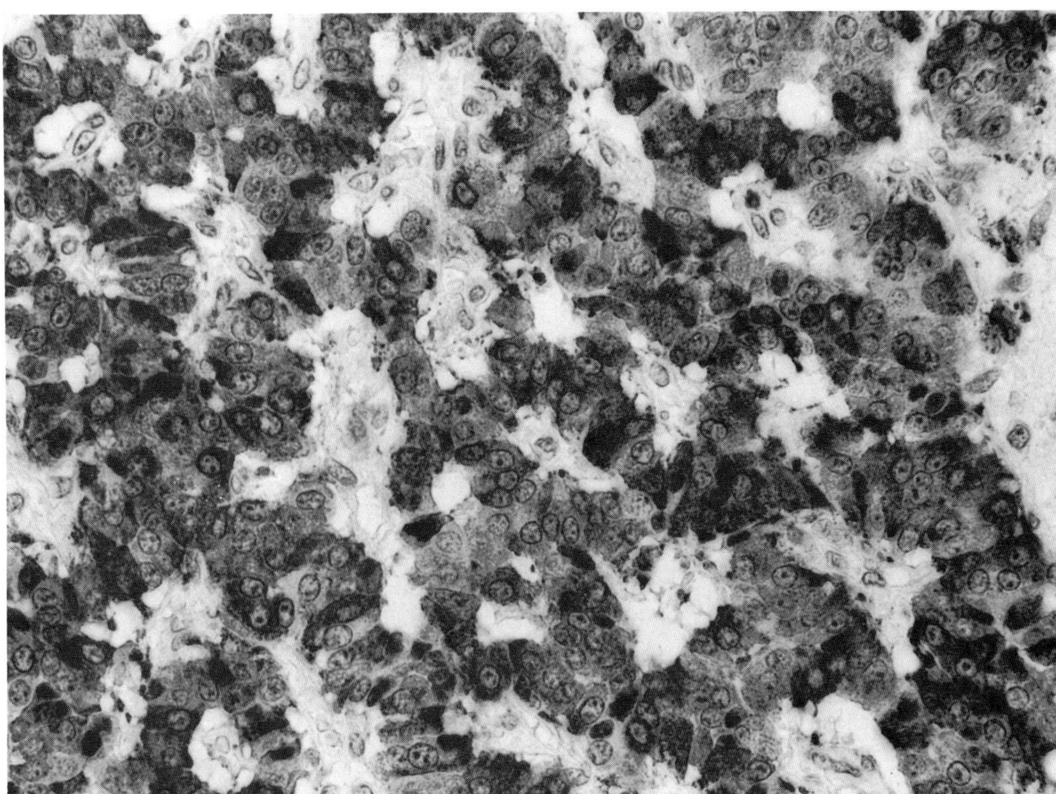

Figure 10–29. Carcinoid. Immunocytochemical preparation shows strong reactivity for chromogranin A.

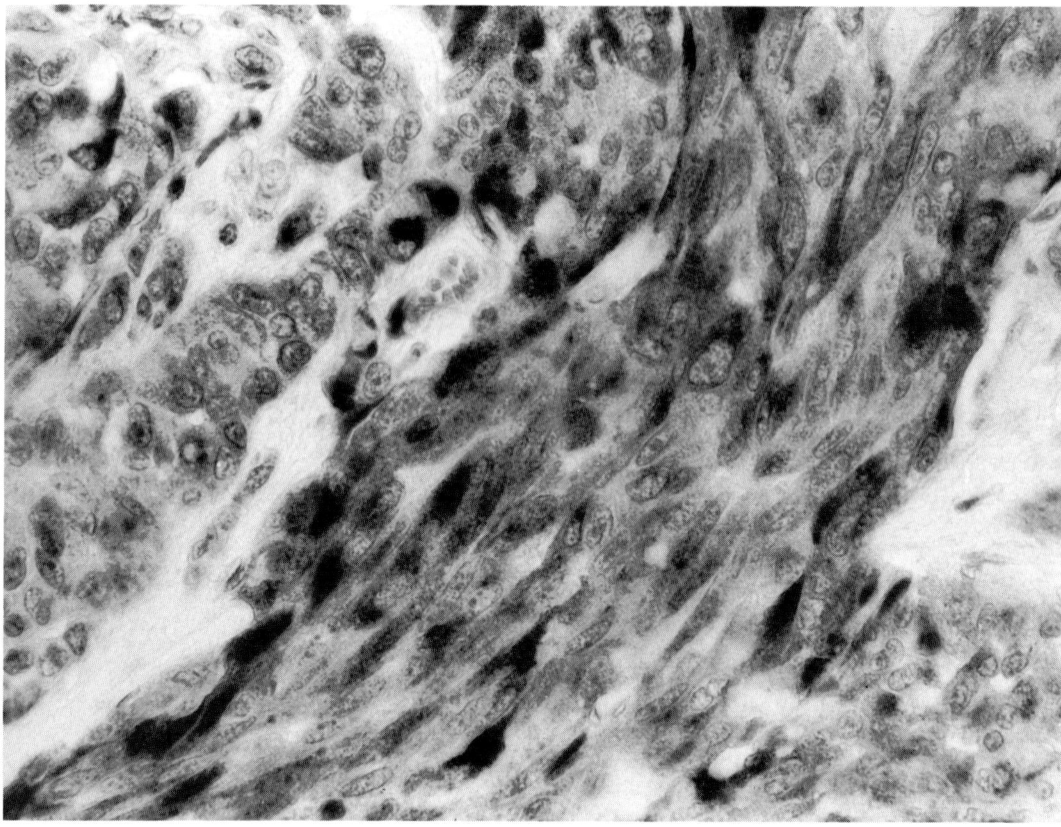

Figure 10–30. Carcinoid. Spindle cell carcinoid reacts with PHE-5 monoclonal antibody.

therefore does not have the diagnostic value that has been reported for small cell carcinoma.[2]

In a study of 46 lung carcinoids, we found reactivity for serotonin in 30 (65%). These results are somewhat lower than were obtained by Warren and co-workers,[178] who found it in 9 of their 11 cases (82%). Only one of our patients had symptoms of the carcinoid syndrome, which, as has been noted, is an uncommon clinical finding in patients with lung carcinoids.[140]

ACTH is one of the hormones ectopically expressed by lung carcinoids, and cases of Cushing's syndrome have been reported.[82, 89, 116, 187] We found reactivity for this marker in 6 of 45 cases studied (13%), but higher figures have been reported by others; for example, Warren and co-workers[178] reported ACTH production in 4 of 11 cases (44%).

A variety of other hormones and neuropeptides have been described in lung carcinoids, including prolactin, vasoactive intestinal polypeptide, growth hormone–releasing hormone, calcitonin, human chorionic gonadotropin (hCG), α-melanocyte-stimulating hormone (α-MSH), β-endorphin, and pancreatic polypeptide.[12, 170, 178, 189] Our experience with the immunocytochemical expression of some of these substances is summarized in Table 10–1.

Stellate S-100 protein–positive cells have been detected in lung carcinoids admixed with the tumor cells.[15, 17, 53] They have been called sustentacular or satellite cells because of immunocytochemical and ultrastructural similarities with the sustentacular cells of the carotid body. We have found these cells in 10 of 46 (22%) carcinoids (Fig. 10–31); and in 6 other carcinoids, tumor cells showed S-100 protein immunoreactivity. S-100 protein–positive sustentacular cells have also been reported in carcinoid tumors of the appendix.[125, 183]

On occasion, mucosubstances can be demonstrated in lung carcinoids, indicating the presence of exocrine differentiation.[166] Lee and colleagues[103] have confirmed that a significant number of lung carcinoids react with the 44-3A6 monoclonal antibody, which recognizes a 40,000-M glycoprotein related to exocrine differentiation.

Table 10–1. Expression of Neuroendocrine Markers in Lung Carcinoids

Marker	Total Cases	No. Cases Positive	% Cases Positive
Neuron-specific enolase	64	56	88
Chromogranin A	57	49	86
Bombesin	39	26	67
Serotonin	46	30	65
Leu-enkephalin	44	14	32
Somatostatin	44	11	25
Calcitonin	45	4	9
Vasoactive intestinal polypeptide	45	11	24
β-hCG	28	10	36
Met-enkephalin	44	8	18
ACTH	45	6	13
Pancreatic polypeptide	41	8	20
Substance P	45	9	20
α-Melanocyte-stimulating hormone	28	5	18
Gastrin	45	6	13
β-Endorphin	45	5	11
Cholecystokinin	29	1	3
Vasopressin	28	0	0
Glucagon	45	0	0
Insulin	45	0	0
Prolactin	29	0	0

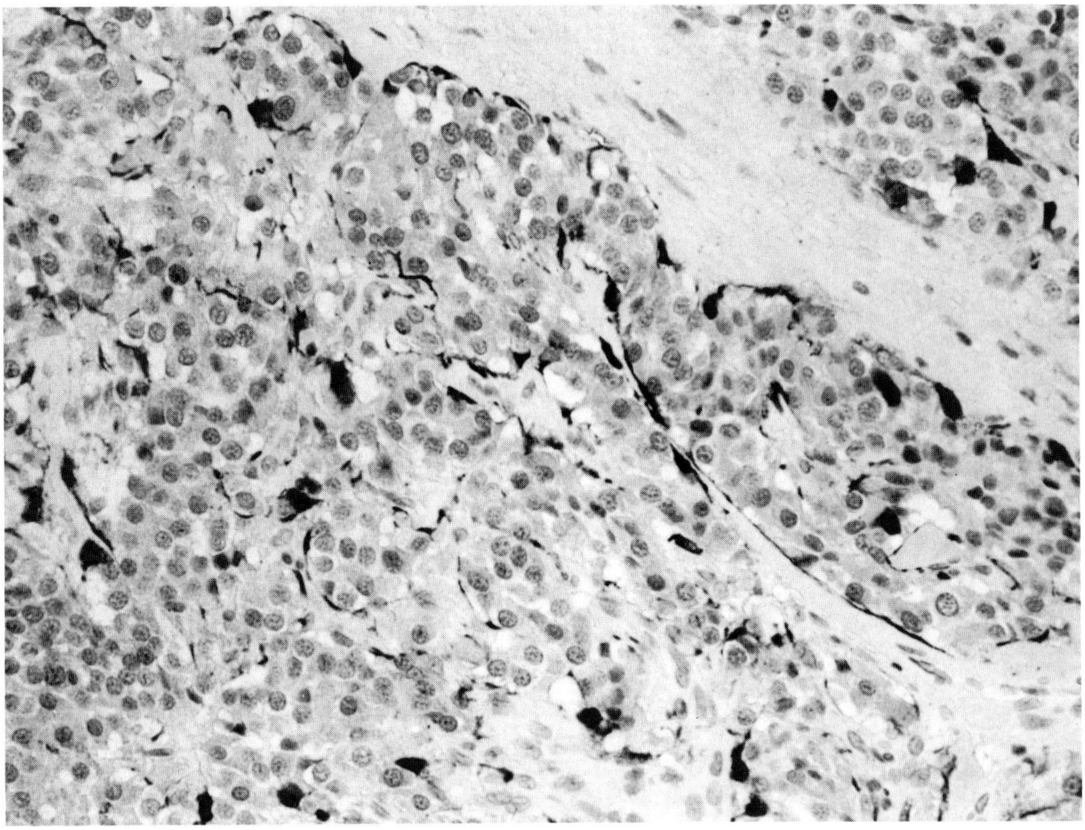

Figure 10–31. Carcinoid. Sustentacular cells are staining for S-100 protein.

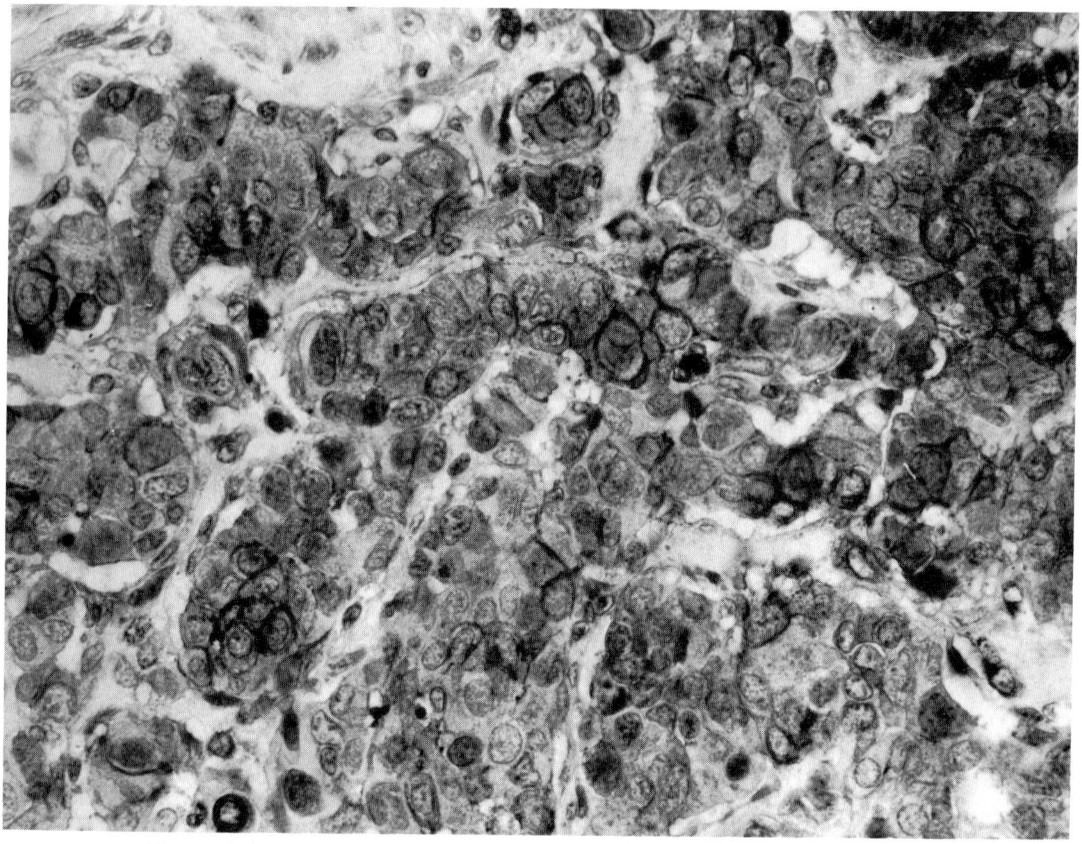

Figure 10–32. Carcinoid showing immunoreactivity for carcinoembryonic antigen.

Carcinoembryonic antigen occurs in approximately one third of lung carcinoids (Fig. 10–32), and positive immunostaining for this marker has been associated with poor prognosis.[24, 80]

ELECTRON MICROSCOPY

The nests of cells in a typical bronchial carcinoid tumor are sharply defined (Fig. 10–33) and bordered by a basal lamina. Cells with the location and fine structure of sustentacular cells (Fig. 10–34) correlate with the immunoreactivity for S-100 protein in slender cells around cell nests. They are flattened cells that lie within the basal lamina, and some smooth muscle myofilaments occupy the subplasmalemmal cytoplasm, so they might reasonably be viewed as myoepithelial cells.

The uniformity of the polygonal cells of a typical carcinoid is illustrated in Figure 10–35. The central nuclei have more coarsely clumped chromatin than that seen in the nuclei of small cell carcinomas, and greater amounts of cytoplasm are visible. The cytoplasmic granules in this tumor are at the upper end of the size range for bronchial carcinoids, accounting for their prominence at low magnification. At higher power (Fig. 10–36), carcinoid secretory granules are mostly round, fairly uniform in caliber in a particular tumor (with occasional exceptions), and bordered by a limiting membrane. In this figure a few short microvilli are sandwiched between the cells. More pleomorphic granules are shown in Figure 10–37. In a morphometric analysis of the granules in 50 carcinoid tumors, we found a range of median diameters between 93 and 383 nm. Four of the tumors had angular, pleomorphic granules. We have not been able to detect a significant correlation between granule caliber and secretory profile and do not anticipate this possibility in view of the frequency with which a tumor elaborates multiple hormonal polypeptides and other products. The endoplasmic reticulum in endocrine cells forms slender cisternae that are often ar-

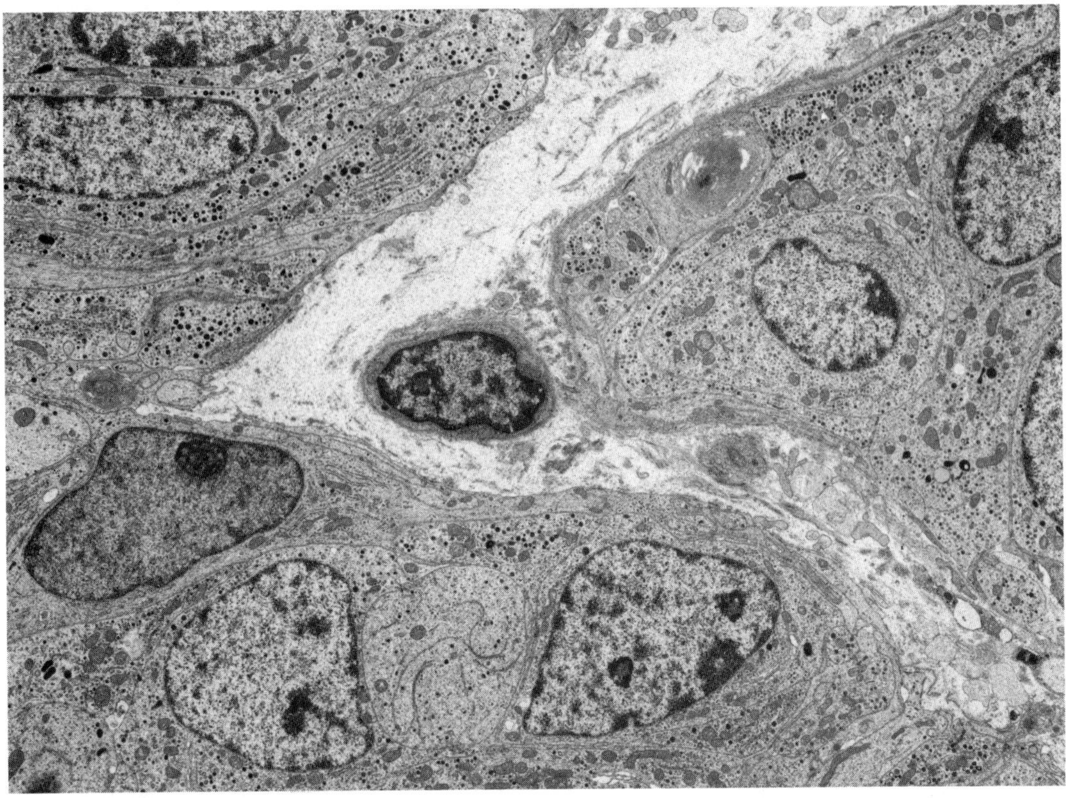

Figure 10–33. Carcinoid. The electron micrograph shows nests of tumor cells abutting on a partition of fibrous connective tissue. (×4,400)

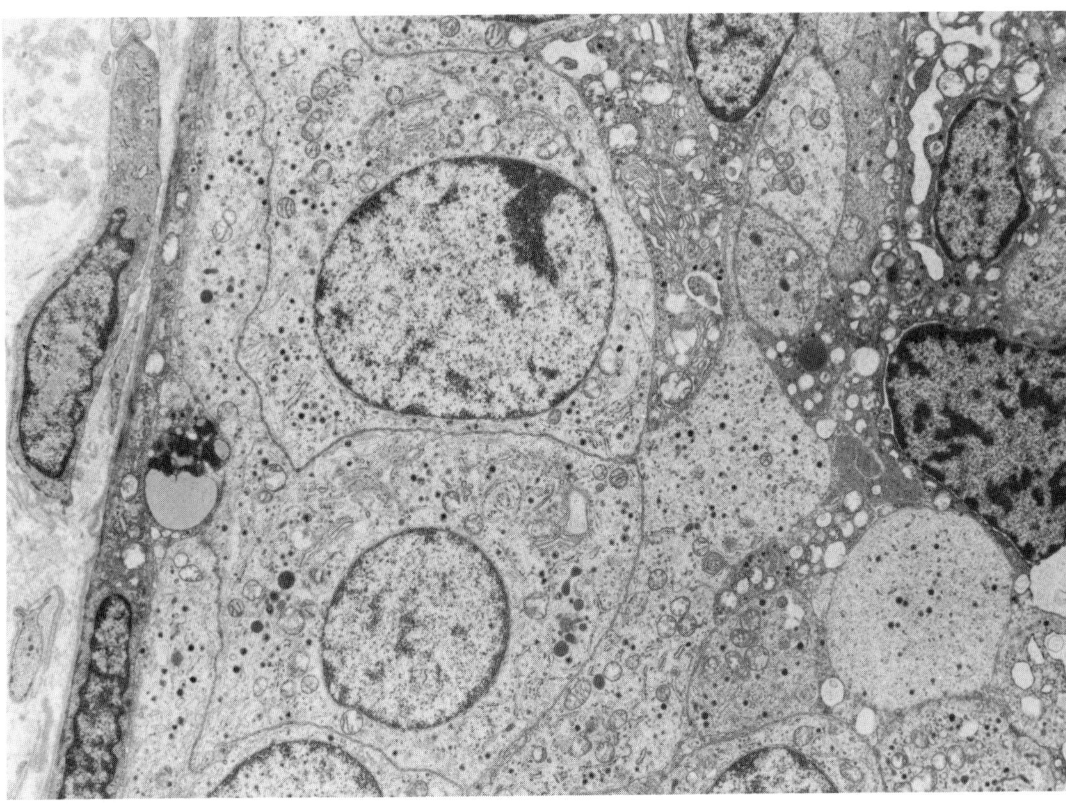

Figure 10–34. Carcinoid. Where the nest of cells contacts the stroma, a slender myoepithelial cell containing slim bundles of smooth muscle myofilaments lies within the basal lamina.

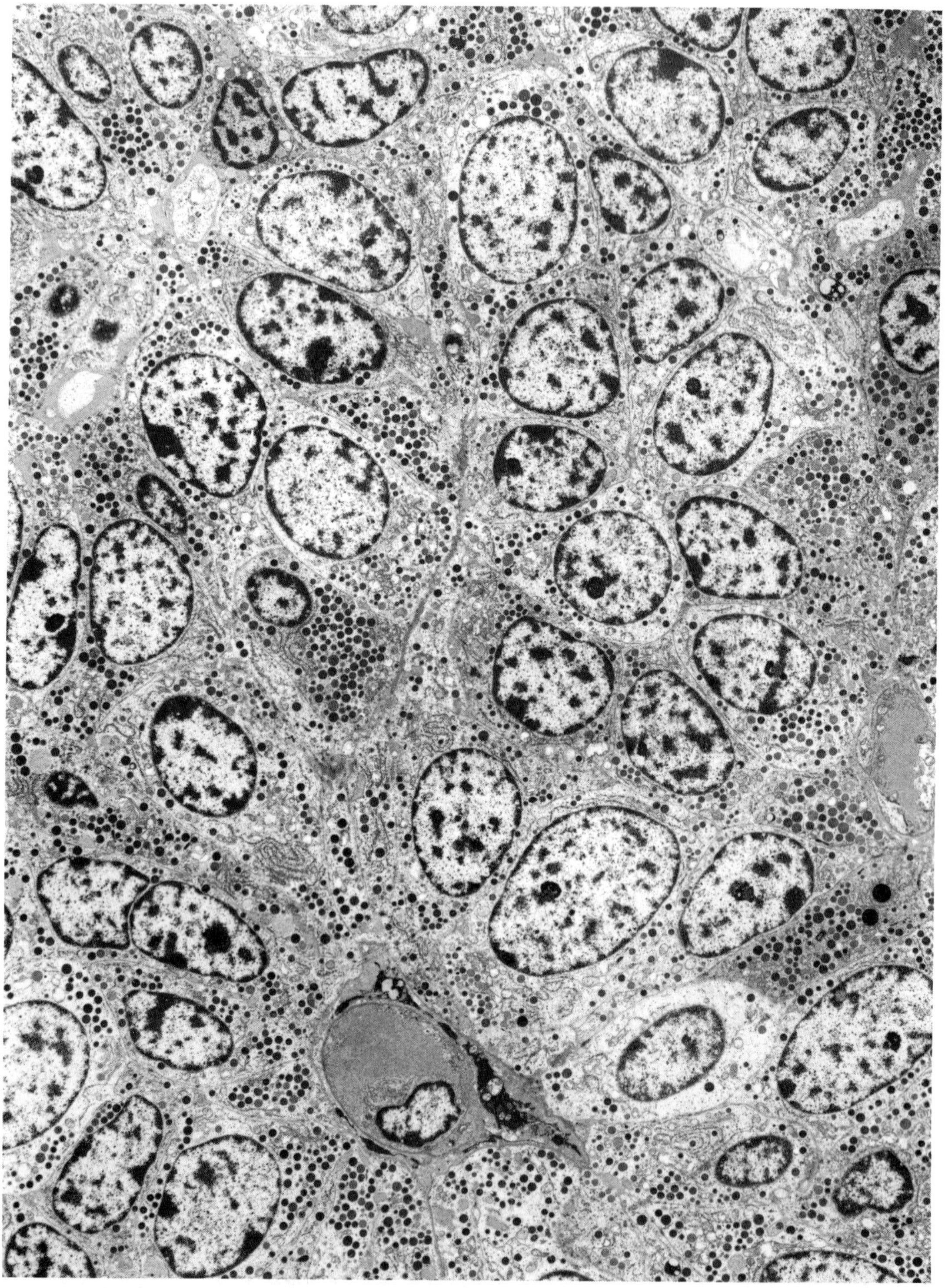

Figure 10–35. Carcinoid. The cells contain numerous granules of relatively large caliber. (×3,200)

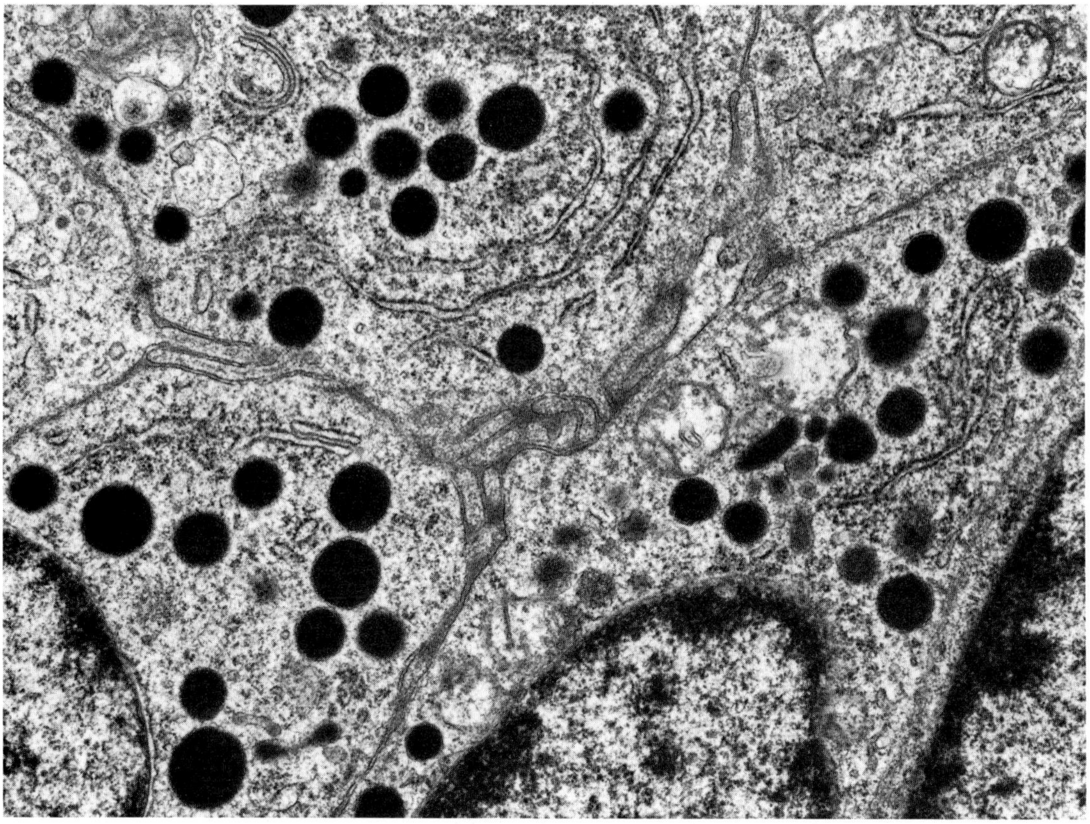

Figure 10–36. Carcinoid. Prominent granules within tumor cells. (×20,000)

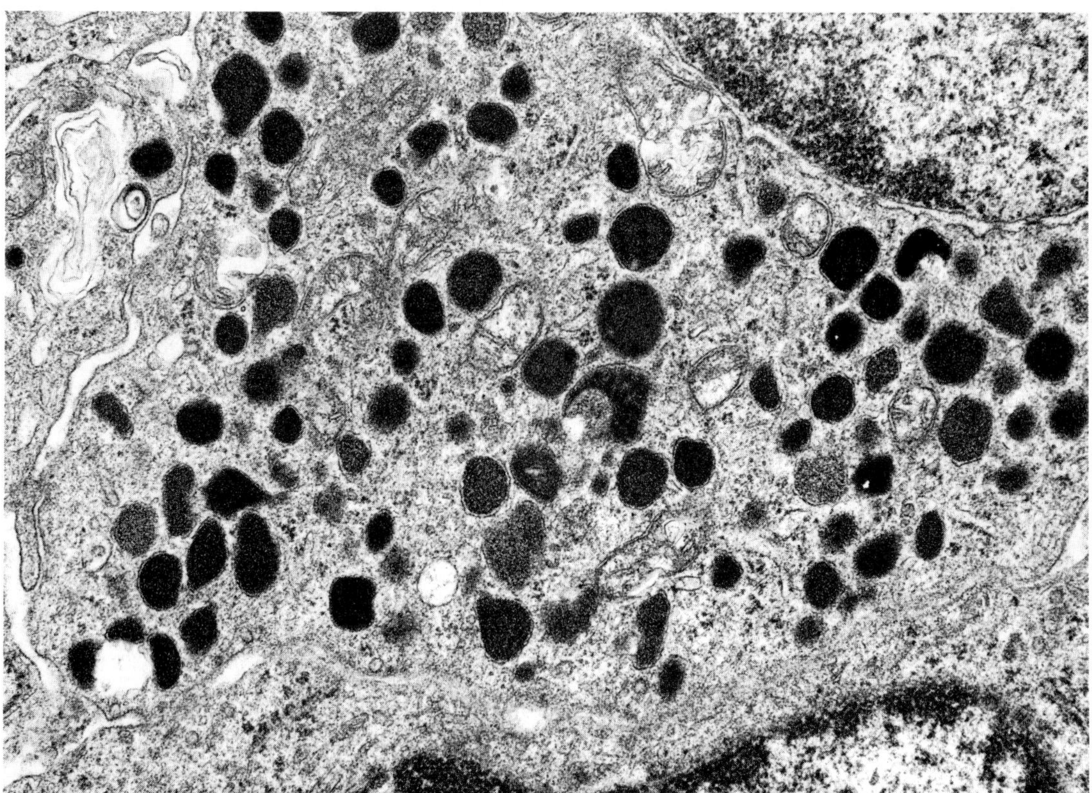

Figure 10–37. Carcinoid. Some pleomorphism of the secretory granules is evident. (×26,000)

ranged in parallel so that stacks or concentric arrays may be seen (Fig. 10–38). The reticulum is unusually prominent in this figure, and the appearance in the cells in Figure 10–39 is more typical.

Because of the range of granule size in bronchial carcinoids,[33] the granules are not always obvious in electron micrographs taken at lower magnifications. This point is illustrated by Figure 10–40. The larger dense bodies in the cytoplasm of the cells are lysosomes, and it might appear that there are no true secretory granules; but they may be made out as tiny dots, and part of a cell with granules of comparable size is shown in Figure 10–41. Intermediate filaments sometimes form discrete aggregates in carcinoid cells[6, 8] (Figs. 10–42 and 10–43), and secretory granules intermingle with the filaments. Glandular differentiation is quite common in bronchial carcinoids,[131] but it is not often well developed. The small acinar lumen with a few microvilli and tight junctions in Figure 10–44 is quite typical, and the lumen may be entirely within the cytoplasm (Fig. 10–45), although tangential slicing through a surface lumen cannot always be ruled out.

No dramatic differences can be seen between the cells of a spindle cell variant of bronchial carcinoid and the tumors with polygonal cells.[45, 63] The granules in spindle cell tumors are generally small to medium in size. They are dwarfed by the lysosomes in Figure 10–46 but are prominent in the elongated cells in Figure 10–47. Geller and Gordon[62] reported a peripheral spindle cell tumor with structures resembling lamellar bodies. When concentric membranous structures are sparse, the possibility of myelin figures must be considered, and immunostaining for surfactant should be performed for confirmation.

Oncocytic transformation in a carcinoid tumor is revealed at the ultrastructural level to be due to an accumulation of mitochondria. Typical[99, 147, 150, 175] and atypical[7] examples have been studied by electron microscopy. The numbers of mitochondria vary,

Text continued on page 277

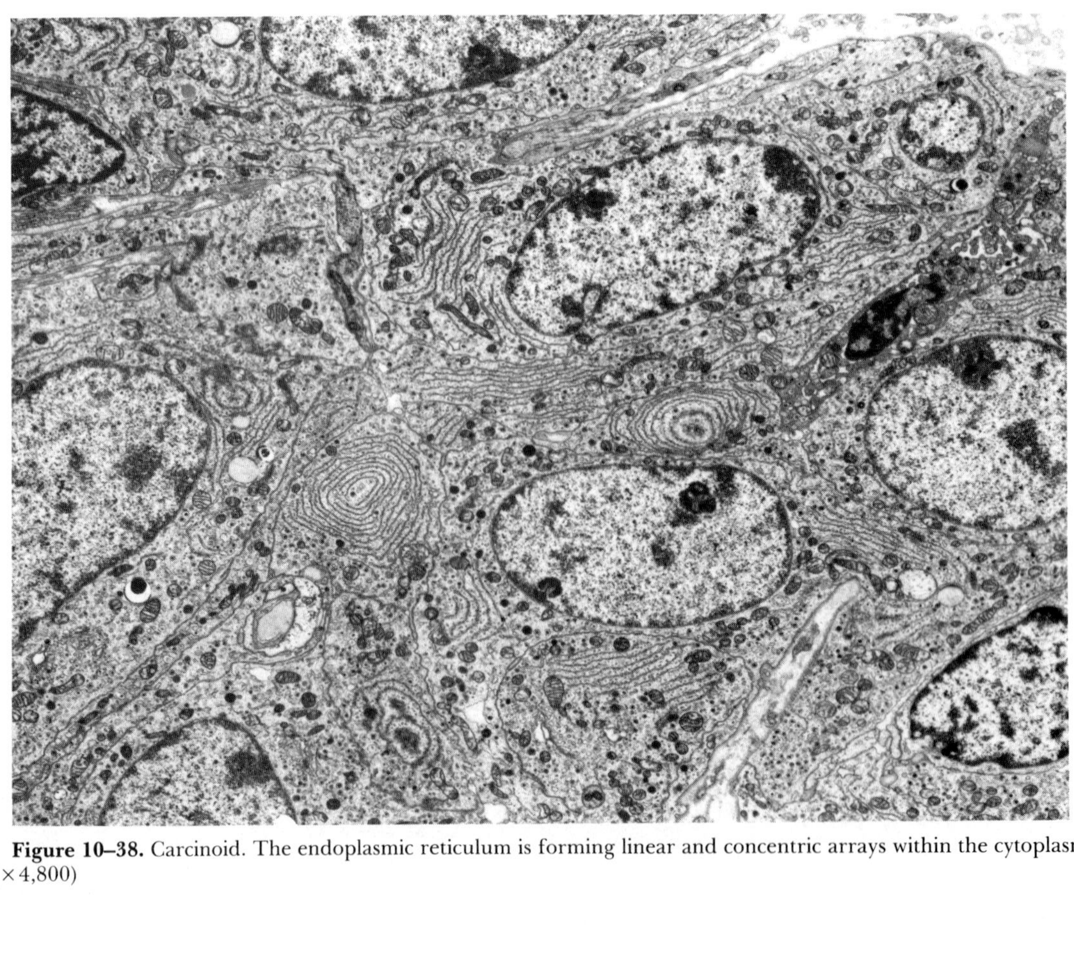

Figure 10–38. Carcinoid. The endoplasmic reticulum is forming linear and concentric arrays within the cytoplasm. (×4,800)

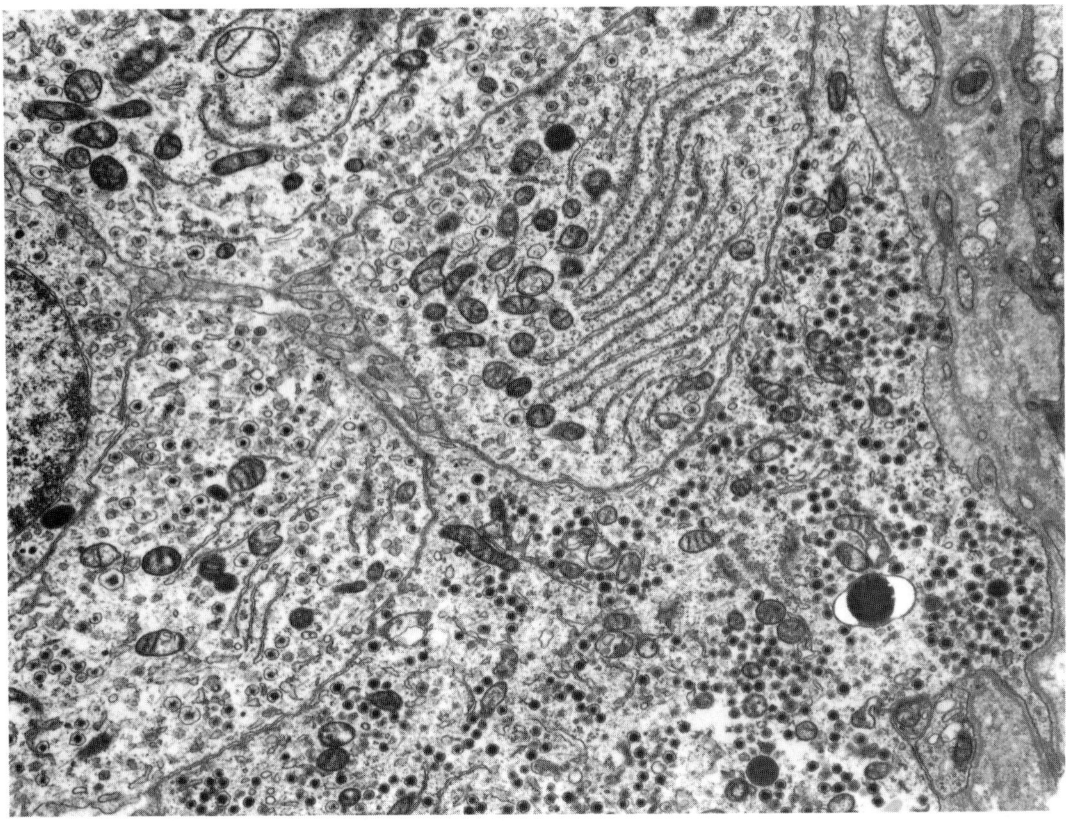

Figure 10–39. Carcinoid. The endoplasmic reticulum is arranged in parallel cisternae. The granules are plentiful but quite small. (×10,800)

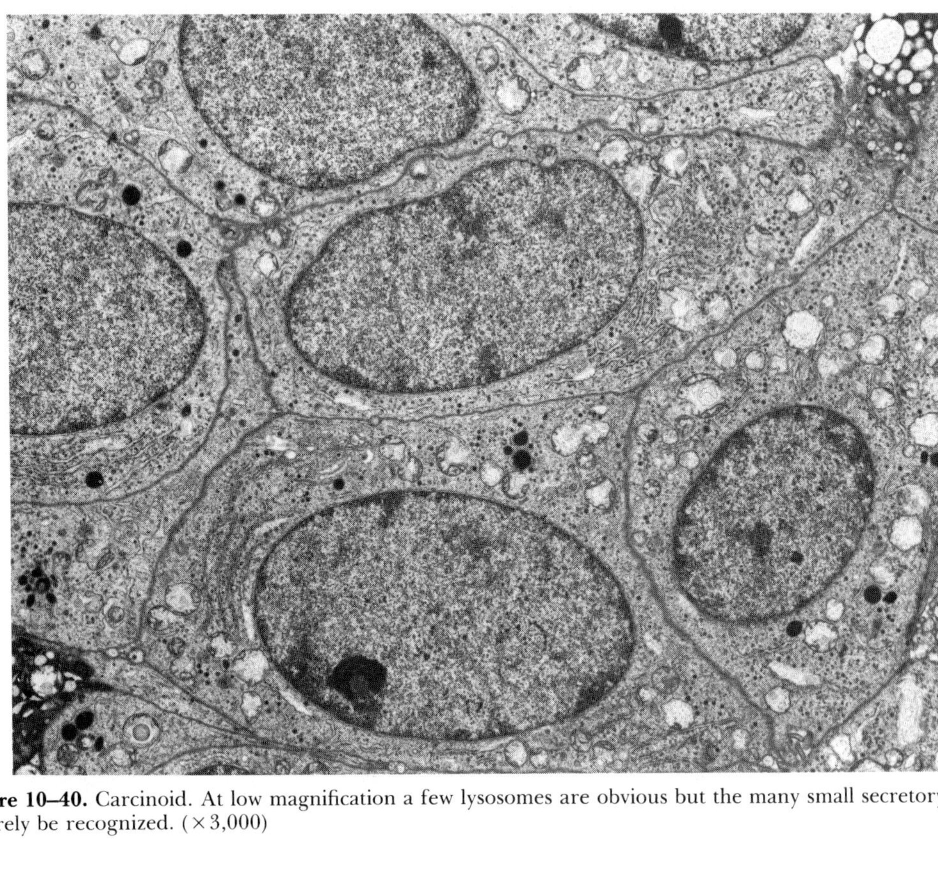

Figure 10–40. Carcinoid. At low magnification a few lysosomes are obvious but the many small secretory granules can barely be recognized. (×3,000)

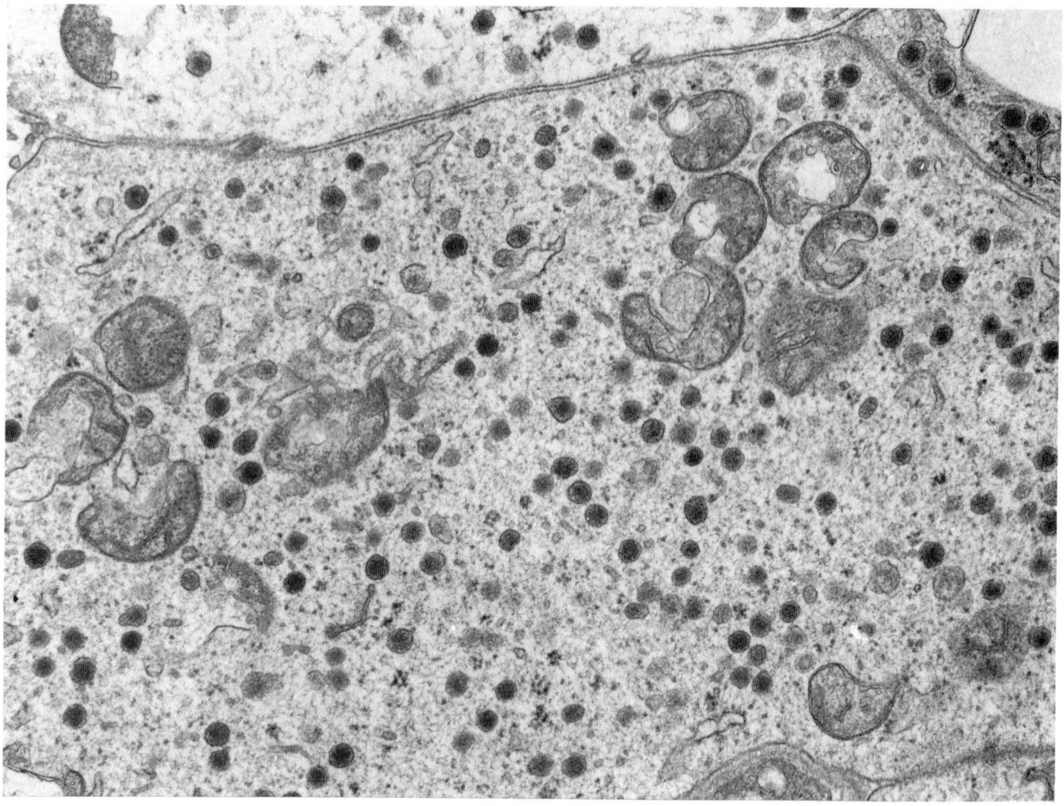

Figure 10–41. Carcinoid. Detail of a small area of the cytoplasm of a tumor cell shows small granules. Contrast their size to that of the mitochondria. (×24,000)

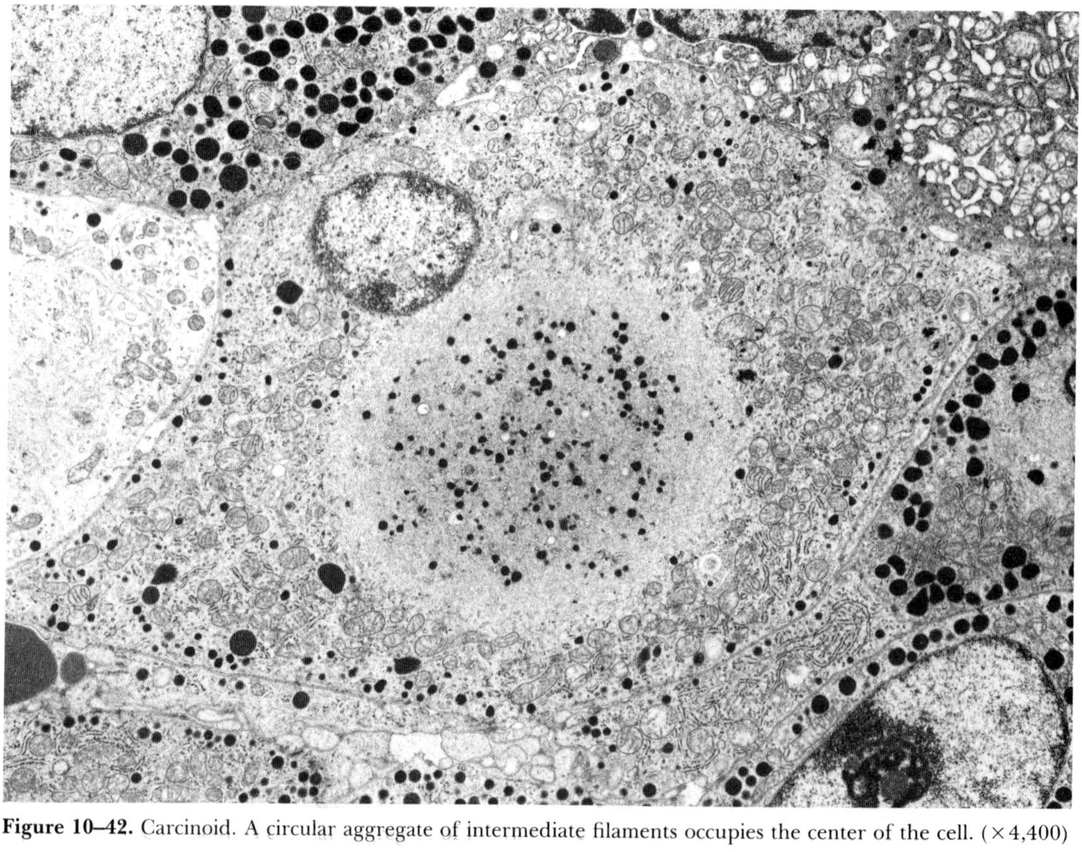

Figure 10–42. Carcinoid. A circular aggregate of intermediate filaments occupies the center of the cell. (×4,400)

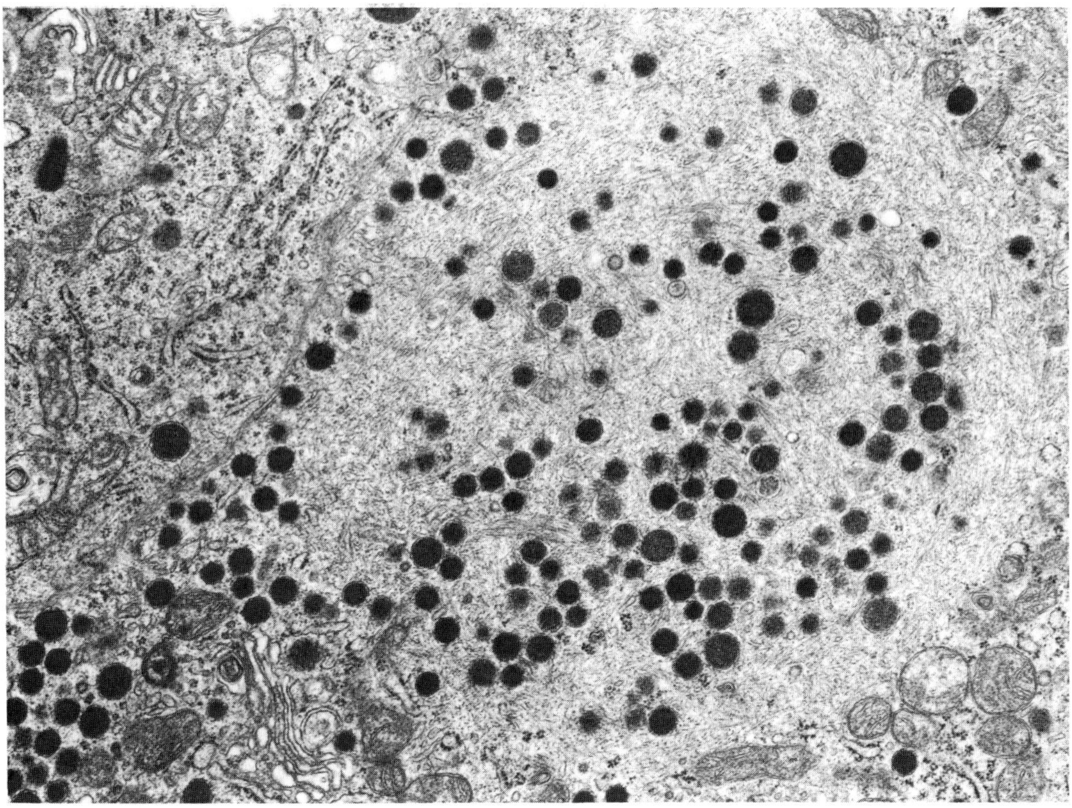

Figure 10–43. Carcinoid. Intermingling of granules and intermediate filaments. (×19,000)

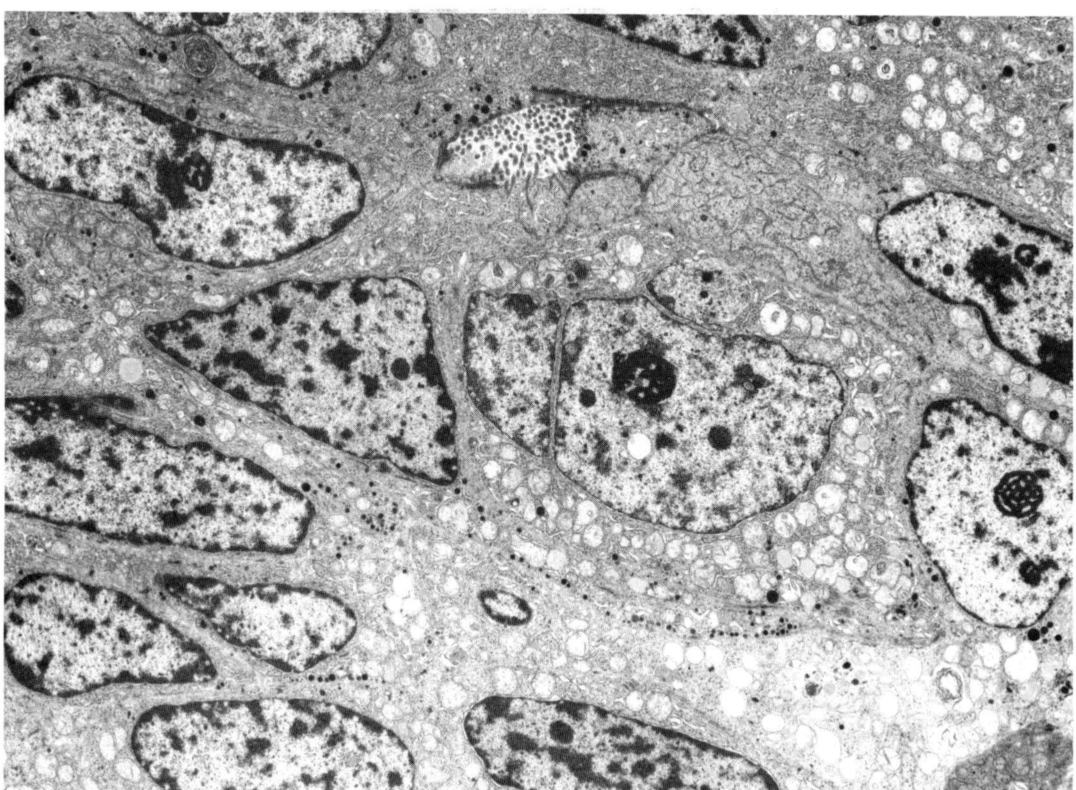

Figure 10–44. Carcinoid. A small lumen containing microvilli is surrounded by tumor cells. (×4,200)

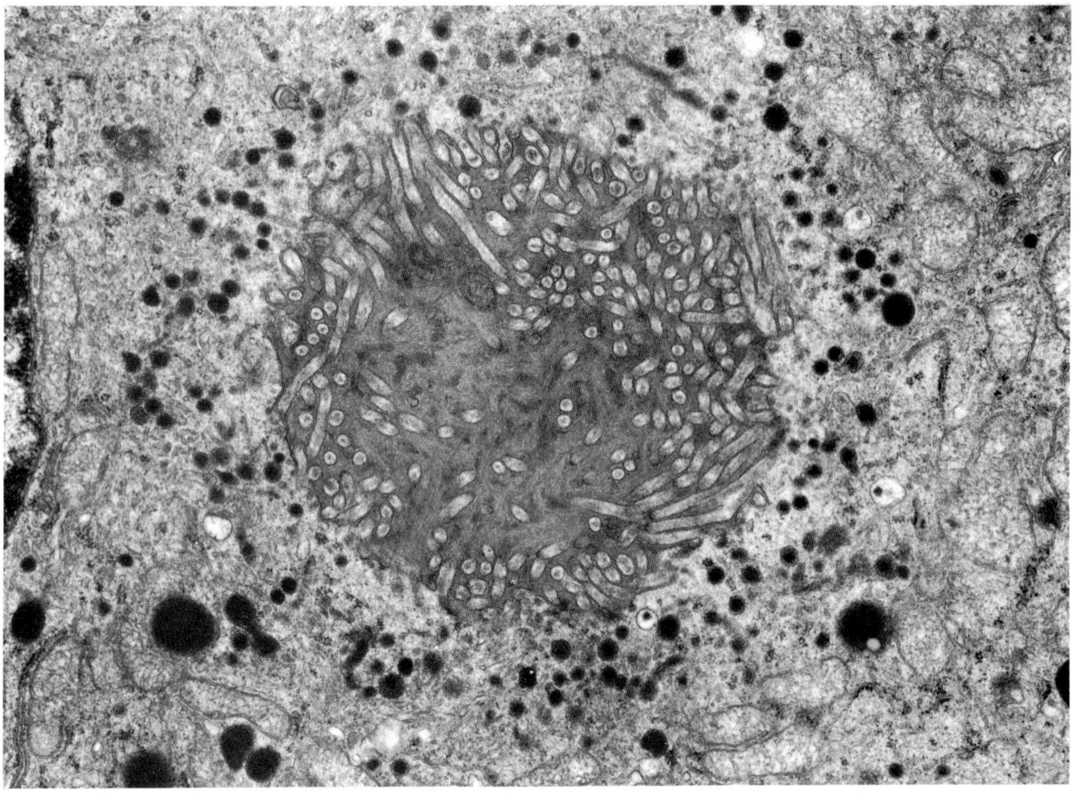

Figure 10–45. Carcinoid. The cell contains an intracytoplasmic lumen with many microvilli. (×17,000)

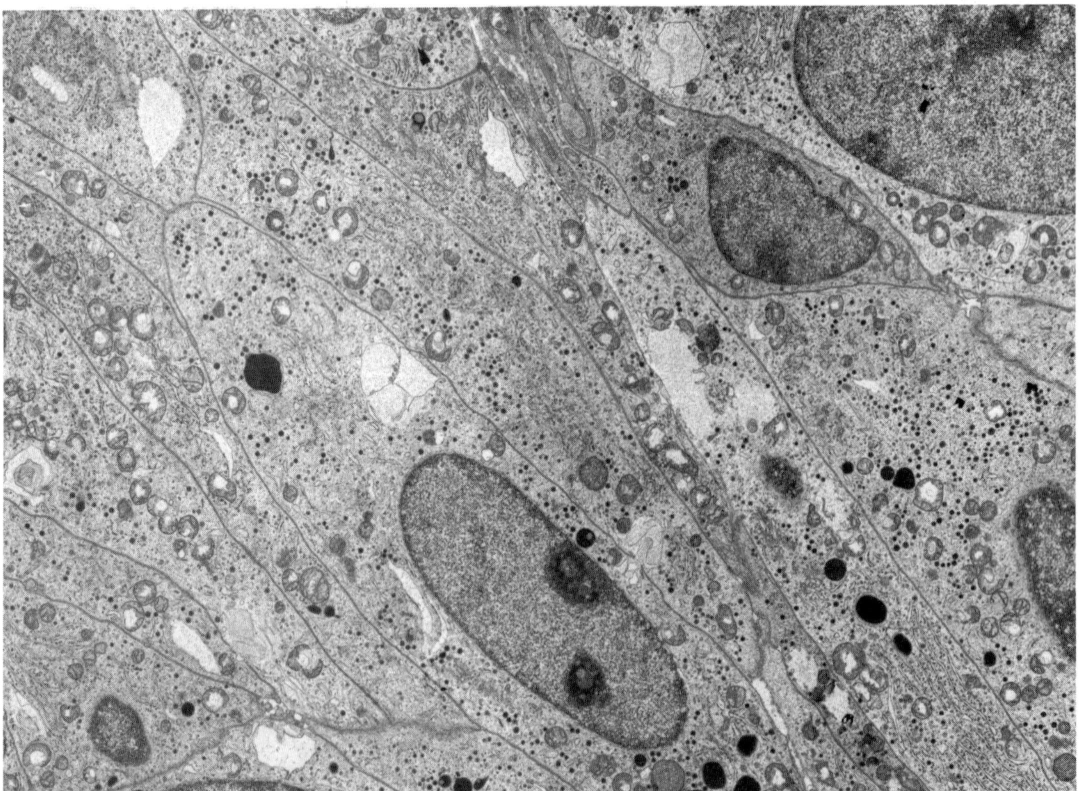

Figure 10–46. Carcinoid, spindle cell variant. The secretory granules are relatively small, but a few larger lysosomes are present. (×5,000)

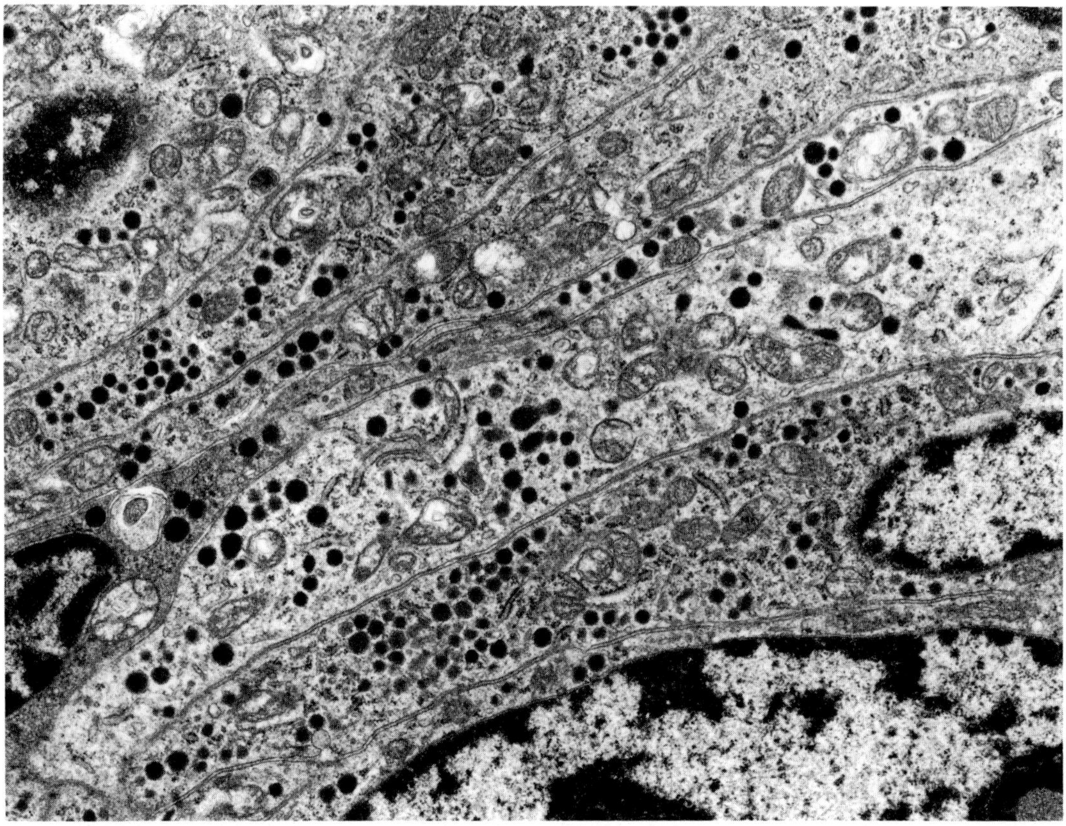

Figure 10–47. Carcinoid, spindle cell variant. The elongated cytoplasm of the tumor cells contains many granules of medium caliber. (×12,000)

and they do not always pack the cytoplasm, nor do they have the altered patterns of cristae that are often seen in salivary gland neoplasms such as Warthin's tumor or in renal oncocytic tumors. It is difficult to gauge the number of mitochondria from the light microscopic appearance. The cells of the tumor shown in Figure 10–48 were markedly eosinophilic in paraffin sections, yet they contain only moderate numbers of mitochondria for an oncocytic neoplasm. When the mitochondria are particularly numerous, it can be difficult to locate dense-core granules. An area of an oncocytic tumor with the typical carcinoid appearance may be present and merge with the oncocytic region through a zone of transitional cells that contain increased numbers of mitochondria and progressively fewer dense-core granules.[147]

ANALYTIC CYTOLOGY

Jones and associates[91] performed flow cytometry on 53 lung carcinoid tumors using material retrieved from paraffin. Twenty-eight tumors were typical and 25 were classified as well-differentiated neuroendocrine carcinomas. Twenty-seven were found to be diploid and 26 aneuploid, and aneuploidy was significantly associated with histologic features of increased malignant potential. In 43 patients with survival data, 19 had diploid tumors and 16 survived 5 years, compared with 14 of 24 patients with aneuploid tumors: the significance is borderline. The authors conclude that although aneuploidy is an indicator of increased malignant potential, it does not provide clinically useful information beyond the findings from conventional histologic examination. Blondal and colleagues[26] found a higher proportion of S-phase cells in small cell carcinomas than in carcinoid tumors.

CARCINOID AND ITS VARIANTS

The term *carcinoid,* applied to a bronchogenic tumor with typical morphology, has a

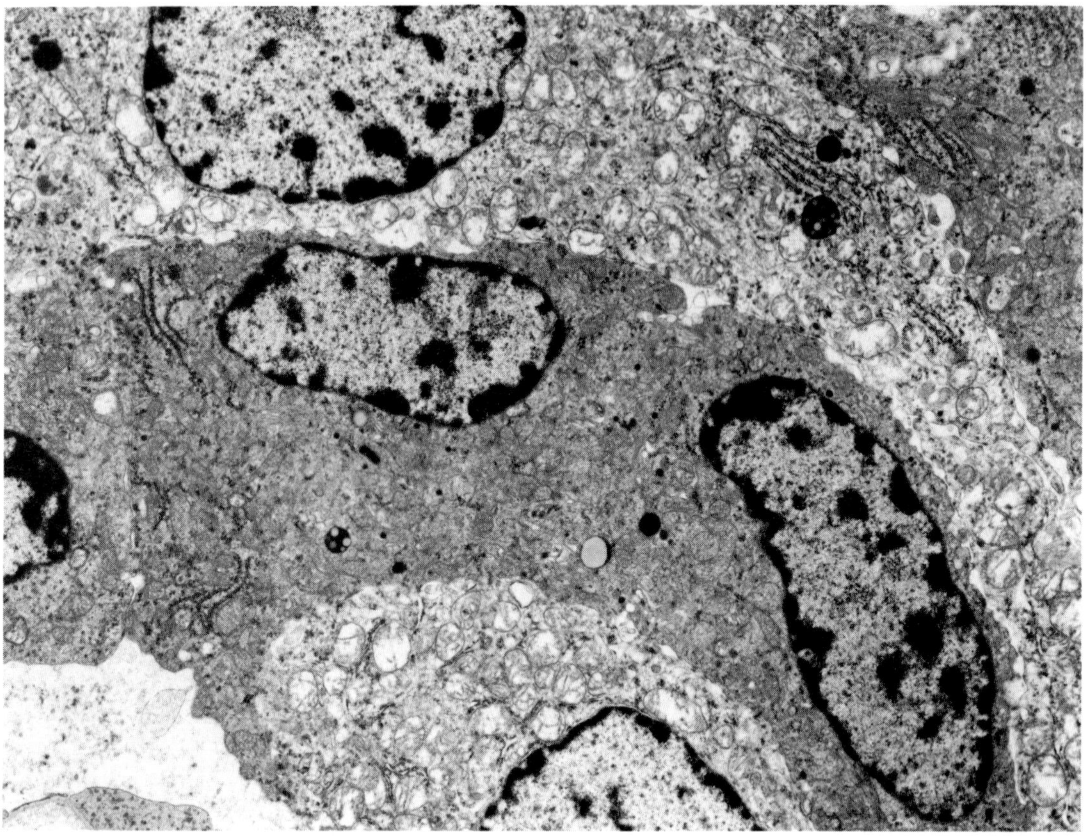

Figure 10–48. Carcinoid, oncocytic variant, with many mitochondria and only scattered granules. (×8,000)

precise connotation to pathologist and clinician. The diagnosis can usually be made with confidence by light microscopy, particularly if a tissue specimen is available, and the prognosis with complete resection is good. If atypical cytologic features are identified, it is appropriate to classify the tumor as an atypical carcinoid: an aggressive and uncertain course can be anticipated, and the need for vigorous management and diligent surveillance is understood. Some atypical carcinoids have metastasized at the time of diagnosis, while others will subsequently give rise to metastases, and it is then reasonable to call the tumor a malignant carcinoid, even though every bronchial carcinoid should be regarded as at least potentially malignant.

It has already been noted that there is overlap in morphology and immunoreactivity between carcinoid tumors and small cell and large cell carcinomas, and this is a source of confusion in diagnosis and uncertainty with regard to terminology. Questions concerning histogenesis are also raised. The overlap reflects similarities in tumor cell structure and common endocrine properties, features that might be traced to embryologic roots or attributed to shared stem cells. Studies on the gut indicate that exocrine and endocrine cells may have a common progenitor capable of multidirectional differentiation.[44, 154] Until more of the variant tumors have been studied and reported, firm conclusions about them are not possible, but it is important to recognize that they exist and to document their features as precisely as possible, and they should be flagged for later clinicopathologic correlation.

Carcinoid is readily distinguished from non–small cell carcinomas with neuroendocrine differentiation when the latter are clearly adenocarcinomas (squamous tumors rarely show this property), but uncertainty may be occasioned when an unusual degree of glandular or papillary structure is present in a carcinoid. A positive mucin stain will strongly favor adenocarcinoma. Separation from undifferentiated large cell carcinoma can be more difficult, although cells of the latter are larger and less uniform; if the nesting pattern of a carcinoid is not found, separation by light microscopy may be impossible.

McDowell and colleagues[120] described 7 malignant peripheral lung tumors that were diagnosed by light microscopy as non–small cell carcinomas. Four of the tumors produced mucin, but 6 contained serotonin and all had dense-core granules. They were designated atypical endocrine tumors. Neal and coworkers[126] found 19 tumors among 205 consecutive primary and metastatic lung cancers that had been diagnosed as small cell carcinomas but contained neuroendocrine granules by electron microscopy and were therefore reclassified as atypical endocrine tumors. Electron microscopy showed glandular differentiation in 12 cases, but none was squamous. The tumors were aggressive, with a median survival of 12 months and a 22% response to combination chemotherapy, and there were no complete responses even though some patients received a small cell carcinoma treatment regimen. Since 8 of the 19 tumors contained mucin and 14 of 19 showed positive periodic acid–Schiff (PAS) staining after diastase digestion, at least some might fall into the category of non–small cell carcinomas with neuroendocrine differentiation.[108, 123]

Mills and co-workers[121] described 17 lung tumors that were histologically intermediate between typical carcinoid and small cell carcinoma. The intermediate-sized, moderately pleomorphic cells did not possess the nuclear molding and dense hyperchromasia of small cell carcinomas, and they formed a distinctive microscopic pattern of nests, trabeculae, and ribbons. Fifteen tumors contained mucin. Electron microscopy was performed on three primary tumors and one metastasis, and dense-core granules and variable degrees of squamous and glandular differentiation were seen. The tumors ranged in size from 2.5 to 20 cm, with a mean size of 4.9 cm. Four patients were treated palliatively and died within 2 to 21 months. The remaining 13 underwent surgical resection (wedge, 2; lobe, 8; lung, 3), and 4 died, while 9 were free of disease after a mean follow-up period of 20 months. Fourteen small cell tumors intermediate between typical carcinoid and small cell carcinoma were reported by Mark and Ramirez.[114] All were peripheral, and 3 were considered low grade and 11 high grade. As with the cases of Mills and co-workers,[121] the behavior was worse than for typical carcinoids but better than that for small cell carcinoma.

The existence of tumors morphologically somewhere between typical carcinoid and small cell carcinoma prompts the assumption that they fall toward the midpoint of a continuous spectrum, but this presupposes a histogenetic relationship that has not as yet been established. There are in fact sufficient differences between carcinoid and small cell carcinoma to support their being regarded as separate entities. The response to combination therapy of small cell carcinoma, the good prognosis of most carcinoids, ultrastructural differences between the tumors, and findings from epidemiologic studies argue for their being different neoplasms, albeit with some similarities. Godwin and colleagues[66] conducted an epidemiologic comparison of 124 carcinoids and 2,751 small cell carcinomas and pointed out that the male to female ratio for carcinoid was 0.85 as against 3.67 for small cell carcinoma. Risk factors identified with small cell carcinoma that have not been observed for carcinoid are cigarette smoking, occupation (*e.g.*, uranium mining), and urban dwelling. Carcinoid tumors may form part of the multiple endocrine neoplasia syndrome, indicating a hereditary connection with other neuroectodermal cells. Extrapulmonary small cell carcinomas occur, but they are uncommon; in the gastrointestinal tract, where carcinoids are seen frequently, small cell carcinoma is a rarity.

These observations call into question the value of attempts to devise a terminology for a spectrum of tumors with carcinoid tumor at one end, small cell carcinoma the opposite extreme, and a place in between for intermediate tumors. Gould and co-workers[68, 177] classified the tumors into four types and introduced the term well-differentiated neuroendocrine carcinoma, which would encompass atypical carcinoids[178] and might be diagnosed from its cytological features,[92] although electron microscopy is clearly useful to establish a precise diagnosis.[56, 76] Paladugu and co-workers[135] suggested the term bronchopulmonary Kulchitsky cell carcinoma, which assumes that the common cell of origin is the bronchial endocrine cell that has been given this and many other names (see Chapter 1). Forster and colleagues[59] applied this classification in a study of 31 tumors.

In conclusion, we would reiterate that there are clear differences between typical lung carcinoids and small cell carcinomas, and careful study of well-preserved tissue or cytology specimens will allow a confident diagnosis in most instances. Intermediate variants do occur, and the name that is applied to them is less important than ensuring that clinicians are aware that they are likely to be aggressive tumors that may not respond to combination chemotherapy. Until more is known about the nature of these intermediate forms, a designation of neuroendocrine carcinoma with an explanatory comment is a convenient if less than ideal compromise.

REFERENCES

1. Abdi EA, Goel R, Bishop S et al: Peripheral carcinoid tumours of the lung: A clinicopathological study. J Surg Oncol 39:190, 1988.
2. Addis BJ, Hamid Q, Ibrahim NBN et al: Immunohistochemical markers of small cell carcinoma and related neuroendocrine tumors of the lung. J Pathol 153:137, 1987.
3. Ahlman H: Serotonin and carcinoid tumors. J Cardiovasc Pharmacol 7:S79, 1985.
4. Al-Kaisi N, Abdul-Karim FW, Mendelsohn G et al: Bronchial carcinoid tumor with amyloid stroma. Arch Pathol Lab Med 112:211, 1988.
5. Altschuler M, Warner RRP, Kirschner PA: Resection of mediastinal metastasis of malignant bronchial carcinoid 32 years after pneumonectomy. NY State J Med 78:2205, 1978.
6. Alvarez-Fernandez E: Intracytoplasmic fibrillary inclusions in bronchial carcinoid. Cancer 46:144, 1980.
7. Alvarez-Fernandez E, Folque-Gomez E: Atypical bronchial carcinoid with oncocytoid features: Its ultrastructure, with special reference to its granular content. Arch Pathol Lab Med 105:428, 1981.
8. An T: Cytoplasmic inclusions in bronchial carcinoid. Hum Pathol 9:241, 1978.
9. Anastasi A, Erspamer V, Bucci M: Isolation and structure of bombesin and alytesin, two analogous active peptides from the skin of European amphibians *Bombina* and *Alytes*. Experientia 27:166, 1971.
10. Arrigoni MG, Woolner LB, Bernatz PE: Atypical carcinoid tumors of the lung. J Thorac Cardiovasc Surg 64:413, 1972.
11. Arrigoni MG, Woolner LB, Bernatz PE: Typical carcinoid tumors of the lung. J Thorac Cardiovasc Surg 79:532, 1980.
12. Asa SL, Kovacs K, Thorner MO et al: Immunohistological localization of growth hormone–releasing hormone in human tumors. J Clin Endocrinol Metabol 60:423, 1985.
13. Ashraf MH: Bronchial carcinoid with osteoblastic metastases. Thorax 32:509, 1977.
14. Attar S, Miller JE, Hankins J et al: Bronchial adenoma: A review of 51 patients. Ann Thorac Surg 40:126, 1985.
15. Barbareschi M, Ferrero S, Frigo B et al: Bronchial carcinoid with S-100 positive sustentacular cells. Tumori 74:705, 1988.
16. Barbareschi M, Frigo B, Cristina S et al: Bronchial carcinoid with paranuclear fibrillary inclusions related to cytokeratins and vimentin. Virchows Arch [A] 415:31, 1989.
17. Barbareschi M, Mauri MF, Muscara M et al: S-100 protein in human lung neuroendocrine neoplasms: Immunohistochemical study of 14 cases and review of the literature. Histol Histopathol 2:185, 1987.
18. Basso-Ricci S, Bertario L, Piva L et al: Pulmonary carcinoid tumors: Report on 19 cases. Int Surg 68:131, 1983.
19. Battifora H, Silva EG: The use of antikeratin antibodies in the immunohistochemical distinction between neuroendocrine (Merkel cell) carcinoma of the skin, lymphoma, and oat cell carcinoma. Cancer 58:1040, 1986.
20. Beaujeu de JM, Chavrier Y, Allantaz F: Les tumeurs broncho-pulmonaires primitives de l'enfant: A propos de 25 cas. Pediatrie 5:419, 1979.
21. Becker KL, Monaghan KG, Silva OL: Immunocytochemical localization of calcitonin in Kulchitsky cells of human lung. Arch Pathol Lab Med 104:196, 1980.
22. Berger G, Berger F, Bejui F et al: Bronchial carcinoid with fibrillary inclusions related to cytokeratins: An immunohistochemical and ultrastructural study with subsequent investigation of 12 foregut APUDomas. Histopathology 8:245, 1984.
23. Bertelsen S, Aasted A, Lund C et al: Bronchial carcinoid tumours: A clinicopathologic study of 82 cases. Scand J Thorac Cardiovasc Surg 19:105, 1985.
24. Bishopric GA, Ordonez NG: Carcinoembryonic antigen in primary carcinoid tumors of the lung. Cancer 58:1316, 1986.
25. Blobel GA, Gould VE, Moll R et al: Coexpression of neuroendocrine markers and epithelial cytoskeletal proteins in bronchopulmonary neuroendocrine neoplasms. Lab Invest 52:39, 1985.
26. Blondal T, Arnorsson, Bengtsson A et al: Nuclear DNA in carcinoid tumours of the lung. Eur J Respir Dis 64:298, 1983.
27. Blondal T, Grimelius L, Now E et al: Argyrophil carcinoid tumors of the lung: Incidence, clinical study and follow-up of 46 patients. Chest 78:840, 1980.
28. Bonikos DS, Archibald R, Bensch KG: Origin of the so-called tumorlets of lung. Hum Pathol 7:461, 1976.
29. Bostwick DG, Bensch KG: Gastrin-releasing peptide in human neuroendocrine tumors. J Pathol 147:237, 1985.
30. Brandt B, Heintz SE, Rose EF et al: Bronchial carcinoid tumors. Ann Thorac Surg 38:63, 1984.
31. Briselli M, Mark GJ, Grillo HC: Tracheal carcinoids. Cancer 42:2870, 1978.
32. Brown BL, Scharifker DA, Gordon R et al: Bronchial carcinoid tumor with ovarian metastasis: A light microscopic and ultrastructural study. Cancer 46:543, 1980.
33. Capella C, Gabrielli M, Polak JM et al: Ultrastructural and histological study of 11 bronchial carcinoids. Virchows Arch [A] 381:313, 1979.
34. Carter D, Yesner R: Carcinomas of the lung with neuroendocrine differentiation. Semin Diagn Pathol 2:235, 1985.
35. Caya JG, Tieu TM, Wollenberg NJ et al: Psam-

moma bodies in malignant carcinoid tumor metastases. Am J Clin Pathol 81:372, 1984.
36. Cebelin MS: Melanocytic bronchial carcinoid tumor. Cancer 46:1843, 1980.
37. Choplin RH, Kawamoto EH, Dyer RB et al: Atypical carcinoid of the lung: Radiographic features. AJR 146:665, 1986.
38. Christen B, Trojanowski JQ, Pietra GG: Immunohistochemical demonstration of phosphorylated and nonphosphorylated forms of human neurofilament subunits in human pulmonary carcinoids. Hum Pathol 18:997, 1987.
39. Churg A: Large spindle cell variant of peripheral bronchial carcinoid tumor. Arch Pathol Lab Med 101:216, 1977.
40. Churg A, Warnock MD: Pulmonary tumorlet: A form of peripheral carcinoid. Cancer 37:1469, 1976.
41. Cookson PJ: Delayed osteoblastic metastases from a childhood bronchial carcinoid tumor. Hum Pathol 5:493, 1974.
42. Cooney T, Sweeney EC, Luke D et al: Pulmonary carcinoid tumours: A comparative regional study. J Clin Pathol 32:1100, 1979.
43. Cooper PH, Warkel RL: Ultrastructure of the goblet cell type of adenocarcinoid of appendix. Cancer 42:2687, 1978.
44. Cox WF, Pierce GB: The endodermal origin of the endocrine cells of an adenocarcinoma of the colon of the rat. Cancer 50:1530, 1982.
45. Craig ID, Finley RJ: Spindle-cell carcinoid tumor of lung. Cytologic, histopathologic and ultrastructural features. Acta Cytol 26:495, 1982.
46. Cutz E, Chan W, Track NS: Bombesin, calcitonin and Leu-enkephalin immunoreactivity in endocrine cells of human lung. Experientia 37:765, 1981.
47. D'Agati VD, Perzin KH: Carcinoid tumorlets of the lung with metastasis to a peribronchial lymph node: Report of a case and review of the literature. Cancer 55:2472, 1985.
48. Dayer AM, DeMey J, Will JA: Localization of somatostatin-, bombesin-, and serotonin-like immunoreactivity in the lung of fetal rhesus monkeys. Cell Tissue Res 239:621, 1985.
49. DeCaro LF, Paladugu R, Benfield JR et al: Typical and atypical carcinoids within the pulmonary APUD tumor spectrum. J Thorac Cardiovasc Surg 86:528, 1983.
50. Dehesdin D, Andrieu-Guitrancourt J, Crenn JY: Carcinoid bronchial cancer in children (a case report). J Fr Otol Rhinol Laryngol 33:15, 1984.
51. De Lellis RA, Dayal Y, Wolfe HJ: Carcinoid tumors: Changing concepts and new perspectives. Am J Surg Pathol 8:295, 1984.
52. De Stephano DB, Lloyd RV, Schteingart DE: Cushing's syndrome produced by a bronchial carcinoid tumor. Hum Pathol 15:890, 1984.
53. El-Salhy M, Lundqvist M, Wilander E: Bronchial carcinoids and pheochromocytomas: A comparative study with special emphasis on S-100 protein, serotonin and neuron-specific enolase (NSE) immunoreactivity. Acta Pathol Microbiol Scand [A] 94:229, 1986.
54. Elhassani NB: Bronchial carcinoid tumors. Ann Saudi Med 8:35, 1988.
55. Engelbreth-Holm J: Benign bronchial adenoma. Acta Chir Scand 90:383, 1944.
56. Erlandson RA: Carcinoid and atypical carcinoid (well-differentiated neuroendocrine carcinoma) of the lung. Ultrastruct Pathol 13:333, 1989.
57. Farhangi M, Taylor J, Havey A et al: Neuroendocrine (carcinoid) tumor of the lung and type I multiple endocrine neoplasia. South Med J 80:1459, 1987.
58. Fechner RE, Bentinck BR: Ultrastructural of bronchial oncocytoma. Cancer 31:1451, 1973.
59. Forster BB, Muller NL, Miller RR et al: Neuroendocrine carcinomas of the lung: Clinical, radiologic, and pathologic correlation. Radiology 170:441, 1989.
60. Frierson HF, Covell JL, Mills SE: Fine-needle aspiration cytology of atypical carcinoid of the lung. Acta Cytol 31:471, 1987.
61. Fu YS, McWilliams NB, Stratford TP et al: Bronchial carcinoid with choroidal metastasis in an adolescent: Case report and ultrastructural study. Cancer 33:707, 1974.
62. Geller SA, Gordon RE: Peripheral spindle cell carcinoid tumor of the lung with type II pneumocyte features: An ultrastructural study with comments on possible histogenesis. Am J Surg Pathol 8:145, 1984.
63. Gillespie JJ, Luiger A, Callaway LA et al: Peripheral spindled carcinoid tumor: A review of its ultrastructure, differential diagnosis, and biologic behavior. Hum Pathol 10:601, 1979.
64. Givens CD, Marini JJ: Transbronchial needle aspiration of a bronchial carcinoid tumor. Chest 88:152, 1985.
65. Gloor E, Campiche M, Libanska C et al: Bronchopulmonary carcinoid tumours: Pathological study of 37 cases. Arch Anat Cytol Pathol 26:19, 1978.
66. Godwin JD, Brown CC: Comparative epidemiology of carcinoid and oat cell tumors of the lung. Cancer 40:1671, 1977.
67. Gould VE, Lee I, Warren WH: Immunohistochemical evaluation of neuroendocrine cells and neoplasms of the lung. Pathol Res Pract 183:200, 1988.
68. Gould VE, Linoila RI, Memoli VA: Neuroendocrine cells and neuroendocrine neoplasms of the lung. Pathol Annu 18:287, 1983.
69. Gould VE, Memoli VA, Dardi LE et al: Neuroendocrine carcinomas with multiple immunoreactive peptides and melanin production. Ultrastruct Pathol 2:199, 1981.
70. Gould VE, Wiedenmann B, Lee I et al: Synaptophysin expression in neuroendocrine neoplasms as determined by immunocytochemistry. Am J Pathol 126:243, 1987.
71. Grazer R, Cohen SM, Jacobs JB et al: Melanin-containing peripheral carcinoids of the lung. Am J Surg Pathol 6:73, 1982.
72. Greenberg RS, Baumgarten DA, Clark WS et al: Prognostic factors for gastrointestinal and bronchopulmonary carcinoid tumors. Cancer 60:2476, 1987.
73. Greengard O, Head JF, Goldberg SL et al: Pulmonary carcinoid tumors: Enzymic discriminants, growth rate, and early age of inception. Cancer Res 46:2600, 1986.
74. Grote TH, Macon WR, Davis FB et al: Atypical carcinoid of the lung: A distinct clinicopathologic entity. Chest 93:370, 1988.
75. Hajdu SI, Winawer SJ, Myers WP: Carcinoid tu-

mors: A study of 204 cases. Am J Clin Pathol 61:521, 1974.
76. Hammond ME, Sause WT: Large cell neuroendocrine tumors of the lung: Clinical significance and histopathologic definition. Cancer 56:1624, 1985.
77. Hamperl H: Uber gutartige Bronchialtumoren (Cylindrome und Carcinoide). Virchows Arch [A] 300:46, 1937.
78. Harrist TJ, Kalisher L: Breast metastasis: An unusual manifestation of a malignant carcinoid tumor. Cancer 40:3102, 1977.
79. Hartman GE, Shochet SJ: Primary pulmonary neoplasms of childhood: A review. Ann Thorac Surg 36:108, 1983.
80. Hasleton PS, Al-Saffar N: The histological spectrum of bronchial carcinoid tumours. Appl Pathol 7:205, 1989.
81. Hausman DH, Weinmann RB: Pulmonary tumorlet with hilar lymph node metastases: Report of a case. Cancer 20:1515, 1967.
82. Hearn PR, Reynolds CL, Johansen K: Lung carcinoid with Cushing's syndrome: Control of serum ACTH and cortisol levels using SMS 201-995 (Sandostatin). Clin Endocrinol 28:181, 1988.
83. Heitz PU: Neuroendocrine tumor markers. Curr Top Pathol 77:279, 1987.
84. Hepper NG, Payne WS, Sheps SG et al: Unilateral hypoperfusion of the lung and carcinoid syndrome due to bronchial carcinoid tumor. Am Rev Respir Dis 115:351, 1977.
85. Herrlinger JD, Euler HH, Kleine L et al: Successful conservative treatment of bronchial carcinoid with Cushing's syndrome due to ectopic ACTH production. Dtsch Med Wochenschr 108:1200, 1983.
86. Hoog A, Gould VE, Grimelius L et al: Tissue fixation methods alter the immunohistochemical demonstrability of synaptophysin. Ultrastruct Pathol 12:673, 1988.
87. Horan DC, Bonfiglio TA, Patten SF et al: Fineneedle aspiration cytopathology of bronchial carcinoid tumor: An analytical study of the cells. Anal Quant Cytol 4:105, 1982.
88. Hurt R, Bates M: Carcinoid tumours of the bronchus: A 33-year experience. Thorax 39:617, 1984.
89. Imura H, Matsukura S, Yamamoto H: Studies of ectopic ACTH-producing tumors. Cancer 35:1430, 1975.
90. Isawa T, Okubo K, Konno K et al: Cushing's syndrome caused by recurrent malignant bronchial carcinoid: Case report with 12 years' observation. Am Rev Respir Dis 108:1200, 1973.
91. Jones DJ, Hasleton PS, Moore M: DNA ploidy in bronchopulmonary carcinoid tumours. Thorax 43:195, 1988.
92. Jordan AG, Predmore L, Sullivan MM et al: The cytodiagnosis of well-differentiated neuroendocrine carcinoma: A distinct clinicopathologic entity. Acta Cytol 31:464, 1987.
93. Kaminski PF, Tavassoli FA: Plexiform tumorlet: A clinical and pathologic study of 15 cases with ultrastructural observations. Int J Gynecol Pathol 3:124, 1984.
94. Keane J, Fretzin DF, Jao W et al: Bronchial carcinoid metastatic to skin. J Cutan Pathol 7:43, 1980.
95. Keller KM, Helwig H: Carcinoid tumor of the lung in childhood: Review and case report. Klin Pediatr 193:355, 1981.
96. Kim K, Mah C, Dominguez J: Carcinoid tumors of the lung: Cytologic differential dignosis in fineneedle aspirates. Diagn Cytopathol 2:343, 1986.
97. Kramer R: Adenoma of bronchus. Ann Otol Rhinol Laryngol 39:689, 1930.
98. Krawisz BR, Ludwig J: Multiple bronchial carcinoid tumors. Am J Surg Pathol 4:309, 1980.
99. Kuwahara T, Maruyama K, Mochizuki S et al: Oncocytic carcinoid of the lung: An ultrastructural observation. Acta Pathol Jpn 34:355, 1984.
100. Laennec RTH: Traite de l'Auscultation Mediate et des Maladies des Poumons et du Coeur, 3rd ed, vol 1, p 250. Paris, Chaude, 1831.
101. Lawson RM, Ramanathan L, Hurley G et al: Bronchial adenoma: Review of an 18-year experience at the Brompton Hospital. Thorax 31:245, 1976.
102. Leader M, Collins M, Patel J et al: Anti–neuronspecific enolase staining reactions in sarcomas and carcinomas: Its lack of neuroendocrine specificity. J Clin Pathol 39:1186, 1986.
103. Lee I, Radosevich JA, Ma YX et al: Immunocytochemical analysis of human pulmonary carcinomas using monoclonal antibody 44-3A6. Cancer Res 45:5813, 1985.
104. Lehto VP, Miettinen M, Dahl D et al: Bronchial carcinoid cells contain neural-type intermediate filaments. Cancer 54:624, 1984.
105. Lehto VP, Miettinen M, Virtanen I: A dual expression of cytokeratin and neurofilaments in bronchial carcinoid cells. Int J Cancer 35:421, 1985.
106. Leonhardt P, Gosse H: Value of cytologic diagnosis of pulmonary carcinoid tumors: A morphologicoclinical analysis. Zentralbl Allg Pathol 133:285, 1987.
107. Lewin KJ, Layfield L, Cheng L: Disseminated bombesin-producing carcinoid tumor of pulmonary origin. Am J Surg Pathol 9:129, 1985.
108. Linnoila RI, Mulshine JL, Steinberg SM et al: Neuroendocrine differentiation in endocrine and nonendocrine lung carcinomas. Am J Clin Pathol 90:641, 1988.
109. Lovett JV, Manalo PB, Barcia TC et al: Diagnosis of pulmonary masses by fine-needle aspiration. Am J Surg 156:441, 1988.
110. Lozowski W, Hajdu SI, Melamed MR: Cytomorphology of carcinoid tumors. Acta Cytol 23:360, 1979.
111. Lubarsch O: Ueber den primaren Krebs des Ileum nebst Bemerkungen uber das gleichzeitige Vorkommen Von Krebs und Tuberculose. Virchows Arch [A] 111:280, 1888.
112. Magid D, Siegelman SS, Eggleston JC et al: Pulmonary carcinoid tumors: CT assessment. J Comput Assist Tomogr 13:244, 1989.
113. Mark EJ, Quay SC, Dickersin GR: Papillary carcinoid tumor of the lung. Cancer 48:316, 1981.
114. Mark EJ, Ramirez JF: Peripheral small-cell carcinoma of the lung resembling carcinoid tumor: A clinical and pathologic study of 14 cases. Arch Pathol Lab Med 109:263, 1985.
115. Marks C, Marks PH: Bronchial carcinoids and hormonal disorders. South Med J 71:108, 1978.
116. Mason AMS, Ratcliffe JG, Buckle RM et al: ACTH secretion by bronchial carcinoid tumors. Clin Endocrinol 1:3, 1972.
117. May EE, Perentes E: Anti-Leu-7 immunoreactivity with human tumors: Its value in the diagnosis

of prostatic adenocarcinoma. Histopathology 11:295, 1987.
118. McCaughan BC, Martin N, Bains MS: Bronchial carcinoids: Review of 124 cases. J Thorac Cardiovasc Surg 89:8, 1985.
119. McDonald TJ, Jörnvall H, Nilsson G et al: Characterization of gastrin-releasing peptide from porcine non-antral tissue. Biochem Biophys Res Commun 90:227, 1979.
120. McDowell EM, Wilson TS, Trump BF: Atypical endocrine tumors of the lung. Arch Pathol Lab Med 105:20, 1981.
121. Mills SE, Cooper PH, Walker AN et al: Atypical carcinoid tumor of the lung: A clinicopathologic study of 17 cases. Am J Surg Pathol 6:643, 1982.
122. Minamino N, Kangawa K, Matsuo H et al: Neuromedin C: A bombesin-like peptide identified in porcine spinal cord. Biochem Biophys Res Commun 119:14, 1984.
123. Mooi WJ, Dewar A, Springall D et al: Non–small cell lung carcinomas with neuroendocrine features: A light microscopic, immunohistochemical and ultrastructural study of 11 cases. Histopathology 13:329, 1988.
124. Mueller H: Sur Entstehungsgeschichte der Bronchialerweiterungen. Ermsleben, East Germany, Busch, 1882.
125. Nakajima T, Watanabe S, Sato Y et al: An immunoperoxidase study of S-100 protein distribution in normal and neoplastic tissues. Am J Surg Pathol 6:715, 1982.
126. Neal MA, Kosinski R, Cohen P et al: Atypical endocrine tumors of the lung: A histologic, transmission electron microscopic and clinical study of 19 cases. Am J Clin Pathol 85:386, 1986.
127. Nielsen AL: Malignant bronchial oncocytoma: Case report and review of the literature. Hum Pathol 16:852, 1985.
128. Nishikawa A, Nakamura A, Nishikawa H et al: Exfoliative cytopathology of atypical pulmonary carcinoid: A case report. Jpn J Clin Oncol 16:413, 1986.
129. Oates JA: The carcinoid syndrome. N Engl J Med 315:702, 1986.
130. Obendorfer A: Karzinoide tumoren des Dunndarms. Frankfurt A Pathol 1:426, 1907.
131. Ohtsuki H, Midorikawa O, Okada H et al: Pulmonary atypical carcinoid tumor with marked alpha-fetoprotein production and features of an adenocarcinoma differentiation. Pathol Res Pract 184:86, 1988.
132. Okike N, Bernatz PE, Woolner LB: Carcinoid tumors of the lung. Ann Thorac Surg 22:270, 1976.
133. Olurin EO, Sofowora O, Afonja AO et al: Cushing's syndrome and bronchial carcinoid tumor. Cancer 31:1514, 1973.
134. Pagel W: Uber den Zusammengang von ungewohnlichen Wucherungen atypischen und ortsfremden Epithels der Bronchien mit Bronchiesktasien. Virchows Arch [A] 262:583, 1926.
135. Paladugu RR, Benfield JR, Pak HY et al: Bronchopulmonary Kulchitzky cell carcinomas: A new classification scheme for typical and atypical carcinoids. Cancer 55:1303, 1983.
136. Radke R: Carcinoid of the distal trachea. Z Erkr Atmungsorgane 159:221, 1982.
137. Ranchod M: The histogenesis and development of pulmonary tumorlets. Cancer 39:1135, 1978.
138. Ranchod M, Levine GD: Spindle cell carcinoid tumors of the lung: A clinicopathologic study of 35 cases. Am J Surg Pathol 4:315, 1980.
139. Reeve JR, Walsh JH, Chew P et al: Amino acid sequences of three bombesin-like peptides from canine intestine extracts. J Biol Chem 258:5582, 1983.
140. Ricci C, Patrassi N, Massa R: Carcinoid syndrome in bronchial adenoma. Am J Surg 126:671, 1973.
141. Riddell K, Tippens D, Gown AM: PHE-5, a new monclonal antibody to a unique neuroendocrine granule protein. Lab Invest 56:64A, 1987.
142. Rodgers-Sullivan RF, Weiland LH, Palumbo PJ et al: Pulmonary tumorlets associated with Cushing's syndrome. Am Rev Respir Dis 117:799, 1978.
143. Rodriguez FH, Sarma DP, Lunseth JH: Goblet cell carcinoid of the appendix. Hum Pathol 13:286, 1982.
144. Rusthoven JJ, Robinson JB, Kolin A et al: The natural killer cell–associated HNK-1 (Leu-7) antibody reacts with hypertrophic and malignant prostatic epithelium. Cancer 56:289, 1985.
145. Saeed uz Zafar M, Mellinger RC, Fine G, et al: Acromegaly associated with a bronchogenic carcinoid tumor: Evidence for ectopic production of growth hormone–releasing activity. J Clin Endocrinol Metab 48:66, 1979.
146. Said JW, Vimadalal S, Nash G et al: Immunoreactive neuron-specific enolase, bombesin, and chromogranin as markers for neuroendocrine lung tumors. Hum Pathol 16:236, 1985.
147. Sajjad SM, Mackay B, Lukeman JM: Oncocytic carcinoid tumor of the lung. Ultrastruct Pathol 1:171, 1980.
148. Salyer DC, Salyer WR, Eggleston JC: Bronchial carcinoid tumors. Cancer 36:1522, 1975.
149. Santos-Briz A, Terron J, Sastre R et al: Oncocytoma of the lung. Cancer 40:1330, 1977.
150. Scharifker D, Marchevsky A: Oncocytic carcinoid of lung: An ultrastructural analysis. Cancer 47:530, 1981.
151. Scheithauer BW, Carpenter PC, Bloch B et al: Ectopic secretion of a growth hormone–releasing factor: Report of a case of acromegaly with bronchial carcinoid tumor. Am J Med 76:605, 1984.
152. Shaw JH, Canal A: Carcinoid tumours in Auckland, New Zealand. Aust NZ J Surg 59:229, 1989.
153. Sibley RK, Dahl D: Primary neuroendocrine (Merkel cell?) carcinoma of the skin: II. An immunocytochemical study of 21 cases. Am J Surg Pathol 9:109, 1985.
154. Sidhu GS: The endodermal origin of digestive and respiratory tract APUD cells: Histopathologic evidence and a review of the literature. Am J Pathol 96:5, 1979.
155. Siwersson U, Kindblom LG: Oncocytic carcinoid of the nasal cavity and carcinoid of the lung in a child. Pathol Res Pract 178:562, 1984.
156. Skinner C, Ewen SWB: Carcinoid lung: Diffuse pulmonary infiltration by a multifocal bronchial carcinoid. Thorax 31:212, 1976.
157. Sklar JL, Churg A, Bensch KG: Oncocytic carcinoid tumor of the lung. Am J Surg Pathol 4:287, 1980.
158. Soga J, Tazawa K, Aizawa O et al: Argentaffin cell adenocarcinoma of the stomach: An atypical carcinoid. Cancer 28:999, 1971.

159. Springall DR, Lackie P, Levene MM et al: Immunostaining of neuron-specific enolase is a valuable aid to the cytological diagnosis of neuroendocrine tumours of the lung. J Pathol 143:259, 1984.
160. Sukumaran M, Wilkinson ZS, Christianson L et al: Acute carcinoid syndrome: A complication of flexible fiberoptic bronchoscopy. Ann Thorac Surg 34:702, 1982.
161. Suzuki K, Kimula Y, Ogata T et al: Bronchial carcinoid with multiple aerogenous implanted foci. J Surg Oncol 34:211, 1987.
162. Sweeney EC, Cooney T: Mucin producing atypical bronchial carcinoid. J Clin Pathol 31:1218, 1978.
163. Szyfelbein WM, Ross JS: Carcinoids, atypical carcinoids, and small-cell carcinomas of the lung: Differential diagnosis of fine-needle aspiration biopsy specimens. Diagn Cytopathol 4:1, 1988.
164. Talerman A: Multiple foci of atypical epithelial hyperplasia (tumourlets) in irradiated human lungs. Br J Radiol 46:464, 1973.
165. Tamai S, Kameya T, Yamaguchi K et al: Peripheral lung carcinoid tumor producing predominantly gastrin releasing peptide (GRP): Morphological and hormonal studies. Cancer 52:273, 1983.
166. Terzakis JA: Bronchial adenocarcinoid tumor metastatic to skin. Hum Pathol 15:1188, 1984.
167. Tesluk H, Dajee A: Pulmonary oncocytoma. J Surg Oncol 29:173, 1985.
168. Thunnissen FB, Van-Eijk J, Baak JP et al: Bronchopulmonary carcinoids and regional lymph node metastases: A quantitative pathologic investigation. Am J Pathol 132:119, 1988.
169. Todd TR, Cooper JD, Weissberg D et al: Bronchial carcinoid tumors: Twenty years' experience. J Thorac Cardiovasc Surg 79:532, 1980.
170. Tsutsumi Y, Osamura RY, Watanabe K et al: Immunohistochemical studies on gastrin releasing peptide and adrenocorticotropic hormone–containing cells in human lung. Lab Invest 48:623, 1983.
171. Van der Veen F, Van den Bosch JMM, Wagenaar SS et al: Bronchial carcinoid: Discussion of 51 cases. Ned Tijdschr Geneeskd 125:217, 1981.
172. Viard H, Cayot M: Carcinoid tumors of the bronchi: Fifteen cases. Ann Chir 33:537, 1979.
173. Vinores SA, Bonnin JM, Rubinstein LJ et al: Immunohistochemical demonstration of neuron-specific enolase in neoplasms of the CNS and other tissues. Arch Pathol Lab Med 108:536, 1984.
174. Wahab ZA, Wright GL Jr: Monoclonal antibody (anti-Leu-7) directed against natural killer cells reacts with normal, benign and malignant prostate tissues. Int J Cancer 36:677, 1985.
175. Walter A, Walter P: Bronchial oncocytic carcinoid: Histological, histochemical and ultrastructural studies. Arch Anat Cytol Pathol 27:63, 1979.
176. Warner TFCS: Bronchial carcinoid appearing as a breast mass. Arch Pathol Lab Med 104:531, 1980.
177. Warren WH, Faber LP, Gould VE: Neuroendocrine neoplasms of the lung: A clinicopathologic update. J Thorac Cardiovasc Surg 98:321, 1989.
178. Warren WH, Memoli VA, Gould VE: Immunohistochemical and ultrastructural analysis of bronchopulmonary neuroendocrine neoplasms: II. Well-differentiated neuroendocrine carcinomas. Ultrastruct Pathol 7:185, 1984.
179. Warthon J, Polak JM, Bloom SR et al: Bombesin-like immunoreactivity in the lung. Nature 273:769, 1978.
180. Watanabe H, Kobayashi H, Honma K et al: Diffuse panbronchiolitis with multiple tumorlets: A quantitative study of the Kulchitsky cells and the clusters. Acta Pathol Jpn 35:1221, 1985.
181. Weiler R, Feichtinger H, Schmid KW et al: Chromogranin A and B and secretogranin II in bronchial and intestinal carcinoids. Virchows Arch [A] 412:103, 1987.
182. Whitwell F: Tumourlets of the lung. J Pathol Bacteriol 70:529, 1955.
183. Wilander E, Lundqvist M, Movin T: S-100 protein in carcinoid tumours of appendix. Acta Neuropathol 66:306, 1985.
184. Wilkins EW, Grillo HC, Moncure AC et al: Changing times in surgical management of bronchopulmonary carcinoid tumor. Ann Thorac Surg 38:339, 1984.
185. Wise WS, Bonder D, Aikawa M et al: Carcinoid tumor of lung with varied histology. Am J Surg Pathol 6:261, 1982.
186. Wisniewski M, Fayemi AO: Bronchial carcinoid: A malignant tumor. Chest 62:760, 1972.
187. Yamashina M: An 18-year history of a corticotropin-secreting spindle cell carcinoid of the lung. Arch Pathol Lab Med 109:673, 1985.
188. Yamashina M, Flinner RA: Concurrent occurrence of adenocarcinoma and carcinoid tumor in the stomach: A composite tumor or collision tumors? Am J Clin Pathol 83:233, 1985.
189. Yang K, Ulich T, Taylor I et al: Pulmonary carcinoids: Immunohistochemical demonstration of brain–gut peptides. Cancer 52:819, 1983.
190. Yellin A, Benfield JR: The pulmonary Kulchitsky cell (neuroendocrine) cancers. Curr Probl Cancer 9:1, 1985.
191. Zanetta G, Zanoni M, Colombo F: Argentaffin pulmonary tumorlets. Tumori 65:761, 1979.

Chapter

11

UNCOMMON LUNG TUMORS

Compared with the common types of lung carcinoma, the tumors discussed in this chapter occur infrequently, and a number are distinctly rare. Collectively they make up perhaps 2% of all primary lung neoplasms. A few are intriguing because their histogenesis is not well understood, and while some are almost always benign, others are aggressive, so it is important to know the criteria for their identification and be able to anticipate how they are likely to behave. In the case of lymphomas and melanoma, it may not be possible to establish that the tumor is arising within the lung, and a search for extrapulmonary involvement is always necessary.

Although benign tumors can mimic carcinomas and nonneoplastic lesions on radiography, not more than 15% of solitary pulmonary nodules turn out to be benign neoplasms.[246] Multiple lesions on radiography or computed tomography are more likely to be metastatic; this was the case in 73% of 114 patients studied with computed tomography by Gross and co-workers.[119] The authors noted that malignant nodules were statistically larger, more numerous, and more rounded, whereas calcification was significantly associated with benign disease.

The pathology of most of the uncommon tumors that arise in the lung is reviewed briefly here, but a liberal number of recent references are included. The authoritative review by Dail[61] is detailed and superbly illustrated and is recommended for further reading.

HAMARTOMA

Solitary hamartomas of the adult type[206, 337] are the most common benign tumors of the lung, and they are found in about 0.25% of patients at autopsy. Albrecht defined a hamartoma as a congenital abnormal mixing of the normal components of an organ.[4] Since cartilage is usually the predominant component, the lesion has also been called a chondromatous hamartoma or hamartochondroma. Although pulmonary hamartomas are rarely aggressive, it is necessary to establish the diagnosis and exclude other lesions that can be simulated radiologically. DeRooij and colleagues[69] advocate conservative investigative techniques (chest radiograph, computed tomography, fine-needle aspiration) but recommend exploratory thoracotomy when the lesion is larger than 2.5 cm or is obviously growing. Most of the lesions are peripheral and beyond the reach of the bronchoscope, and cytologic smears of sputum are consistently negative. If the diagnosis can be established by transbronchial bronchoscopic biopsy, the need for a more invasive procedure will be obviated,[254] but bronchoscopy often fails to yield a diagnosis; in one series of 154 cases only 12 were endobronchial and the remaining 142 were parenchymal. It was not successful in any of the 49 patients of Ramirez-Chavez and colleagues, 43 of whom had a rounded peripheral opacity.[270] Steen-Hansen and associates[308] advocate the use of fine-needle aspiration: in their hands, it was diagnostic in 31 of 33 patients and surgical biopsy was avoided in 29 patients. With this technique, Hamper and co-workers[124] made the diagnosis in 12 of 14 patients, and in 8, a single procedure sufficed.

A hamartoma is generally asymptomatic, although a central lesion will occasionally produce obstructive symptoms. The great majority of hamartomas are detected on a routine chest radiograph as round, well-circumscribed solid nodules smaller than 4 cm in diameter. A cystic form has been described.[71] Fine calcifications may be present, and popcorn calcification has been suggested as a diagnostic aid, but Crouch and colleagues[58] confirmed pathologically that calcification was absent in 19 resected tumors. Computed tomographic findings are described by Siegelman and associates:[297] their criteria include a diameter of 2.5 cm or less, a smooth edge, and focal collections of fat or fat alternating with areas of calcification.

Multiple hamartomas have been reported.[22] Occasionally a hamartoma grows to a large size.[261] The average patient age is about 50, and in some series there has been no obvious predilection for either sex; however, among the 154 cases reviewed by Van den Bosch and co-workers[337] there were 116 male and 38 female patients. The peak incidence was in the sixth decade, and only 3 patients were younger than 20. There was a slight preponderance in the left upper lobe, but all lobes were involved. In 55 patients, the tumor first appeared during adult life, and in 53 patients it progressively increased in size. The authors consider that the lesion is a benign neoplasm rather than a true hamartoma and suggest that mesenchymoma would be a more appropriate designation. Twenty-eight of the 49 patients reviewed by Ramirez-Chavez and colleagues[270] were male and 21 were female, and the mean age was 49.8 years. Most had incidental findings on chest radiographs, although 6 patients had obstructive changes. The lesion is rare in children, but Yamazaki and co-workers[361] reported an asymptomatic hamartoma of the adult type in the right upper lobe of an 11-year-old boy.

Hamartomas grow slowly. Hackl[121] calculated that typical lesions have a doubling time of about 14 years. Sarcomatous transformation is unusual,[129] but Basile and associates[17] reported this occurrence in a long-standing, clinically silent lesion shortly after it was resected. A small number have been accompanied by a carcinoma. Mompoint and colleagues[222] reported the coexistence of bronchioloalveolar adenocarcinoma distal to an endobronchial hamartoma in a 60-year-old man. In 4 of 52 cases reviewed by Karasik and co-workers,[163] carcinoma developed in the lobe from which the hamartoma had previously been resected.

Microscopically, most hamartomas are made up of mixtures of cartilage, fat cells, and undifferentiated mesenchymal cells, and they usually contain entrapped slender clefts lined by a single layer of cuboidal or columnar epithelial cells. Ultrastructurally, these epithelial cells are the types found in the distal respiratory passages, and many are hyperplastic type II pneumocytes. Pleomorphism in a hamartoma is unusual.[114] In some lesions, the mesenchymal cells predominate, and terminology may become arbitrary: a lesion containing fat and cartilage could be considered a lipomatous hamartoma or a lipoma with a cartilaginous component. A lipomatous hamartoma in the same lobe but separate from a typical chondromatous hamartoma was reported by Palvio and colleagues.[252] Tomashefski[326] compared 17 benign endobronchial tumors with 147 intraparenchymal hamartomas and concluded that the two were similar mesenchymal neoplasms occurring at different loci within the bronchial tree. Mark[212] discusses five symptomatic patients with a distinct entity that he terms mesenchymal cystic hamartoma of the lung. In four cases, the disease was multifocal and bilateral. The nodules were composed of primitive mesenchymal cells and became cystic when they reached a diameter of about 1 cm. Although the behavior was on the whole indolent, erosion of vessels, pneumothorax from rupture of a subpleural cyst, and malignant transformation of one tumor were noted.

The ultrastructural features[309, 258] of hamartoma are largely predictable from the light microscopy. Mature cartilage cells are accompanied by varying numbers of undifferentiated mesenchymal cells, and transitional forms can be recognized. Unusual stellate smooth muscle cells have been found in areas of loose myxoid tissue.[258] The epithelial components of a hamartoma have an intact basal lamina and the fine structure of terminal bronchiolar cells and type II pneumocytes.

MUCOEPIDERMOID TUMOR

Mucoepidermoid tumor is identical microscopically to its counterpart in the salivary glands. It appears to arise from the excretory duct reserve cells[228] and is composed of mixtures of mucus-forming and epidermoid cells with intermediate forms. The earliest cases recognized in the tracheobronchial tree were believed clinically and histologically to be benign, and they were called bronchial adenomas.[16] When instances of metastasis to bronchial and mediastinal nodes were reported, it was realized that they were part of a spectrum of mucoepidermoid tumors that included a more aggressive form with a propensity for spreading. It was further appreciated that the histology cannot always be an accurate prognostic indicator.

Turnbull and co-workers[332] found 12 mucoepidermoid tumors at Memorial Hospital among approximately 5,500 lung tumors accessioned between 1949 and 1968, making up one third of all the cases recorded at that time. By 1979, about 80 cases had been reported in bronchi and a few involved the trachea.[26] Mucoepidermoid tumors have occurred in patients from 4 to 76 years of age, but about two thirds are older adults and fewer than 15% are children. The childhood tumors have mainly been of low grade.[329] Regadera and associates[271] reported a case in an 8-year-old boy who had been suspected for 18 months of having tuberculosis: the patient was doing well 9 years after lobectomy. The tumor in a 4-year-old boy reported by Seo and colleagues[292] was aggressive and produced nodal metastases. Cutaneous[219] and intracranial[357] metastases have been recorded. Factors affecting prognosis are discussed by Conlan and co-workers.[50] Breyer and associates[30] and Leonardi and colleagues[196] discuss therapy: conservative management is recommended[30] with preservation of as much lung parenchyma as possible.

Most mucoepidermoid carcinomas arise from main or segmental bronchi, and a polypoid tumor may grow within the bronchial lumen and cause obstructive symptoms. Higher grade tumors are more inclined to infiltrate the surrounding lung parenchyma. The tumors are composed of solid nests and tubular structures formed by squamous, mucous, and intermediate cells (Fig. 11–1). Cytokeratin can be demonstrated immunocytochemically, but keratinization is not usually pronounced. The glandular pattern tends to predominate throughout much of the tumor, so adequate sampling may be needed to distinguish it from a pure adenocarcinoma, and the glandular areas merge imperceptibly with the squamous foci. Cytologic preparations may show the epithelial or glandular components or both (Figs. 11–2 through 11–4). Higher grade, infiltrative tumors contain more extensive solid areas with cytologic atypia and pleomorphic cells, foci of necrosis, and greater mitotic activity. An oncocytic variant was reported by Stafford and colleagues.[307] Adenosquamous carcinoma contrasts to mucoepidermoid carcinoma in frequently being peripheral, and it more consistently infiltrates the lung parenchyma.

There have been a number of ultrastructural studies of mucoepidermoid carcinomas in the lung, and they and the salivary tumors are comparable in their fine structure.[65, 173, 176, 259, 328] Tonofibrils and mucin granules can be seen in largely epidermoid tumors,[259] but some cells have extensive mucin and few or no tonofibrils reflecting the multipotentiality of the neoplastic cells; transitional forms are frequent.[173]

ADENOID CYSTIC CARCINOMA

Adenoid cystic carcinoma of the tracheobronchial passages differs from mucoepidermoid carcinoma in that roughly one third occur in the trachea and children are hardly ever affected. Van der Veen and associates[338] made the diagnosis in 11 patients (six men and five women) during a 15-year period, and three tumors were located in the trachea and eight occurred in the main bronchi. It can also involve the larynx.[248] The synonym cylindroma is attributed to Billroth.

The ages in reported cases range from 18 to 65 years, but the average is between 45 and 50. The tumor forms a firm nodule that is centrally located in approximately 90% of cases,[107] and it is generally between 1 and 5 cm in diameter at the time it is resected. Adenoid cystic carcinoma has a tendency to spread along and encircle the bronchus from which it arises as well as neighboring bronchi and vessels. Obstructive symptoms and hemoptysis are consequently common clinical findings. A unique example was a tumor secreting ACTH and growth hormone–re-

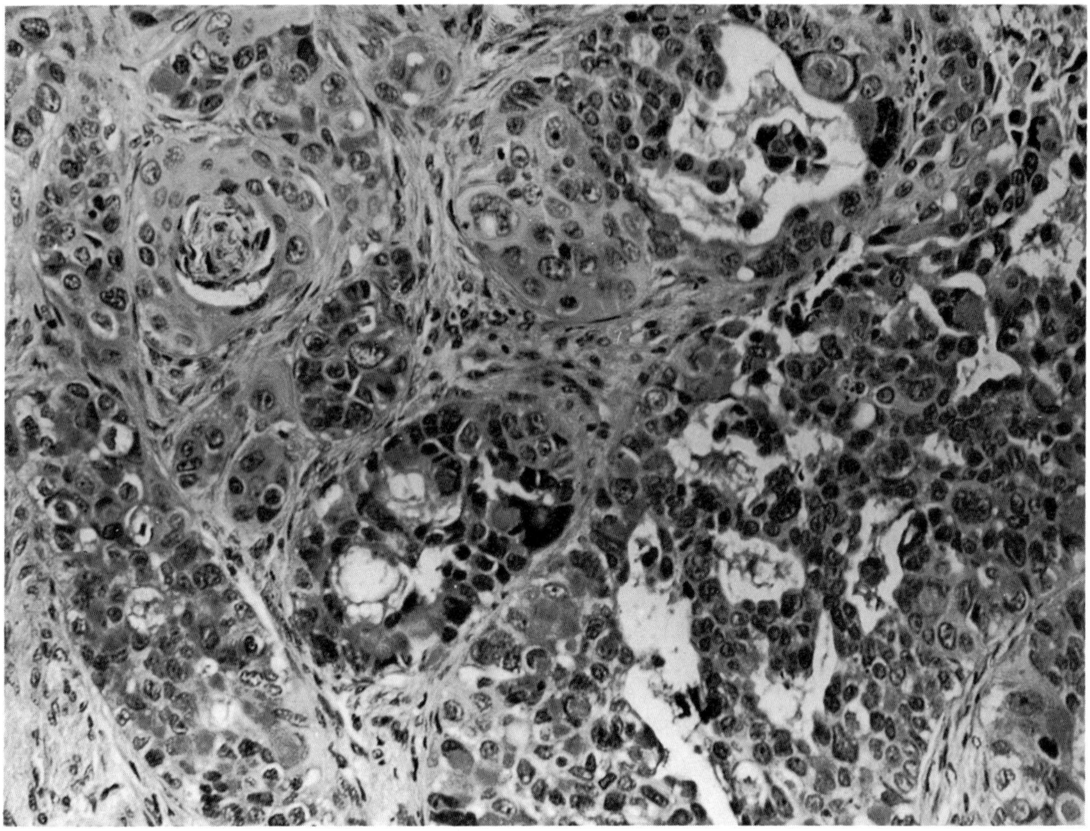

Figure 11–1. Mucoepidermoid carcinoma. Groups of closely packed cells with squamous features merge with glandular structures.

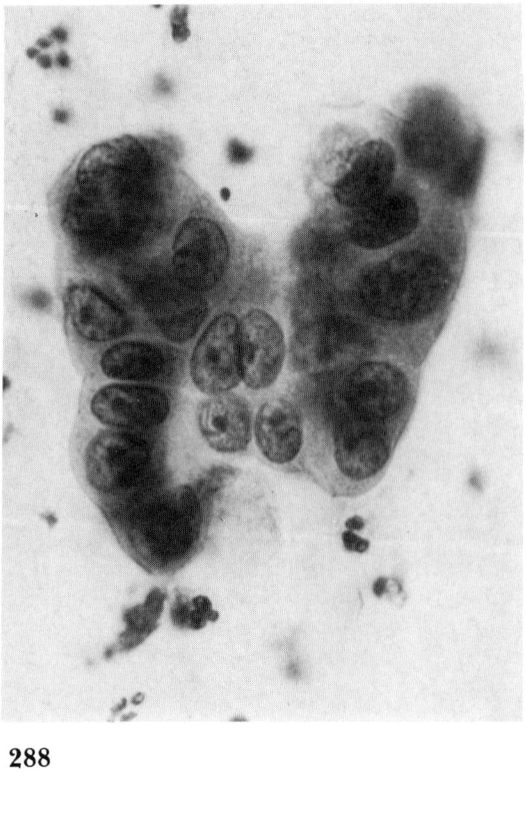

Figure 11–2. Mucoepidermoid carcinoma. Cytology of the epidermoid component.

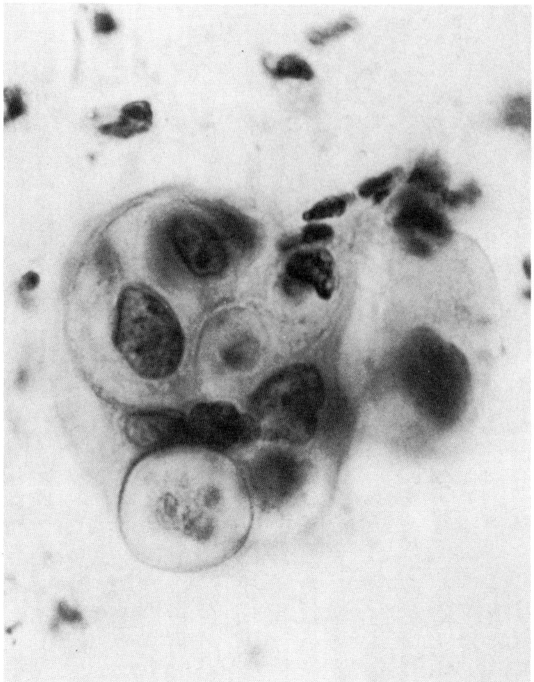

Figure 11–3. Mucoepidermoid carcinoma. Cytology of the glandular component.

leasing hormone reported in a 23-year-old male patient with acromegaly.[301] Many patients survive for at least 10 years, but recurrences are a problem and can occur many years after the primary tumor has been resected. Gallagher and co-workers report a woman who developed multiple lung nodules 11 years after the original tumor had been resected.[107] A few tumors metastasize, initially to regional lymph nodes and infrequently to distant sites.[107] A solitary renal metastasis after 23 years has been recorded.[190]

The microscopic appearance is identical to that of adenoid cystic carcinomas in other locations, and a metastatic adenoid cystic carcinoma in the lung, a much more frequent occurrence, cannot be distinguished from a lung primary lesion. A distinctive cribriform pattern is created by the rather uniform cells, which have round hyperchromatic nuclei and inconspicuous nucleoli (Fig. 11–5). Mingled in this basic architecture are solid clusters, cords, and ductlike structures. The cells in the cribriform areas encircle zones of stroma to create round pseudocysts that mimic glandular lumens by light microscopy, but electron microscopy shows that they are circular zones of stroma containing replicated basal lamina (Fig. 11–6). Smaller true lumens into which microvilli project are also present. The mucin in the pseudocysts is acidic mucopolysaccharide, while the mucin in the true lumens is neutral mucin. As the tumors infiltrate the surrounding lung parenchyma, they may grow along perineural spaces.

Adenoid cystic carcinomas co-express keratin and vimentin,[269] and cells containing intermediate filaments can be seen by electron microscopy. It is postulated that adenoid cystic carcinoma arises in the collecting duct–acinar region of the bronchial glands since both myoepithelial cells and lining (secretory) cells are present in this location.

ACINIC CELL TUMOR

Very occasionally the serous cells of the mixed bronchial glands give rise to an acinic cell tumor that appears identical to its counterpart in the salivary gland. Ultrastructurally the cells have large cytoplasmic granules of the exocrine type.[88] Tracheal involvement has also been reported.[131]

MIXED BRONCHIAL GLAND TUMORS

A 1965 report of two cases from the Mayo Clinic[256, 257] appears to be the first account of

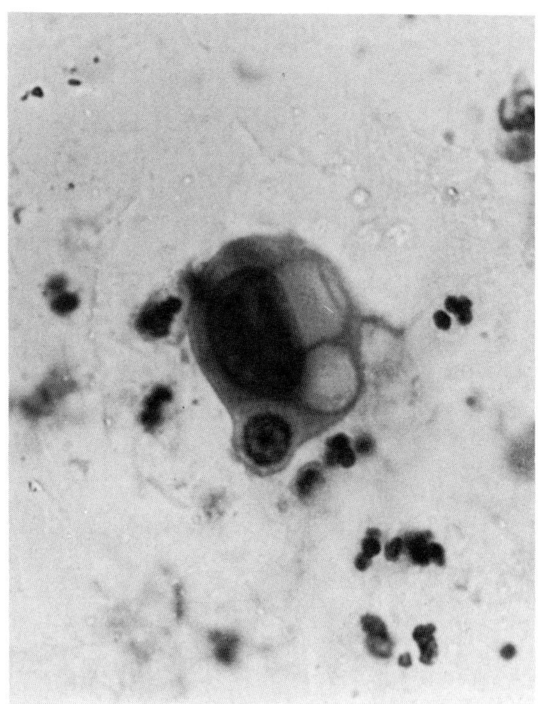

Figure 11–4. Mucoepidermoid carcinoma. Cytology showing a cell with markedly vacuolated cytoplasm.

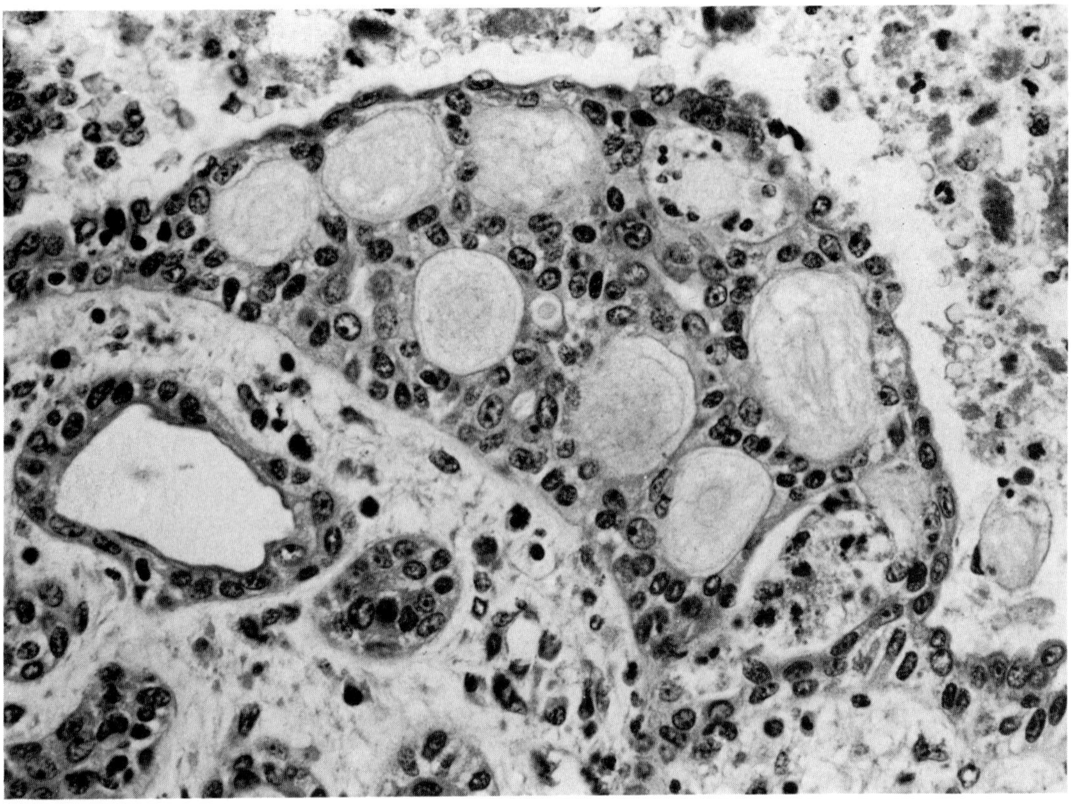

Figure 11–5. Adenoid cystic carcinoma. The typical pattern with many round cystic spaces surrounded by the polygonal tumor cells.

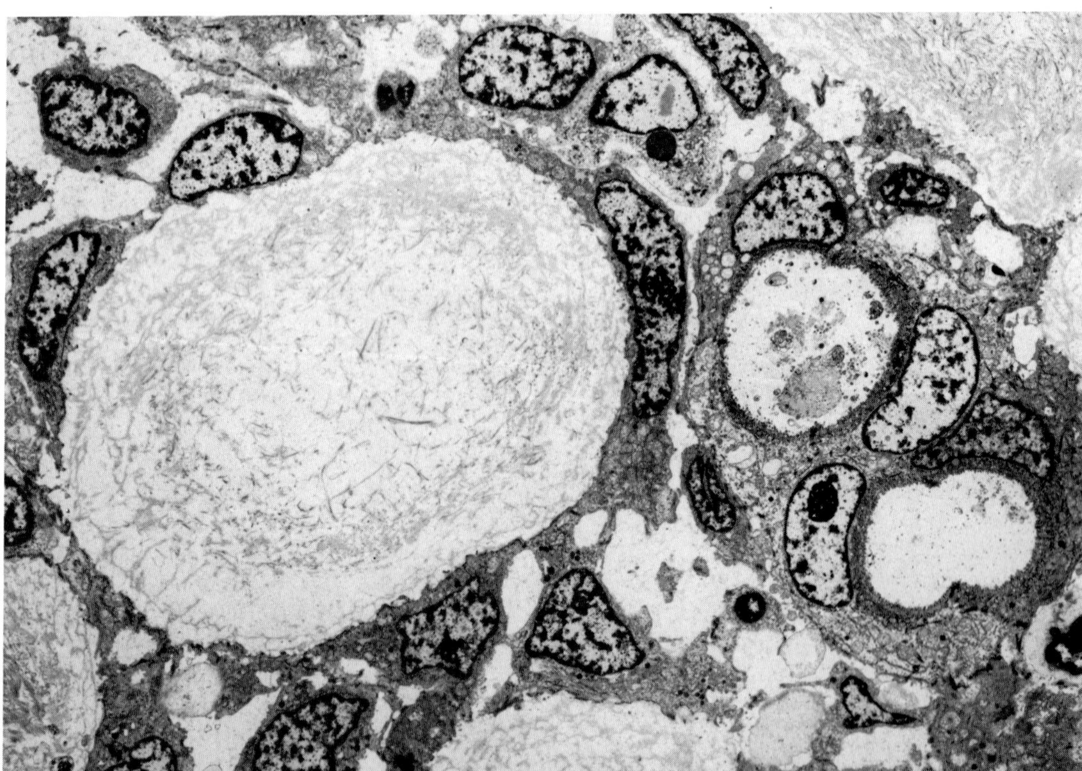

Figure 11–6. Adenoid cystic carcinoma. Electron micrograph showing a cystic space containing some replicated basal laminar material, together with two small lumens into which microvilli project. (×2,500)

mixed tumors of salivary gland type presenting as primary lesions of bronchus. Pleomorphic adenomas can also arise in the trachea.[203, 282] A bronchial mixed tumor[67, 81, 291, 359] usually forms a polypoid endobronchial lesion, but a few grow out into the lung parenchyma as a round nodule. The overlying bronchial mucosa may be intact, and cytologic specimens can therefore be negative. All the histologic variations that characterize salivary tumors of this type are seen, including anastomosing strands of epithelial cells; focal squamous metaplasia; myxoid, stellate, and spindle cells; and chondroid metaplasia. A more cellular variant also occurs.

A malignant pleomorphic adenoma arising in the trachea of a 65-year-old woman formed a polypoid submucosal tumor and metastasized to the lung and chest wall 11 years after it had first been resected.[133] This tumor contained myoepithelial cells as well as glandular structures and a myxochondroid stroma.

ONCOCYTOMA

Some oncocytic lung tumors are carcinoids, but nonendocrine mitochondrion-rich cells occur in the ducts of the bronchial glands and occasionally a true oncocytic tumor devoid of neuroendocrine features is formed in the lung.[89, 93, 283, 322] These uncommon lesions are rarely larger than 4 cm, and the few that have been reported have behaved in benign fashion. The cells in paraffin sections have eosinophilic, finely granular cytoplasm, and electron microscopy reveals the numerous mitochondria, some with atypical arrangements of their cristae. Secretory granules are sparse in the cells of oncocytic carcinoids, so confirmation of a true oncocytoma requires careful ultrastructural analysis of well-preserved material. Immunostaining for chromogranin may also be helpful.

CHEMODECTOMA

Small chemodectoma-like bodies occur in the lungs, and Dail[61] suggests that a diligent prosector may detect them in at least 2% of patients at autopsy. Fourteen of the 19 examples described by Korn and associates[178] were in women, and almost all were found during routine microscopic examination of sections of the lungs. The cells are commonly round with central nuclei and moderate amounts of rather pale cytoplasm, but they may have a spindle shape, and they can form a solid nodule or permeate thickened alveolar septa. They may present a meningothelial-like appearance.[105] The zellballen pattern that is seen in a paraganglioma is not prominent.[125] The chemodectoma-like lesions are often intimately related to veins. In a study of 26 cases, Churg and Warnock[42] found that 23% were associated with pulmonary thromboemboli and many patients had cardiac and other pathology that had caused pulmonary injury. Electron microscopy does not reveal neural elements or neuroendocrine granules, and the absence of neuroendocrine granules distinguishes chemodectoma-like bodies from tumorlets.[56, 186] The cells contain many intermediate filaments, and neighboring cells are intimately apposed and connected by desmosomes.

SQUAMOUS CELL PAPILLOMA

Spencer and colleagues[304] reviewed 19 papillary, noninvasive tumors not including carcinoids. Eight were solitary papillomas, and squamous epithelium was the most common, but three were covered by a mixture of epithelial types. Laryngeal squamous cell papillomas in children may be multiple, and they infrequently extend into the bronchi.[5, 75] They are rare in the lower respiratory tract of adults in the absence of laryngeal disease. A condylomatous papilloma of the bronchus was reported by Trillo and Guha.[331] Solitary papillomas in adults may show varying degrees of cytologic atypia. The proliferation of squamous cells can continue into bronchial glands, and frank invasion has occurred in adults and in children.[90, 276, 296] Al-Saleem and associates[5] collected 11 cases of multiple papillomatosis in the respiratory tract seen over a 50-year period at one hospital, and they included tracheal and bronchial lesions without associated laryngeal disease and two cases in which only the bronchi were involved.

BRONCHIAL ADENOMAS

The term bronchial adenoma[10, 57] has been used to encompass a variety of monomorphic benign neoplasms arising from the cells of the respiratory passages, and carcinoid tumors have made up around 90% of the total in reported series. When carcinoids are excluded, monomorphic adenomas of the bronchus are distinctly uncommon. Pleomorphic adenomas resembling the mixed tumors of the salivary glands have already been mentioned.

Mucous Gland Adenoma

Mucous gland adenomas[7, 80, 83, 303] are also termed cystadenomas of the bronchus, and an endobronchial lesion may be referred to as an adenomatous polyp. The majority have been smaller than 2 cm in diameter and confined to the wall of the bronchus where they are amenable to bronchoscopic biopsy. The overlying bronchial epithelium is usually intact. Obstructive symptoms can be produced, but transmural expansion into the surrounding lung parenchyma rarely occurs.

Well-differentiated mucus-forming cells surround a mucin-filled cystic space that may also contain small concretions. Cuboidal or flattened cells are present in the larger cysts. Dail recognizes three patterns: tubular glands lined by a single layer of columnar mucus-producing cells, papillary and cystic adenomas, and a type that resembles low-grade mucoepidermoid tumors.[61] Heard and associates describe the ultrastructural features.[130]

Clara Cell Adenoma

Benign tumors composed of cuboidal to columnar cells with Clara cell granules have been described in mice,[166, 251, 285] but they are rare in humans.[86, 240] There were two possibilities among the 19 surface tumors reviewed by Spencer and co-workers.[304] Type II pneumocyte differentiation can also be present, a situation similar to that seen in bronchioloalveolar adenocarcinomas. The histogenesis is discussed by Kauffman.[167]

Alveolar Adenoma

Six tumors with this designation were reported by Yousem and Hochholzer.[365] Five

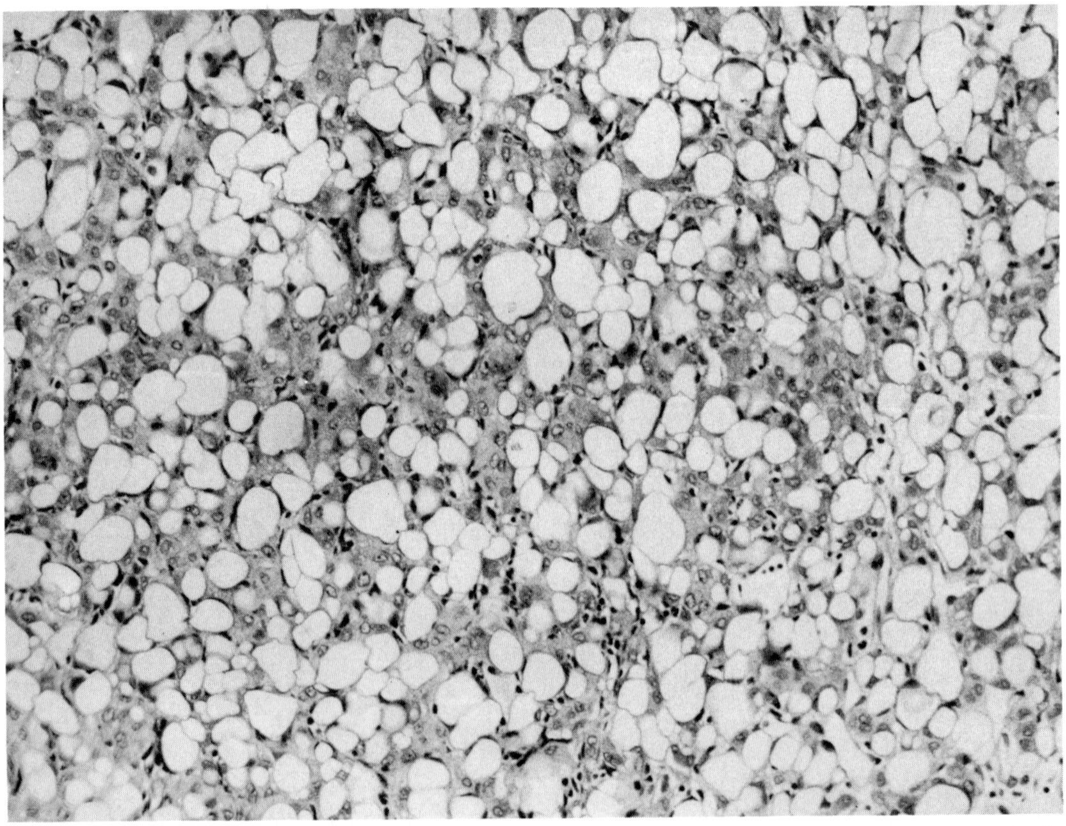

Figure 11–7. A peculiar solitary vacuolated lesion from the lung of a 32-year-old male. The impression by light microscopy was that the cells were histiocytes and fat cells.

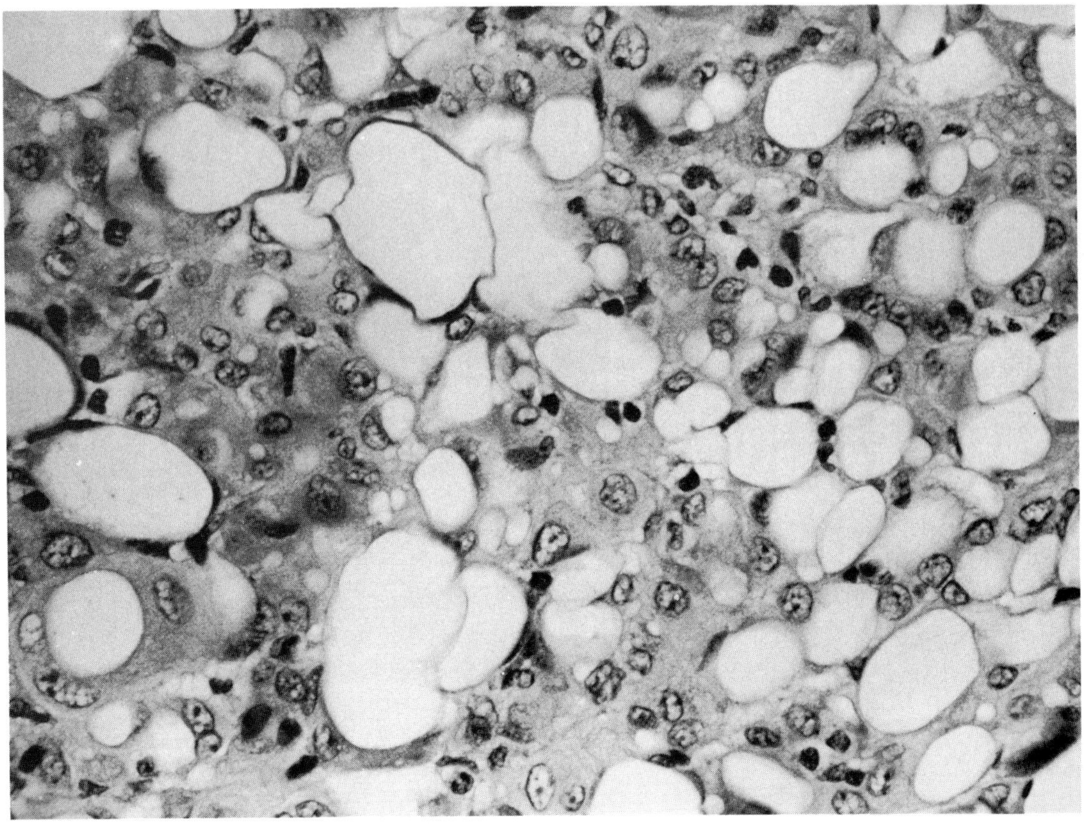

Figure 11–8. Greater detail of the tumor shown in Figure 11–7.

were peripheral solitary coin lesions under 2 cm in average size. The many cysts within the lesions were lined by flattened cells. Pneumocyte differentiation was suspected in a peculiar vacuolated lung lesion that we saw some years ago (Figs. 11–7 through 11–9), but the evidence was not conclusive.[43]

Benign Clear Cell Tumor

Although a "sugar tumor" is included in many differential diagnoses of lung lesions, we have not seen a convincing example at our hospital and believe that it is exceedingly uncommon. Twelve cases were reported in 1971 by Liebow and Castleman,[198] and Andrion and associates[9] stated that there were only 10 more examples in the world literature by 1985. Sale and Kulander referred to 23 published cases in 1988.[281] Kung and colleagues[187] reported a clear cell tumor of the trachea. Most of Liebow and Castleman's cases were in middle-aged adults whose ages ranged from 28 to 64 years, but a case has been reported in an 8-year-old girl.[101] Any lobe of the lung can be involved, and there are usually no symptoms: the lesion is detected as an incidental finding on routine chest radiography. Aspiration biopsy cytology has been described.[238] The tumor forms a sharply circumscribed mass that measures up to 7 cm in diameter and separates readily from the surrounding lung parenchyma. There is not a consistent relationship to vessels or bronchi.

The cells are polygonal with central bland nuclei and clear cytoplasm, and they form sheets and possibly clusters or cords within sharply demarcated islands (Figs. 11–10 and 11–11) containing thin-walled vessels.[233] Mitotic figures are rare.

Immunostaining[232] has been negative for actin and other markers. By electron microscopy, the cells have abundant free and rosette glycogen. Some interdigitation of cell membranes is evident, and a few microvilli are sandwiched between neighboring cells.[137]

The lesion appears to be almost always benign, and resection is considered curative.

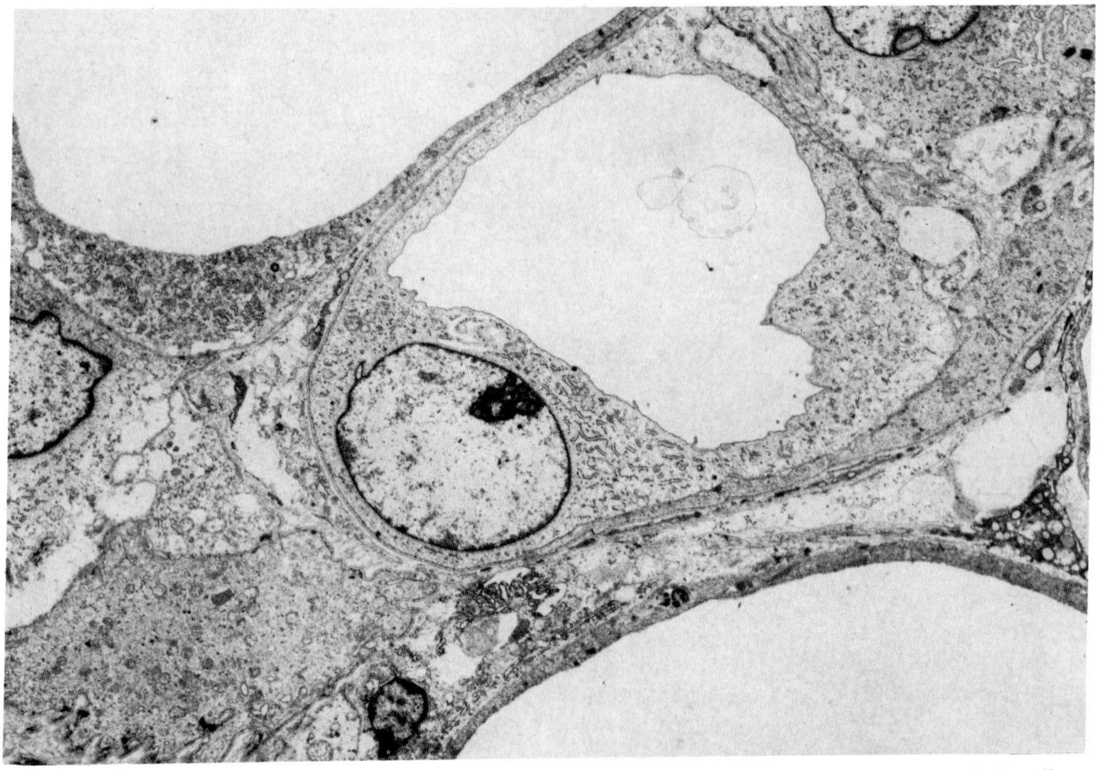

Figure 11–9. The tumor shown in Figures 11–7 and 11–8 was examined by electron microscopy. A single cell type appeared to be present containing vacuoles of varying size, some with attenuated cytoplasm. The cells were in groups bordered by a basal lamina. (×3,900)

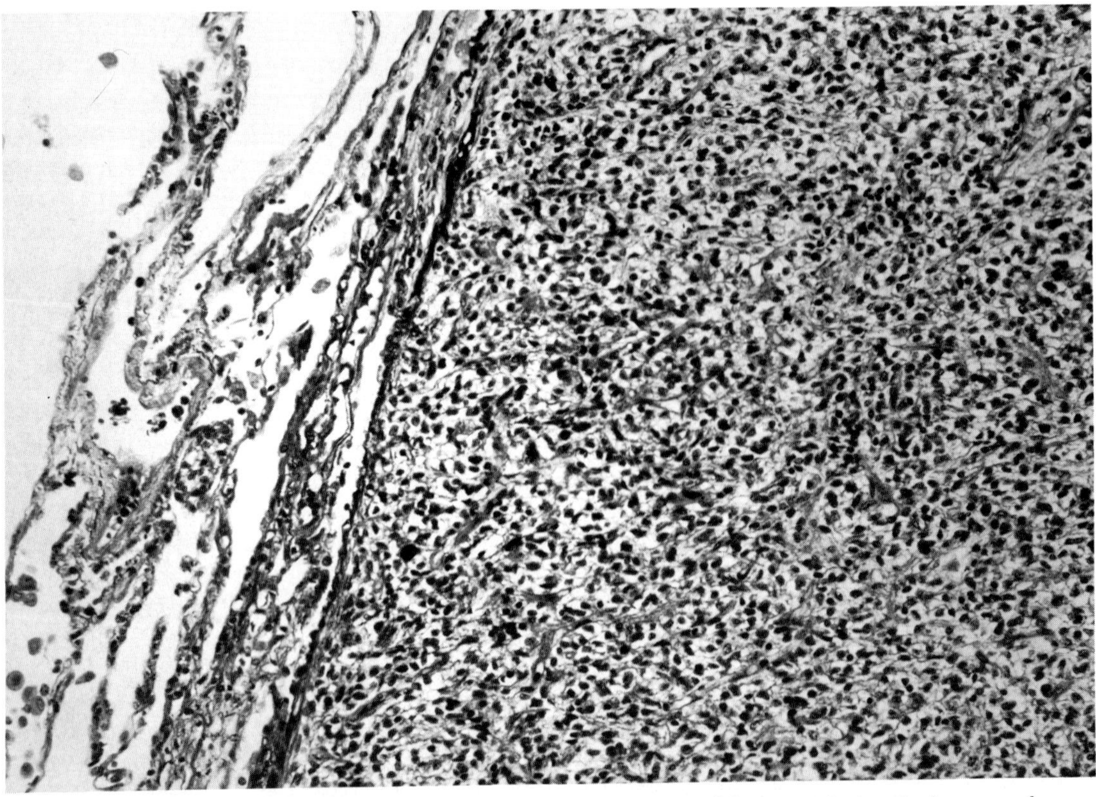

Figure 11–10. Benign clear cell tumor of the lung. The periphery of the tumor is sharply demarcated.

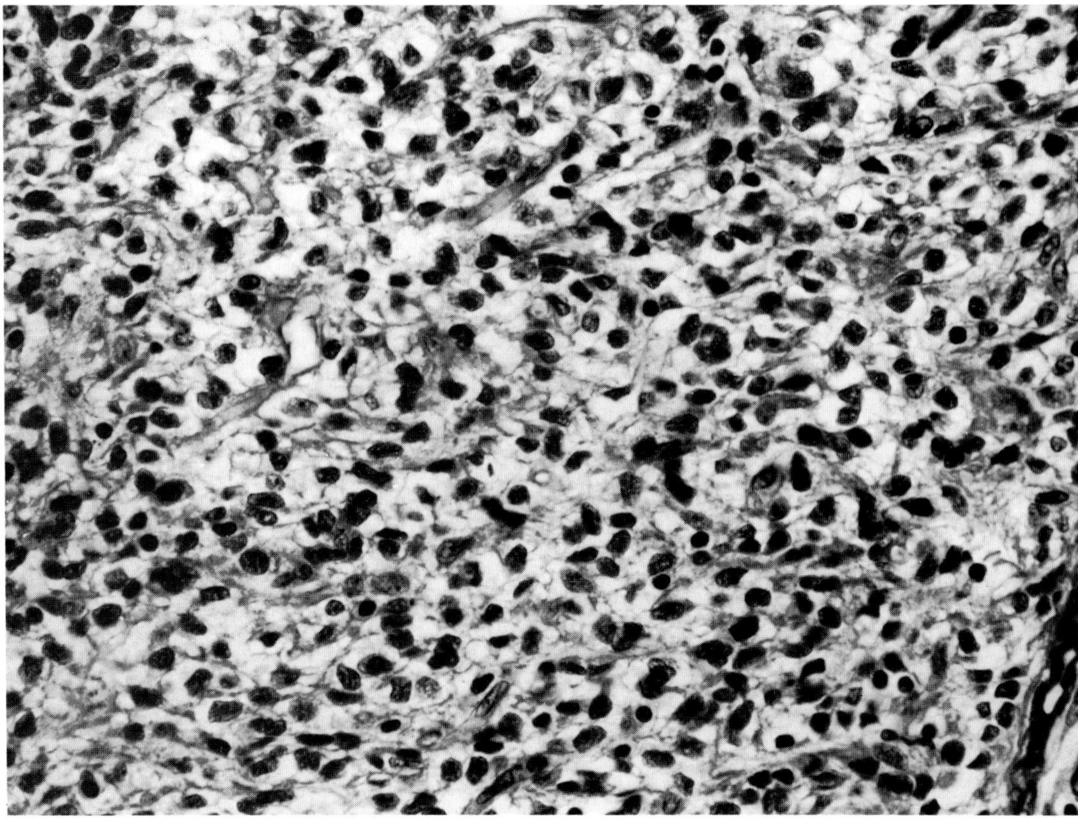

Figure 11–11. Benign clear cell tumor. The cells are more or less round with clear cytoplasm reflecting the large amounts of glycogen.

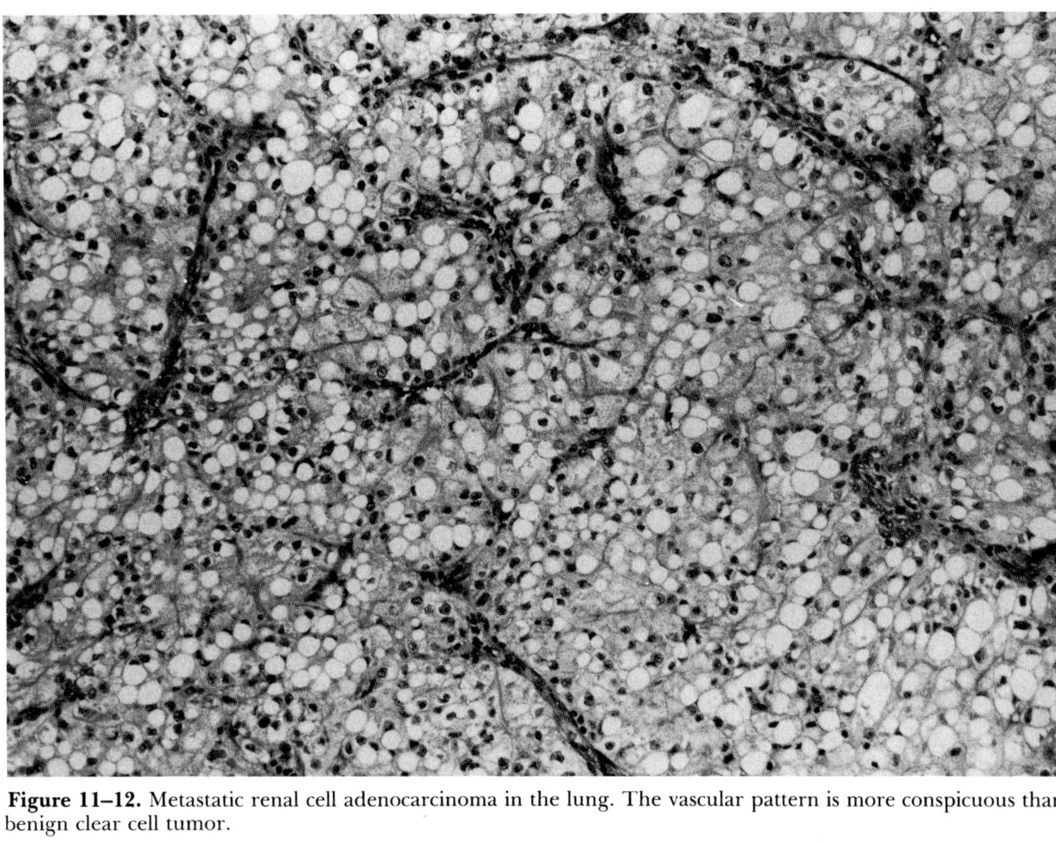

Figure 11–12. Metastatic renal cell adenocarcinoma in the lung. The vascular pattern is more conspicuous than in a benign clear cell tumor.

The case reviewed by Sale and Kulander[281] raised the possibility that exceptions exist: in this patient, hepatic and peritoneal metastases developed 10 years after removal of the primary lung tumor and the patient died 17 years after diagnosis. However, the original tumor contained areas of necrosis and focal columnar cell arrangement and Dail[59] considers it atypical. The differential diagnosis of benign clear cell tumor must include the much more common metastatic renal cell adenocarcinoma, and abundant glycogen is not helpful in making the distinction. Renal cell carcinoma has a more sturdy vascular component (Fig. 11–12), the cells may show more nuclear pleomorphism, mitotic activity is obvious, ultrastructurally microvilli are more numerous and organized, and the cells generally contain many lipid droplets.

INFLAMMATORY PSEUDOTUMOR

Inflammatory pseudotumor has been reported under various names, including histiocytoma, fibroxanthoma, and plasma cell granuloma.[23, 150] It can mimic a neoplasm, particularly if it is angioinvasive.[344] Although most have been reported in adults, it also occurs in children.[290] Typically the patient is asymptomatic and the lesion is smaller than 3 cm in diameter. There may be a history of pneumonia[213] or trauma.[98] Microscopically, a proliferation of mature plasma cells and lymphocytes is present within a framework of fibrosis and granulation tissue. Some mast cells can usually be identified, and there may be aggregates of large histiocytes with foamy cytoplasm (xanthoma cells). The ultrastructure of a myxomatous variant has been described.[39]

SOFT TISSUE TUMORS

Benign soft tissue tumors arising in the lung can produce pressure effects and bronchial obstruction, and when they are multiple they cause confusion radiologically with metastatic carcinoma.

As is the case in soft tissues, pure fibromas are infrequently diagnosed in the lung,[52, 174] but they have been responsible for atelectasis.[72] A mixture of mature fibroblasts with more primitive mesenchymal cells in a myxoid stroma may be called a fibromyxoma or, if the entire tumor is myxoid, a myxoma.[201] A pronounced storiform pattern will suggest the designation of fibrous histiocytoma.[279] Tan-Liu and associates describe seven invasive tumors of the tracheobronchial tree composed of fibroblasts that resembled but also differed from fibrous histiocytomas.[318]

Leiomyomas are the most common soft tissue tumors of the lung.[106, 341, 354, 360, 362] Leiomyomatosis with endobronchial extension and cyst formation has been reported.[335] Bilateral multiple smooth muscle nodules in the lungs of women who have undergone hysterectomy for leiomyomas may be interpreted as metastasis despite their bland histologic appearance.[36, 141, 358]

Bronchial lipomas are submucosal lesions that protrude into the bronchus and if sufficiently large cause obstructive symptoms.[77, 148, 288] Most of the reported cases have been in males. Multiple cavernous hemangiomas were reported by Mori and colleagues.[226] Endobronchial schwannomas have been described by light microscopy,[91, 207] and the trachea can also be involved.[140, 278] Neurofibromas occur in the lung as part of a systemic neurofibromatosis[334] and have been associated with arteriovenous shunts and hypoxemia.[244] A pulmonary chondroma in association with gastric leiomyosarcoma and extra-adrenal paraganglioma constitutes Carney's triad.[268]

Granular cell tumors, formerly termed myoblastomas and now more appropriately also called schwannomas, are almost invariably benign, although rare malignant granular cell tumors have been reported.[175] A coin lesion may be the presentation.[289] The lesions occur in the larger bronchi where they produce an elevation that is amenable to bronchoscopic biopsy, and cytologic preparations may be positive.[103, 323] A granular cell tumor of the bronchus may coexist with other lung pathology including carcinoma,[104, 145] and identification of a granular cell tumor in a bronchoscopic biopsy specimen of a large mass should not be allowed to obscure the possibility of carcinoma: a fine-needle aspiration biopsy specimen from the mass may reveal different histology. Most bronchial granular cell tumors are smaller than 2 cm, but multiple lesions are seen in at least 10% of patients. Squamous metaplasia, hyperplasia, and atypia are common in the overlying mucosa.

Sarcomas arising in the lung[234] are infrequent, sometimes large, solitary lesions, whereas metastatic sarcomas are common and often form multiple small nodules. As in the extremities, the most common subtype among primary sarcomas of the lung is malignant fibrous histiocytoma.[19, 27, 40, 160, 171, 194, 217, 340, 366] The findings on fine-needle aspiration have been described.[142, 168] A myxoid form was reported by Silverman and Coalson.[298] Fibrosarcoma[115, 262] is less often diagnosed than leiomyosarcoma:[21, 34, 70, 221, 355] a cystic leiomyosarcoma has been reported,[199] and the tumor has been recorded in childhood.[158] Liposarcoma has been reported within the lung[192, 287] and involving the pleura.[120] Sarcomas of the pulmonary artery[13, 28, 241, 255, 295] cannot usually be subtyped from their microscopic appearance. Primary chondrosarcoma[156, 225, 274, 315, 363] requires an adequate biopsy specimen to allow confident separation from a bronchial mixed tumor. Rhabdomyosarcoma is a rare lesion when only the lung is involved.[6, 11, 84, 195, 293, 324]

Angiosarcoma of the lung[249, 364] may cause intractable hemorrhage.[253, 306] Kaposi's sarcoma is now being encountered with some frequency in the lungs of patients with the acquired immunodeficiency syndrome (AIDS)[96, 113, 211, 218, 236, 266, 310, 371] and may present as pulmonary disease[179, 235, 275] and be diagnosed with fiberoptic bronchoscopy.[123, 126] Hemangiopericytoma is a difficult diagnosis in any site since the distinctive histologic pattern can be present in other sarcomas,[205] and a generous biopsy or resection specimen is needed to confirm its presence.[27, 48, 135, 154, 277, 294, 336, 367] This tumor has been reported in a child.[73] Primary osteosarcoma of the lung is a rare event, and the differential diagnosis of carcinosarcoma should be considered.[44]

The postoperative prognosis associated with soft tissue sarcomas involving the lung is discussed by Gebauer, who reviewed 435 case reports in the literature from 1957 to 1972 and 41 of his own cases,[108] including those of primary sarcomas. The prognosis associated with the sarcomas appeared to be related to the degree of differentiation but was also influenced by their location and was less favorable than with similar tumors arising in the chest wall.

LYMPHANGIOLEIOMYOMATOSIS

In lymphangioleiomyomatosis there is a proliferation of smooth muscle in the walls of lymphatic vessels, and several organs are usually involved, including the thoracic duct and lung.[55, 76, 189, 300] There may be an association with tuberous sclerosis.[35] Response to progesterone has been reported.[216]

GLOMUS TUMOR

There have been reports of a glomus tumor arising in the trachea,[85, 131, 172] but this type of tumor is hardly ever encountered in the lung.[320] Malignant glomus tumors are exceptionally rare, but we have seen one that presented in the lung as a coin lesion, probably from a primary lesion in the buttock.[205]

SCLEROSING HEMANGIOMA

A benign lesion, sclerosing hemangioma is misnamed: its histogenesis is not known, but endothelial origin has been ruled out by immunocytochemistry and electron microscopy. Particularly in a small biopsy specimen, it is possible to confuse a sclerosing hemangioma with a carcinoid or carcinoma, but the lesion is readily identified in a resection specimen. It was described by Liebow and Hubbel in 1956.[197] Katzenstein and colleagues reviewed 51 cases.[164]

At least 80% of the reported patients have been female. They may be any age from adolescence to the eighth decade. The tumor is more common in the lower lobes, and 5% involve multiple tumors.[159, 239] The lesion is usually peripheral and solitary, the patient is asymptomatic, and the radiologic appearance is nonspecific. The nodules grow slowly and resection is curative. Tanaka and coworkers[319] reported a case in a 22-year-old Japanese man in whom a single hilar lymph node was involved.

The tumor usually measures less than 5 cm, and it is sharply demarcated from the surrounding lung parenchyma but not encapsulated. The cut surface is firm to the touch, and hemorrhagic foci are visible. A number of histologic patterns can be found,[305, 319] although one generally predominates. The cells are round to polygonal when they are forming sheets and cuboidal when they clothe papillary structures (Figs. 11–13 and 11–14). The central round nucleus is surrounded by a moderate amount of rather pale cytoplasm. Mitotic figures are not usually numerous. The fibrous component

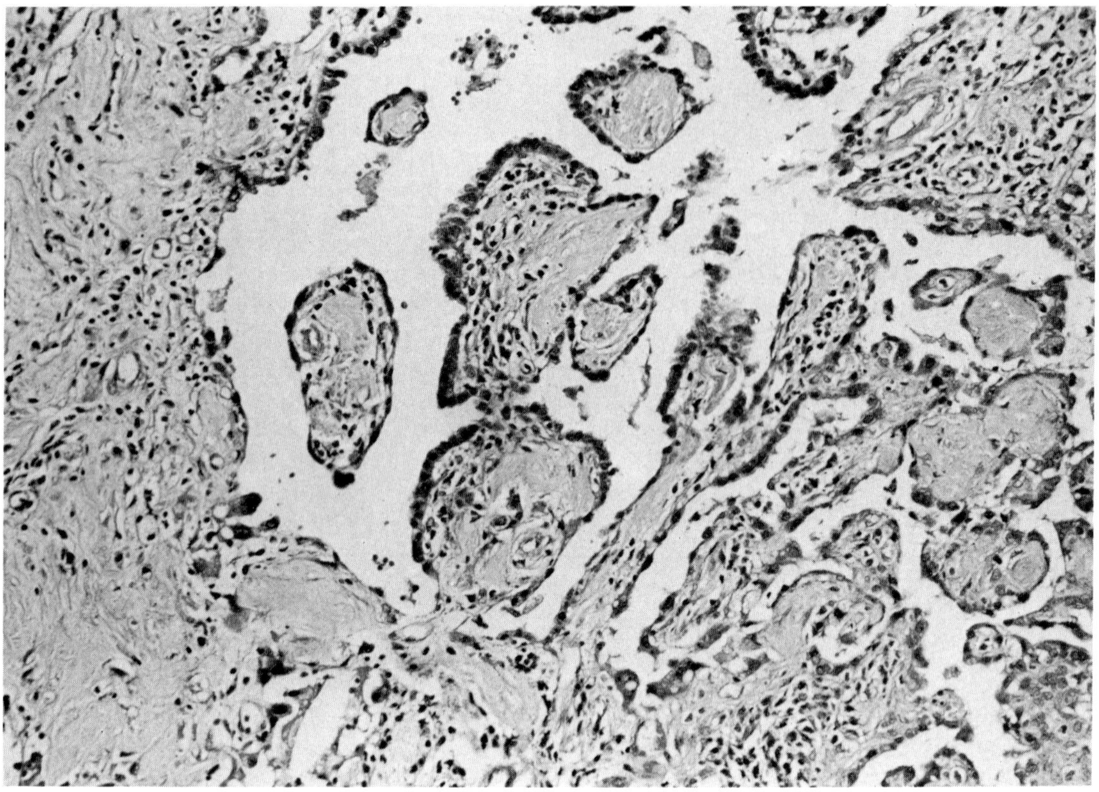

Figure 11–13. Sclerosing hemangioma. Fibrous cores covered by a single layer of cells create a papillary architecture.

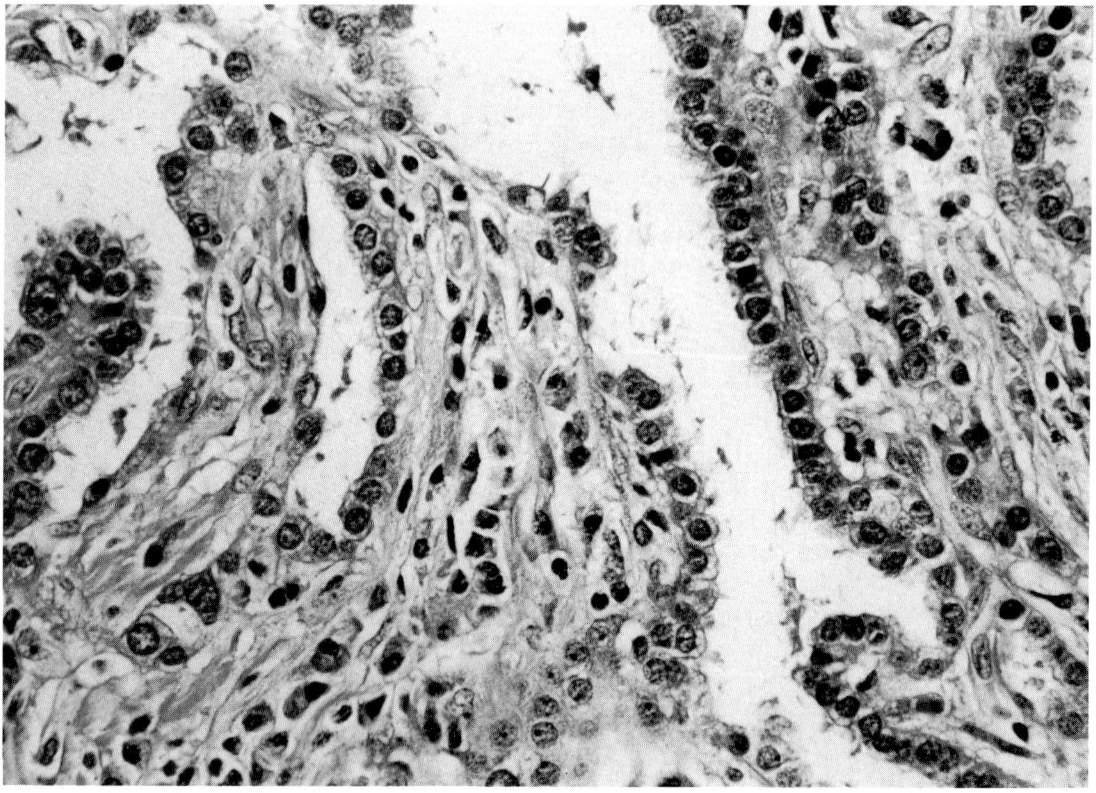

Figure 11–14. Sclerosing hemangioma. The single layer of cuboidal cells covers the papillary structures within the tumor.

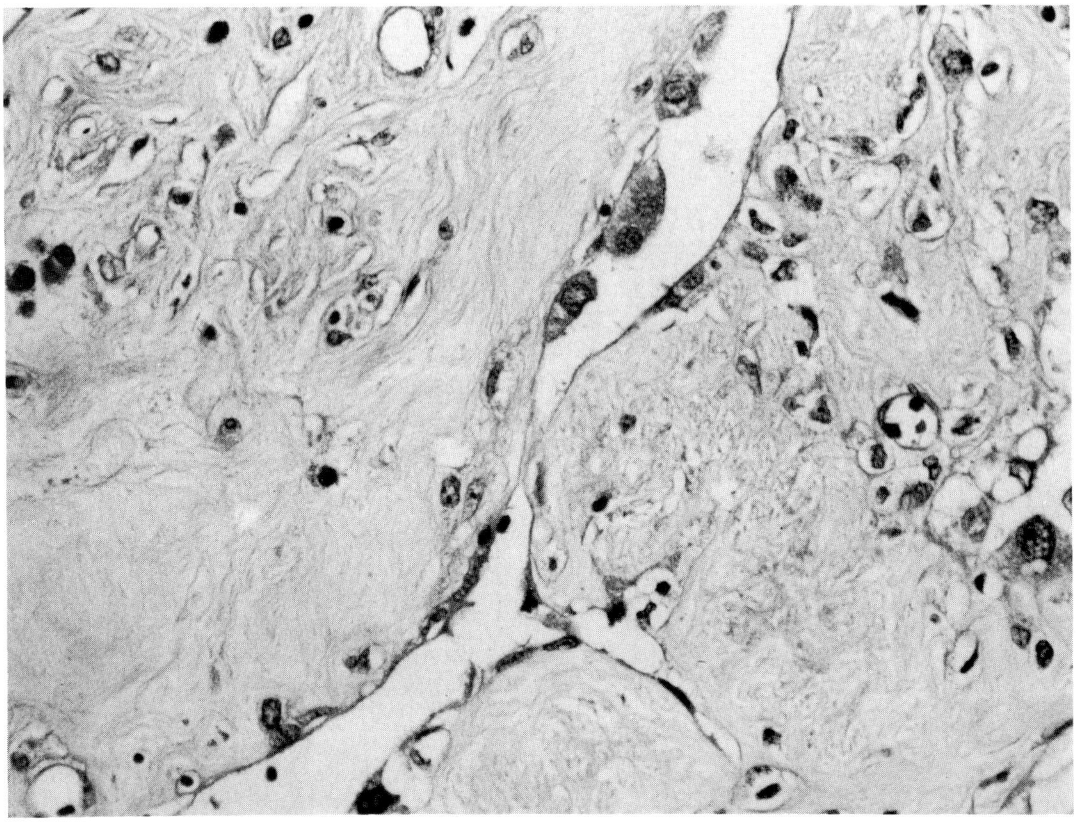

Figure 11–15. Sclerosing hemangioma showing some of the extensive fibrous component.

(Fig. 11–15) is typically extensive, and it forms the cores of the papillary structure. Dilated vascular spaces filled with blood cells (Fig. 11–16) can be surrounded by tumor cells or fibrous tissue. Foci of hemosiderin and macrophages are common. Sclerosing hemangioma must be distinguished from the sclerosing vascular variant of plasma cell granuloma.[327]

Debate on the histogenesis has centered on whether the lesion is endothelial, and the possibility has now been excluded since immunostaining is consistently negative for endothelial markers.[8, 100, 122, 147, 286] A number of reports have confirmed the presence of surfactant apoprotein in the cells,[3, 230, 231, 299, 369] suggesting that they are derived from pulmonary epithelial cells.

Observations from electron microscopy[100, 136, 250, 286, 319] do not support endothelial cell differentiation. The cells can be closely apposed with interdigitating cell membranes, but more often they are slightly separated, revealing many slender filopodia at the cell margin (Figs. 11–17 and 11–18). The cytoplasm shows no specific features. Organelles are not numerous, and there is no clear resemblance to any of the cells of the respiratory passages. However, Tanaka and associates[319] reported large polygonal foamy cells forming tubular or papillary structures that contained lamellar bodies and reacted with antisurfactant apoprotein. Mesothelial differentiation has been suggested,[165] but the ultrastructural features are not similar to those of normal mesothelium or epithelial mesotheliomas.

EPITHELIOID HEMANGIOENDOTHELIOMA

Epithelioid hemangioendothelioma is an uncommon lesion that was recognized by Dail and Leibow in 1975[62] and has been more recently reviewed by Dail.[60, 61, 63] Eggleston[82] pointed out that two cases had been reported under other names before Dail and Leibow described this tumor as an intravascular bronchioloalveolar tumor.[62] The initial

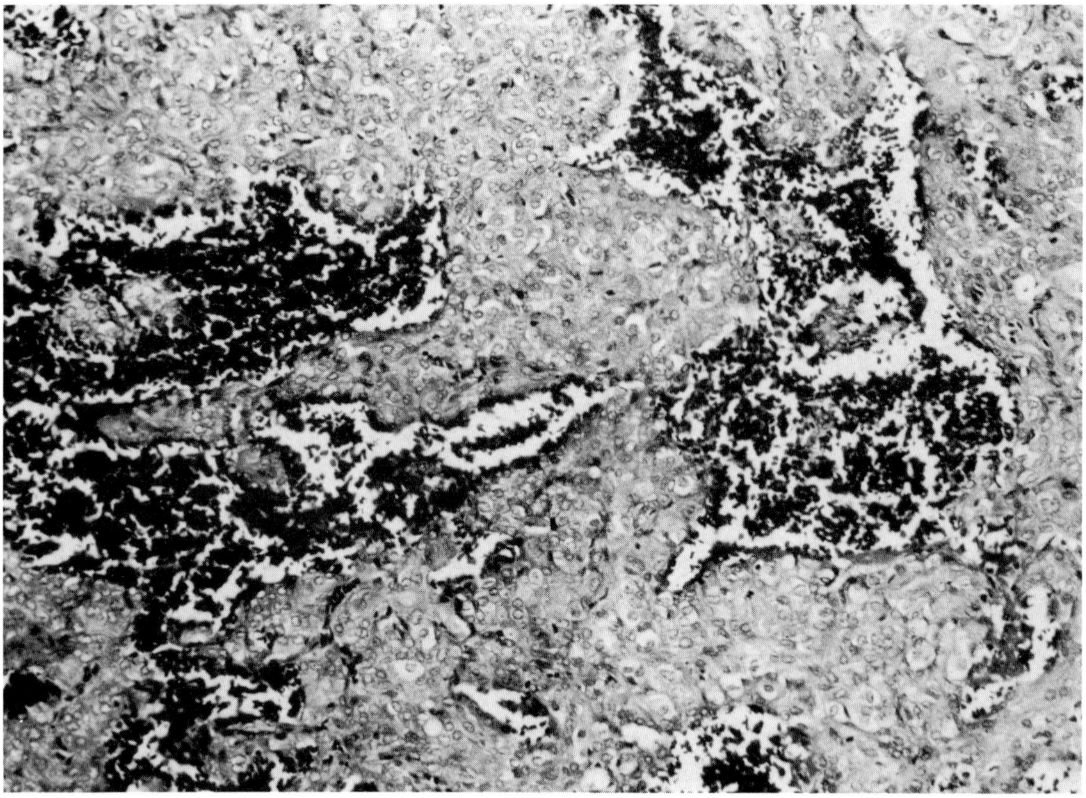

Figure 11–16. Sclerosing hemangioma. Dilated blood-filled spaces are surrounded by sheets of tumor cells.

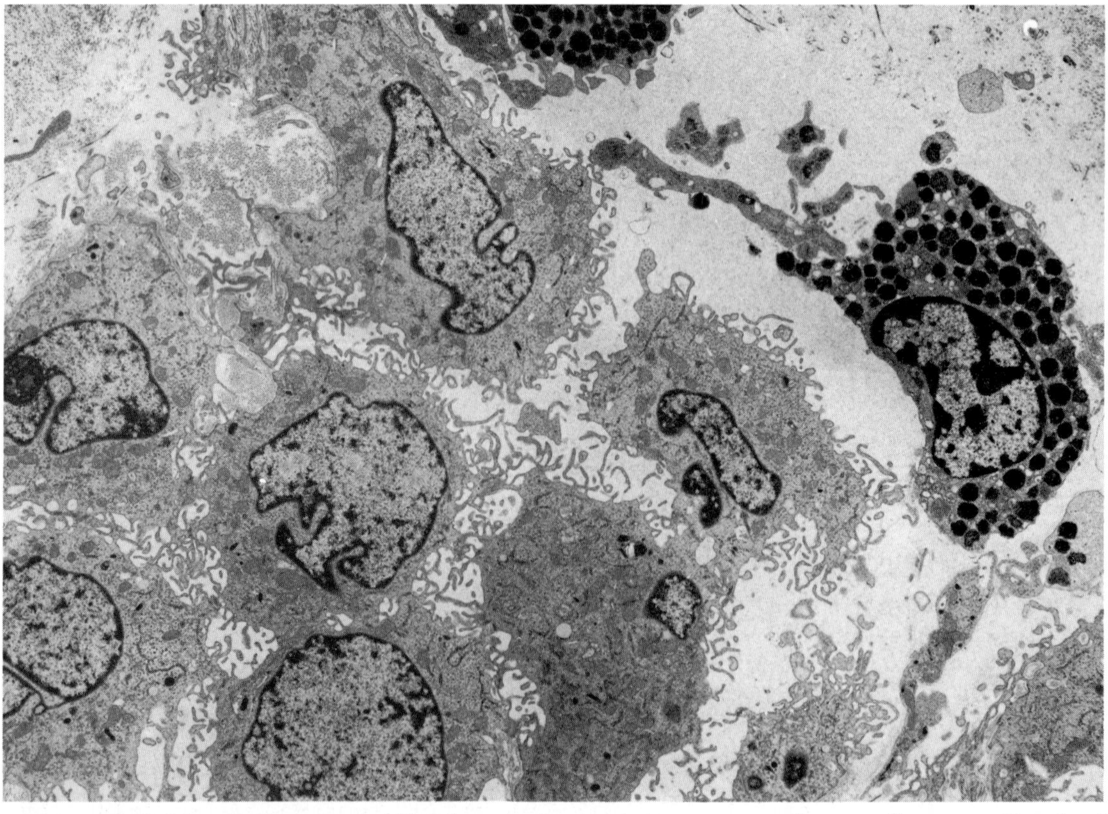

Figure 11–17. Sclerosing hemangioma. The electron micrograph shows a group of tumor cells separated by a basal lamina from the collagenous stroma. Mast cells are also present. (×4,000)

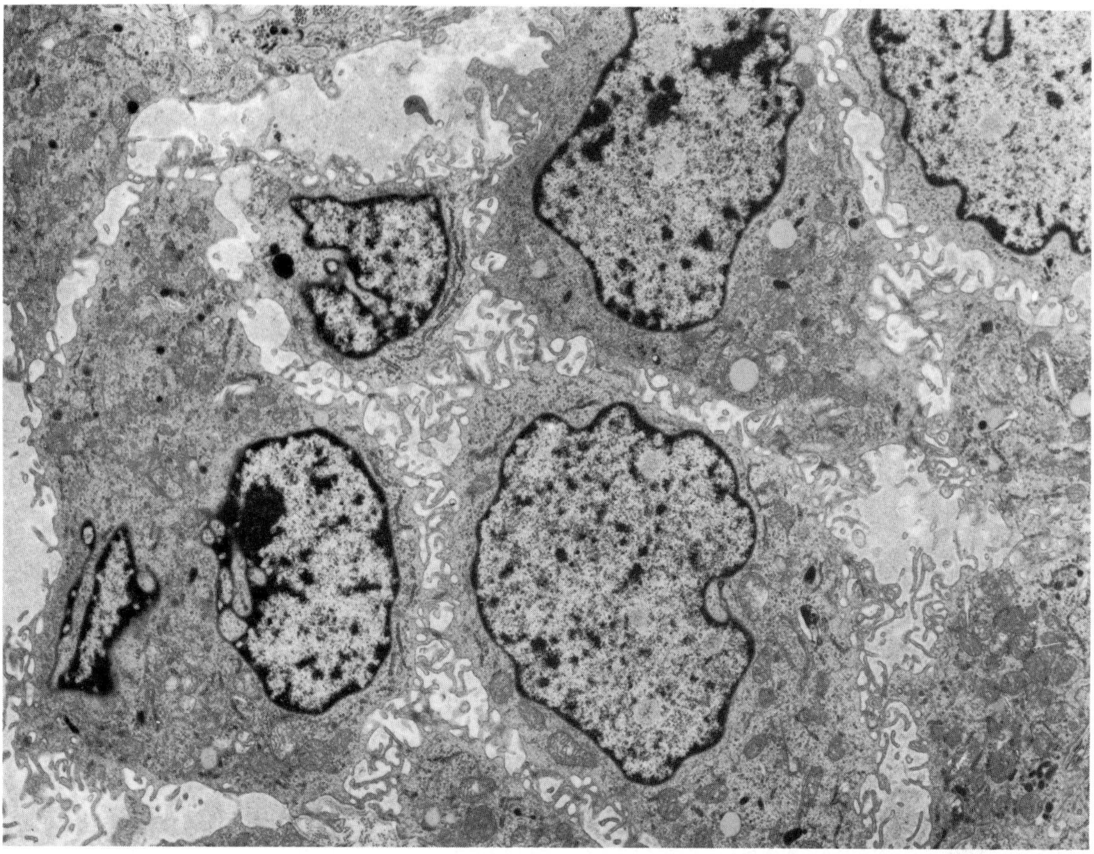

Figure 11–18. Sclerosing hemangioma showing the tumor cells in greater detail than in Figure 11–17. They are connected by a few desmosomes, and many filopodia clothe their surfaces. Dense bodies can be seen in the cytoplasm, and from their paucity and irregular profiles, they are probably lysosomes. (×5,700)

impression of a bronchioloalveolar carcinoma spreading through vessels within the lung was revised following the demonstration that the tumor cells stained with endothelial cell markers[25, 79, 220, 263, 353] and with support from reports of ultrastructural observations.[53, 54, 263, 352] Electron microscopy reveals that adjacent cells are closely apposed, and they have many pinocytotic vesicles. The lesion resembles epithelioid hemangioendotheliomas in other locations, and this is currently the preferred term for the lung tumor.[350, 351] Metastasis from an extrapulmonary source can mimic the primary lung lesion.[342]

About 80% of these tumors occur in women, many of whom are young adults. It has not been recorded in young children. A patient may be free of symptoms, but cough and dyspnea are sometimes complaints. Sputum cytology is rarely contributory, but fine-needle aspiration may suggest the diagnosis. The nodules are not usually larger than 3 cm, and they grow slowly, but half of the patients have died of their tumor. Spread beyond the lungs is uncommon, although the hilar lymph nodes may be involved and pleural extension can occur.

The tumor nodules are round and firm, and some contain small areas of calcification. They do not have a capsule. Within a nodule, a slender peripheral band is composed of round cells with eosinophilic cytoplasm forming cords and nests within a fibrous stroma, and the cells tail off into the surrounding alveoli. Many cells have vacuolated cytoplasm (Figs. 11–19 and 11–20). The central area is acellular and often myxoid. Immunocytochemical studies demonstrate reactivity for factor VIII–related antigen (Fig. 11–21).

PULMONARY BLASTOMA

The tumor was first described in 1945,[15] and in 1952 the term embryoma was suggested.[14] Spencer reviewed the entity in

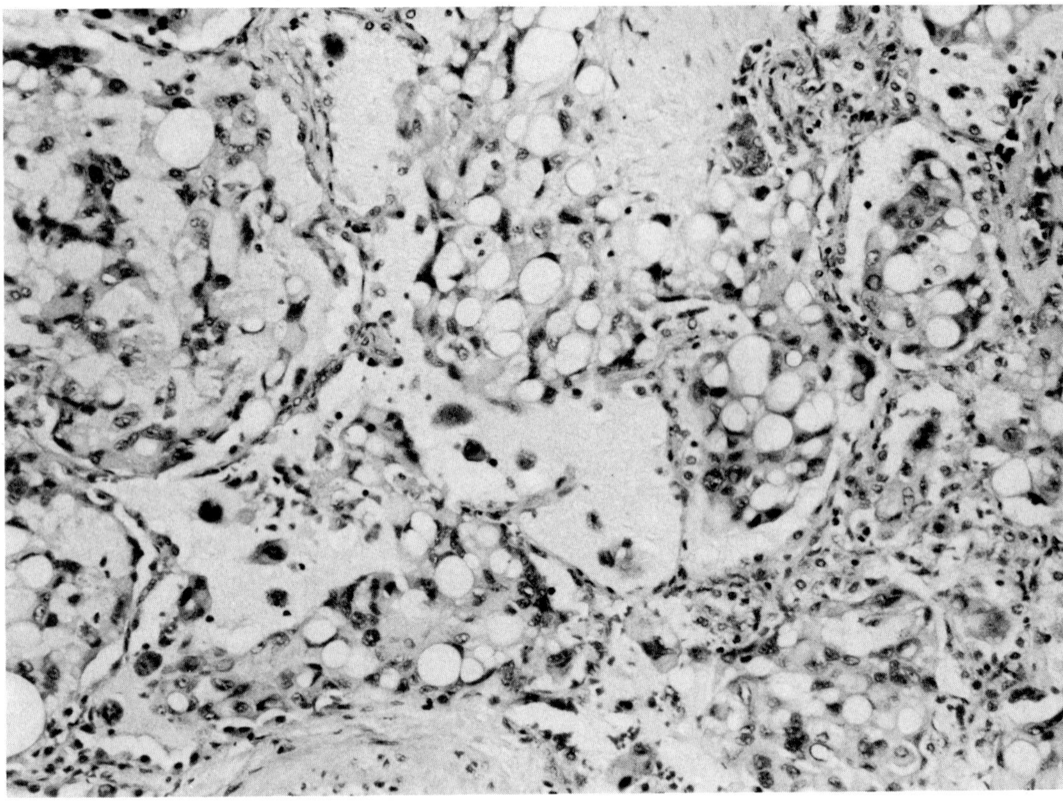

Figure 11–19. Epithelioid hemangioendothelioma. The tumor cells are growing through the alveolar spaces.

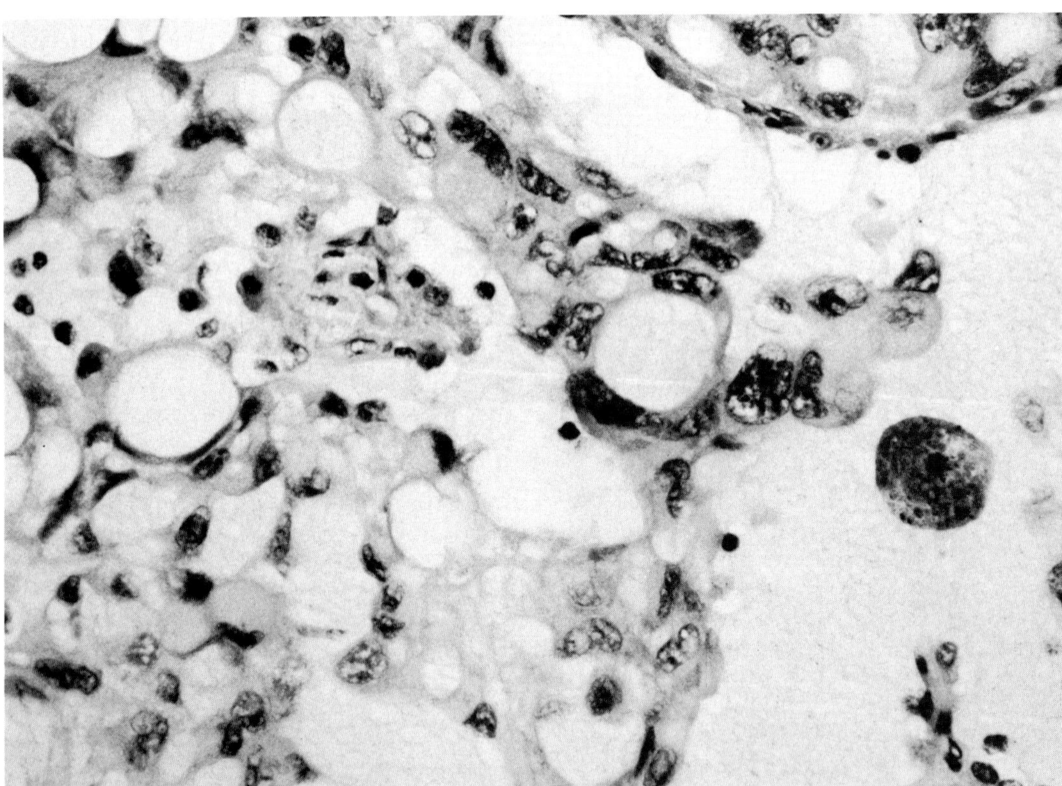

Figure 11–20. Epithelioid hemangioendothelioma. Many of the cells have vacuolated cytoplasm. Some nuclear pleomorphism is evident.

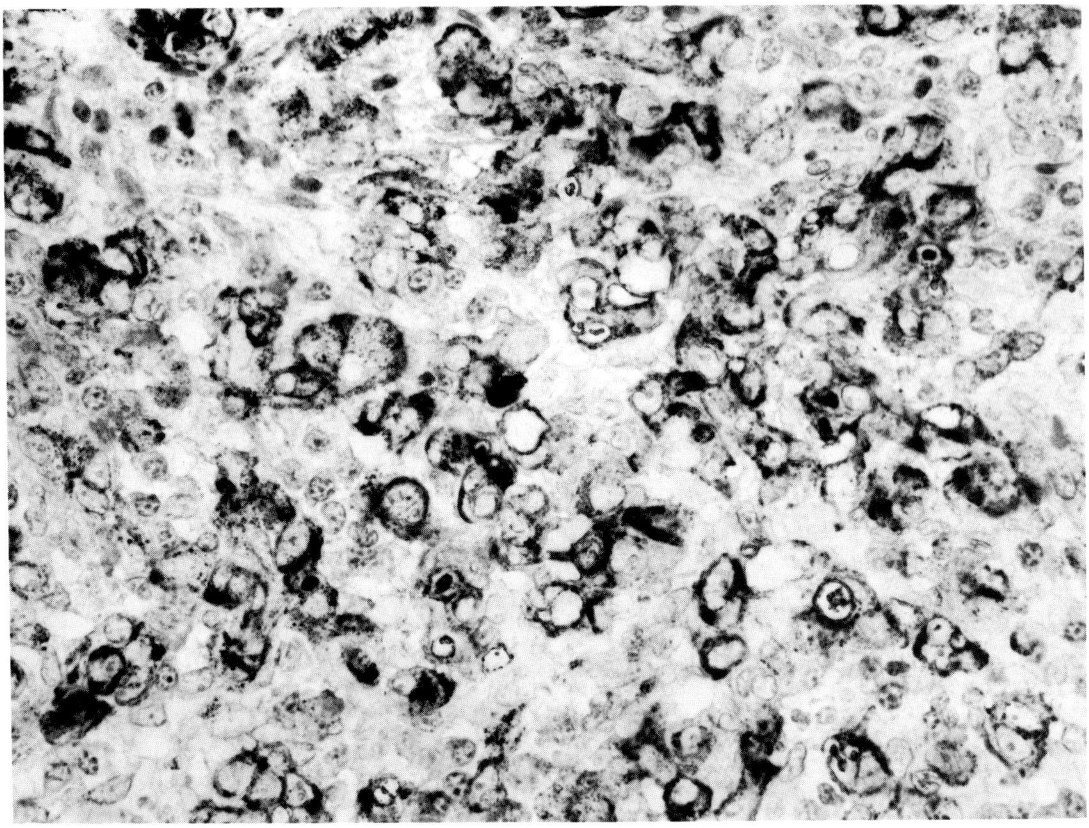

Figure 11–21. Epithelioid hemangioendothelioma showing reactivity for factor VIII–related antigen.

1961[302] when he described three new cases, and he recommended that the tumor be called a blastoma because of similarity with Wilms' tumor. The tumor is not common.[348] A similar lesion has been observed in the larynx.[78]

Pulmonary blastomas occur in children, but there is a second peak in the seventh decade.[61, 127, 157, 208] In the review by Francis and Jacobsen of 72 published and 11 personal cases,[97] 20% of the patients were under the age of 20; the 5-year survival was 15.7% and seven (8.4%) survived 10 years. Long survival with lymph node metastasis is recorded by Gibbons and co-workers.[111]

The tumors can be central or peripheral, but some are extensive and their localization is not possible. Areas of necrosis are common. In microscopic sections, the appearance is striking. A mixture of epithelial and mesenchymal components is usual, although one or the other may predominate and occupy considerable areas of the tumor. It is questionable whether pure epithelial or mesenchymal forms of blastoma exist, but their presence is theoretically possible. A blastoma with mesenchymal predominance may be particularly difficult to diagnose on a small biopsy specimen. The epithelial component is well differentiated. Tall columnar cells line glandular spaces (Fig. 11–22). The nuclei may be basal, but generally they are positioned at differing levels, creating an impression of stratification (Fig. 11–23). The cytoplasm is pale, and mucin and glycogen can be demonstrated. Merging with the glandular component there are compact groups of cells (Fig. 11–24) that have a squamoid or even a chondroid appearance. Foci of cartilage can also be present. The stromal component is typically made up of small stellate or spindle-shaped cells (Fig. 11–25) that may be loosely distributed within a myxoid or, in some areas, a collagenous matrix. Of the three cases reported by Dienemann and colleagues,[74] two were mixed epithelial and mesenchymal tumors and the third was a monomorphic tumor of blastomatous character. A resemblance to fetal lung in the pseudoglandular stage has been noted in a number of the reported cases.[177,

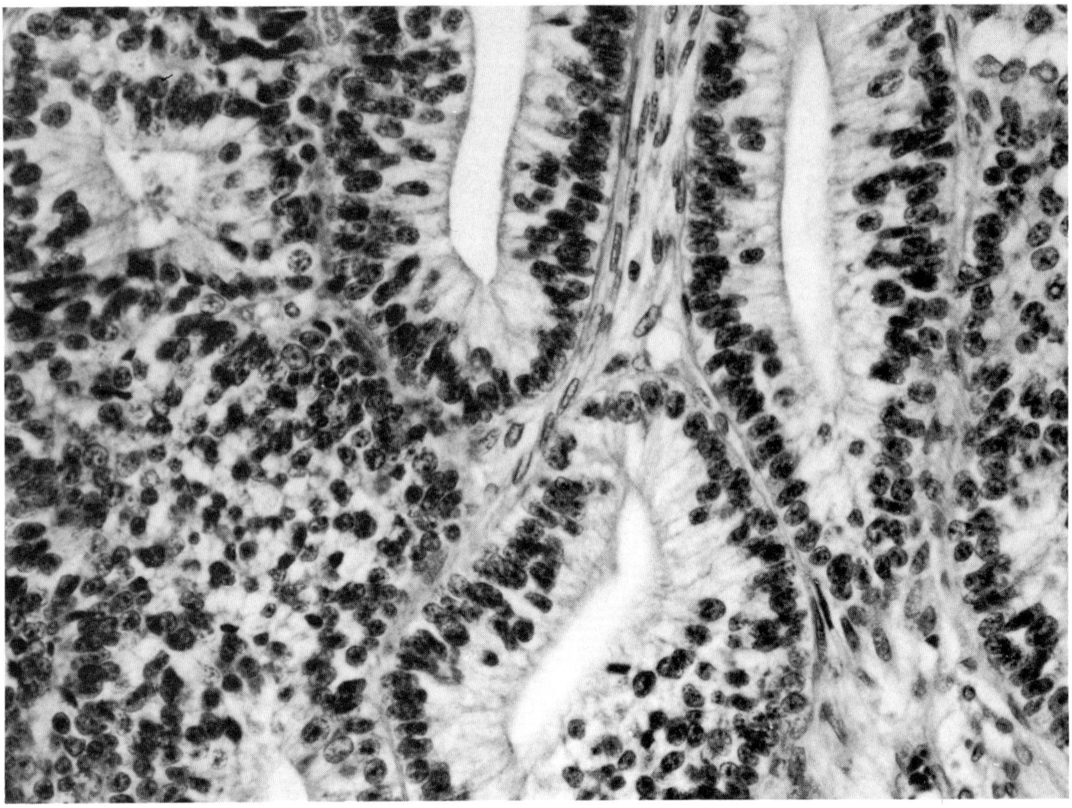

Figure 11–22. Pulmonary blastoma. The orderly architecture of the epithelial component is illustrated.

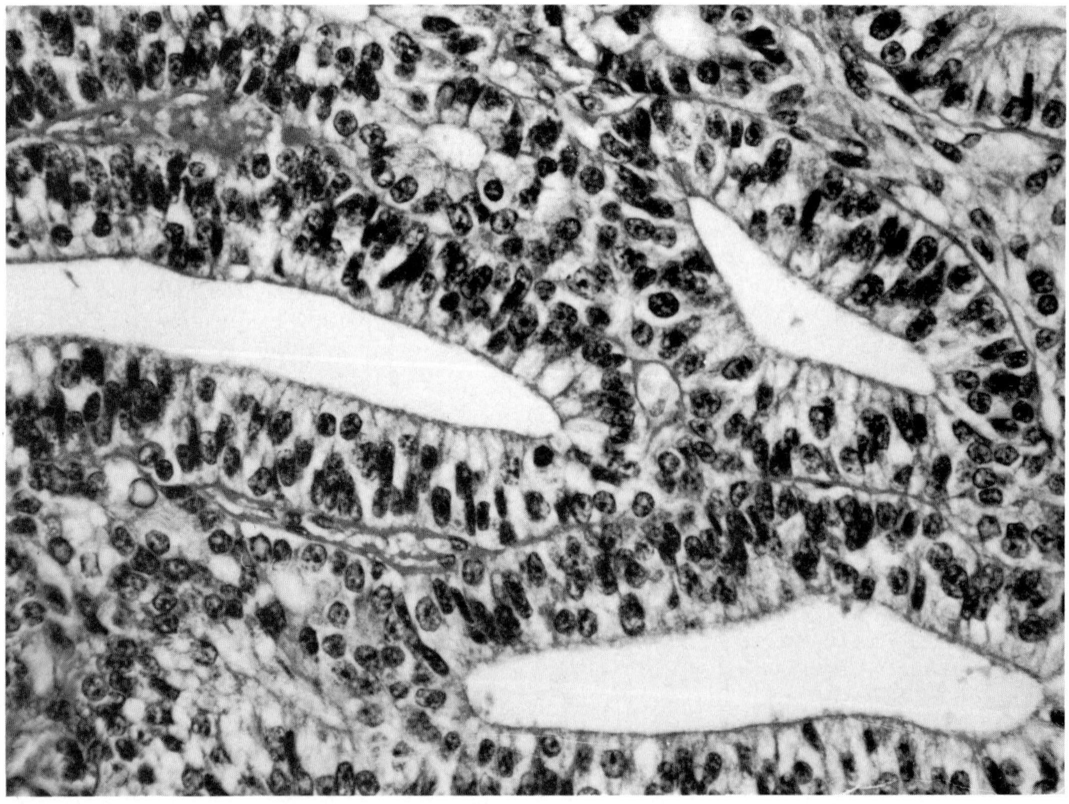

Figure 11–23. Pulmonary blastoma. Nuclei are at varying levels within the columnar cells, creating an impression of stratification.

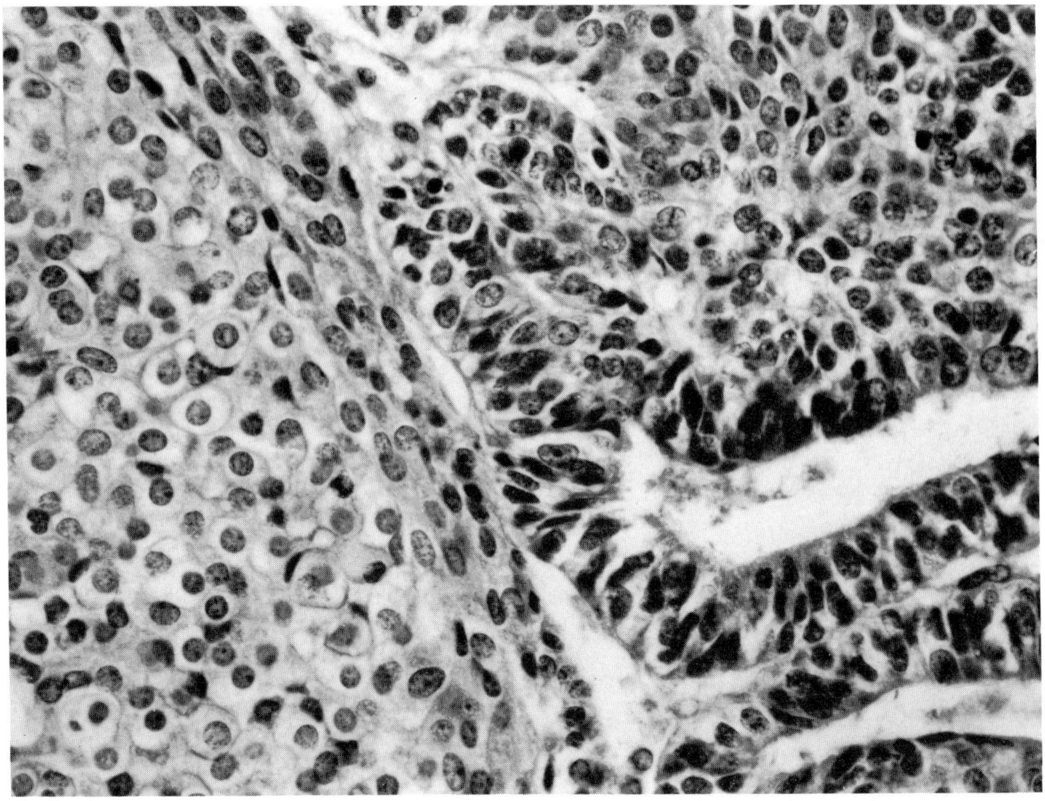

Figure 11–24. Pulmonary blastoma. A solid nest of cells abuts on a glandular area.

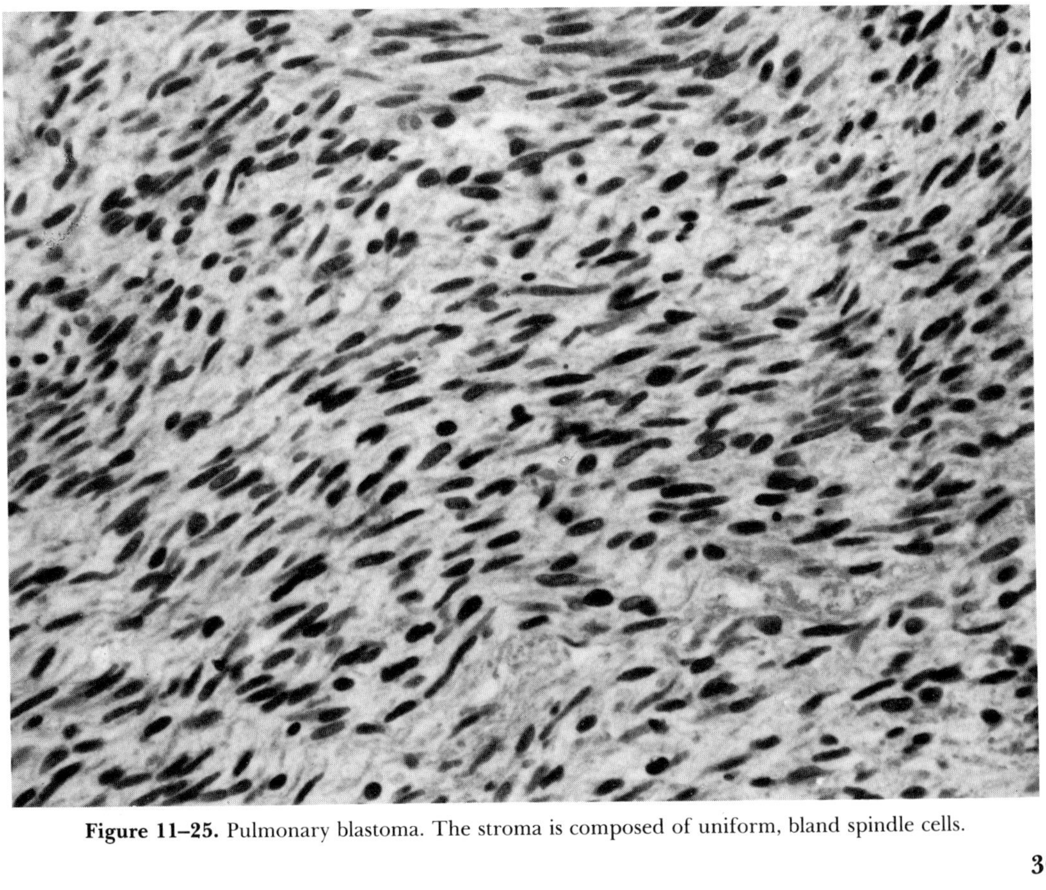

Figure 11–25. Pulmonary blastoma. The stroma is composed of uniform, bland spindle cells.

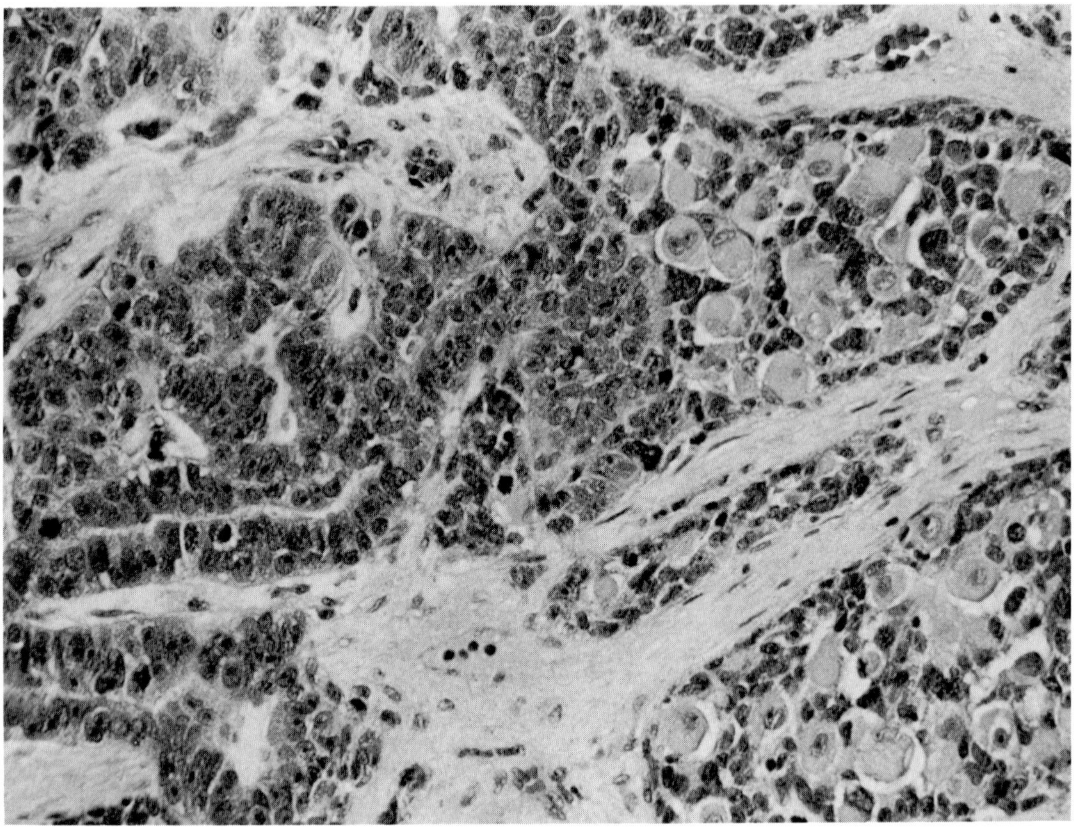

Figure 11–26. Pulmonary blastoma containing rhabdomyoblasts.

[209, 227] Rhabdomyoblasts may be identified[132] (Figs. 11–26 and 11–27), as may argyrophil cells, and myofilaments and neuroendocrine granules have been confirmed by electron microscopy.[184]

Immunocytochemical staining[1, 24] shows that reactivity to epithelial markers is confined to the epithelial cells. Antibodies against low-molecular-weight keratin proteins react with the glandular areas, especially along the apices of the cells, whereas those against high-molecular-weight keratin proteins show strong reactivity in the squamoid areas of the tumor (Figs. 11–28 and 11–29). Immunostaining for chromogranin helps to identify endocrine cells (Fig. 11–30), while immunostaining for myoglobin or desmin can assist in the recognition of rhabdomyoblastic differentiation (Fig. 11–31). Reactivity for S-100 protein occurs in the chondroid areas that are present in some tumors (Fig. 11–32).

Electron microscopy[102, 153, 184, 215] shows typical glandular features with junctional complexes and sparse microvilli in the epithelial component (Fig. 11–33), and lakes of glycogen in many of the cells. The stromal component contains cells with smooth muscle myofilaments, and lipid droplets are seen in fibroblast-like cells (Fig. 11–34). Electron microscopy has confirmed the presence of skeletal muscle myofilaments and of granules, some of them of neuroendocrine caliber[184] but others are large and of uncertain nature.[153] Tamai and associates transplanted one tumor into nude mice[317] and illustrated the ultrastructural features of the xenografted cells.

CARCINOSARCOMA

Carcinosarcoma derives its name from the mixture of malignant epithelial and mesenchymal components. As is the case when this tumor occurs in other organs, distinction from a sarcomatoid carcinoma[144] can be a problem. Moore[223] reviewed 13 pulmonary carcinosarcomas, and Kakos and co-workers, in 1971,[162] provided a case report and reviewed 19 cases from the literature. In 1985,

Text continued on page 311

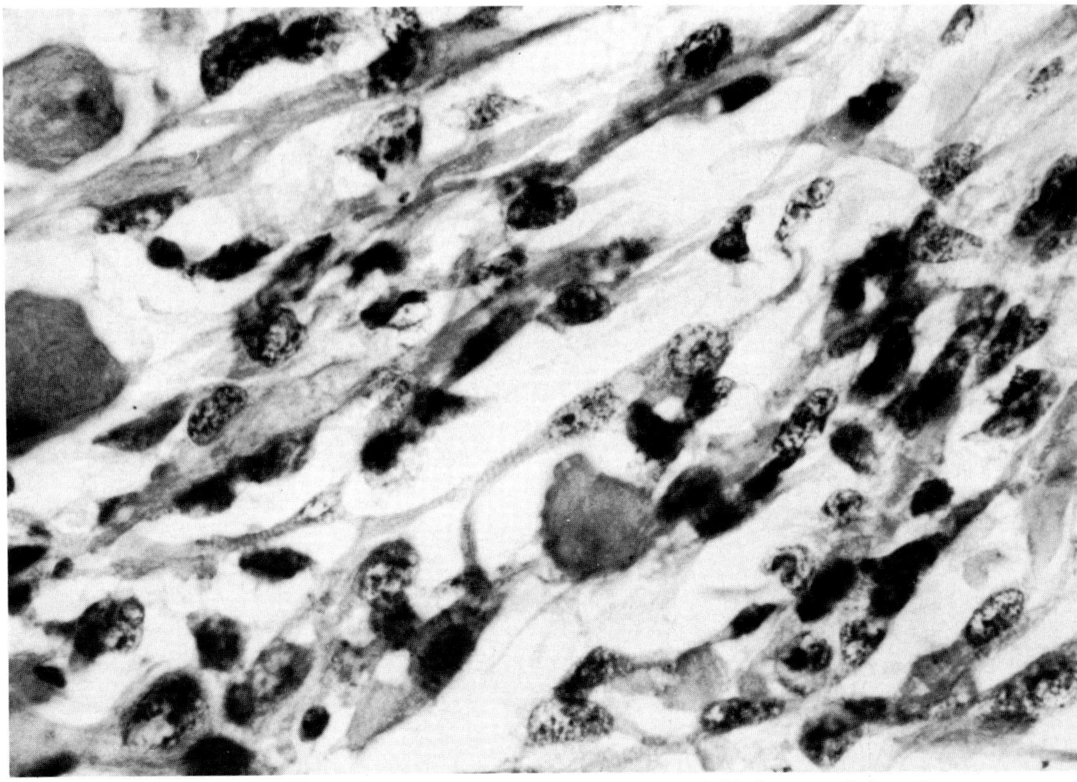

Figure 11–27. Pulmonary blastoma. Cross striations are visible in some of the cells.

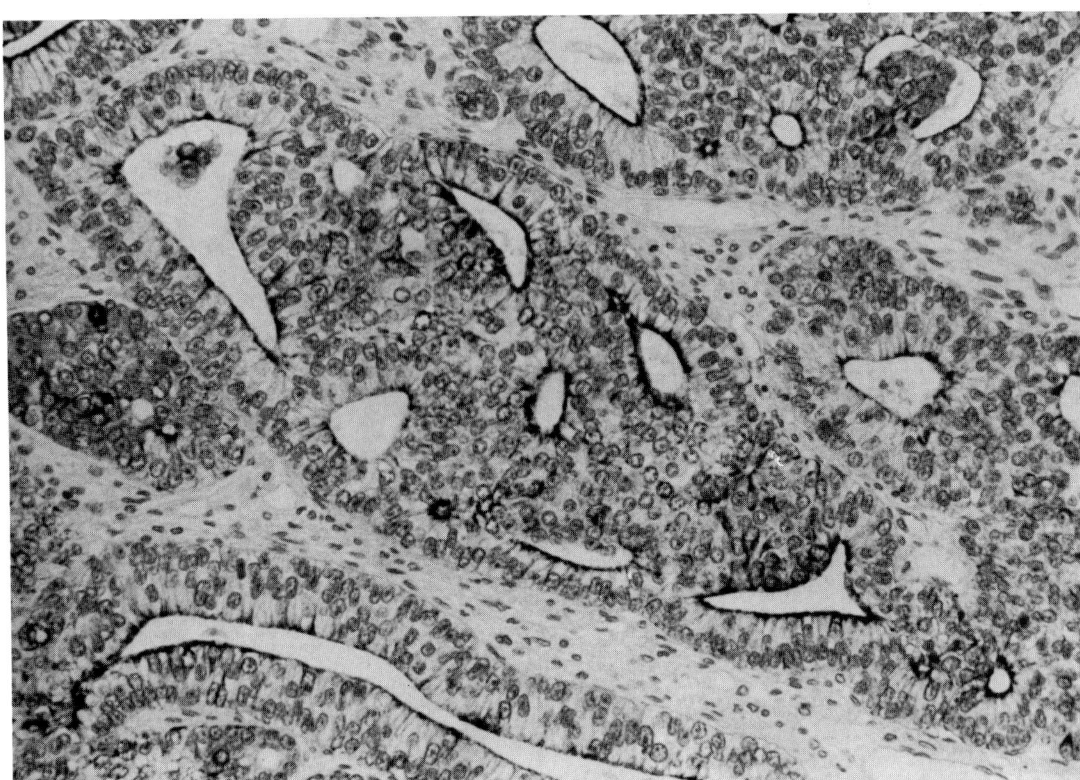

Figure 11–28. Pulmonary blastoma. Glandular component reacting with a low-molecular-weight keratin antibody.

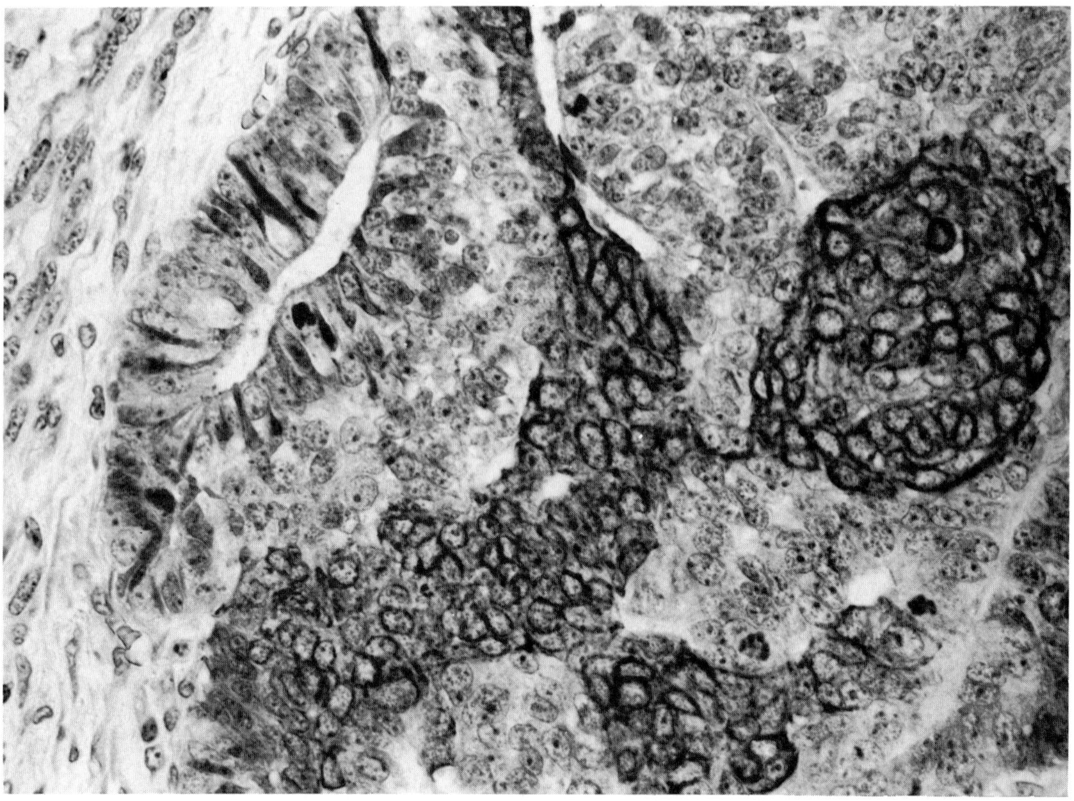

Figure 11–29. Pulmonary blastoma. Squamoid area reacting with a high-molecular-weight keratin antibody.

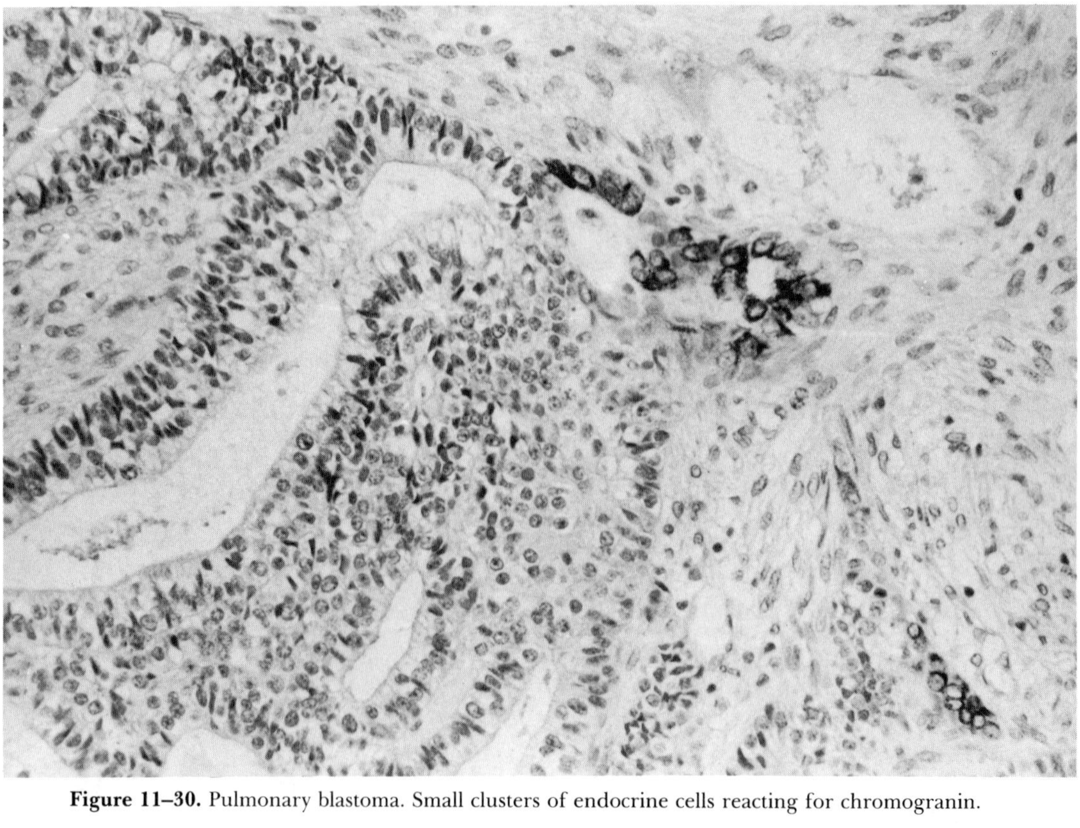

Figure 11–30. Pulmonary blastoma. Small clusters of endocrine cells reacting for chromogranin.

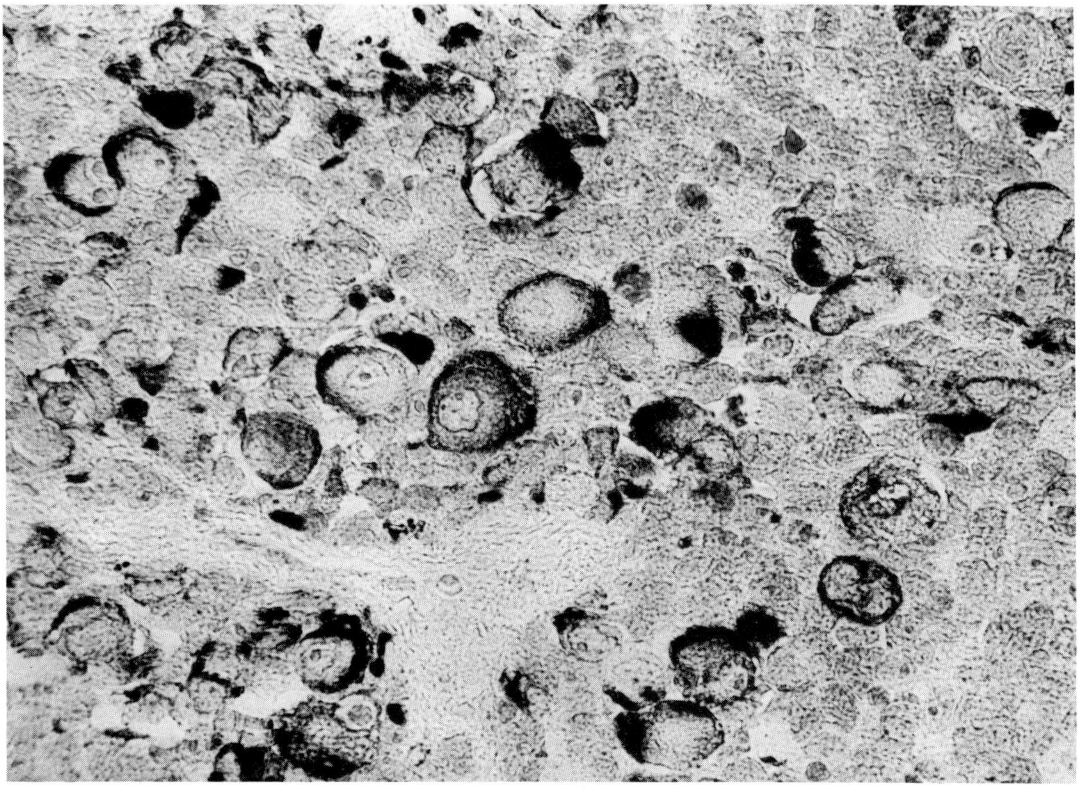

Figure 11–31. Pulmonary blastoma showing numerous rhabdomyoblasts reacting for desmin.

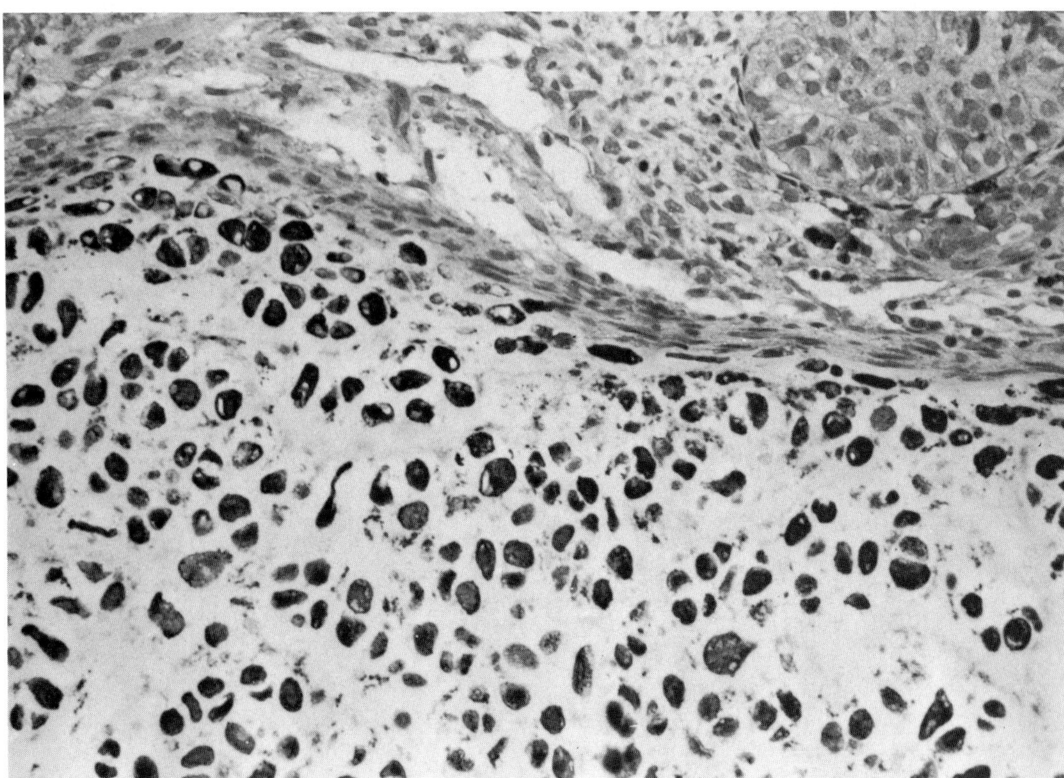

Figure 11–32. Pulmonary blastoma. Chondroid areas reacting for S-100 protein.

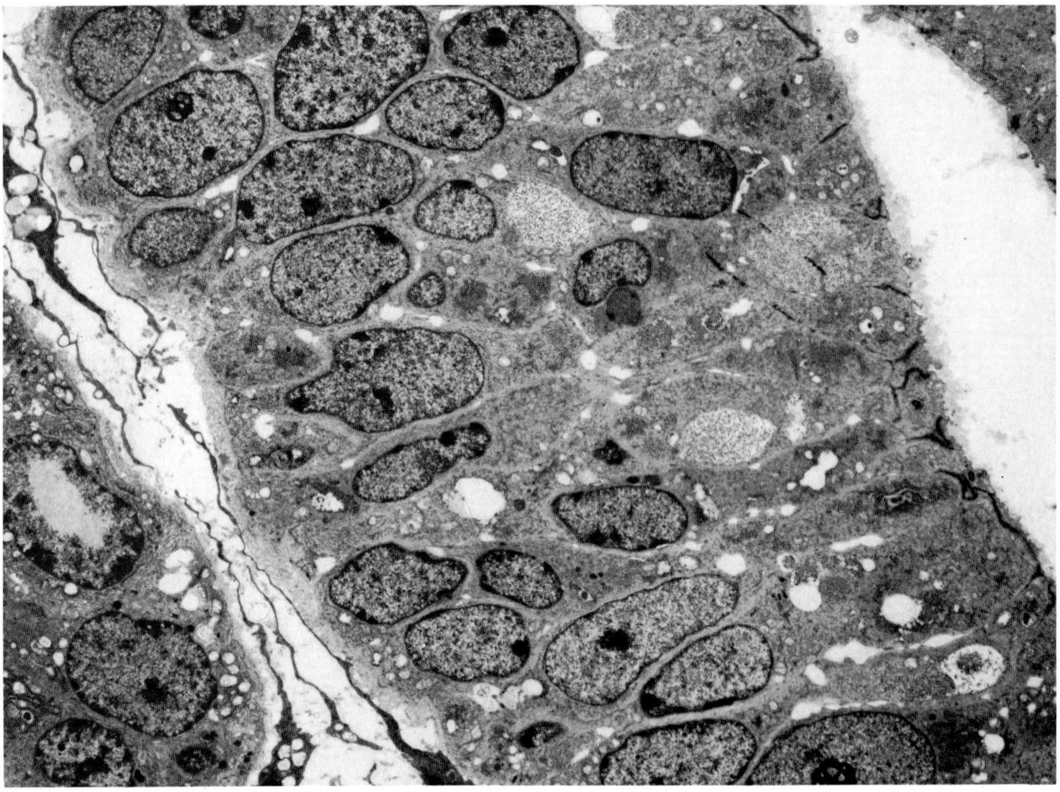

Figure 11–33. Pulmonary blastoma. Ultrastructure of the epithelial component. Tight junctions unite the apical regions of the cells. (×3,000)

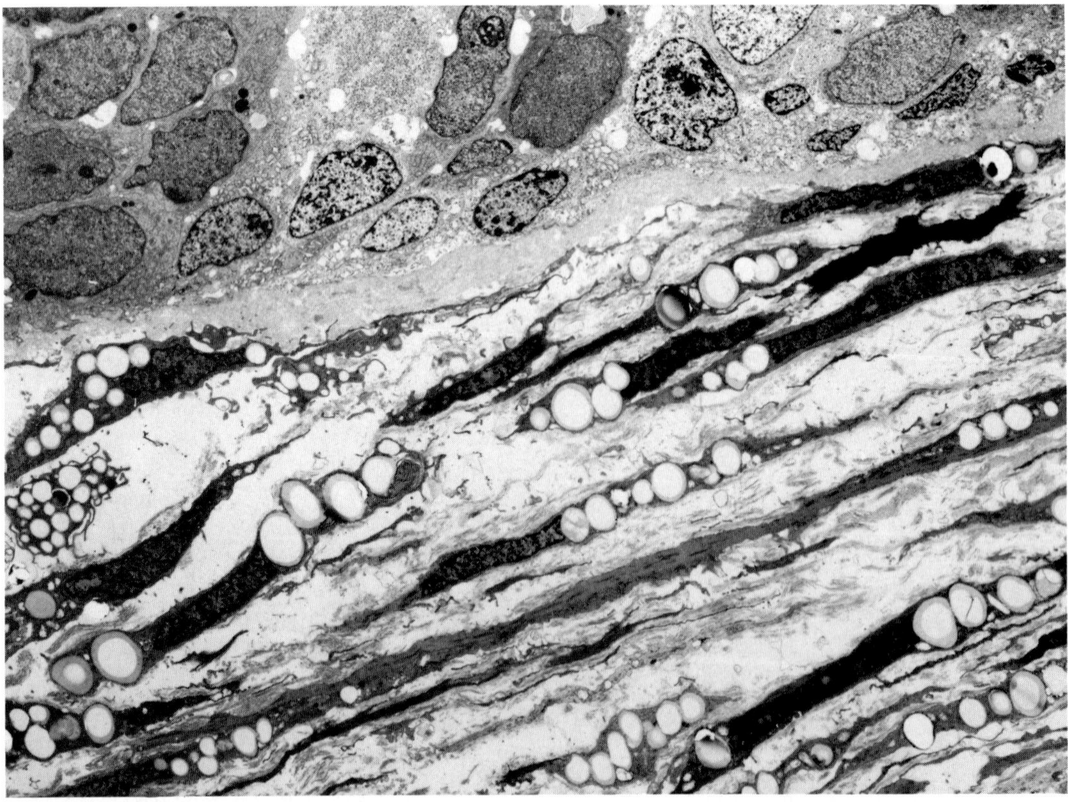

Figure 11–34. Pulmonary blastoma. The spindle cells in the stroma contain many lipid droplets. (×3,000)

Cabarcos and colleagues[32] reviewed 48 cases. Most of the patients are older men, and the male to female ratio is as high as 5:1. No cases appear to have been recorded in children. The upper lobes are more frequently involved. The tumor may be central or peripheral, and the peripheral lesions in particular can be large with extensive necrosis. The tumors are aggressive, and metastases may be present at the time of diagnosis. Spread is initially to hilar lymph nodes, and the tumor may grow through the pleura into the chest wall or penetrate the mediastinum.

The epithelial component is usually squamous cell carcinoma. Approximately 20% of tumors have adenocarcinoma and 10% have large cell undifferentiated carcinoma. Frequently it is not possible to subtype the mesenchymal components, and it may simply be designated fibrosarcoma or, if more pleomorphic cells are present, malignant fibrous histiocytoma. There may be areas of cartilage or osteoid formation, or rhabdoid differentiation can occur.[151] The two components are occasionally sharply separated, but more frequently they merge through zones of transitional cells.

Ultrastructural study helps to distinguish the tumor from a sarcomatoid carcinoma, but if the cells are poorly differentiated there may not be sufficiently distinctive features to allow classification. Immunostaining is therefore more appropriate.[1, 146] It is probable that with immunocytochemical studies, the frequency of carcinosarcoma will drop and many of these tumors will be recognized to be sarcomatoid sarcomas.

INTRAPULMONARY LYMPH NODES

Lymph nodes are not often noticed within surgical specimens of the lung more distal than the fourth bifurcation of the bronchial tree, although they have been demonstrated in 18% of autopsy lungs.[330] Occasionally one is detected on a radiograph as a coin lesion.[118, 183] Intraparenchymal lymph nodes are usually subpleural, and they can be multiple. They contain dust-laden histiocytes and may, by polarized light, be found to contain birefringent crystals of silica, suggesting that they are stimulated to develop by exposure to dusts.[183]

THYMOMA

Rarely, intrapulmonary occurrence of a thymoma is recorded.[117] A mediastinal thymoma may extend into the pleural space or invade the lung directly.

LYMPHOMA

Involvement of the lung parenchyma by a lymphoma[45, 47, 134, 180, 188, 193, 349] is uncommon when compared with the frequency with which other extranodal locations are affected, and it is not usually found to be limited to the lung after a complete staging procedure has been carried out.[87, 343] It is, however, being seen more often in patients with AIDS,[112] and has been reported following long-standing pyothorax.[152] The majority of primary lymphomas of the lung are of B-cell origin.[149] The history and findings on physical examination are not specific,[260] but the diagnosis may be reached by bronchial cytology,[20, 68, 202, 229, 245] facilitated by immunocytochemical procedures.[110, 116, 345] Patients with lymphoma are at increased risk to develop infectious processes in the lung, and open lung biopsy may provide information on the nature of discrete masses seen on chest radiography.[214]

Kennedy and co-workers[170] separated 64 patients with pulmonary lymphoid lesions into three groups. In 32 patients, the proliferating cell was a small mature-appearing lymphocyte. This was a heterogeneous group that included small lymphocytic lymphoma, lymphoid interstitial pneumonia, and lymphoid hyperplasia or pseudolymphoma. In 13 of the 32 patients with similar histologic findings but with a higher incidence of plasmacytoid features and mast cell infiltration, the findings of monoclonality and progressive disease in other locations led to the diagnosis of small lymphocytic lymphoma; large cell lymphoma subsequently developed in 4 of these patients. The remaining two groups of patients had various forms of malignant lymphoma other than the small lymphocytic type.

In 40% of the 47 patients with primary well-differentiated lymphoma of the lung studied by Turner and co-workers,[333] the diagnosis was supported by ancillary findings, including involvement of other organs, monoclonal immunologic markers, or a monoclonal serum gammopathy; follow-up of 33 cases revealed only one death. Burkitt's lymphoma may present as an endobronchial lesion[272] or produce an infiltrative pattern.[243]

Lymphoma has been found coexisting with a primary lung carcinoid.[161] A prominent lymphoid infiltrate associated with an undifferentiated lung carcinoma can produce a lymphoepithelioma-like appearance and simulate lymphoma.[31] Lymphoid hyperplasias,[182] lymphoid interstitial pneumonia,[2] pseudolymphoma,[92, 182, 210] and the granulomatoses[29, 181, 347] enter into the differential diagnosis of pulmonary lymphoma. A solitary mast cell tumor of the lung has been reported.[185]

HISTIOCYTOSIS

When the lung is involved by a disorder in the histiocytosis X spectrum, it may be part of a systemic disease, but in many patients it is limited to the lung.[18, 46, 99] Bilateral involvement is usual. The process may be associated with lymphoma[237] or Hodgkin's disease[280] and can be confused histologically with other lung disorders.[264] Patients are usually young, but some adults are affected. Basset and coworkers found a 4:1 male to female ratio among 78 patients.[18] The lesions are small and multiple, and they can be asymptomatic or cause cough, dyspnea, or a febrile disorder. If they are subpleural, pneumothorax may be produced. Children often respond to treatment, but otherwise the lesions may cavitate and ultimately fibrose, creating a honeycomb lung. In histologic sections there are many eosinophils and plasma cells in addition to the histiocytes, which mark for S-100 protein and HLA-DR antigen[95, 346] and contain Langerhans' granules.

HODGKIN'S DISEASE

Primary pulmonary Hodgkin's disease[139, 366, 372] is rare, but the lung may be involved as part of more widespread disease. Usually the parenchymal involvement is associated with lymphadenopathy in the hilar or mediastinal regions,[313] but this is not always the case.[368] Sarcoidosis may be mimicked.[64] Bronchial washings may lead to the diagnosis,[224, 356] which can also be obtained in some cases by fine-needle aspiration.[94] In open-lung biopsies on 41 patients known to have the disease who developed pulmonary infiltrates, Catterall and colleagues[38] obtained a specific diagnosis in 19 (46%), and in 12 it was Hodgkin's disease. Patients treated for Hodgkin's disease can develop other tumors involving the lung.[49, 200, 247, 265, 339]

GERM CELL TUMORS

Three cases of germ cell tumors were reported by Nozaki and associates.[242] Teratomas presenting in the lung are uncommon lesions.[138, 284] Some of the reported cases were probably mediastinal teratomas that infiltrated contiguous lung. The diagnosis may be suggested by radiology, although the features are not specific. The tumors can present in young adults, and they may contain thymic tissue.[138, 155] The lung is a rare site for primary choriocarcinoma.[267, 314, 321]

NODULAR AMYLOIDOSIS

The respiratory tract is sometimes involved as part of systemic amyloidosis. A solitary lung nodule can occur[128] and can produce massive hilar lymphadenopathy.[325] Multiple nodules can also be present in the lungs,[191] but it is rare to encounter extensive bilateral involvement. Hui and associates reported 48 cases.[143] Lesions generally occur in older adults and may be mistaken for carcinoma on chest radiography.

MELANOMA

Since a cutaneous or mucosal melanoma can spontaneously regress, it is generally impossible to establish beyond doubt that a focus of melanoma within the lung is primary at that site unless the lesion is confined to the bronchial epithelium.[12, 33, 37, 109, 273, 316] Metastatic melanoma frequently involves the lung.[66]

MENINGIOMA

Primary meningiomas have been described within the lung.[41, 169, 311, 370] Since ectopic meningiomas can occur in other extracranial locations, it is conceivable that they might occasionally arise within the lung, but meningiomas can closely resemble peripheral nerve sheath tumors and the enigmatic pulmonary chemodectoma. Confirmation by electron microscopy is always desirable. Undulating cell processes and prominent desmosomes are seen by electron microscopy.[41, 169] Accounts of metastatic meningiomas involving the lung are more common.[312] Lung carcinoma on occasion metastasizes to a primary intracranial meningioma.[51]

REFERENCES

1. Addis BJ, Corrin B: Pulmonary blastoma, carcinosarcoma and spindle cell carcinoma: An immunohistochemical study of keratin intermediate filaments. J Pathol 147:291, 1985.
2. Addis BJ, Hyjek E, Isaacson PG: Primary pulmonary lymphoma: A re-appraisal of its histogenesis and its relationship to pseudolymphoma and lymphoid interstitial pneumonia. Histopathology 13:1, 1988.
3. Aiba M, Hirayama A, Sakurada M et al: So-called sclerosing hemangioma of the lung with nuclear inclusion bodies: Immunohistochemical study of a case. Acta Pathol Jpn 38:873, 1988.
4. Albrecht E: Ueber hamartome. Verhandl Dtsch Pathol Gesselsch 7:153, 1904.
5. Al-Saleem T, Peale AR, Norris CM: Multiple papillomatosis of the lower respiratory tract: Clinical and pathologic study of eleven cases. Cancer 22:1173, 1968.
6. Allan BT, Day DL, Dehner LP: Primary pulmonary rhabdomyosarcoma of the lung in children: Report of two cases presenting with spontaneous pneumothorax. Cancer 59:1005, 1987.
7. Allen MS, Marsh WL, Geissinger WT: Mucus gland adenoma of the bronchus. J Thorac Cardiovasc Surg 67:966, 1974.
8. Alvarez-Fernandez E, Carretero-Albinana L et al: Sclerosing hemangioma of the lung: An immunohistochemical study of intermediate filaments and endothelial markers. Arch Pathol Lab Med 113:121, 1989.
9. Andrion A, Mazzucco G, Gugliotta P et al: Benign clear cell (sugar) tumor of the lung: A light microscopic, histochemical, and ultrastructural study with a review of the literature. Cancer 56:2657, 1985.
10. Attar S, Miller JE, Hankins J et al: Bronchial adenoma: A review of 51 patients. Ann Thorac Surg 40:126, 1984.
11. Avagnina A, Elsner B, De Marco L et al: Pulmonary rhabdomyosarcoma with isolated small bowel metastasis: A report of a case with immunohistochemical and ultrastructural studies. Cancer 53:1948, 1984.
12. Bagwell SP, Flynn SD, Cox PM et al: Primary malignant melanoma of the lung. Am Rev Respir Dis 139:1543, 1989.
13. Baker PB, Goodwin RA: Pulmonary artery sarcomas: A review and report of a case. Arch Pathol Lab Med 109:35, 1985.
14. Barnard WG: Embryoma of lung. Thorax 7:299, 1952.
15. Barett NR, Barnard WG: Some unusual thoracic tumours. Br J Surg 32:447, 1945.
16. Barsky SH, Martin SE, Matthews M et al: Low-grade mucoepidermoid carcinoma of the bronchus with high-grade biological behavior. Cancer 51:1505, 1983.
17. Basile A, Gregoris A, Antoci B et al: Malignant change in a benign pulmonary hamartoma. Thorax 44:232, 1989.
18. Basset F, Corrin B, Spencer H et al: Pulmonary histiocytosis X. Am Rev Respir Dis 118:811, 1978.
19. Bedrossian CW, Verani R, Unger KM et al: Pulmonary malignant fibrous histiocytoma. Chest 75:186, 1979.
20. Bellotti M, Elsner B, Esteva H et al: Fiberoptic bronchoscopy in the diagnosis of pulmonary lymphomas. Respiration 52:201:1987.
21. Beluffi G, Bertolotti P, Mietta A et al: Primary leiomyosarcoma of the lung in a girl. Pediatr Radiol 16:240, 1986.
22. Bennett LL, Lesar MS, Tellis CJ: Multiple calcified chondrohamartomas of the lung: CT appearance. J Comput Assist Tomogr 9:180, 1985.
23. Berardi RS, Lee SS, Chen HP et al: Inflammatory pseudotumors of the lung. Surg Gynecol Obstet 156:89, 1983.
24. Berean K, Truong LD, Dudley AW et al: Immunohistochemical characterization of pulmonary blastoma. Am J Clin Pathol 89:773, 1988.
25. Bhagavan BS, Dorfman HD, Murthy MSN et al: Intravascular bronchioloalveolar tumor (IVBAT): A low-grade sclerosing epithelioid angiosarcoma of the lung. Am J Surg Pathol 6:41, 1982.
26. Bharani SN, Arbeit JM, Hyde JS et al: Mucoepidermoid tumor of trachea. Chest 70:782, 1976.
27. Bierhoff E, Baum HP, Mildenberger P et al: Hemangiopericytoma of the lung: A rare differential diagnosis of lung tumors. Thorac Cardiovasc Surg 36:292, 1988.
28. Bleisch VR, Kraus FT: Polypoid sarcoma of the pulmonary trunk: Analysis of the literature and report of a case with leptomeric organelles and ultrastructural features of rhabdomyosarcoma. Cancer 46:314, 1980.
29. Bleiweiss IJ, Strauchen JA: Lymphomatoid granulomatosis of the lung: Report of a case and gene rearrangement studies. Hum Pathol 19:1109, 1988.
30. Breyer RH, Dainauskas JR, Jensik RJ et al: Mucoepidermoid carcinoma of the trachea and bronchus: The case for conservative resection. Ann Thorac Surg 29:197, 1980.
31. Butler AE, Colby TV, Weiss L et al: Lymphoepithelioma-like carcinoma of the lung. Am J Surg Pathol 13:632, 1989.
32. Cabarcos A, Gomez Dorronsoro M, Lobo Beristain JL: Pulmonary carcinosarcoma: A case study and review of the literature. Br J Dis Chest 79:83, 1985.
33. Cagle P, Mace ML, Judge DM et al: Pulmonary melanoma: Primary versus metastatic. Chest 85:125, 1984.
34. Capewell S, Webb JN, Crompton GK: Primary leiomyosarcoma of the lung presenting with a persistent pneumothorax. Thorax 41:649, 1986.
35. Capron F, Ameille J, Leclerc P et al: Pulmonary

lymphangioleiomyomatosis and Bourneville's tuberous sclerosis with pulmonary involvement: The same disease. Cancer 52:851, 1983.
36. Carnot F, Riquet M, Desche-Labarthe S et al: Multiple leiomyomatous pulmonary nodules in women: Apropos of 2 cases of metastasizing benign leiomyoma. Rev Pneumol Clin 43:131, 1987.
37. Carstens PHB, Kuhns JG, Ghazi C: Primary malignant melanomas of the lung and adrenal. Hum Pathol 15:910, 1984.
38. Catterall JR, McCabe RE, Brooks RG et al: Open lung biopsy in patients with Hodgkin's disease and pulmonary infiltrates. Am Rev Respir Dis 139:1274, 1989.
39. Chen HP, Lee SS, Berardi RS: Inflammatory pseudotumor of the lung: Ultrastructural and light microscopic study of a myxomatous variant. Cancer 54:861, 1984.
40. Chowdhury LN, Swerdlow MA, Jao W et al: Postirradiation malignant fibrous histiocytoma of the lung: Demonstration of alpha-1-antitrypsin-like material in neoplastic cells. Am J Clin Pathol 74:820, 1980.
41. Chumas JC, Lorelle CA: Pulmonary meningioma: A light and electron microscopic study. Am J Surg Pathol 6:795, 1982.
42. Churg AM, Warnock ML: So-called "minute pulmonary chemodectoma": A tumor not related to paraganglioma. Cancer 37:1759, 1976.
43. Clayton F, Mackay B, Ayala AG et al: Vacuolated epithelial lesion in lung. Ultrastruct Pathol 2:303, 1981.
44. Colby TV, Bilbao JE, Battifora H et al: Primary osteosarcoma of the lung: A reappraisal following immunohistologic study. Arch Pathol Lab Med 113:1147, 1989.
45. Colby TV, Carrington CB: Pulmonary lymphomas: Current concepts. Hum Pathol 14:884, 1983.
46. Colby TV, Lombard C: Histiocytosis X in the lung. Hum Pathol 14:847, 1983.
47. Colby TV, Yousem SA: Pulmonary lymphoid neoplasms. Semin Diagn Pathol 2:183, 1985.
48. Collet P, Loire R, Guerin JC et al: Apparently primary thoracic hemangiopericytoma: Apropos of 12 cases. Rev Pneumol Clin 41:151, 1985.
49. Colman M, Easton DF, Horwich A et al: Second malignancies and Hodgkin's disease: the Royal Marsden Hospital experience. Radiother Oncol 11:229, 1988.
50. Conlan AA, Payne WE, Woolner LB et al: Adenoid cystic carcinoma (cylindroma) and mucoepidermoid carcinoma of bronchus: Factors affecting survival. J Thorac Cardiovasc Surg 76:369, 1978.
51. Conzen M, Sollmann H, Schnabel R: Metastasis of lung carcinoma to intracranial meningioma: Case report and review of the literature. Neurochirurgia 29:206, 1986.
52. Corona FE, Okeson GC: Endobronchial fibroma: An unusual cause of segmental atelectasis. Am Rev Respir Dis 110:350, 1974.
53. Corrin B, Manners B, Millard M et al: Histogenesis of the so-called intravascular bronchioloalveolar tumor. J Pathol 128:163, 1979.
54. Corrin B, Harrison WJ, Wright DH et al: The so-called 'intravascular' bronchioloalveolar tumour of lung (low-grade sclerosing angiosarcoma): Presentation with extrapulmonary deposits. Diagn Histopathol 6:229, 1983.
55. Corrin B, Liebow A, Friedman PJ: Pulmonary lymphangiomyomatosis: A review. Am J Pathol 79:347, 1985.
56. Costero I, Barroso-Moguel R, Martinez-Palomo A: Pleural origin of some of the supposed chemodectomoid structures of the lung. Beitr Pathol 146:351, 1972.
57. Courtin P, Janin A, Sault MC et al: Pure bronchial adenoma: Anatomicoclinical and ultrastructural study of a case. Ann Pathol 7:315, 1987.
58. Crouch JD, Keagy BA, Starek PJ et al: A clinical review of patients undergoing resection for pulmonary hamartoma. Am Surg 54:297, 1988.
59. Dail DH: Benign clear cell ("sugar") tumor of the lung. Arch Pathol Lab Med 113:573, 1989.
60. Dail DH: Intravascular bronchiolar and alveolar tumor (IVBAT) of the lung. ASCP Check Sample (Tumor Diagnosis) 11:4, 1984.
61. Dail DH: Uncommon Lung Tumors. In Dail DH, Hammar SP (eds): Pulmonary Pathology, p 903. New York, Springer-Verlag, 1988.
62. Dail DH, Liebow A: Intravascular bronchioloalveolar tumor (abstr). Am J Pathol 78:6a, 1975.
63. Dail DH, Liebow AA, Gmelich JT et al: Intravascular, bronchiolar, and alveolar tumor of the lung (IVBAT): An analysis of twenty cases of a peculiar sclerosing endothelial tumor. Cancer 51:451, 1983.
64. Daly PA, O'Brian DS, Robinson I et al: Hodgkin's disease with a granulomatous pulmonary presentation mimicking sarcoidosis. Thorax 43:407, 1988.
65. Dardick I, Daya D, Hardie J et al: Mucoepidermoid carcinoma: Ultrastructural and histogenetic aspects. Oral Pathol 13:342, 1984.
66. Das Gupta T, Brasfield R: Metastatic melanoma: A clinicopathologic study. Cancer 17:1323, 1964.
67. Davis PW, Briggs JC, Seal RME et al: Benign and malignant mixed tumors of the lung. Thorax 27:657, 1972.
68. Davis WB, Gadek JE: Detection of pulmonary lymphoma by bronchoalveolar lavage. Chest 91:787, 1987.
69. DeRooij PD, Meijer S, Calame J et al: Solitary hamartoma of the lung: Is thoracotomy still mandatory? Neth J Surg 40:145, 1988.
70. Defraigne JO, Borlee-Hermans G, Honore P et al: Primary pulmonary leiomyosarcoma: Review of the literature apropos of a case. J Chir 124:272, 1987.
71. Deoms TC, Armin A, Chandrasekhar AJ et al: Cystic hamartoma of the lung. J Can Assoc Radiol 34:149, 1983.
72. Desato K, Yoneyama T, Tanimura S et al: A case of bronchial fibroma associated with subsegmental atelectasis. J Clin Oncol 9:285, 1979.
73. Dewandre JM, Hainaut H, Paquot JP et al: Primary pulmonary hemangiopericytoma in children: Apropos of a case. Chir Pediatr 27:226, 1986.
74. Dienemann D, Hartmann CA, Minck C: Pulmonary blastomas: Immunohistochemical investigations of three cases. Pathol Res Pract 184:306, 1989.
75. DiMarco AF: Papillomas of tracheobronchial tree with malignant degeneration. Chest 74:464, 1978.
76. Dishner W, Cordasco EM, Blackburn J et al: Pulmonary lymphangiomyomatosis. Chest 85:796, 1984.

77. Eastridge CE, Young JM, Steplock AL: Endobronchial lipoma. South Med J 77:759, 1984.
78. Eble JN, Hull MT, Bojrab D: Laryngeal blastoma: A light and electron microscopic study of a novel entity analogous to pulmonary blastoma. Am J Clin Pathol 84:378, 1985.
79. Echevarria RA: Angiogenic nature of "intravascular bronchioloalveolar tumor." Arch Pathol Lab Med 105:627, 1981.
80. Edwards CW, Matthews HR: Mucous gland adenoma of the bronchus. Thorax 36:147, 1981.
81. Edwards CW, Saunders AM, Collins F: Mixed malignant tumor of the lung. Thorax 34:629, 1979.
82. Eggleston JG: The intravascular bronchioloalveolar tumor and the sclerosing hemangioma of the lung: Misnomers of pulmonary neoplasia. Semin Diagn Pathol 2:270, 1985.
83. Emory WB et al: Mucous gland adenoma of the bronchus. Am Rev Respir Dis 108:1407, 1973.
84. Ericksson A, Thunell M, Lundqvist G: Pendulating endobronchial rhabdomyosarcoma with fatal asphyxia. Thorax 37:390, 1982.
85. Fabich DR, Hafez GR: Glomangioma of the trachea. Cancer 45:2337, 1980.
86. Fantone JC, Geisinger KR, Appelman HD: Papillary adenoma of the lung with lamellar and electron-dense granules: An ultrastructural study. Cancer 50:2839, 1982.
87. Farquhar DL, Crompton GK, McIntyre MA et al: Non-Hodgkin's lymphoma of the lung. Scott Med J 33:243, 1988.
88. Fechner RE, Bentinck BR, Askew JB: Acinic cell tumor of the lung: A histologic and ultrastructural study. Cancer 29:501, 1972.
89. Fechner R, Bentinck BR: Ultrastructure of bronchial oncocytoma. Cancer 31:1450, 1973.
90. Fechner RE, Fitz-Hugh GS: Invasive tracheal papillomatosis. Am J Surg Pathol 4:79, 1981.
91. Feldhaus RJ, Anene C, Bogard P: A rare endobronchial neurilemmoma (schwannoma). Chest 95:461, 1989.
92. Feoli F, Carbone A, Dina MA et al: Pseudolymphoma of the lung: Lymphoid subsets in the lung mass and in peripheral blood. Cancer 48:2218, 1981.
93. Fernandez MA, Nyssen J: Oncocytoma of the lung. Can J Surg 25:332, 1982.
94. Flint A, Kumar NB, Naylor B: Pulmonary Hodgkin's disease: Diagnosis by fine-needle aspiration. Acta Cytol 32:221, 1988.
95. Flint A, Lloyd RV, Colby TV et al: Pulmonary histiocytosis X: Immunoperoxidase staining for HLA-DR antigen and S-100 protein. Arch Pathol Lab Med 110:930, 1986.
96. Fouret PJ, Touboul JL, Mayoud CM et al: Pulmonary Kaposi's sarcoma in patients with acquired immune deficiency syndrome: A clinicopathologic study. Thorax 42:262, 1987.
97. Francis D, Jacobsen M: Pulmonary blastoma. Curr Top Pathol 73:265, 1983.
98. Freschi P, Pocecco M, Carini C et al: Post-traumatic inflammatory pseudotumor of the lung: Description of a case. Pediatr Med Chir 11:93, 1989.
99. Friedman PJ, Liebow AA, Sokoloff J: Eosinophilic granuloma of the lung. Medicine 60:385, 1981.
100. Fukayama M, Kioke M: So-called sclerosing hemangioma of the lung: An immunohistochemical, histochemical and ultrastructural study. Acta Pathol Jpn 38:627, 1988.
101. Fukuda T, Machinami R, Joshita T et al: Benign clear cell tumor of the lung in an 8-year old girl. Arch Pathol Lab Med 110:664, 1986.
102. Fung CH, Lo JW, Yonan TN et al: Pulmonary blastoma: An ultrastructural study with a brief review of the literature and a discussion of pathogenesis. Cancer 39:153, 1977.
103. Fuzesi L, Hoer PW, Schmidt W: Exfoliative cytology of multiple endobronchial granular cell tumor. Acta Cytol 33:516, 1989.
104. Gabriel JB, Thomas L, Mendoza CB et al: Granular cell tumor of the bronchus co-existing with a bronchogenic adenocarcinoma: A case report. J Surg Oncol 24:103, 1983.
105. Gaffey MJ, Mills SF, Askin FB: Minute pulmonary meningothelial-like nodules: A clinicopathologic study of so-called minute pulmonary chemodectoma. Am J Surg Pathol 12:167, 1988.
106. Gal AA, Brooks JS, Pietra GG: Leiomyomatous neoplasms of the lung: A clinical, histologic, and immunohistochemical study. Mod Pathol 2:209, 1989.
107. Gallagher CG, Stark R, Teskey J et al: Atypical manifestations of pulmonary adenoid cystic carcinoma. Br J Dis Chest 80:396, 1986.
108. Gebauer C: The postoperative prognosis of primary pulmonary sarcomas: A review with a comparison between the histological forms and the other primary endothoracal sarcomas based on 474 cases. Scand J Thorac Cardiovasc Surg 16:91, 1982.
109. Gephardt GN: Malignant melanoma of the bronchus. Hum Pathol 12:671, 1981.
110. Gephardt GN, Tubbs RR, Liu AC et al: Pulmonary lymphoid neoplasms: Role of immunohistology in the study of cellular immunotypes and in differential diagnosis. Chest 89:545, 1986.
111. Gibbons JRP, McKeown F, Field TW: Pulmonary blastoma with hilar lymph node metastases: Survival for 24 years. Cancer 47:152, 1981.
112. Gibson PG, Bryant DH, Harkness J et al: Pulmonary manifestations of the acquired immunodeficiency syndrome. Aust NZ J Med 17:551, 1987.
113. Gill PS, Akil B, Colletti P et al: Pulmonary Kaposi's sarcoma: Clinical findings and results of therapy. Am J Med 87:57, 1989.
114. Gisser SD et al: Pleomorphic pulmonary hamartoma, an apparently unique variant of pulmonary hamartoma. Hum Pathol 10:393, 1979.
115. Goldthorn JF, Duncan MH, Kosloske AM et al: Cavitating primary pulmonary fibrosarcoma in a child. J Thorac Cardiovasc Surg 91:932, 1986.
116. Gouldesbrough DR, McGoogan E: Primary pulmonary lymphoma: A case diagnosed by bronchial cytology and immunocytochemistry. Histopathology 13:465, 1988.
117. Green WR, Pressoir R, Gumbs RV et al: Intrapulmonary thymoma. Arch Pathol Lab Med 111:1074, 1987.
118. Greenberg HB: Benign subpleural lymph nodes appearing as pulmonary "coin" lesions. Radiology 77:97, 1961.
119. Gross BH, Glazer GM, Bookstein FL: Multiple pulmonary nodules detected by computed tomography: Diagnostic implications. J Comput Assist Tomogr 9:880, 1985.
120. Gupta RK, Paolini FA: Liposarcoma of the pleura: Report of a case with review of literature and views on histogenesis. Am Rev Respir Dis 95:298, 1967.

121. Hackl H: Growth rate of hamartomas of the lung. Z Erkr Atmungsorgane 167:261, 1986.
122. Haimoto H, Tsutsumi Y, Nagura H et al: Immunohistochemical study of so-called sclerosing haemangioma of the lung. Virchow Arch [A] 407:419, 1985.
123. Hamm PG, Judson MA, Aranda CP: Diagnosis of pulmonary Kaposi's sarcoma with fiberoptic bronchoscopy and endobronchial biopsy: A report of five cases. Cancer 59:807, 1987.
124. Hamper UM, Khouri NF, Stitik FP et al: Pulmonary hamartoma: Diagnosis by transthoracic needle-aspiration biopsy. Radiology 155:15, 1985.
125. Hangartner JR, Loosemore TM, Burke M et al: Malignant primary pulmonary paraganglioma. Thorax 44:154, 1989.
126. Hanson PJ, Harcourt-Webster JN, Gazzard BG et al: Fiberoptic bronchoscopy in diagnosis of bronchopulmonary Kaposi's sarcoma. Thorax 42:269, 1987.
127. Hartman GE, Shochet SJ: Primary pulmonary neoplasms of childhood: A review. Ann Thorac Surg 36:108, 1983.
128. Hayes WT, Bernhardt H: Solitary amyloid mass of the lung: Report of a case with a 6-year follow-up. Cancer 24:820, 1969.
129. Hayward RH, Carabasi RJ: Malignant hamartoma of the lung: Fact or fiction. J Thorac Cardiovasc Surg 53:457, 1967.
130. Heard BE, Corrin B, Dewar A: Pathology of seven mucous cell adenomas of the bronchial glands with particular reference to ultrastructure. Histopathology 9:687, 1985.
131. Heard BE, Dewar A, Firmin RK et al: One very rare and one new tracheal tumor found by electron microscopy: Glomus tumor and acinic cell tumor resembling carcinoid tumors by light microscopy. Thorax 37:97, 1982.
132. Heckman CJ, Truong LD, Cagle PT et al: Pulmonary blastoma with rhabdomyosarcomatous differentiation: An electron microscopic and immunohistochemical study. Am J Surg Pathol 12:35, 1988.
133. Hemmi A, Hiraoka H, Mori Y et al: Malignant pleomorphic adenoma (malignant mixed tumor) of the trachea: Report of a case. Acta Pathol Jpn 38:1215, 1988.
134. Herbert A, Wright DH, Isaacson PG et al: Primary malignant lymphoma of the lung: Histopathologic and immunologic evaluation of nine cases. Hum Pathol 15:415, 1984.
135. Hercot O, Giron J, Joffre P et al: Pulmonary hemangiopericytoma: Apropos of a case and review of the literature. J Radiol 69:443, 1988.
136. Hill GS, Eggleston JC: Electron microscopic study of so-called "pulmonary sclerosing hemangioma": Report of a case suggesting epithelial origin. Cancer 30:1092, 1972.
137. Hoch WS, Patchefsky AS, Takeda M et al: Benign clear cell tumor of the lung: An ultrastructural study. Cancer 33:1328, 1974.
138. Holt S, Deverall PB, Boddy JE: A teratoma of the lung containing thymic tissue. J Pathol 126:85, 1978.
139. Homan R, Lechner K, Neumann E et al: Primary Hodgkin's disease of the lung: Case report and review of the literature. Blut 47:231, 1983.
140. Horovitz AG, Khalil KG, Verani RR et al: Primary intratracheal neurilemoma. J Thorac Cardiovasc Surg 85:313, 1983.
141. Horstmann JP, Pietra GG, Harman JA et al: Spontaneous regression of pulmonary leiomyomas during pregnancy. Cancer 39:314, 1977.
142. Hsiu JG, Kreuger JK, D'Amato NA et al: Primary malignant fibrous histiocytoma of the lung: Fine needle aspiration cytologic features. Acta Cytol 31:345, 1987.
143. Hui AN et al: Amyloidosis presenting in the lower respiratory tract: Clinicopathologic, radiologic, immunohistochemical, and histochemical studies in 48 cases. Arch Pathol Lab Med 110:212, 1986.
144. Humphrey PA, Scroggs MW, Roggli VL et al: Pulmonary carcinomas with a sarcomatoid element: An immunocytochemical and ultrastructural analysis. Hum Pathol 19:155, 1988.
145. Hurwitz SS, Conlan AA, Gritzman MCD et al: Coexisting granular cell myoblastoma and squamous carcinoma of the bronchus. Thorax 37:292, 1982.
146. Huszar M, Herczeg E, Lieberman Y et al: Distinctive immunofluorescent labeling of epithelial and mesenchymal elements of carcinosarcoma with antibodies specific for different intermediate filaments. Hum Pathol 15:532, 1984.
147. Huszar M, Suster S, Herczeg E et al: Sclerosing hemangioma of the lung: Immunohistochemical demonstration of mesenchymal origin using antibodies to tissue-specific intermediate filaments. Cancer 58:2422, 1986.
148. Iannicello CM, Shoenut JP, Sharma GP et al: Endobronchial lipoma: Report of three cases. Can J Surg 30:430, 1987.
149. Isaacson PG, Spencer J: Malignant lymphoma of mucosa-associated lymphoid tissue. Histopathology 11:445, 1987.
150. Ishida T, Oka T, Nishino T et al: Inflammatory pseudotumor of the lung in adults: Radiographic and clinicopathological analysis. Ann Thorac Surg 48:90, 1989.
151. Ishizuka T, Yoshitake J, Yamada T et al: Diagnosis of a case of pulmonary carcinosarcoma by detection of rhabdomyosarcoma cells in sputum. Acta Cytol 32:658, 1988.
152. Iuchi K, Ichimiya A, Akashi A et al: Non-Hodgkin's lymphoma of the pleural cavity developing from long-standing pyothorax. Cancer 60:1771, 1987.
153. Jackson MD, Albrecht R, Roggli VL et al: Pulmonary blastoma: An ultrastructural and histochemical study. Ultrastruct Pathol 7:259, 1984.
154. Jakob H, Oelert H: Letter: Hemangiopericytoma of the lung: A rare differential diagnosis of lung tumors. Thorac Cardiovasc Surg 37:61, 1989.
155. Jamieson MPG, McGowan AR: Endobronchial teratoma. Thorax 37:157, 1982.
156. Jazy FK, Cormier WJ, Panke TW et al: Primary chondrosarcoma of the lung: A report of two cases. Clin Oncol 10:273, 1984.
157. Jimenez JF: Pulmonary blastoma in childhood. J Surg Oncol 34:87, 1987.
158. Jimenez JF, Uthman EO, Townsend JW et al: primary bronchopulmonary leiomyosarcoma in childhood. Arch Pathol Lab Med 110:348, 1986.
159. Joshi K, Shankar SK, Gopinath N et al: Multiple sclerosing haemangiomas of the lung. Postgrad Med J 56:50, 1980.
160. Juettner FM, Popper H, Sommersgutter K et al:

Malignant fibrous histiocytoma of the lung: Prognosis and therapy of a rare disease: Report of two cases and review of the literature. Thorac Cardiovasc Surg 35:226, 1987.
161. Juettner FM, Fellbaum C, Popper H et al: Synchronous pulmonary carcinoid tumour and non-Hodgkin's lymphoma: Report of two cases. Thorax 44:516, 1989.
162. Kakos GS, Williams TE, Assor D et al: Pulmonary carcinosarcoma: Etiologic, therapeutic, and prognostic considerations. J Thorac Cardiovasc Surg 61:777, 1971.
163. Karasik A, Modan M, Jacob CO et al: Increased risk of lung cancer in patients with chondromatous hamartoma. J Thorac Cardiovasc Surg 80:217, 1980.
164. Katzenstein AL, Gmelich JT, Carrington CB: Sclerosing hemangioma of the lung: A clinicopathologic study of 51 cases. Am J Surg Pathol 4:343, 1980.
165. Katzenstein AL, Weise DL, Fulling K et al: So-called sclerosing hemangioma of the lung: Evidence for mesothelial origin. Am J Surg Pathol 7:3, 1983.
166. Kauffman SL, Alexander L, Sass L: Histologic and ultrastructural features of the Clara cell adenoma of the mouse lung. Lab Invest 40:708, 1979.
167. Kauffman SL: Histogenesis of the papillary Clara cell adenoma. Am J Pathol 103:174, 1981.
168. Kawahara E, Nakanishi I, Kuroda Y et al: Fine-needle aspiration biopsy of primary malignant fibrous histiocytoma of the lung. Acta Cytol 32:226, 1988.
169. Kemnitz P, Spormann H, Heinrich P: Meningioma of the lung: First report with light and electron microscopic findings. Ultrastruct Pathol 3:359, 1982.
170. Kennedy JL, Nathwani BN, Burke JS et al: Pulmonary lymphomas and other pulmonary lymphoid lesions: A clinicopathologic and immunologic study of 64 patients. Cancer 56:539, 1985.
171. Kern WH, Hughes RK, Meyer BW et al: Malignant fibrous histiocytoma of the lung. Cancer 44:1793, 1979.
172. Kim YI, Kim JH, Suh J-S et al: Glomus tumor of the trachea: Report of a case with ultrastructural observations. Cancer 64:881, 1989.
173. Klacsmann PG, Olson JL, Eggleston JC: Mucoepidermoid carcinoma of the bronchus: An electron microscopic study of the low-grade and high-grade variants. Cancer 43:1720, 1979.
174. Kleinert R, Popper H: Giant fibroma of the lung: A morphological study. Virchows Arch [A] 410:363, 1987.
175. Klima M, Peters J: Malignant granular cell tumor. Arch Pathol Lab Med 111:1070, 1987.
176. Kodama T, Shimosato Y, Kameya T: Histology and ultrastructure of bronchogenic and bronchial gland adenocarcinomas (including adenoid cystic and mucoepidermoid carcinomas) in relation to histogenesis. In Shimosato Y, Melamed MR, Nettesheim P (eds): Morphogenesis of Lung Cancer, vol 1, p 147. Boca Raton, FL, CRC Press, 1982.
177. Kodama T, Shimosato Y, Watanabe S et al: Six cases of well-differentiated adenocarcinoma simulating fetal lung tubules in pseudoglandular stage: Comparison with pulmonary blastoma. Am J Surg Pathol 8:735, 1984.
178. Korn D, Bensch K, Liebow AA et al: Multiple minute pulmonary tumors resembling chemodectomas. Am J Pathol 37:641, 1960.
179. Kornfeld H, Axelrod JL: Pulmonary presentation of Kaposi's sarcoma in a homosexual patient. Am Rev Respir Dis 127:248, 1983.
180. Koss MN, Hochholzer L, Nichols PW et al: Primary non-Hodgkin's lymphoma and pseudolymphoma of the lung: A study of 161 patients. Hum Pathol 14:1024, 1983.
181. Koss MN, Hochholzer L, Langloss JM et al: Lymphomatoid granulomatosis: A clinicopathologic study of 42 patients. Pathology 18:283, 1986.
182. Kradin RL, Mark EJ: Benign lymphoid disorders of the lung, with a theory regarding their development. Hum Pathol 14:857, 1983.
183. Kradin RL, Spirn PW, Mark EJ: Intrapulmonary lymph nodes: Clinical, radiologic and pathologic features. Chest 87:662, 1985.
184. Kradin RL, Young RH, Dickersin GR: Pulmonary blastoma with argyrophil cells and lacking sarcomatous features (pulmonary endodermal tumor resembling fetal lung). Am J Surg Pathol 6:165, 1982.
185. Kudo H, Morinaga S, Shimosato Y et al: Solitary mast cell tumor of the lung. Cancer 61:2089, 1988.
186. Kuhn C, Askin FB: The fine structure of so-called minute pulmonary chemodectomas. Hum Pathol 6:681, 1975.
187. Kung M, Landa JF, Lubin J: Benign clear cell tumor ("sugar tumor") of the trachea. Cancer 54:517, 1984.
188. L'Hoste RJ Jr, Filippa DA, Lieberman PH et al: Primary pulmonary lymphomas: A clinicopathologic analysis of 36 cases. Cancer 54:1397, 1984.
189. Lack EE, Dolan MF, Finisio J et al: Pulmonary and extrapulmonary lymphangioleiomyomatosis: Report of a case with bilateral renal angiomyolipomas, multifocal lymphangioleiomyomatosis, and a glial polyp of the endocervix. Am J Surg Pathol 10:650, 1986.
190. Ladefoged C, Bisgaard C, Petri J: Solitary renal metastasis 23 years after extirpation of a bronchial adenoid cystic carcinoma. Scand J Thorac Cardiovasc Surg 18:245, 1984.
191. Laden SA, Cohen ML, Harley RA: Nodular pulmonary amyloidosis with extrapulmonary involvement. Hum Pathol 15:594, 1984.
192. Lagrange AM, Servais B, Wurtz A et al: Lipoblastic liposarcoma of the lung: Ultrastructural study of a case. Ann Pathol 8:152, 1988.
193. Le Tourneau A, Audouin J, Garbe L et al: Primary pulmonary malignant lymphoma: Clinical and pathological findings, immunocytochemical and ultrastructural studies in 15 cases. Hematol Oncol 1:49, 1983.
194. Lee JT, Shelburne JD, Linder J: Primary malignant fibrous histiocytoma of the lung: A clinicopathologic and ultrastructural study of five cases. Cancer 53:1124, 1984.
195. Lee SH, Reganchary SS, Paramesh J: Primary pulmonary rhabdomyosarcoma: A case report and review of the literature. Hum Pathol 12:92, 1981.
196. Leonardi HK, Jung-Legg Y, Legg MA et al: Tracheobronchial mucoepidermoid carcinoma: Clinicopathological features and results of treatment. J Thorac Cardiovasc Surg 76:431, 1978.
197. Liebow AA, Hubbell DS: Sclerosing hemangioma

(histiocytoma, xanthoma) of the lung. Cancer 9:53, 1956.
198. Liebow AA, Castleman B: Benign clear cell ("sugar") tumors of the lung. Yale J Biol Med 43:213, 1971.
199. Lillo-Gil R, Albrechtsson U, Jakobsson B: Pulmonary leiomyosarcoma appearing as a cyst: Report of one case and review of the literature. Thorac Cardiovasc Surg 33:250, 1985.
200. List AF, Doll DC, Greco FA: Lung cancer in Hodgkin's disease: Association with previous radiotherapy. J Clin Oncol 3:215, 1985.
201. Littlefield JB, Drash EC: Myxoma of the lung. J Thorac Cardiovasc Surg 37:745, 1959.
202. Lorenzetti E, Nardi F: Diagnostic value of bronchial washing in a case of primary pulmonary non-Hodgkin lymphoma. Appl Pathol 2:277, 1984.
203. Ma CK, Fine G, Lewis J et al: Benign mixed tumor of the trachea. Cancer 44:2260, 1979.
204. Mackay B, Legha SS, Pickler G: Coin lesion of the lung in a 19-year-old male. Ultrastruct Pathol 2:289, 1981.
205. Mackay B, Ordóñez NG, Huang WL. Ultrastructural and immunocytochemical observations on angiosarcomas. Ultrastruct Pathol 12:97, 1989.
206. Malauzat C, Malauzat F, Petit MA et al: Bronchopulmonary hamartochondroma (apropos of 136 cases, including a homogeneous series of 124 cases). Rev Pneumol Clin 41:163, 1985.
207. Malik SK, Behera D, Kalra S et al: Intrabronchial schwannoma: A case report. Scand J Thorac Cardiovasc Surg 21:281, 1987.
208. Manivel JC, Preist JR, Watterson J et al: Pleuropulmonary blastoma: The so-called pulmonary blastoma of childhood. Cancer 62:1516, 1988.
209. Manning JT, Ordonez NG, Rosenberg HS et al: Pulmonary endodermal tumor resembling fetal lung: Report of a case with immunohistochemical studies. Arch Pathol Lab Med 109:48, 1985.
210. Marchevsky A, Padilla M, Kaneko M et al: Localized lymphoid nodules of lung: A reappraisal of the lymphoma versus pseudolymphoma dilemma. Cancer 51:2070, 1983.
211. Marchevsky A, Rosen MJ, Chrystal G et al: Pulmonary complication of the acquired immunodeficiency syndrome: A clinicopathologic study of 70 cases. Hum Pathol 16:659, 1985.
212. Mark EJ: Mesenchymal cystic hamartoma of the lung. N Engl J Med 315:1255, 1986.
213. Matsubara O, Tan-Liu NS, Kenney RM et al: Inflammatory pseudotumors of the lung: Progression from organizing pneumonia to fibrous histiocytoma or to plasma cell granuloma in 32 cases. Hum Pathol 19:807, 1988.
214. McCabe RE, Brooks RG, Catterall JR et al: Open lung biopsy in patients with non-Hodgkin's lymphoma and pulmonary infiltrates. Chest 96:319, 1989.
215. McCann MP, Fu Y-S, Kay S: Pulmonary blastoma: A light and electron microscopic study. Cancer 38:789, 1976.
216. McCarty KS Jr, Mossler JA, McLelland R et al: Pulmonary lymphangiomyomatosis responsive to progesterone. N Engl J Med 303:1461, 1980.
217. McDonnell T, Kyriakos M, Roper C et al: Malignant fibrous histiocytoma of the lung. Cancer 61:137, 1988.
218. Meduri GU, Stover DE, Lee M et al: Pulmonary Kaposi's sarcoma in the acquired immune deficiency syndrome: Clinical, radiographic and pathologic manifestations. Am J Med 81:11, 1986.
219. Metcalf JS, Mays JC, Shaw AB: Bronchial mucoepidermoid carcinoma metastatic to skin: Report of a case and review of the literature. Cancer 58:2556, 1986.
220. Miettinen M, Collan Y, Halttunen P et al: Intravascular bronchioloalveolar tumor. Cancer 60:2471, 1987.
221. Miller-Pedersen V, Schulze S, Hier-Madsen K et al: Primary pulmonary leiomyosarcoma: Review of the literature and report of a case. Scand J Thorac Cardiovasc Surg 18:251, 1984.
222. Mompoint D, Groussard O, Grenier P: Endobronchial hamartoma associated with bronchioalveolar cell carcinoma. Chest 94:1094, 1988.
223. Moore TC: Carcinosarcoma of the lung. Surgery 50:886, 1961.
224. Morales FM, Matthews JI: Diagnosis of parenchymal Hodgkin's disease using bronchoalveolar lavage. Chest 91:785, 1987.
225. Morgan AD, Salama FD: Primary chondrosarcoma of the lung: Case report and a review of the literature. J Thorac Cardiovasc Surg 64:460, 1972.
226. Mori A, Obata K, Tada T et al: A case of multiple cavernous hemangiomas of the lung. Gan No Rinsho 31:1433, 1985.
227. Muller-Hermelink HK, Kaiserling E: Pulmonary adenocarcinoma of fetal type: Alternating differentiation argues in favour of a common endodermal stem cell. Virchows Arch [A] 409:195, 1986.
228. Mullins JD, Barnes RP: Childhood bronchial mucoepidermoid tumors: A case report and review of the literature. Cancer 44:315, 1979.
229. Myers JL, Fulmer JD: Bronchoalveolar lavage in the diagnosis of pulmonary lymphomas. Chest 91:642, 1987.
230. Nagata N, Dairaku M, Sueishi K et al: Sclerosing hemangioma of the lung: An epithelial tumor composed of immunohistochemically heterogeneous cells. Am J Clin Pathol 88:552, 1987.
231. Nagata N, Masashi D, Ishida T et al: Sclerosing hemangioma of the lung: Immunohistochemical characterization of its origin as related to surfactant apoprotein. Cancer 55:116, 1985.
232. Nakamura T, Muramoto Y, Sato E et al: Benign clear cell tumor of the lung: A study of immunohistochemistry. Gan No Rinsho 32:1466, 1986.
233. Nakanishi K, Kawai T, Suzuki M: Benign clear cell tumor of the lung: A histopathologic study. Acta Pathol Jpn 38:515, 1988.
234. Nascimento AG, Unni KK, Bernatz PE: Sarcomas of the lung. Mayo Clin Proc 57:355, 1982.
235. Nash G, Fligiel S: Kaposi's sarcoma presenting as pulmonary disease in the acquired immunodeficiency syndrome: Diagnosis by lung biopsy. Hum Pathol 15:999, 1984.
236. Neidt GW, Schinella RA: Acquired immunodeficiency syndrome: Clinicopathologic study of 56 cases. Arch Pathol Lab Med 109:727, 1985.
237. Neumann MP, Frizzera G: The co-existence of Langerhans' cell granulomatosis and malignant lymphoma may take different forms: Report of seven cases with a review of the literature. Hum Pathol 17:1060, 1986.
238. Nguyen GK: Aspiration biopsy cytology of benign clear cell ("sugar") tumor of the lung. Acta Cytol 33:511, 1989.

239. Noguchi M, Kodama T, Morinaga S et al: Multiple sclerosing hemangiomas of the lung. Am J Surg Pathol 10:429, 1986.
240. Noguchi M, Kodama T, Shimosato Y et al: Papillary adenoma of type 2 pneumocytes. Am J Surg Pathol 10:134, 1986.
241. Nonomura A, Kurumaya H, Kono N et al: Primary pulmonary artery sarcoma: Report of two autopsy cases studied by immunohistochemistry and electron microscopy and review of 110 cases reported in the literature. Acta Pathol Jpn 38:883, 1988.
242. Nozaki M, Mitsuhashi N, Takahashi I et al: Three cases of primary lung and mediastinal malignant germ cell tumors: Clinical and pathologic studies. Gan No Rinsho 30:1314, 1984.
243. Nzeh DA: Atypical intrathoracic manifestations of Burkitt's lymphoma. Pediatr Radiol 18:411, 1988.
244. O'Donohue WJ Jr, Edland J, Mohiuddin SM et al: Multiple pulmonary neurofibromas with hypoxemia: Occurrence due to pulmonary arteriovenous shunts within the tumors. Arch Intern Med 146:1618, 1986.
245. Oka M, Kawano K, Kanda T et al: Bronchoalveolar lavage in primary pulmonary lymphoma with monoclonal gammopathy. Am Rev Respir Dis 137:957, 1988.
246. Oldham HN: Benign tumors of the lung and bronchus. Surg Clin North Am 60:825, 1980.
247. Oliphant L, McFadden RG: Lung cancer following therapy for Hodgkin's disease. Can Med Assoc J 132:533, 1985.
248. Olofsson J, van Nostrand AWP: Adenoid cystic carcinoma of the larynx: A report of four cases and a review of the literature. Cancer 40:1307, 1977.
249. Ott RA, Eugene J, Kollin J et al: Primary pulmonary angiosarcoma associated with multiple synchronous neoplasms. J Surg Oncol 35:269, 1987.
250. Palacios JJN, Escribano PM, Toledo J et al: Sclerosing hemangioma of the lung: An ultrastructural study. Cancer 44:949, 1979.
251. Palmer KC: Clara cell adenomas of the mouse lung: Interaction with alveolar type 2 cells. Am J Pathol 120:455, 1985.
252. Palvio D, Egebald K, Paulsen SM: Atypical lipomatous hamartoma of the lung. Virchows Arch [A] 405:253, 1985.
253. Palvio DH, Paulsen SM, Henneberg EW: Primary angiosarcoma of the lung presenting as intractable hemoptysis. Thorac Cardiovasc Surg 35:105, 1987.
254. Panos RJ, Chang SW: Diagnosis of pulmonary hamartoma by bronchoscopic transbronchial biopsy. J Natl Med Assoc 81:460, 1989.
255. Paulsen SM, Egeblad K: Sarcoma of the pulmonary artery: A light and electron microscopic study. J Submicrosc Cytol 15:811, 1983.
256. Payne WS, Fontana RS, Woolner LB: Bronchial tumors originating from mucous glands: Current classification and unusual manifestations. Med Clin North Am 48:945, 1968.
257. Payne WS, Schier J, Woolner LB: Mixed tumors of the bronchus (salivary gland type). J Thorac Cardiovasc Surg 49:663, 1965.
258. Perez-Atayde AR, Seiler MW: Pulmonary hamartoma: An ultrastructural study. Cancer 53:485, 1984.
259. Perrone TL, Dickersin GR: Ultrastructure of a bronchial mucoepidermoid carcinoma. Hum Pathol 14:1011, 1983.
260. Peterson H, Snider HL, Yam LT et al: Primary pulmonary lymphoma: A clinical and immunohistochemical study of six cases. Cancer 56:805, 1985.
261. Petheram IS, Heard BE: Unique massive pulmonary hamartoma: Case report with review of hamartomata treated at Brompton Hospital in 27 years. Chest 75:95, 1979.
262. Pettinato G, Manivel JC, Saldana MJ et al: Primary bronchopulmonary fibrosarcoma of childhood and adolescence: Reassessment of a low-grade malignancy: Clinicopathologic study of five cases and review of the literature. Hum Pathol 20:463, 1989.
263. Pilotti S, Rilke F, Lombardi L et al: Immunohistochemistry and electron microscopy of intravascular bronchioloalveolar tumor of the lung. Tumori 69:283, 1983.
264. Pomeranz SJ, Proto AV: Histiocytosis X: Unusual-confusing features of eosinophilic granuloma. Chest 89:88, 1989.
265. Prior P, Pope DJ: Hodgkin's disease: Subsequent primary cancers in relation to treatment. Br J Cancer 58:512, 1988.
266. Purdy LJ, Colby TV, Yousem SA et al: Pulmonary Kaposi's sarcoma: Premortem histologic diagnosis. Am J Surg Pathol 10:301, 1986.
267. Pushchak MJ, Farhi DC: Primary choriocarcinoma of the lung. Arch Pathol Lab Med 111:477, 1987.
268. Raafat F, Salman WD, Roberts K et al: Carney's triad: Gastric leiomyosarcoma, pulmonary chondroma and extra-adrenal paraganglioma in young females. Histopathology 10:1325, 1986.
269. Ramaekers F, Broers J, Rot MK et al: Detection of epithelial and neural type of intermediate filament proteins in human lung tumors. Acta Histochem Suppl (Jena) 34:45, 1987.
270. Ramirez-Chavez G, Celard P, Gamondes JP et al: Pulmonary hamartoma: Apropos of 49 surgically treated cases. Sem Hop Paris 60:1181, 1984.
271. Regadera JF, Rodriguez JI, Perera A et al: Infantile pulmonary mucoepidermoid tumor: Clinical and pathological study of one case and review of the literature. An Esp Pediatr 16:249, 1982.
272. Richert-Boe KE, Bagby GC: Burkitt's lymphoma presenting as an endobronchial lesion. Am J Med 85:864, 1988.
273. Robertson AJ, Sinclair DJM, Sutton PP et al: Primary melanocarcinoma of the lower respiratory tract. Thorax 35:158, 1980.
274. Rocca M, Vanel D, Couanet D et al: Pulmonary mesenchymatous chondrosarcoma in children: Report of 2 cases and review of the literature. J Radiol 69:329, 1988.
275. Rucker L, Meador J: Kaposi's sarcoma presenting as homogeneous pulmonary infiltrates in a patient with acquired immunodeficiency syndrome. West J Med 142:831, 1985.
276. Runckel D, Kessler S: Bronchogenic squamous carcinoma in nonirradiated juvenile laryngotracheal papillomatosis. Am J Surg Pathol 3:293, 1980.
277. Rusch VW, Shuman WP, Schmidt R et al: Massive pulmonary hemangiopericytoma: An innovative approach to evaluation and treatment. Cancer 64:1928, 1989.

278. Rutledge JN, Harolds JA: Intratracheal neurofibroma. South Med J 76:1063, 1983.
279. Sajjad SM, Begin LR, Dail DH et al: Fibrous histiocytoma of lung: A clinicopathologic study of two cases. Histopathology 5:325, 1981.
280. Sajjad SM, Luna MA: Primary pulmonary histiocytosis X in two patients with Hodgkin's disease. Thorax 37:110, 1982.
281. Sale GE, Kulander BG: Benign clear-cell tumor (sugar tumor) of the lung with hepatic metastases ten years after resection of pulmonary primary tumor. Arch Pathol Lab Med 112:1177, 1988.
282. Sano T, Hirose T, Hizawa K et al: A case of pleomorphic adenoma of the trachea. Jpn J Clin Oncol 14:93, 1984.
283. Santos-Briz A, Terron J, Sastre R et al: Oncocytoma of the lung. Cancer 40:1330, 1977.
284. Saruk M, Stern H, Tronic BS et al: Intrapulmonary benign cystic teratoma. Conn Med 44:687, 1980.
285. Satoh T, Kauffman SL: A scanning electron microscopic study of the type II and Clara cell adenoma of the mouse lung. Lab Invest 40:28, 1980.
286. Sato Y, Tsuchiya E, Weng S-Y et al: Pulmonary sclerosing hemangioma of the lung: A type II pneumocytoma by immunohistochemical and immunoelectron microscopic studies. Cancer 64:1310, 1989.
287. Sawamura K, Hashimoto T, Nanjo S et al: Primary liposarcoma of the lung: report of a case. J Surg Oncol 19:243, 1982.
288. Schraufnagel DE et al: Endobronchial lipoma. Chest 75:97, 1979.
289. Schulster PL, Khan FA, Azueta V: Asymptomatic pulmonary granular cell tumor presenting as a coin lesion. Chest 68:256, 1975.
290. Scott L, Blair G, Taylor G et al: Inflammatory pseudotumors in children. J Pediatr Surg 23:755, 1988.
291. Seal RME, Gibbs AR: Mixed tumors of the lung: Morphogenesis of lung cancer. In Shimosato Y, Melamed MR, Nettesheim P (eds): Morphogenesis of Lung Cancer, vol 2, p 67. Boca Raton, FL, CRC Press, 1982.
292. Seo IS, Warren J, Mirkin LD et al: Mucoepidermoid carcinoma of the bronchus in a 4-year-old child: A high-grade variant with lymph node metastasis. Cancer 53:1600, 1984.
293. Shariff S, Thomas JA, Shetty N et al: Primary pulmonary rhabdomyosarcoma in a child, with a review of the literature. J Surg Oncol 38:261, 1988.
294. Shin MS, Ho KJ: Primary hemangiopericytoma of lung: Radiology and pathology. Am J Radiol 133:1077, 1979.
295. Shmookler BM, Marsh HB, Roberts WC: Primary sarcoma of the pulmonary trunk and/or right or left main pulmonary artery: A rare cause of obstruction of right ventricular outflow. Am J Med 63:263, 1977.
296. Siegel SE et al: Malignant transformation of tracheobronchial juvenile papillomatosis without prior radiotherapy. Ann Otol Rhinol Laryngol 88:192, 1979.
297. Siegelman SS, Khouri NF, Scott WW Jr et al: Pulmonary hamartoma: CT findings. Radiology 160:313, 1986.
298. Silverman JF, Coalson JJ: Primary malignant myxoid fibrous histiocytoma of the lung: Light and ultrastructural examination with review of the literature. Arch Pathol Lab Med 108:49, 1984.
299. Singh G, Katyal SL, Ordonez NG et al: Type II pneumocytes in pulmonary tumors: Implications for histogenesis. Arch Pathol Lab Med 108:44, 1984.
300. Sobonya RE, Quan SF, Fleishman JS: Pulmonary lymphangioleiomyomatosis: Quantitative analysis of lesions producing airflow limitation. Hum Pathol 16:1122, 1985.
301. Southgate HJ, Archibald GP, el Sayed ME et al: Ectopic release of GHRH and ACTH from an adenoid cystic carcinoma resulting in acromegaly and pituitary infarction. Postgrad Med J 64:145, 1988.
302. Spencer H: Pulmonary blastomas. J Pathol Bacteriol 82:161, 1961.
303. Spencer H: Bronchial mucous gland tumours. Virchows Arch [A] 383:101, 1979.
304. Spencer H, Dail DH, Arneaud J: Noninvasive bronchial epithelial papillary tumours. Cancer 45:1486, 1980.
305. Spencer H, Nambu S: Sclerosing haemangiomas of the lung. Histopathology 10:477, 1986.
306. Spragg RG, Wolf PL, Haghighi P et al: Angiosarcoma of the lung with fatal pulmonary hemorrhage. Am J Med 74:1072, 1983.
307. Stafford JR, Pollock WJ, Wenzel BC: Oncocytic mucoepidermoid tumor of the bronchus. Cancer 54:94, 1984.
308. Steen-Hansen E: The diagnostic value of chest x-ray combined with fine-needle aspiration biopsy in patients suspected for pulmonary hamartomas. Rontgenblatter 40:321, 1987.
309. Stone FJ, Churg AM: The ultrastructure of pulmonary hamartoma. Cancer 39:1064, 1977.
310. Stover DE, White DA, Romano PA et al: Spectrum of pulmonary diseases associated with the acquired immune deficiency syndrome. Am J Med 78:429, 1985.
311. Striklam CV, Golembiewski RS, Celko DA et al: Primary pulmonary meningioma. Surg Neurol 29:410, 1988.
312. Stroller JK, Kavuru M, Mehta AC et al: Intracranial meningioma metastatic to the lung. Cleve Clin J Med 54:521, 1987.
313. Strum SB, Weiss A, McDermed JE et al: Intrathoracic Hodgkin's disease: A case presentation with multiple pulmonary nodules in the absence of mediastinal or hilar node disease. Cancer 56:1953, 1985.
314. Sullivan LG: Primary choriocarcinoma of the lung in a man. Arch Pathol Lab Med 113:82, 1989.
315. Sun CCJ, Kroll M, Miller JE: Primary chondrosarcoma of the lung. Cancer 50:1864, 1982.
316. Taboada CF, McMurray JD, Jordan RA et al: Primary melanoma of the lung. Chest 62:629, 1972.
317. Tamai S, Kameya T, Shimosato Y et al: Pulmonary blastoma: An ultrastructural study of a case and its transplanted tumor in athymic nude mice. Cancer 46:1389, 1980.
318. Tan-Liu NS, Matsubara O, Grillo HC et al: Invasive fibrous tumor of the tracheobronchial tree: Clinical and pathologic study of seven cases. Hum Pathol 20:180, 1989.
319. Tanaka I, Inoue M, Matsui Y et al: A case of pneumocytoma (so-called sclerosing heman-

gioma) with lymph node metastasis. Jpn J Clin Oncol 16:77, 1986.
320. Tang CK, Toker C, Foris NP et al: Glomangioma of the lung. Am J Surg Pathol 2:103, 1978.
321. Tanimura A, Natsuyama H, Kawano M et al: Primary choriocarcinoma of the lung. Hum Pathol 16:1281, 1985.
322. Tesluk H, Dajee A: Pulmonary oncocytoma. J Surg Oncol 29:173, 1985.
323. Thomas L, Risbud M, Gabriel JB et al: Cytomorphology of granular cell tumor of the bronchus: A case report. Acta Cytol 28:129, 1984.
324. Thomas WJ, Koenig HM, Ellwanger FR et al: Primary pulmonary rhabdomyosarcoma in childhood. Am J Dis Child 135:469, 1981.
325. Thompson PJ, Jewkes J, Corrin B et al: Primary bronchopulmonary amyloid tumour with massive hilar lymphadenopathy. Thorax 38:153, 1983.
326. Tomashefski JF: Benign endobronchial mesenchymal tumors: Their relationship to parenchymal pulmonary hamartomas. Am J Surg Pathol 6:531, 1982.
327. Tomita T, Dixon A, Watanabe I et al: Sclerosing vascular variant of plasma cell granuloma. Hum Pathol 11:197, 1980.
328. Tomita T, Lotuaco L, Talbott L et al: Mucoepidermoid carcinoma of the subglottis: An ultrastructural study. Arch Pathol Lab Med 101:145, 1977.
329. Torres AM, Ryckman FC: Childhood tracheobronchial mucoepidermoid carcinoma: A case report and review of the literature. J Pediatr Surg 23:367, 1988.
330. Trapnell DH: Recognition and incidence of intrapulmonary lymph nodes. Thorax 19:44, 1964.
331. Trillo A, Guha A: Solitary condylomatous papilloma of the bronchus. Arch Pathol Lab Med 112:731, 1988.
332. Turnbull AD, Huvos AG, Goodner JT et al: Mucoepidermoid tumors of bronchial glands. Cancer 28:539, 1971.
333. Turner RR, Colby TV, Doggett RS: Well-differentiated lymphocytic lymphoma: A study of 47 patients with primary manifestation in the lung. Cancer 54:2088, 1984.
334. Unger PD, Geller SA, Anderson PJ: Pulmonary lesions in a patient with neurofibromatosis. Arch Pathol Lab Med 108:654, 1984.
335. Uyama T, Monden Y, Harada K et al: Pulmonary leiomyomatosis showing endobronchial extension and giant cyst formation. Chest 94:644, 1988.
336. Van Assendelft AH, Strengell Usanov L: Pulmonary haemangiopericytoma with multiple metastases. Eur J Respir Dis 65:380, 1984.
337. Van den Bosch JM, Wagenaar SS, Corrin B et al: Mesenchymoma of the lung (so called hamartoma): A review of 154 parenchymal and endobronchial cases. Thorax 42:790, 1987.
338. Van der Veen F, Van den Bosch JMM, Wagenaar S et al: Adenoid cystic carcinoma of the main air passages. Ned Tijdschr Geneeskd 126:712, 1982.
339. Van Leeuwen FE, Somers R, Taal BG et al: Increased risk of lung cancer, non-Hodgkin's lymphoma, and leukemia following Hodgkin's disease. J Clin Oncol 7:1046, 1989.
340. Venn GE, Gellister J, DaCosta PE et al: Malignant fibrous histiocytoma in thoracic surgical practice. J Thorac Cardiovasc Surg 91:234, 1986.
341. Vera-Roman JM, Sobonya RE, Gomez-Garcia JL et al: Leiomyoma of the lung: Literature review and case report. Cancer 52:936, 1983.
342. Verbeken E, Beyls J, Moerman P et al: Lung metastasis of malignant epithelioid hemangioendothelioma mimicking a primary intravascular bronchioloalveolar tumor: A histologic, ultrastructural, and immunohistochemical study. Cancer 55:1741, 1985.
343. Verdiani P, Di Carlo S, Sforza V et al: Non-Hodgkin's lymphoma primarily involving the bronchial tree. Tumori 73:593, 1987.
344. Warter A, Satge D, Roeslin N: Angioinvasive plasma cell granulomas of the lung. Cancer 59:435, 1987.
345. Watanabe J, Yamaguchi K, Sugiyama Y et al: Primary pulmonary lymphoma demonstration of monoclonality by lymphocyte surface marker study. Jpn J Med 26:377, 1987.
346. Webber D, Tron V, Askin F et al: S-100 staining in the diagnosis of eosinophilic granuloma of the lung. Am J Clin Pathol 84:447, 1985.
347. Weisbrod GL: Pulmonary angiitis and granulomatosis: A review. J Can Assoc Radiol 40:127, 1989.
348. Weisbrod GL, Chamberlain DW, Tao LC: Pulmonary blastoma, report of three cases and a review of the literature. J Can Assoc Radiol 39:130, 1988.
349. Weiss LM, Yousem SA, Warnke RA: Non-Hodgkin's lymphomas of the lung: A study of 19 cases emphasizing the utility of frozen section immunologic studies in differential diagnosis. Am J Surg Pathol 9:480, 1985.
350. Weiss SW, Enzinger FM: Epithelioid hemangioendothelioma: A vascular tumor often mistaken for a carcinoma. Cancer 50:970:1982.
351. Weiss SW, Ishak KG, Dail DH et al: Epithelioid hemangioendothelioma and related lesions. Semin Diagn Pathol 3:259, 1986.
352. Weldon-Linne CM, Victor TA, Christ ML et al: Angiogenic nature of the "intravascular bronchioloalveolar tumor" of the lung: An electron microscopic study. Arch Pathol Lab Med 105:174, 1981.
353. Weldon-Linne CM, Victor TA, Christ ML: Immunohistochemical identification of factor VIII–related antigen in the intravascular bronchioloalveolar tumor the lung. Arch Pathol Lab Med 105:628, 1981.
354. White SH, Ibrahim NB, Forrester-Wood CP et al: Leiomyomas of the lower respiratory tract. Thorax 40:306, 1985.
355. Wick MR, Scheithauer BW, Piehler JM et al: Primary pulmonary leiomyosarcomas: A light and electron microscopic study. Arch Pathol Lab Med 106:510, 1982.
356. Wisecarver J, Ness MJ, Rennard SI et al: Bronchoalveolar lavage in the assessment of pulmonary Hodgkin's disease. Acta Cytol 33:527, 1989.
357. Wolf KM, Mehta D, Claypool WD: Mucoepidermoid carcinoma of the lung with intracranial metastases. Chest 94:435, 1988.
358. Wolff M, Silva F, Kaye G: Pulmonary metastases (with admixed epithelial elements) from smooth muscle neoplasms: Report of nine cases, including three males. Am J Surg Pathol 3:325, 1979.
359. Wright ES, Pike E, Couves CM: Unusual tumours of the lung. J Surg Oncol 24:23, 1983.
360. Yamada H, Katoh O, Yamaguchi T et al: Intra-

bronchial leiomyoma treated by localized resection via bronchotomy and bronchoplasty. Chest 91:283, 1987.

361. Yamazaki Y, Yasukawa S, Mizuno R et al: The adult type pulmonary hamartoma in an 11-year-old boy. Z Kinderchir 41:109, 1986.
362. Yellin A, Rosenman Y, Lieberman Y: Review of smooth muscle tumours of the lower respiratory tract. Br J Dis Chest 78:337, 1984.
363. Yellin A, Schwartz L, Hersho E et al: Chondrosarcoma of the bronchus. Chest 84:224, 1983.
364. Yousem SA: Angiosarcoma presenting in the lung. Arch Pathol Lab Med 110:112, 1986.
365. Yousem SA, Hochholzer L: Alveolar adenoma. Hum Pathol 17:1066, 1986.
366. Yousem SA, Hochholzer L: Malignant fibrous histiocytoma of the lung. Cancer 60:2532, 1987.
367. Yousem SA, Hochholzer L: Primary pulmonary hemangiopericytoma. Cancer 59:549, 1987.
368. Yousem SA, Weiss LM, Colby TV: Primary pulmonary Hodgkin's disease: A clinicopathologic study of 15 cases. Cancer 57:1217, 1986.
369. Yousem SA, Wick MR, Singh G et al: So-called sclerosing hemangioma of lung: An immunocytochemical study supporting a respiratory epithelial origin. Am J Surg Pathol 12:582, 1988.
370. Zhang FL, Cheng XR, Zhang YS et al: Lung ectopic meningioma: A case report. Chin Med J 96:309, 1983.
371. Zibrak JD, Silverstri RC, Costello P et al: Bronchoscopic and radiologic features of Kaposi's sarcoma involving the respiratory system. Chest 90:476, 1986.
372. Zulian GB, Jaco-des-Combes E, Aapro MS: Primary pulmonary Hodgkin's disease and the dilemma of E stage. Eur J Surg Oncol 12:307, 1986.

Chapter

12

TUMORS OF THE PLEURA AND CHEST WALL

THE PLEURA

The body cavity of the embryo is divided into thoracic and abdominal compartments by the septum transversum, the primordium of the diaphragm, which unites with the pleuroperitoneal folds that separate the pericardial from the pleural cavities. The lung buds grow into the pleural cavities. The parietal pleural membranes are derived from somatic mesoderm and the visceral pleural membranes from splanchnic mesoderm, and they both become covered by a layer of mesothelial cells. The visceral pleura extends to the base of the fissures, and the visceral and parietal pleurae meet around the hilum. Arterial blood reaches the visceral pleura from the bronchial and pulmonary vessels, while the parietal pleura is supplied by branches of the intercostal, internal mammary, and phrenic arteries. Lymphatics[14] form an elaborate network immediately beneath the pleural surface, and most drain toward the hilum, although there is also some passage of lymph from the lung outward to the visceral pleura. The lymphatics of the parietal pleura run to the intercostal drainage system, and those from the lower parietal pleura run to the upper peritoneum. From the diaphragmatic pleura, lymph drains into nodes in the lower mediastinum.

Normal mesothelium[141] is a single layer of flattened cells that appear inconspicuous by light microscopy. Delicate elastic laminae are present in the supporting connective tissue. The thin surface cells are highly susceptible to drying, and it is difficult to obtain good preparations if the tissue is not fixed as soon as it is exposed. Electron microscopy reveals that the mesothelial cells rest on a basal lamina and that their microvilli are long, slender, and sinuous. The pleural space is less than 20 μm wide, and the scanty pleural fluid contains protein, cells (macrophages, a few lymphocytes, and some desquamated mesothelial cells), and mucopolysaccharides, including hyaluronic acid, which diminish rough contacts between the apposed layers. Small quantities of fluid are absorbed from the pleural cavity into lymphatic and vascular capillaries in the submesothelial connective tissue of the visceral and parietal pleura. Some may diffuse through the attenuated cytoplasm of the surface cells, but their lateral cell membranes are separated by small gaps, and fluid and molecules can pass between the cells.[41, 167] Since there is no directional flow in serous fluid, it is possible that the action of the microvilli may promote the transport of fluid and molecules across the mesothelial surface.[6]

Mesothelial cells respond to injurious stimuli by increasing in size from their usual flat configuration to become round and plump. The reactive cells may form papillary projections or become detached and float, singly or in little clusters, within the pleural fluid. The proliferative process produces a diffuse sheet of thickened mesothelium or one or multiple nodules on the pleural surface. A section through the reactive mesothelium may give the impression that some of the cells are infiltrating the underlying connective tissue, and it is possible to mistake nodular mesothelial hyperplasia, which is sometimes seen in a hernia sac,[138] for a neoplastic process. Hyperplastic mesothelial cells infrequently become spindle shaped, and squamous metaplasia occasionally occurs on a serous surface.

Regeneration following damage to a mesothelial surface was formerly believed to be effected by free-floating cells from the pleural fluid settling and spreading on the denuded surface and developing microvilli, but it now appears likely that the cells that were being described were macrophages. More recent studies[19, 20] have shown that the subserosal mesenchymal cells, which look like fibroblasts and express vimentin, proliferate to repair damage to the overlying surface epithelium. Among the cells participating in the reparative process, a continuum of ultrastructural features can be seen from the multipotential subserosal cells, which mark for low-molecular-weight cytokeratin, to newly formed epithelial lining cells, which lose vimentin and express high-molecular-weight keratin.

TUMORS OF THE PLEURA

Benign Fibrous Tumors

Fibrous tumors of the pleura[24, 25, 82, 121, 144, 171] are also referred to as pleural fibromas and localized benign mesotheliomas. Proliferation of the subserosal fibroblasts produces a small nodule, usually on the visceral pleura. As it grows, it either remains sessile or protrudes as an exophytic lesion into the pleural cavity,[56, 104, 115] and it may attach to the opposite pleural surface. Most are discovered on routine chest radiography, and one can be mistaken for a primary pulmonary tumor.[154] Benign fibrous pleural tumors are usually asymptomatic, but some grow to a considerable size before being detected.[114] Large tumors can cause dyspnea, incite a pleural effusion, and rarely be associated with hypoglycemia or hypertrophic pulmonary osteoarthropathy.[7, 102] Occasionally a localized tumor will invade the lung[175] or chest wall and even erode ribs. About 20% recur, especially the infiltrating lesions, often years after excision.[162]

The spindle cells are loosely distributed within a fibrous stroma (Fig. 12–1), but the degree of cellularity varies (Fig. 12–2) and the cells can form intersecting bundles (Fig. 12–3). Palisading of nuclei may be evident, and a well-defined storiform pattern is a common finding. Areas of the lesion can be very vascular. Entrapped mesothelial cells or

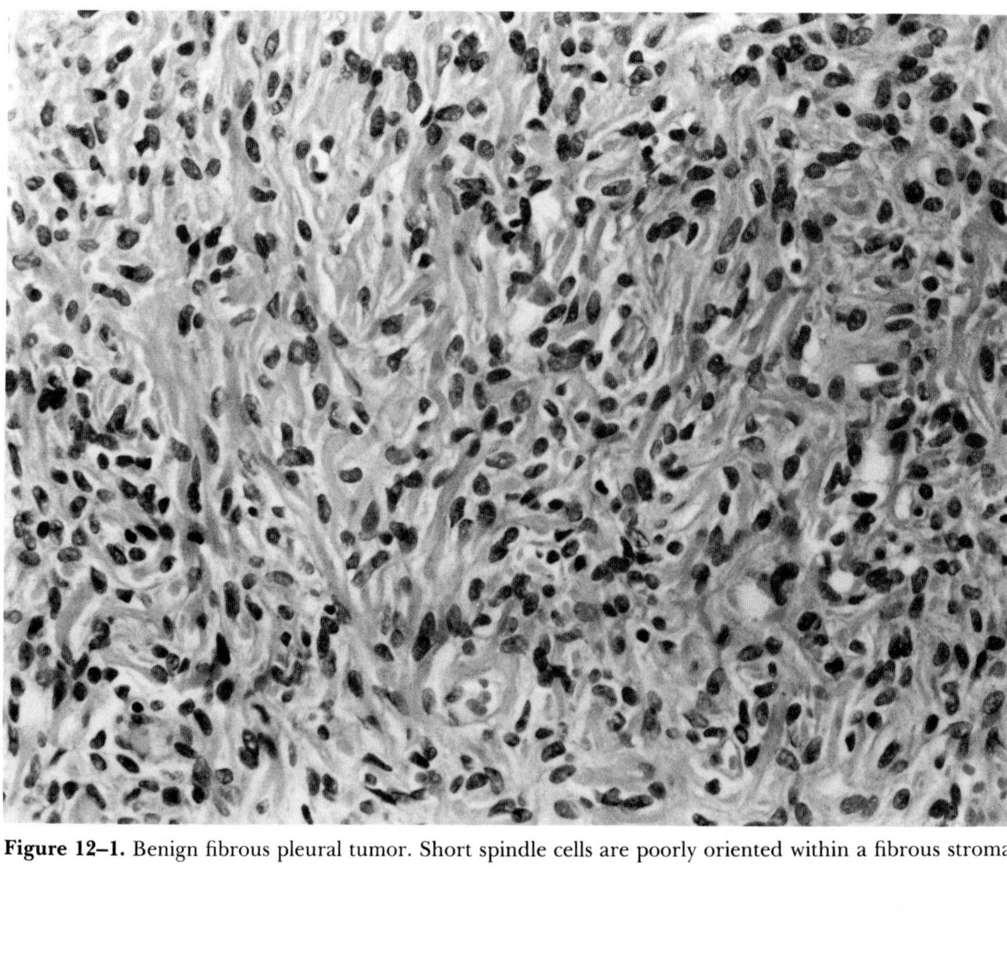

Figure 12–1. Benign fibrous pleural tumor. Short spindle cells are poorly oriented within a fibrous stroma.

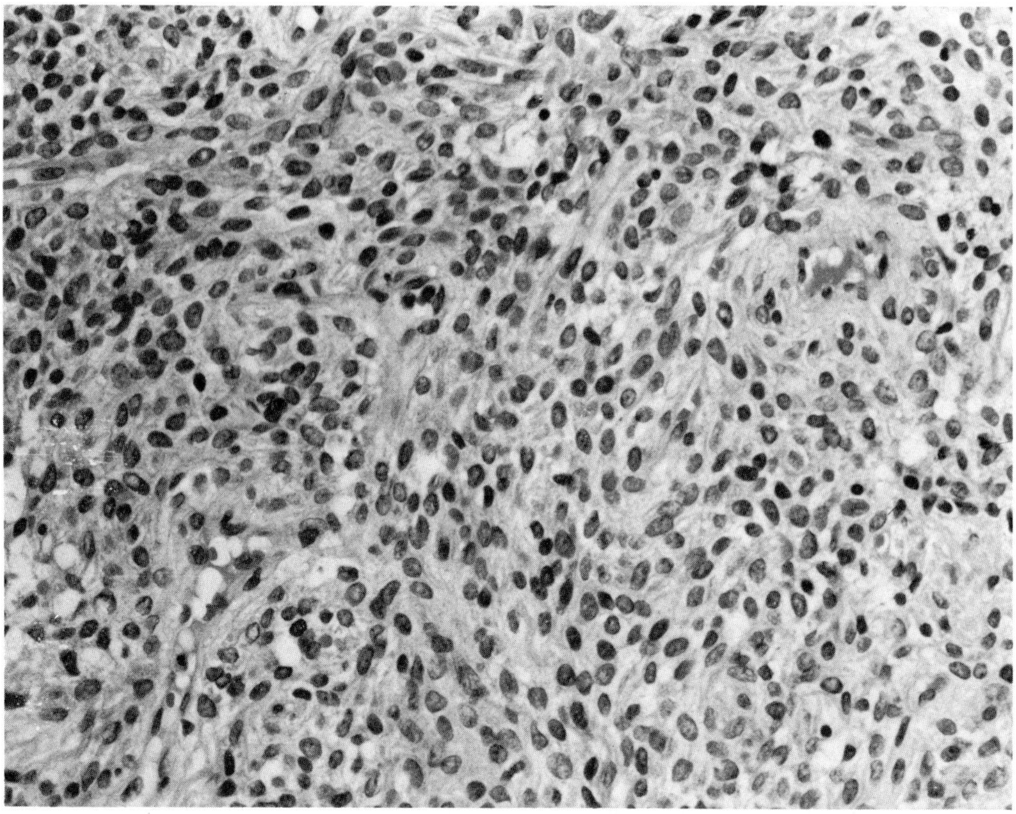

Figure 12–2. Benign fibrous pleural tumor. The tumor is more cellular than in Figure 12–1.

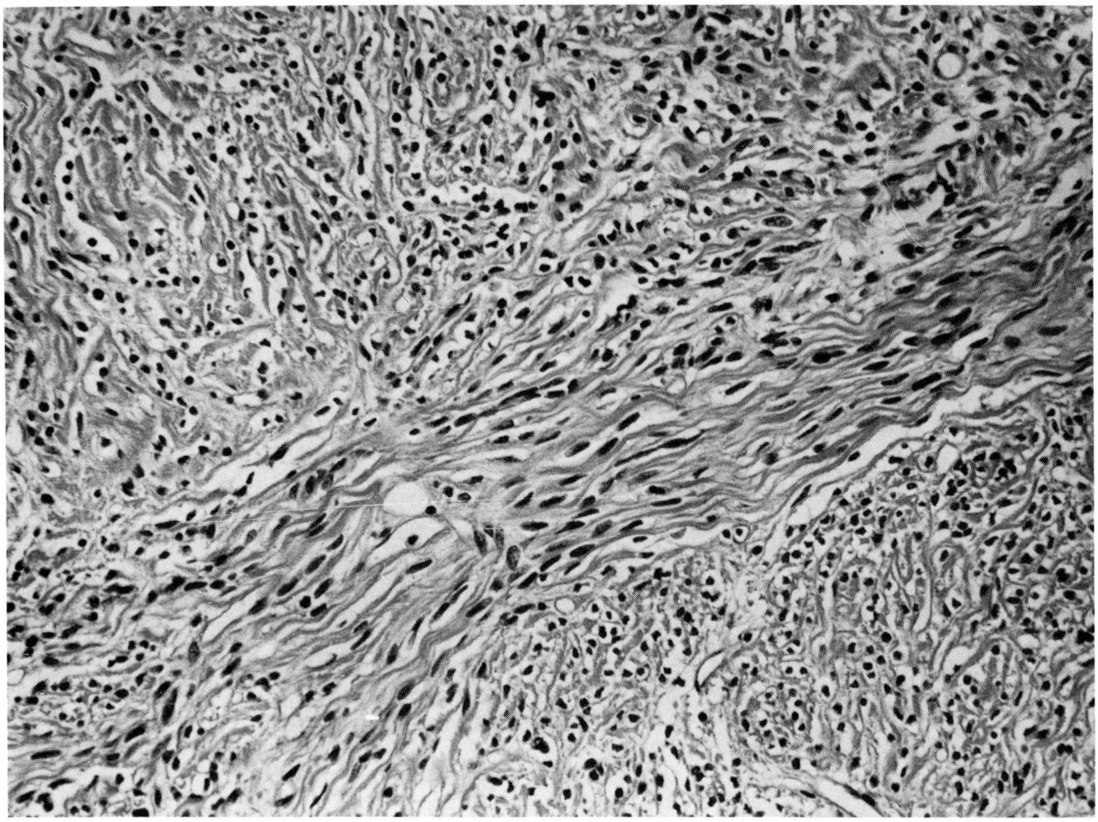

Figure 12–3. Benign fibrous pleural tumor composed of intersecting fascicles of spindle cells.

pneumocytes forming solid nests, glandular inclusions, or papillary structures are on occasion sufficiently abundant to create a biphasic pattern.[93] Mitotic figures can usually be found, but the cells are cytologically benign.

The spindle cells in most benign fibrous pleural tumors are keratin negative.[142] Carter and Otis reported their immunocytochemical findings on 17 fibrous tumors of the pleura[32]: eight were benign and localized and all were keratin negative, and one histologically malignant tumor that recurred three times in 12 years was consistently keratin negative. However, 8 diffuse malignant tumors were intensely keratin positive. The spindle cells of three intrapulmonary fibromas[175] that were histologically identical to localized fibrous tumors of the pleura did not express keratin or other markers apart from vimentin.

The spindle cells have the fine structure of fibroblasts or myofibroblasts, and they lie within a dense collagenous stroma.[30, 73, 128] In cellular tumors, many of the cells are more ovoid than spindle shaped and they form small groups within which neighboring cells are linked by primitive junctions (Fig. 12–4).

Mesotheliomas

Pleural mesotheliomas account for fully two thirds of all reported mesotheliomas, and approximately 75% are diffuse malignant mesotheliomas. The proportion of pleural to peritoneal tumors is 80% to 20% in the United States. In England, figures of 88% and 12% have been reported.[102] In Legha and Muggia's compilation of 559 pleural tumors, the male to female ratio ranged from less than 2:1 to 3:1.[102] Roughly two thirds of the patients are between the ages of 40 and 70 years, and the median age is between 50 and 60 in different series. Any age of patient can be involved, but malignant tumors of the pleura are rare in children[15, 23, 157]: 6 of the 192 patients reported by Hochberg (cited by Legha and Muggia[102]) were in the first decade, 6 in the second decade, and 21 (6.2%)

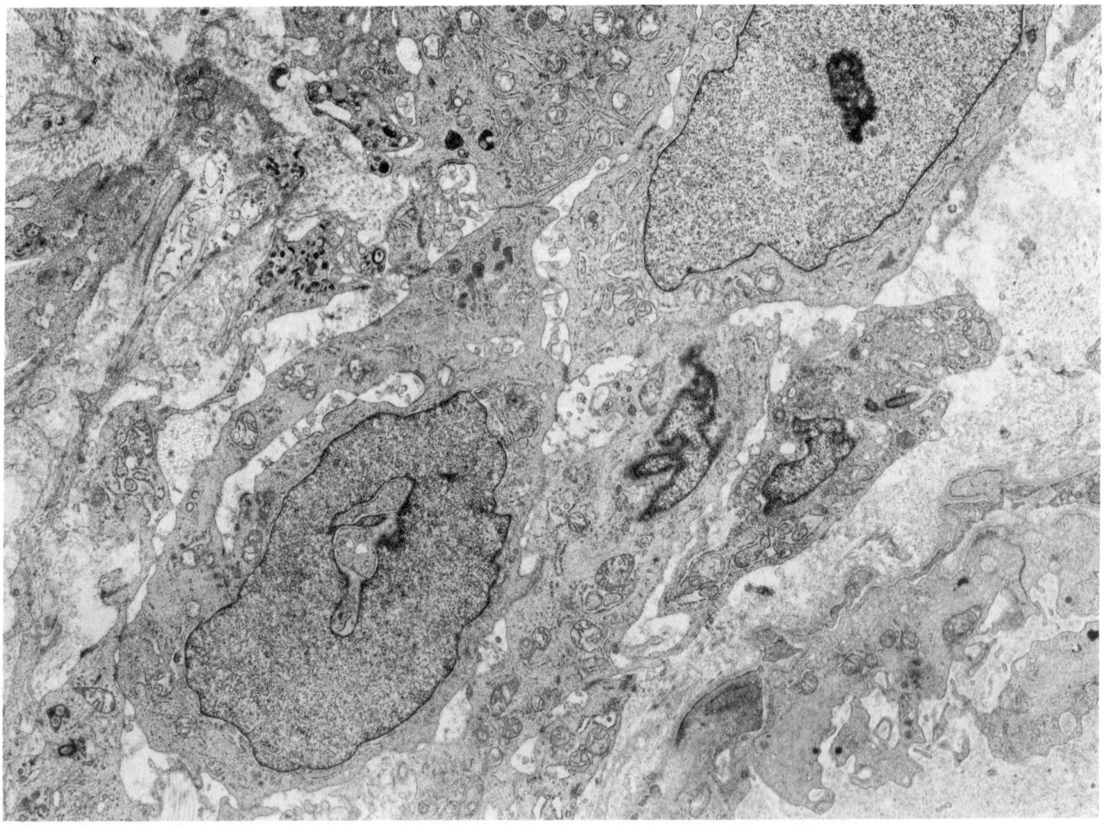

Figure 12–4. Benign fibrous pleural tumor. The ovoid cells are loosely clustered, and primitive cell attachments are present. The cytoplasm contains a moderate number of cisternae. (×4,300)

in the third decade. Familial cases have been recorded.[69]

More than 1,000 new cases of mesothelioma can be anticipated in the United States each year.[164] Spirtas and co-workers found the incidence in males to be between 7 and 13 new cases per million per year.[151] In a study of malignant mesothelioma in four regions of Texas between 1976 and 1980, the age-adjusted incidence of the 88 cases was 5.8 per million for males and 2.1 per million in females.[172]

Churg[35] found an incidence of mesothelioma in British Columbia in 1982 of 17 per million in men and 1.9 per million in women. The rate for men had increased nearly six times compared with the period 1969 to 1975 but had remained roughly the same for women. In Great Britain during the period 1968 to 1983, deaths from mesothelioma among men increased from 114 to 467 and among women from 38 to 90.[86] In 1983, the crude death rates in Great Britain were 17.5 per million and 3.2 per million for men and women, respectively. The annual mortality from malignant mesothelioma of the pleura in Australian men aged 30 and older reached 21 per million in 1983.[173] The rate in Australian women in that year was 3 per million.

Epidemiology

In 1960, Wagner and associates[163] established the relationship of mesothelioma to asbestos, and it is now widely accepted that the prevalence of mesothelioma is related to the level of the industrial use of asbestos. Fourteen of the 15 male cases in Churg's study could be linked to asbestos exposure.[35] However, there are frequent regional variations in the incidence that are not associated with industries in particular areas, and as many as one third of malignant pleural mesotheliomas cannot be attributed to a specific etiologic factor. Many patients develop mesothelioma after minimal exposure,[33] and others are not aware that they have been exposed, although some may unwittingly have undergone at least minimal exposure. Antman[7] notes that a threshold of exposure below which there is no risk of developing mesothelioma has not been determined. Other causative factors that have been implicated include chronic inflammation involving the pleura[76] and a history of prior irradiation.[16, 42]

The literature on asbestos and its pathologic effects is extensive.[89, 103] Asbestos is a family of fibrous hydrated silicates, the composition of which differs from one geographical area to another. The fibers vary considerably in thickness and length. Over 90% of the asbestos in industries in western countries is chrysotile, which may be used alone for insulation and many other products but is sometimes blended with crocidolite and amosite. The physical properties of the asbestos fibers are important. They are smaller than most man-made fibers, and the thinner the fibers, the more deeply they are carried into the respiratory passages. Adamson and Bowden found in the mouse lung that smaller fibers did not elicit the fibrosis that formed in response to larger fibers.[4, 5] Some asbestos fibers can be broken down in the body into smaller fragments and removed by phagocytosis or in the secretions of the respiratory passages, but long amphibole fibers do not disintegrate and will continue to accumulate in the exposed person.

Recognition of the dangers of asbestos has dramatically curtailed its industrial applications, but it continues to be used in floor and ceiling tiles, automobile brake linings, and a variety of other products. There is a latent period of at least 20 years between exposure to asbestos and the development of mesothelioma, but exceptions have been recorded.[1] Trends in the use of asbestos and in age- and sex-specific death rates suggest that the annual number of deaths from mesothelioma in the United States will continue to increase until close to the end of the century. Based on exposures in 1940 and around 1970 when industrial precautions were first instituted, the number of new cases is likely to peak sometime in the 1990s, and thereafter the tumor can be anticipated to become less common.[9] In Australian men, the figures can be related to the increased use of asbestos in that country during and after World War II. It reached its maximum in 1958, and the peak mortality from pleural mesothelioma can be expected in the 1990s.[173] In Great Britain, future cases will mostly be in men, since exposure to asbestos among women was greatest during the war when many worked in factories and annual deaths in British women have probably already peaked.

Clinical Features

The onset of symptoms is usually gradual[8] with mild pleuritic chest pain and dyspnea.

Cough and loss of weight occur later. Once the tumor infiltrates the chest wall, pain becomes localized. A common finding is a unilateral pleural effusion, which may be drained and recur before the diagnosis is established. The effusion can be extensive, and it is often blood stained. The pleura is thickened, and it frequently has a nodular appearance. These changes are more apparent toward the base of the lung. As the disease progresses, adhesions develop between the two pleural layers and the pleural space becomes obliterated, but small spaces containing fluid can persist. Thrombocytosis has been described in patients with malignant mesothelioma,[119] but Oleson and Thorsaughe[125] did not find it more frequent or marked than in other pleural malignancies. Hypertrophic pulmonary osteoarthropathy and intermittent hypoglycemia occur more often with benign fibrous mesotheliomas.[7, 102]

The diagnosis is often reached or suspected when smears of thoracentesis fluid or a fine-needle aspirate are examined, but an open biopsy specimen is obtained for confirmation in about two thirds of cases. In the early stages, thoracoscopy may be helpful.[22, 131] Herbert[72] advocates increased use of thoracoscopy, arguing that it provides a definite diagnosis in most cases and that seeding on the needle track has not proved to be a major problem. Law and co-workers[99, 100] also consider thoracoscopy a useful diagnostic alternative to thoracotomy and believe that, since skin deposits of tumor do not cause pain or other clinical problems, the risk of seeding should not be a reason for witholding diagnostic and therapeutic procedures.

The tumor extends late in its course to mediastinal and less often axillary, cervical, or upper abdominal lymph nodes. Vascular spread is more common than is often realized, and by this route the tumor may reach the opposite lung, the liver and other abdominal viscera, and bone. Blood-borne metastases can be found in about half of the patients at autopsy, but it is the local spread of the tumor that is important clinically and death results from complications produced by the primary lesion. Adams and Unni[2] found distant metastases in 12 of 16 diffuse malignant mesotheliomas, but the lesions were clinically occult in 11. Their distribution was contralateral pleura (6), pericardium (7), bones of thorax (6), lymph nodes (5), liver (4), peritoneum (7), and brachial plexus and neck (3). Direct spread to the pericardium or opposite lung or through the diaphragm is a late event.

In the Butchart staging system,[31] modified by Antman,[7] stage 1 tumors are confined to ipsilateral pleura and lung; stage 2 tumors involve the chest wall, mediastinum, pericardium, or contralateral pleura; a stage 3 tumor is present in both thorax and abdomen or in extrathoracic lymph nodes; and distant blood-borne metastases indicate a stage 4 lesion.

Survival

The results of therapy for diffuse malignant mesothelioma are disappointing. Other than the palliative effect of radiation, treatment does not alter the median survival of approximately 1 year seen in untreated patients. Among patients who survive for longer periods, a few have remained disease-free for over 5 years after intensive treatment. Patients with epithelial tumors appear to live longer than those with sarcomatous lesions.

Pathology

In addition to the three main types of malignant mesothelioma, epithelial, sarcomatous, and biphasic or mixed, an undifferentiated form is recognized[46] but is difficult to diagnose by routine light microscopy. Like Hammar and Bolen,[70] we do not recognize a benign epithelial mesothelioma, agreeing with their reasoning that lesions so designated represent hyperplasias rather than true neoplasms. Differentiation of serosal hyperplasia from mesothelioma is discussed by McCaughey and Al-Jabi.[112] In one review of 382 pleural mesotheliomas,[102] 54% had been classified as epithelial, 21% as sarcomatous, and 25% as mixed. Among 92 tumors in Mayo Clinic patients, 42 tumors were purely epithelial, 21 were sarcomatous, and 29 were mixed.[3] The mixed cellular type is seen more frequently at autopsy, when extensive sampling is possible, than in small surgical biopsy specimens.

The diagnosis of malignant mesothelioma is often difficult. Kannerstein and colleagues sum it up thus:[90] "It would appear that diagnostic assessment of the individual case of possible diffuse mesothelioma must depend on the weighing of a variety of evidential factors, clinical as well as pathologic, and the rendering in some cases of a less than definite opinion."

Early mesotheliomas may be seen at thoracoscopy as whitish or red, elevated, smooth or rough nodules. The lesions coalesce as the tumor extends over the surface of the pleura, forming a sheet that thickens as it expands. It may contain nodular areas and small papillary foci. The pleural thickening is more obvious toward the base of the lung. Diffuse malignant mesotheliomas are usually solid, and cystic spaces are uncommon. With growth, the underlying lung may be infiltrated, but it is usually not extensively involved. The pleural cavity is eventually obliterated. Once the parietal pleura is involved, either primarily or by expansion of a tumor of the visceral pleura, the intercostal spaces and ribs are liable to be invaded. Growth through the mediastinal pleura will reach the pericardium, and through the diaphragm the liver can become involved. Lymph node and distant blood-borne metastases are late events.

LIGHT MICROSCOPY

There is a broad range of microscopic appearances, and the histologic variants include solid, myxoid, tubulopapillary, desmoplastic, sarcomatous, and biphasic forms. In the common form of epithelial mesothelioma, cuboidal or polygonal cells form tubules or papillary structures (Figs. 12–5 and 12–6) or line branching spaces (Fig. 12–7). Cords of cells can divide and connect to create a meshwork (Fig. 12–8). Usually the cells have a central nucleus with a smooth or slightly irregular profile and at least moderate amounts of cytoplasm. Solid areas are common, and a papillary architecture can abut on the diffuse pattern (Fig. 12–9). The stroma is sometimes loose and myxoid, but more frequently it is densely fibrous, enveloping clusters and sheets of uniform cells (Fig. 12–10). Scrutiny of these apparently solid foci will often reveal glandlike arrangements formed by cuboidal cells (Fig. 12–11), facilitating the diagnosis. The presence of

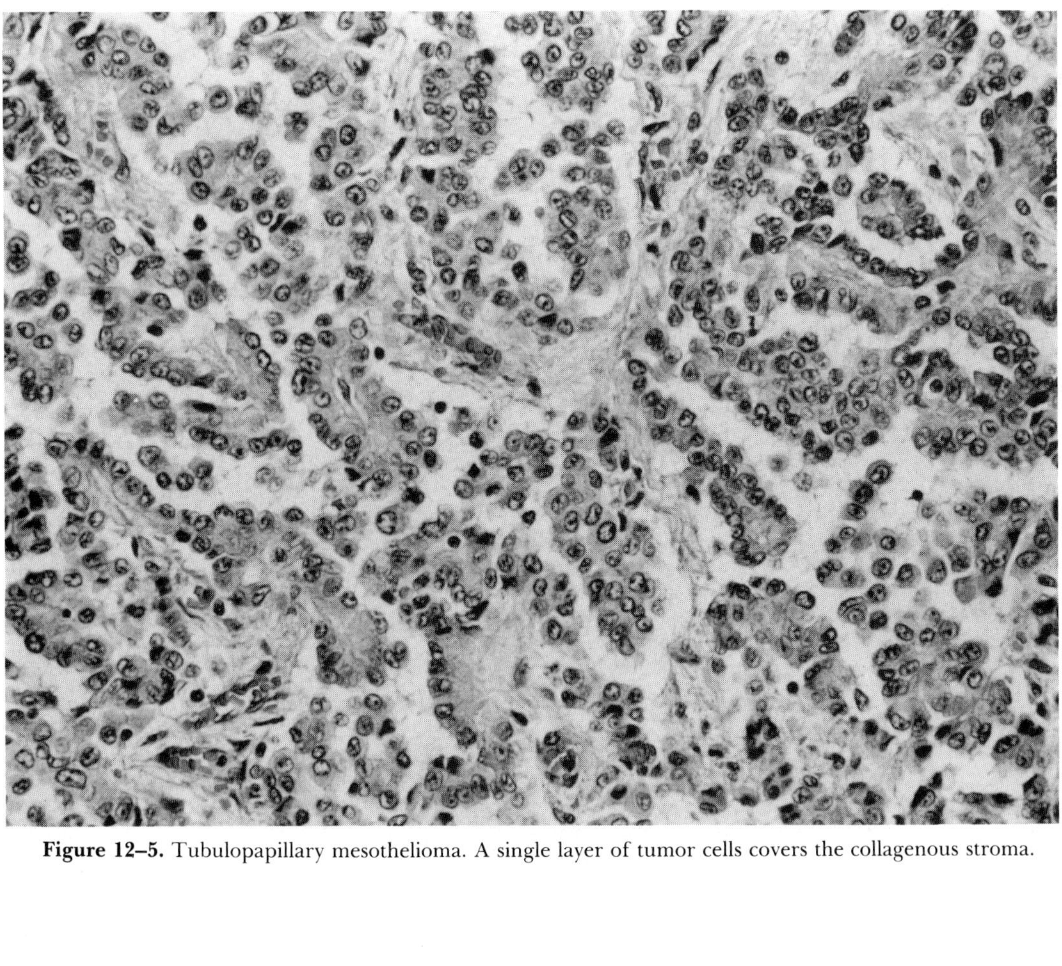

Figure 12–5. Tubulopapillary mesothelioma. A single layer of tumor cells covers the collagenous stroma.

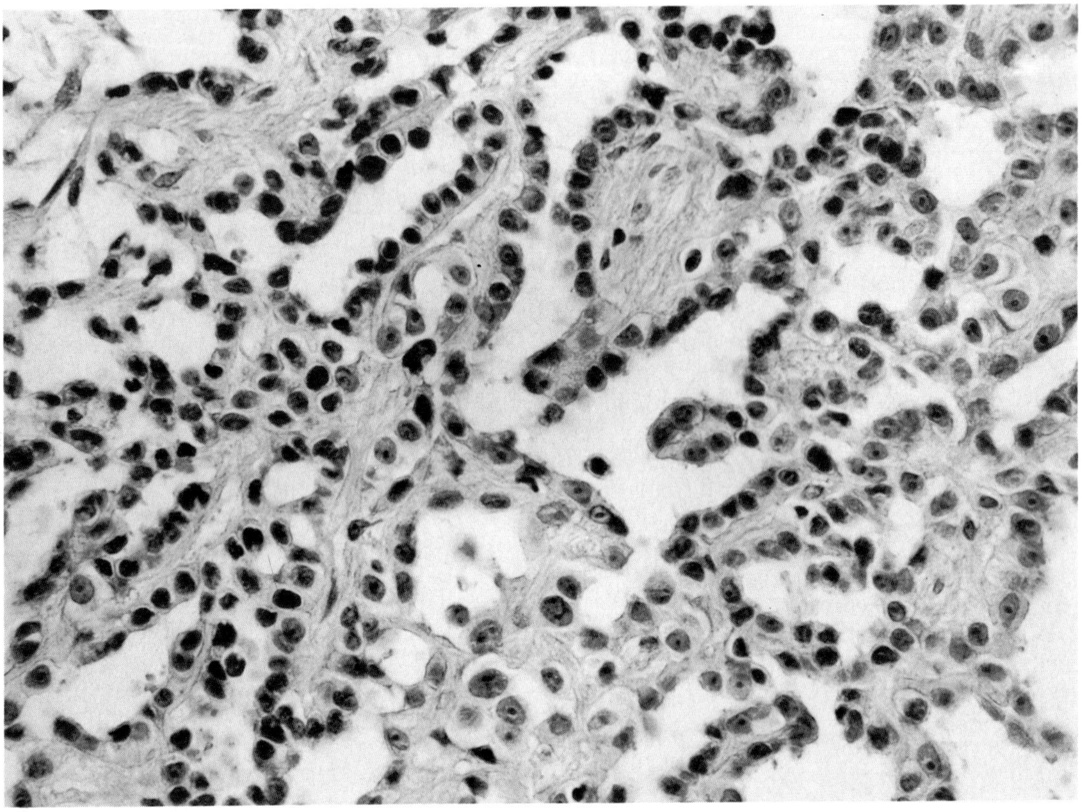

Figure 12–6. Tubulopapillary mesothelioma. The cells are cuboidal and uniform, but some nucleoli are evident.

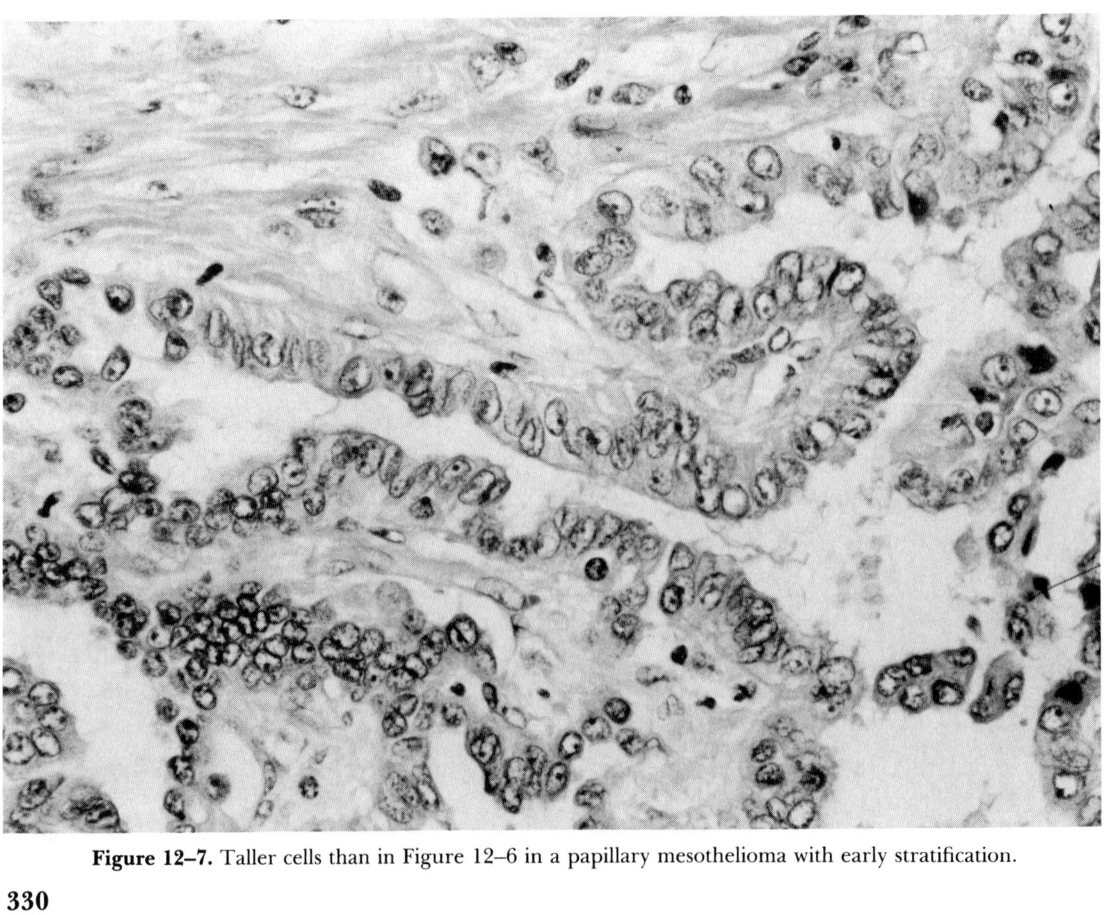

Figure 12–7. Taller cells than in Figure 12–6 in a papillary mesothelioma with early stratification.

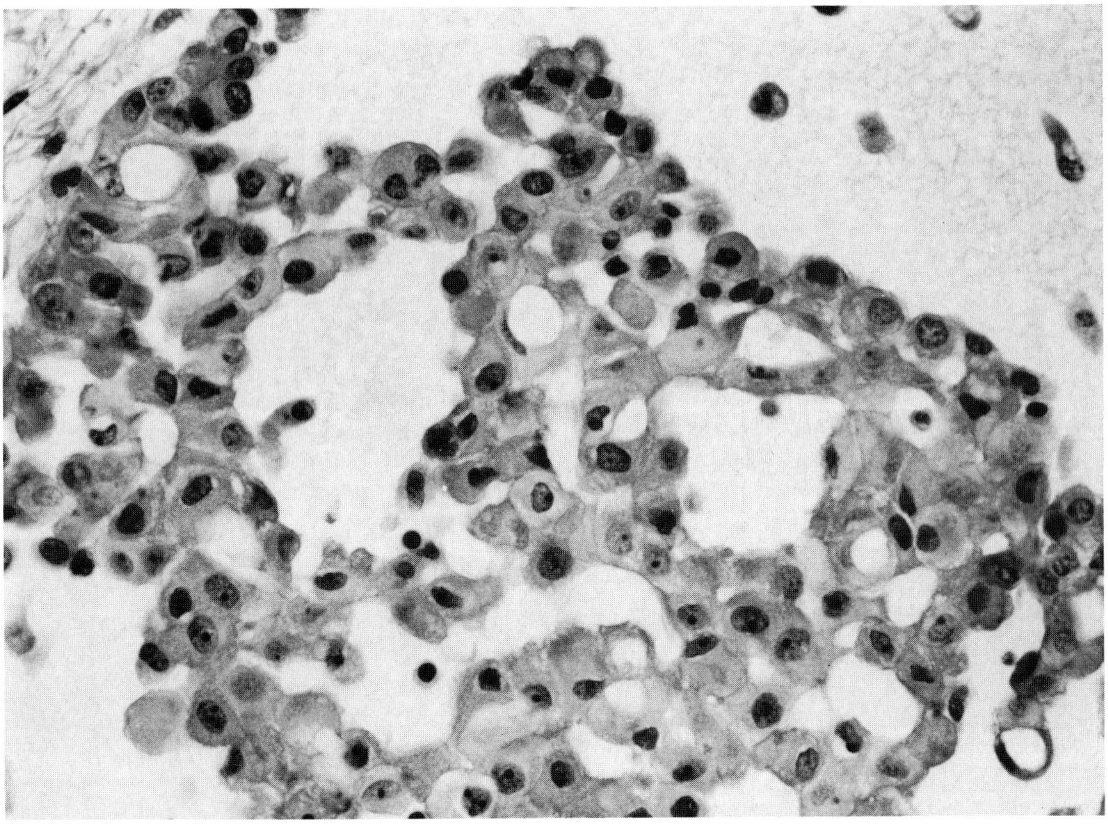

Figure 12–8. Branching cords of mesothelioma cells, some of them vacuolated, create a meshwork.

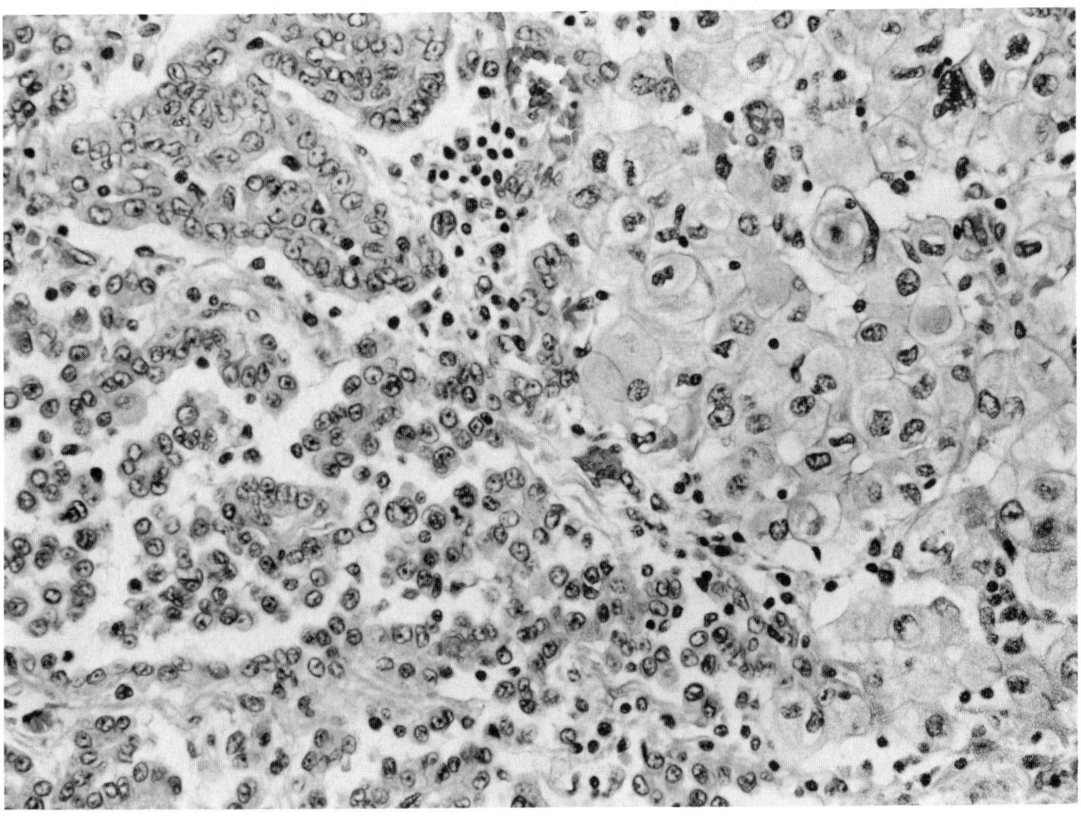

Figure 12–9. Mesothelioma. A papillary area abuts on a solid zone of larger cells.

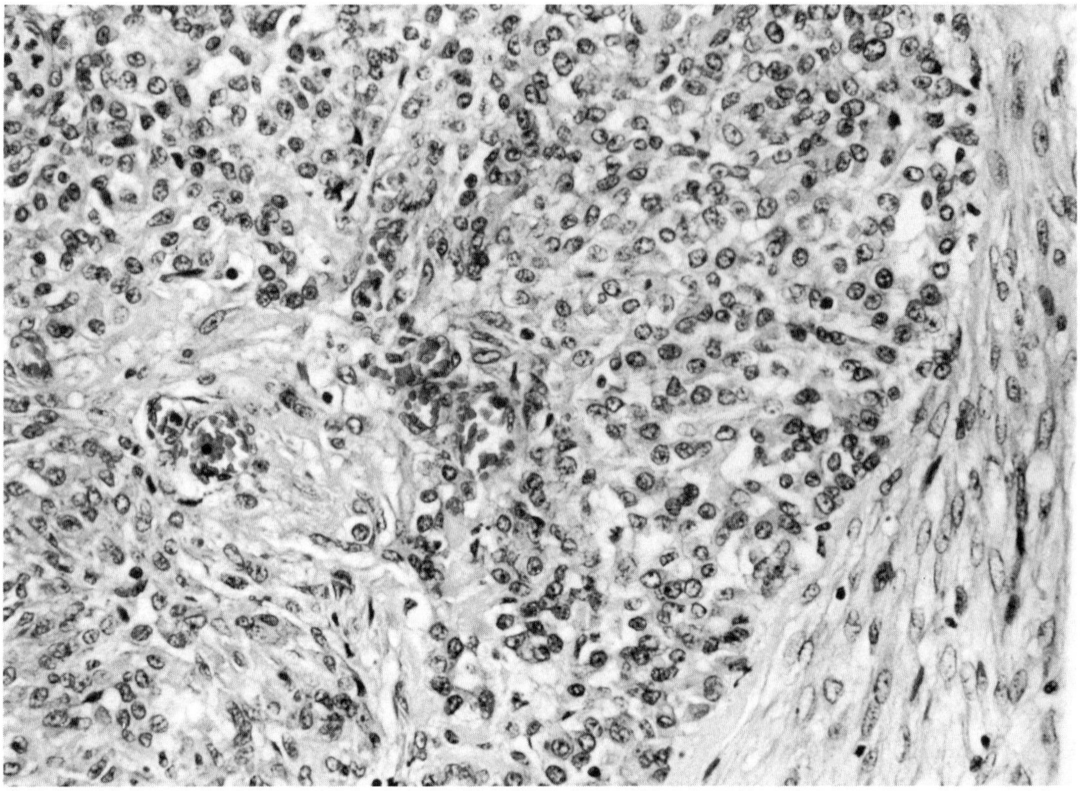

Figure 12–10. Mesothelioma. Cellular stroma borders a large solid nodule of tumor cells.

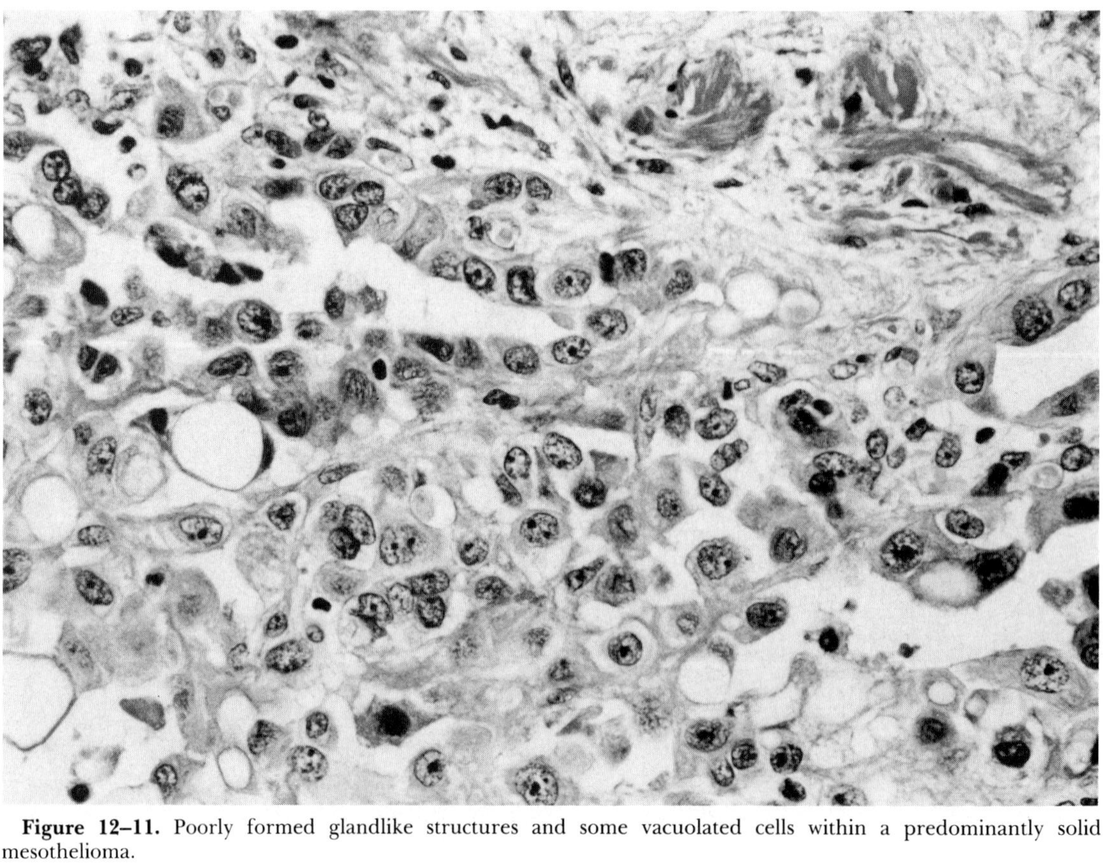

Figure 12–11. Poorly formed glandlike structures and some vacuolated cells within a predominantly solid mesothelioma.

microvilli on the apical surfaces of the cells lining these glandlike spaces can be detected in paraffin sections, and it is consequently worth examining them at high power. When adjacent cells are closely packed (Fig. 12–12), their polygonal outlines are highlighted by the luxuriant surface covering of microvilli that serves to slightly separate the cells from one another (Figs. 12–13 and 12–14). A similar appearance can be seen in cytologic preparations containing clusters of cells (Fig. 12–15).

Most mesotheliomas are composed of uniform cells, but the nuclei can show varying degrees of atypia and the appearance often changes from one region of a tumor to another. Figures 12–16 through 12–21 illustrate a spectrum of cell and nuclear irregularity among several tumors. Atypia is evident in Figures 12–16 through 12–18, and mitoses are present. Markedly irregular cells (Fig. 12–19), and bizarre and multinucleated cells (Fig. 12–20), may give rise to concern that the tumor is a sarcoma, particularly after examination of a small biopsy specimen or fine-needle aspirate, and immunostaining and electron microscopy are then indicated. In an occasional pleomorphic mesothelioma, large vacuoles within cells simulate a signet-ring appearance (Figs. 12–11, 12–15, 12–21, and 12–22), but the cells with attenuated cytoplasm are also keratin positive and electron microscopy shows that they have many microvilli. The cystic form of mesothelioma seen in the peritoneum[91, 116, 148] does not occur in the pleura. Squamous cell carcinoma arising in the pleura has been described,[139] but it is a rare event.

The stroma sometimes contains psammoma bodies. Calcification is not common, but it can occur: Nichols and Johnson[22] described extensive calcification in a rapidly growing malignant mixed mesothelioma from a patient with a lengthy history of asbestos exposure and chronic renal failure. Osseous and cartilaginous differentiation has been reported.[174]

In biphasic tumors (Figs. 12–23 and 12–24), the relative proportions of the two components vary. Since entrapped cells, from

Text continued on page 340

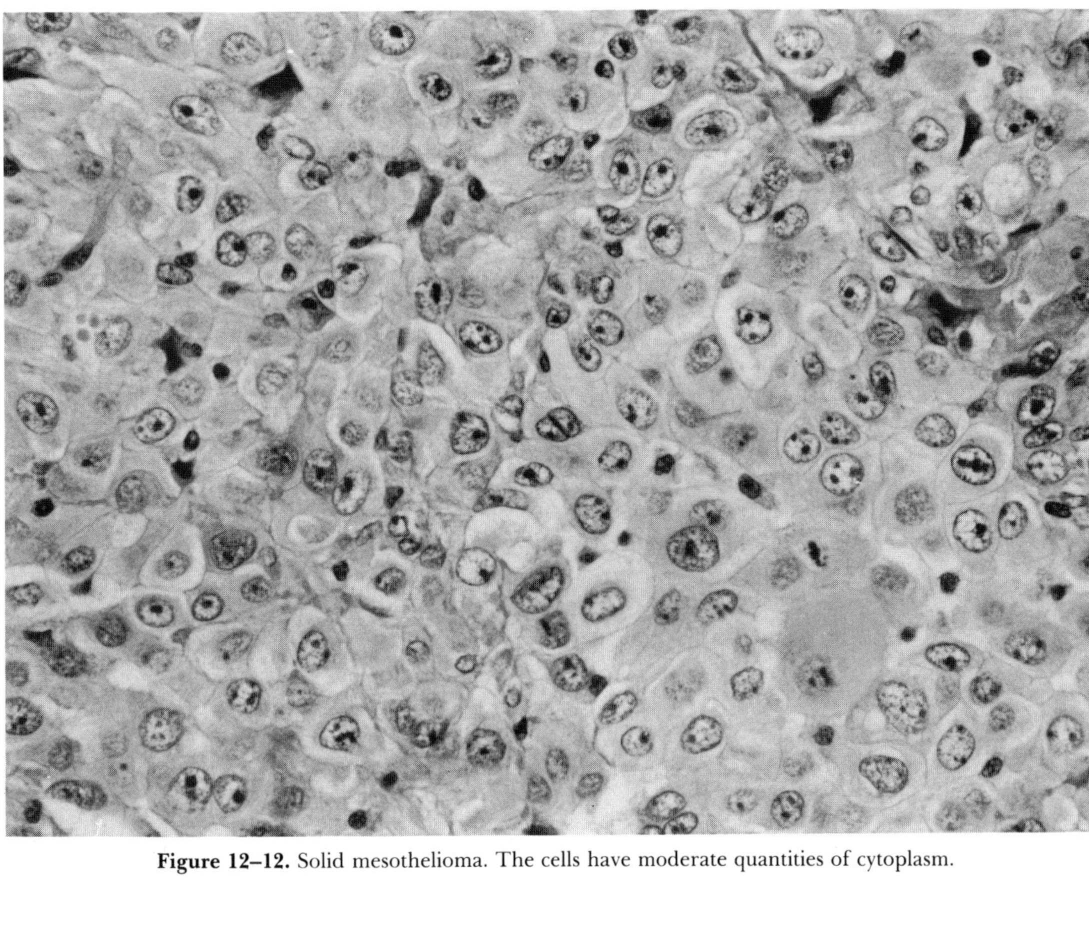

Figure 12–12. Solid mesothelioma. The cells have moderate quantities of cytoplasm.

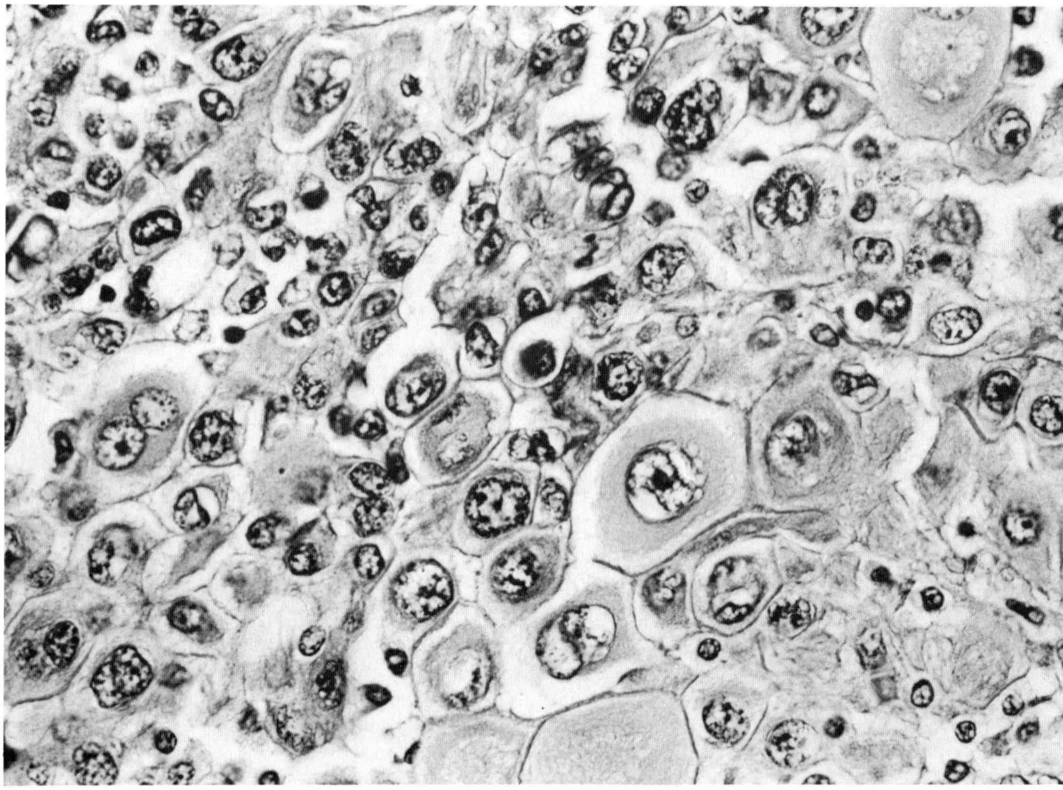

Figure 12–13. The polygonal outlines of the mesothelioma cells can be identified.

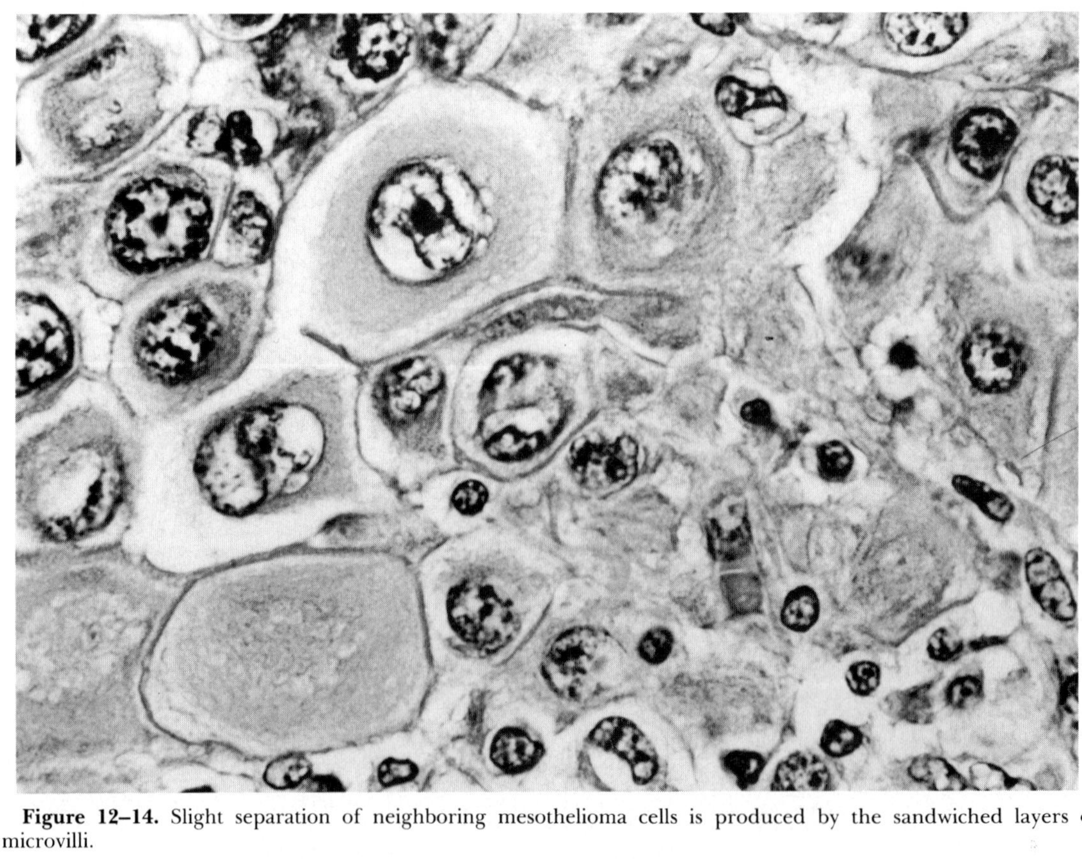

Figure 12–14. Slight separation of neighboring mesothelioma cells is produced by the sandwiched layers of microvilli.

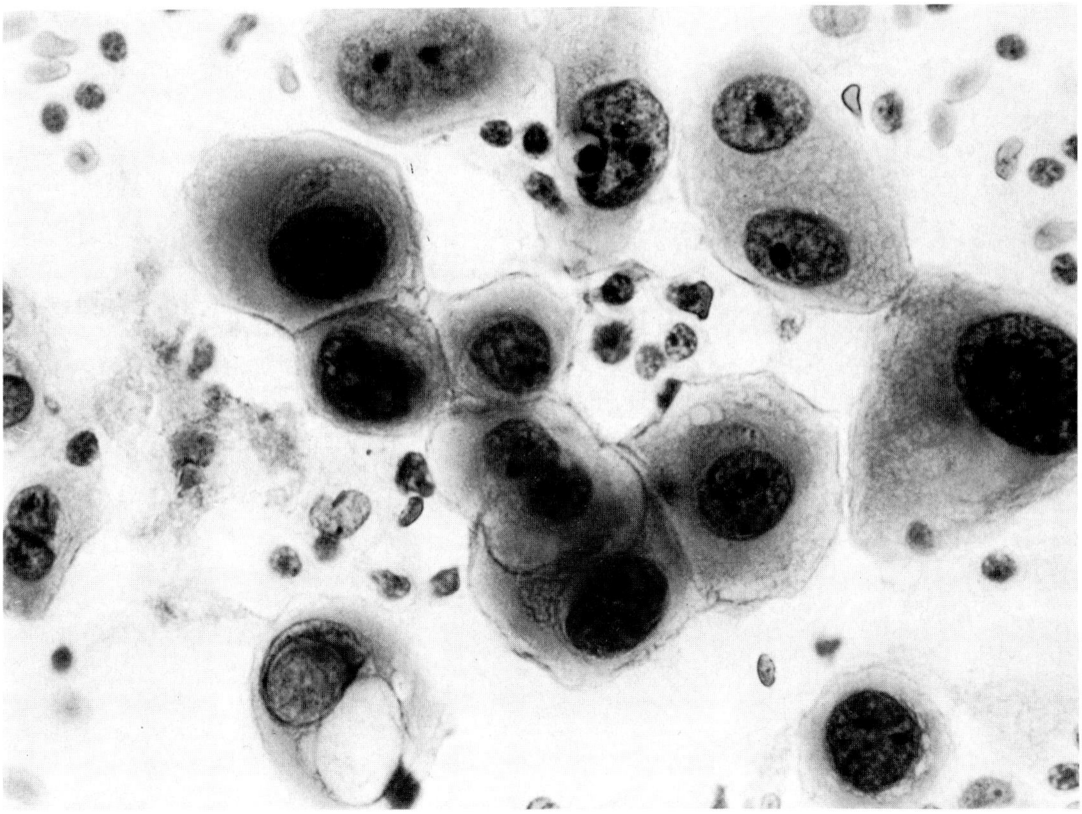

Figure 12–15. A similar appearance to that in Figure 12–14 in a smear from a fine-needle aspirate.

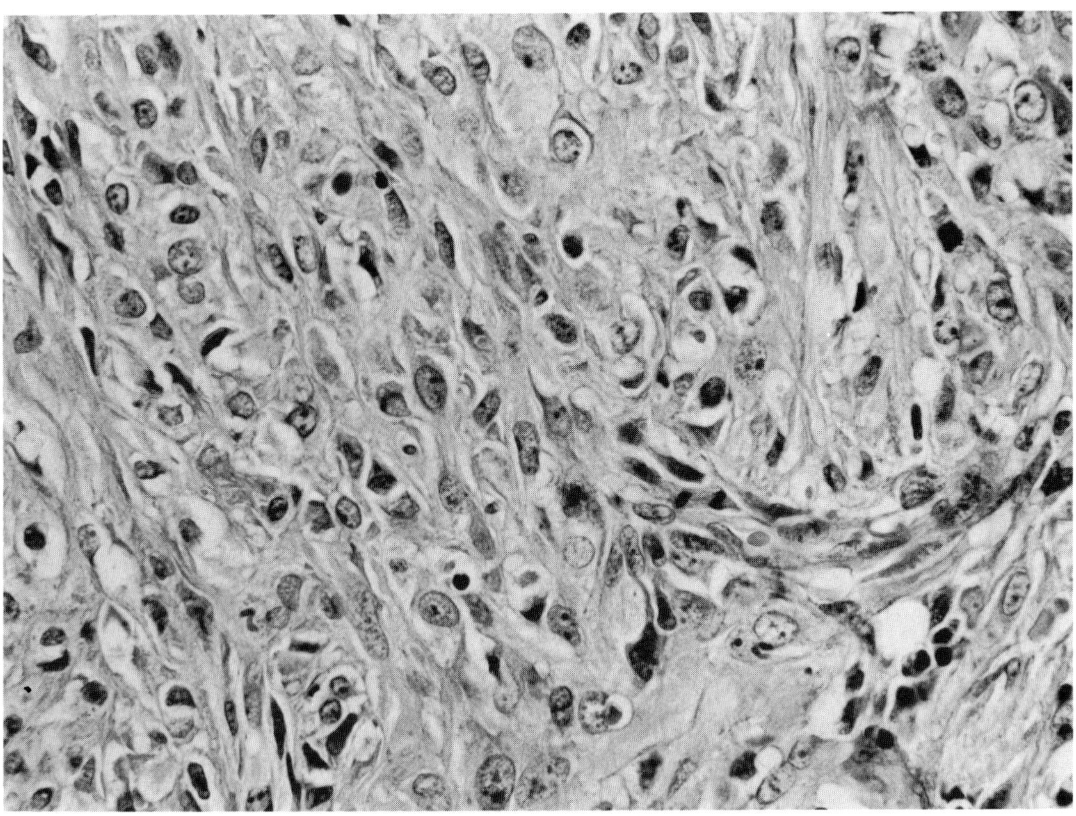

Figure 12–16. A suggestion of spindling in a solid mesothelioma.

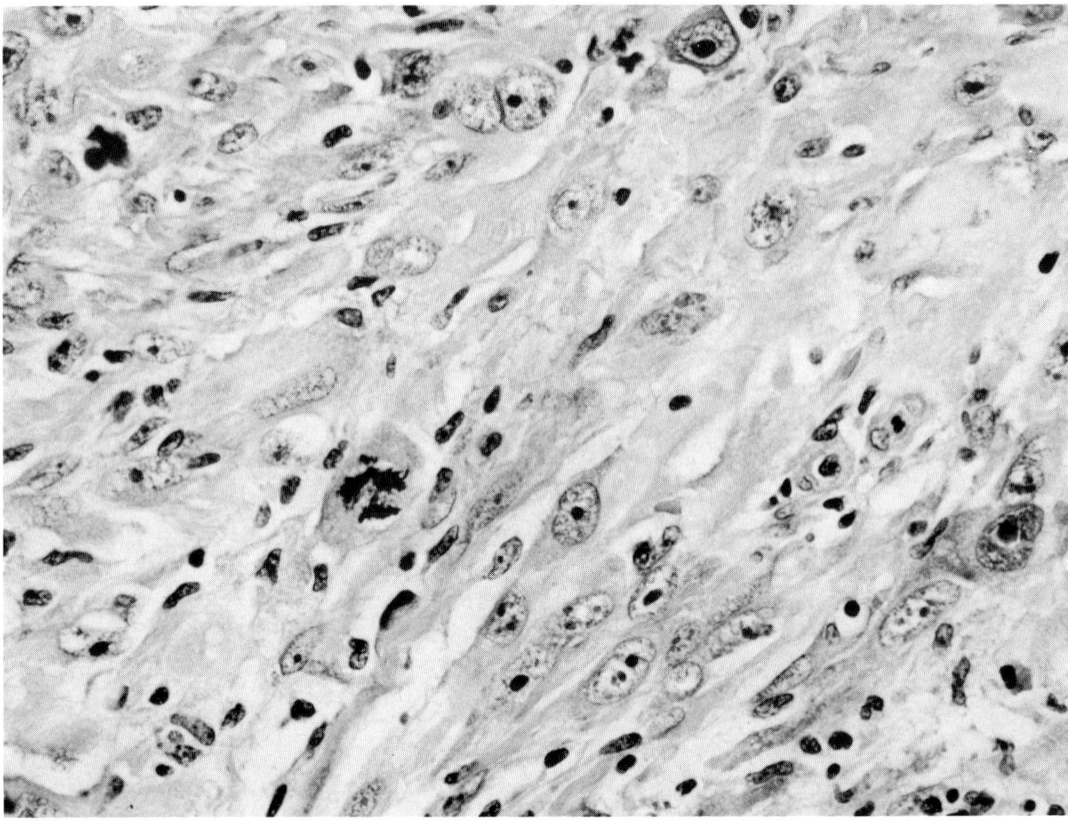

Figure 12–17. Some pleomorphism in a solid mesothelioma with bizarre mitoses and prominent nucleoli.

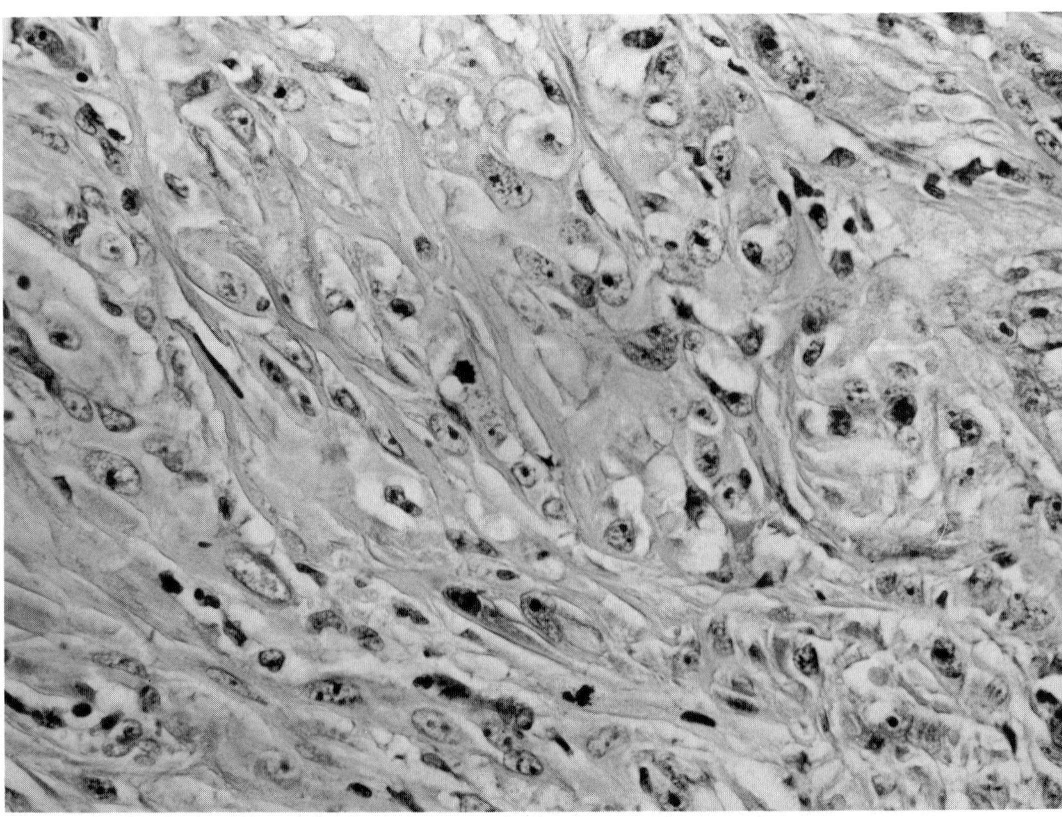

Figure 12–18. Fusiform and irregular cells in a mesothelioma with fibrous stroma.

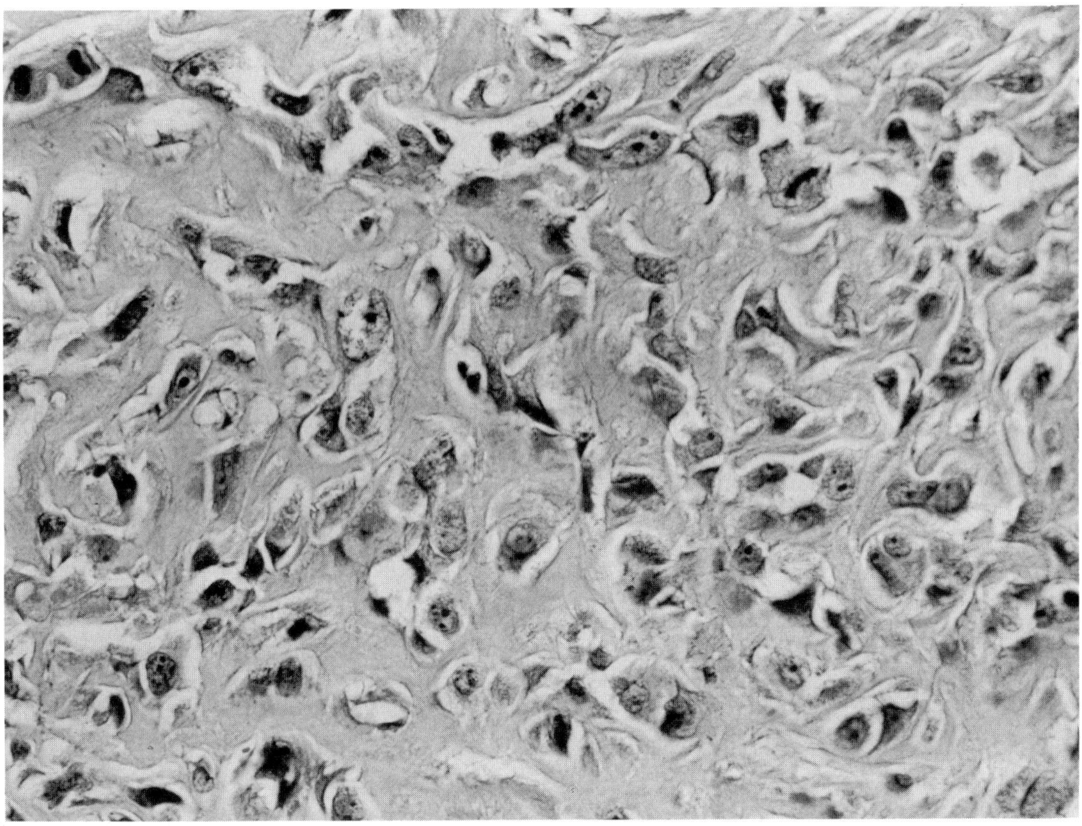

Figure 12–19. Mesothelioma cells with marked variability of cell and nuclear profiles.

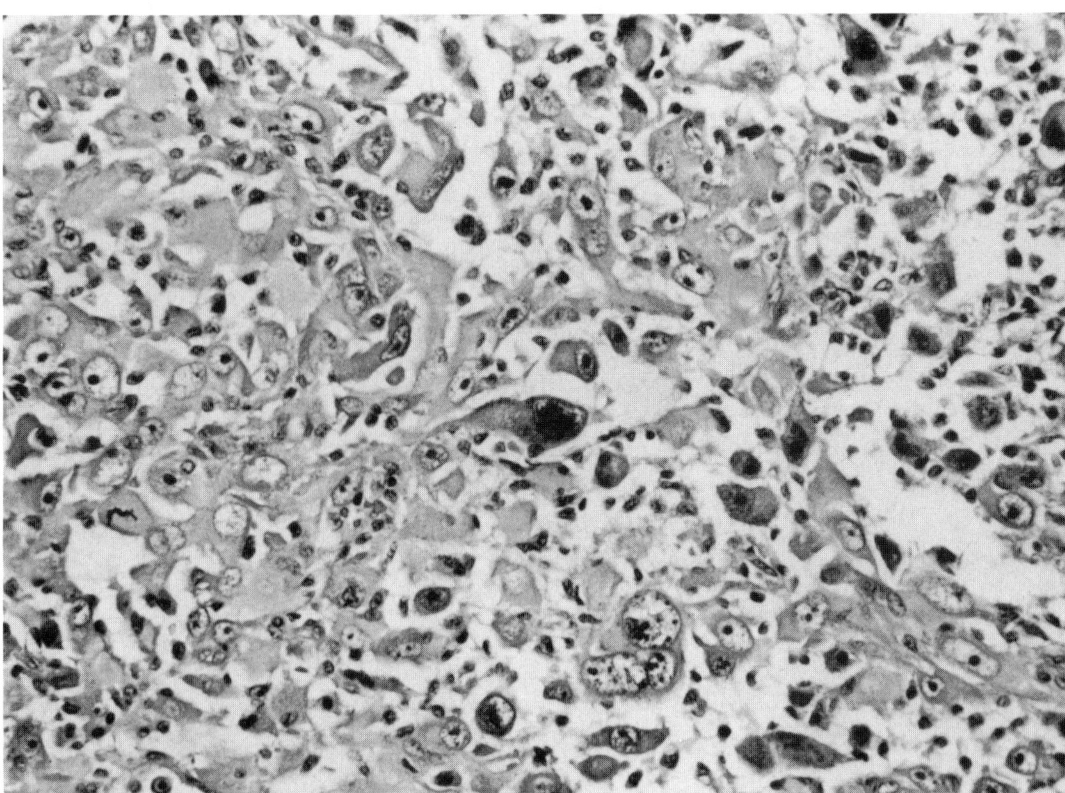

Figure 12–20. Anaplastic mesothelioma with bizarre cells.

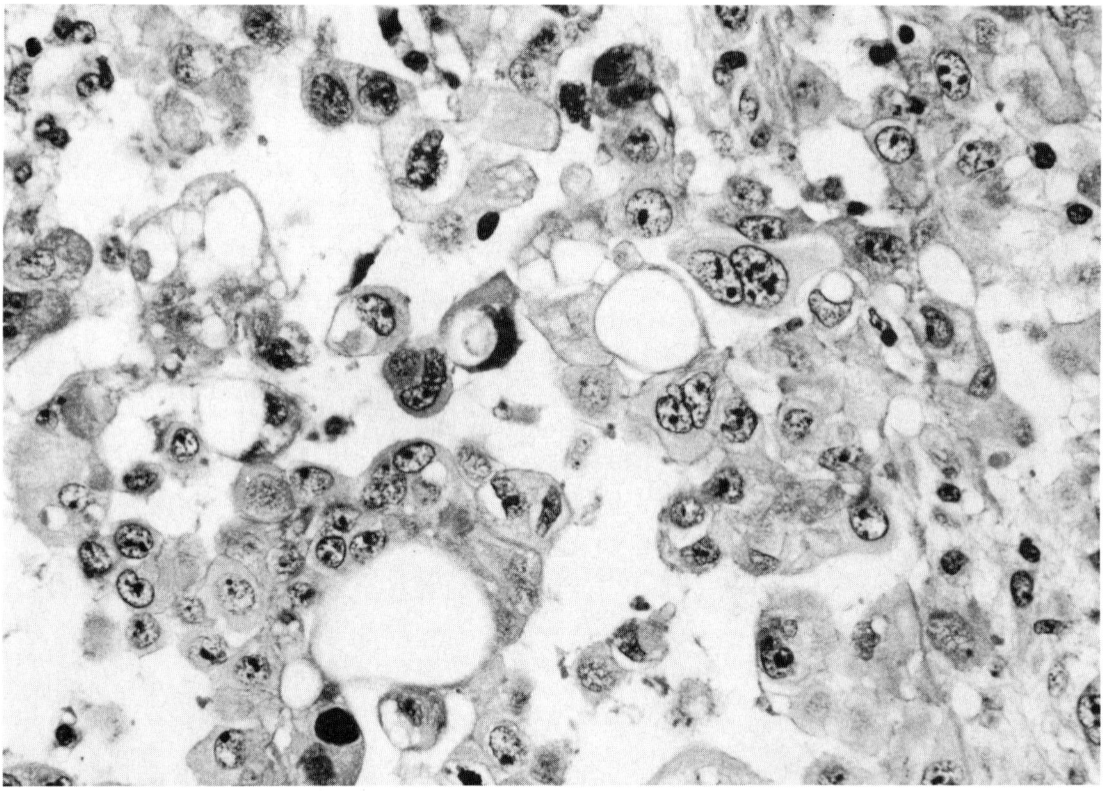

Figure 12–21. Cytoplasmic vacuoles of varying sizes in a pleomorphic mesothelioma.

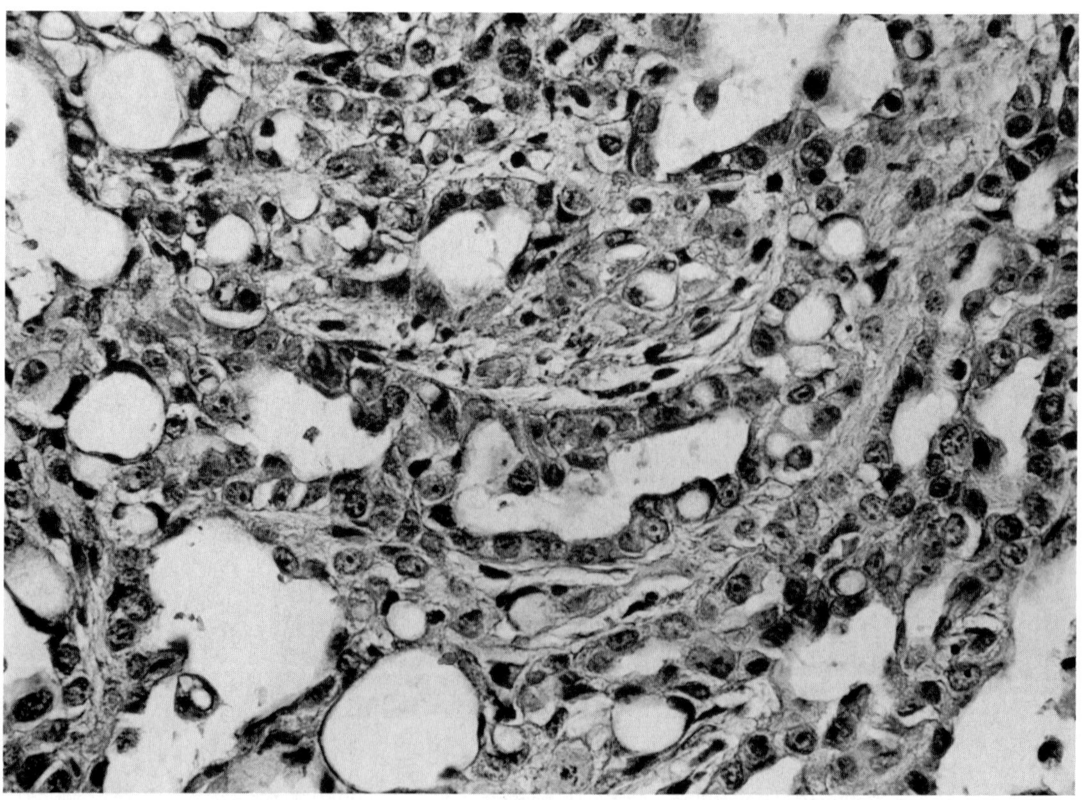

Figure 12–22. The cells of this mesothelioma are more uniform than in Figure 12–21, but small and large vacuoles are evident.

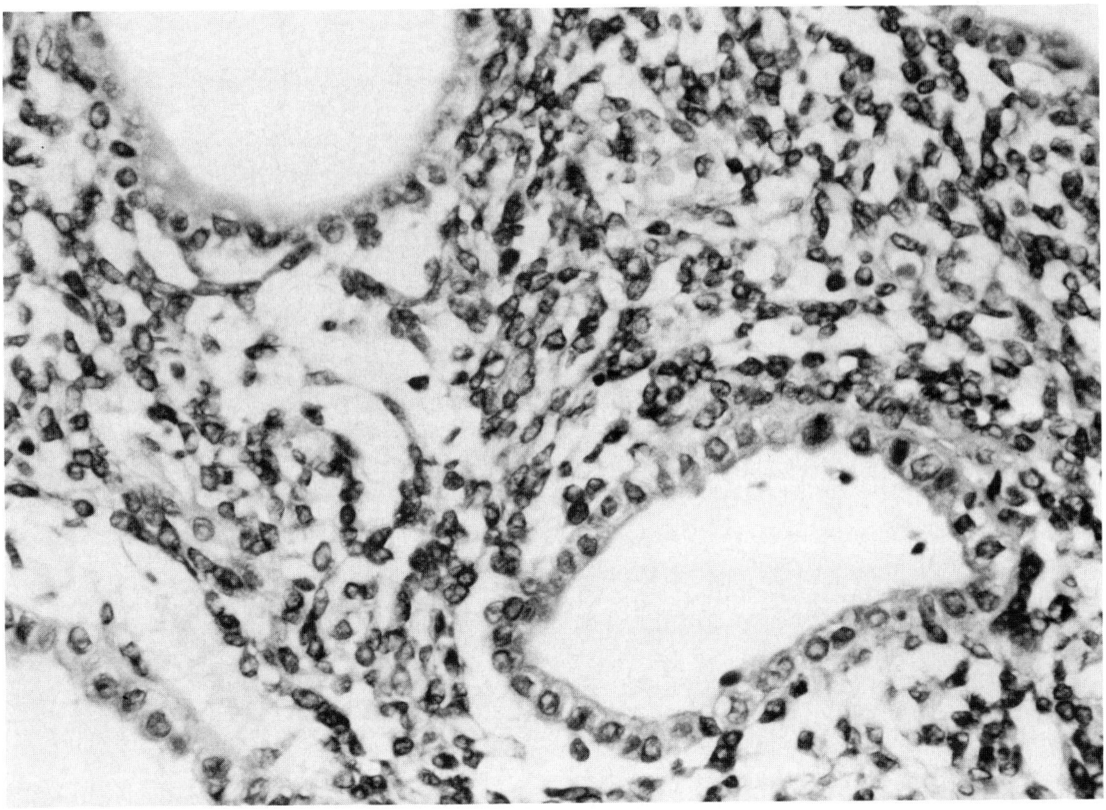

Figure 12–23. Biphasic mesothelioma. Cuboidal epithelial cells are lining spaces within a spindle cell component.

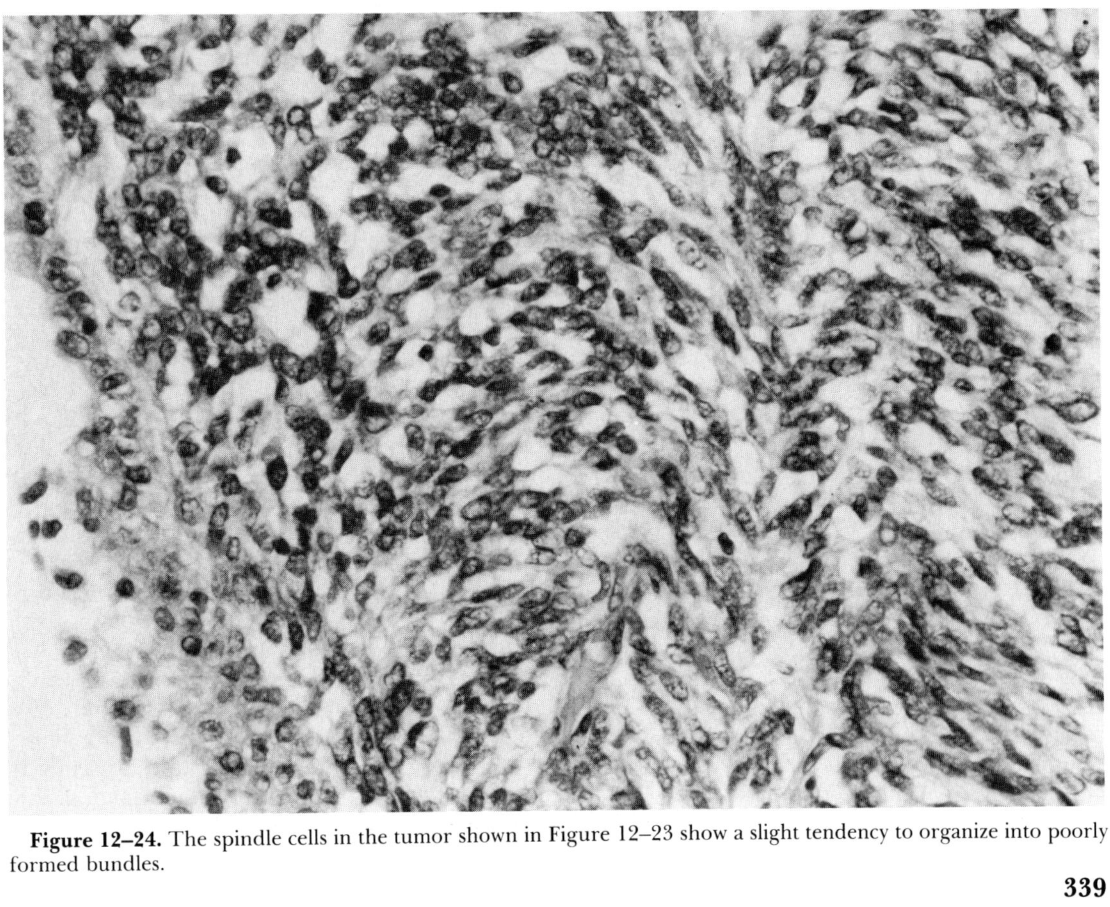

Figure 12–24. The spindle cells in the tumor shown in Figure 12–23 show a slight tendency to organize into poorly formed bundles.

either the mesothelium or underlying lung, are a common finding in spindle cell lesions of the pleura, a tumor should not be designated a mixed mesothelioma unless both components are clearly neoplastic. Transitional forms between the epithelial and spindle cells occur,[70] and they can be identified more reliably by electron microscopy than in light microscopic sections. Donna and Betta[51] reported a biphasic tumor with foci of sarcomatous cartilaginous differentiation and osteoid formation reproducing an embryonal pattern of enchondral ossification.

CYTOLOGY

The microscopic features that are used to identify cells of a mesothelioma in cytologic preparations are similar to those seen in tissue sections. It is not always easy to separate reactive pleural cells in cytologic smears (Figs. 12–25 and 12–26) from mesothelioma cells (Figs. 12–27 and 12–28) or to distinguish between mesothelioma (Fig. 12–29) and metastatic adenocarcinoma.[160] Ehya[55] observes that the cells in effusions have optically dense cytoplasm with lacy peripheral vacuoles, intercellular spaces may be visualized, and cell clusters have scalloped borders, but no feature is pathognomonic. Nevertheless, the rapidity and ease with which cytologic preparations can be obtained inevitably results in their being preferred to a cutting-needle biopsy, and cytologic analysis has a higher sensitivity than needle biopsy for diagnosing malignant pleural effusions,[134] although more than one aspiration may be needed. The operator performing a thoracentesis on a patient with mesothelioma may notice that greater force than usual is required to persuade the needle to enter the pleural cavity.

Prakash and Reiman[134] compared the results of thoracentesis and needle biopsy of the pleura in a series of 414 patients with pleural effusions at the Mayo Clinic between 1973 and 1982. Pleural biopsy failed to provide adequate tissue in 55 patients (13.3%). Malignant disease was present in 281 patients (67.9%), and the diagnosis was established by cytologic study in 162 (57.6%) and by needle biopsy in 123 (43%). A positive biopsy with negative cytology was encountered in only 7.1%. Thoracotomy was necessary to confirm the diagnosis in 60.9% of the patients.

Frierson and co-workers[59] examined the DNA content of 19 mesotheliomas and pleural effusions and reported that 53% were aneuploid. However, Burmer and associates[26] investigated 46 malignant pleural mesotheliomas with flow cytometry and concluded that the tumors frequently display diploid DNA contents (65% in their study) and low proliferative rates despite their clinically aggressive behavior.

Ayres and associates[11] describe an argyrophil method for staining nucleolar organizer regions. In a study of pleural specimens, the number increased in inflammatory conditions compared with normal, and in 23 patients with mesothelioma the technique separated reactive pleural disease from mesothelioma with a high degree of confidence.

HISTOCHEMISTRY

Histochemical stains are of little value in the distinction of mesothelioma from adenocarcinoma. Positive staining for epithelial (neutral) mucosubstances in cells of a pleural tumor does not rule out the possibility of mesothelioma since a few mesothelioma cells also stain.[57] Hammar and Bolen[70] state that approximately 20% of epithelial mesotheliomas produce highly acidic mucosubstances such as hyaluronic acid, which can be identified with the alcian blue or colloidal iron stain (the staining is abolished by pretreatment with hyaluronidase). Stromal staining should be disregarded since reactive fibroblasts can produce hyaluronic acid. Sixty-five to 70% show intracytoplasmic staining for neutral or weakly acidic mucosubstance that can be identified with the periodic acid–Schiff or mucicarmine stain.[70] Kannerstein and co-workers[90] point out that the appearance of staining for mucosubstances should be taken into consideration: a diffuse coarse granularity in the cytoplasm suggests adenocarcinoma. Some glycogen can be found in as many as 50% of mesotheliomas.

The principal glycosaminoglycans in mesotheliomas are hyaluronic acid and chondroitin sulfate. Identification of hyaluronic acid within the tumor cells or documentation of its elevation in pleural fluid is of some help in diagnosis,[10, 44, 45, 137] although the level can also be raised in metastatic carcinoma. Nakano and colleagues[120] found that mesotheliomas on average contained almost eight times the amount of glycosaminoglycans in adenocarcinomas, while hyaluronic acid and chondroitin sulfate levels in the pleural fluid were, respectively, 40 to 230 times and 11 to 87

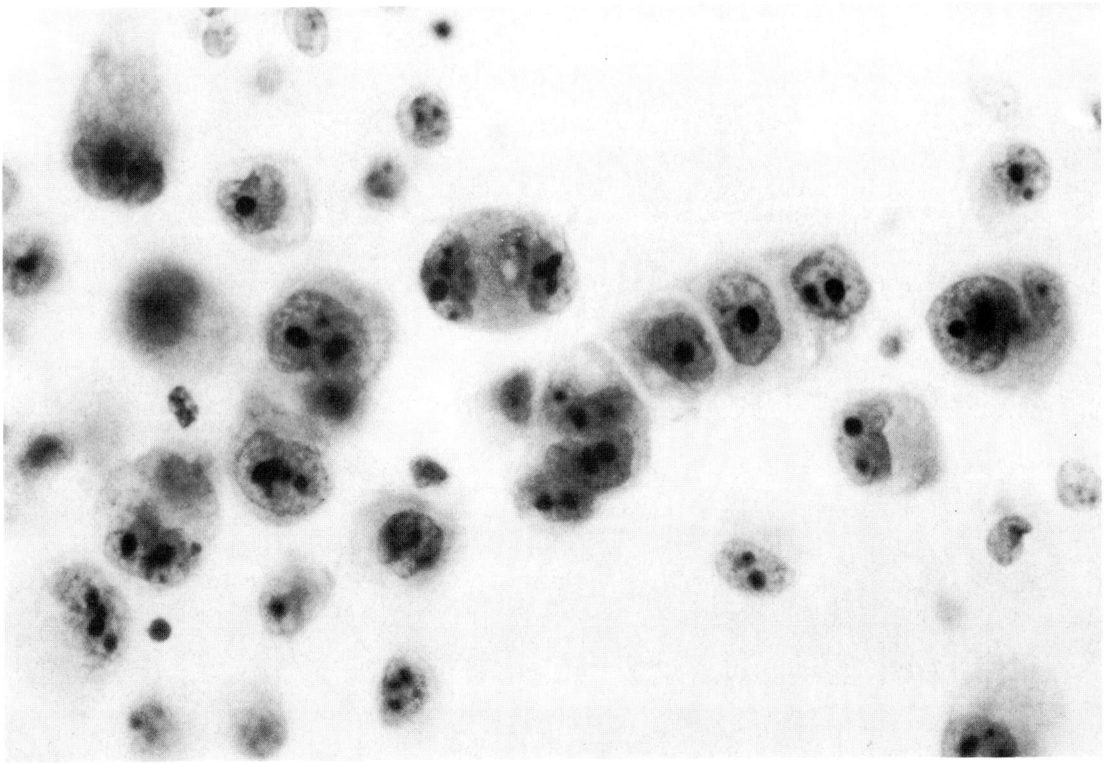

Figure 12–25. Reactive mesothelial cells in bloody chest fluid following lobectomy for squamous cell carcinoma.

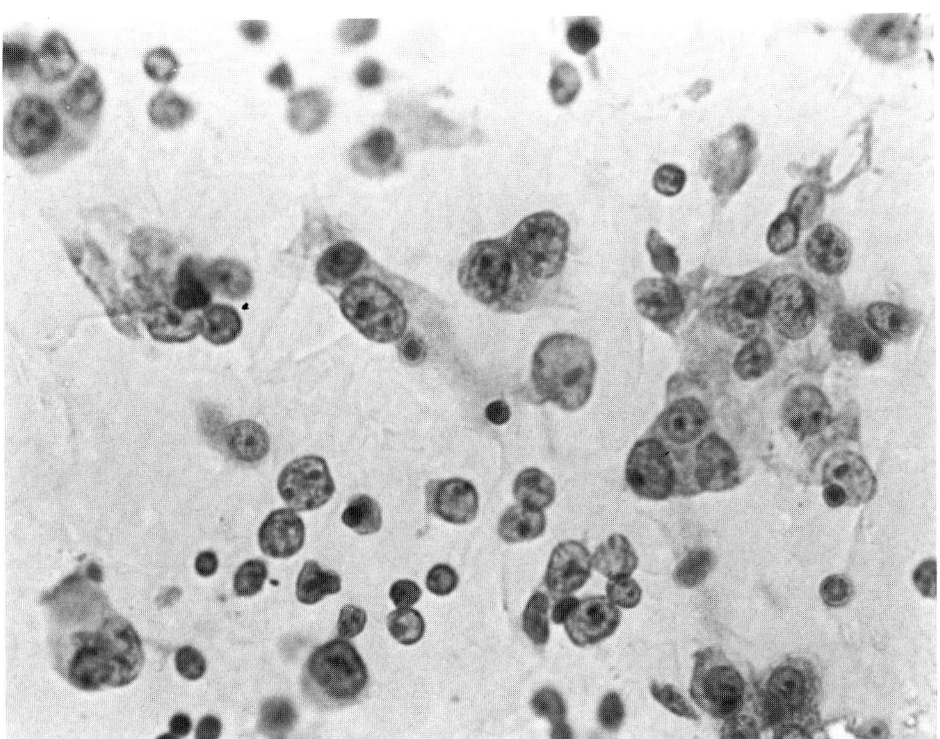

Figure 12–26. Reactive mesothelial cells forming small aggregates in chronic recurrent pleuritis, post-Ficoll treatment. There was no evidence of carcinoma in this patient.

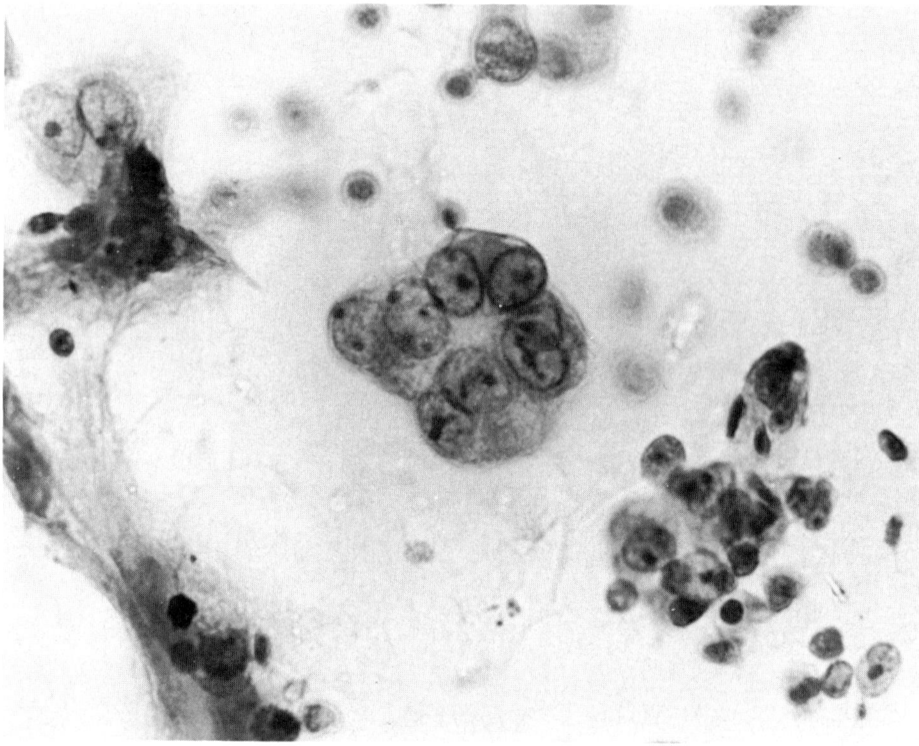

Figure 12–27. Mesothelioma. A characteristic cluster of cells in pleural fluid. Cytoplasmic swelling and some granularity can be noted. Nucleoli are visible, and subplasmalemmal vacuolation is present.

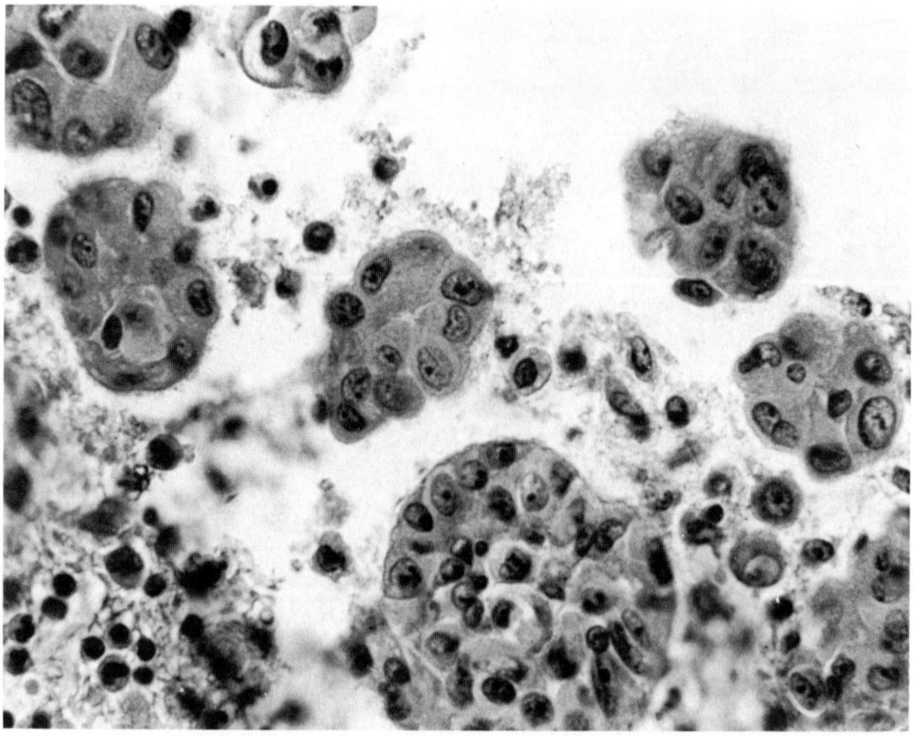

Figure 12–28. Mesothelioma. Note the large aggregates of tumor cells with no evidence of a basement membrane. There is some variation in nuclear size, but nucleoli are not conspicuous.

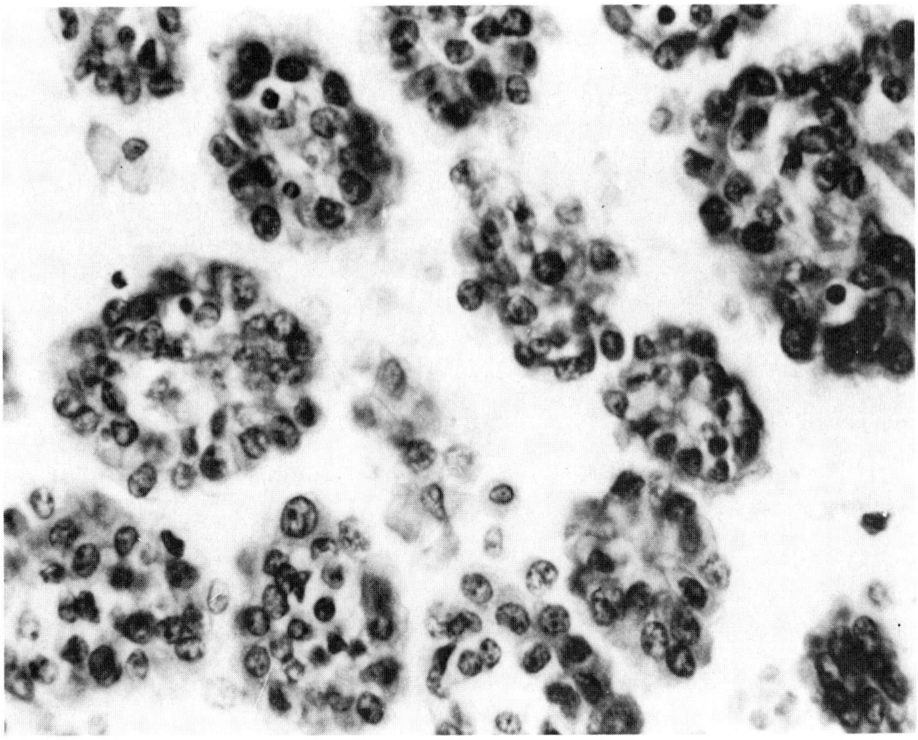

Figure 12–29. Mesothelioma. Numerous small clusters in this cytospin preparation simulate metastatic adenocarcinoma.

times higher. Kawai and co-workers[92] also found that the total quantity of glycosaminoglycans in mesotheliomas was significantly greater than in lung adenocarcinomas.

IMMUNOCYTOCHEMISTRY

Numerous studies have implied that it is possible to differentiate mesothelioma from pulmonary adenocarcinoma by the immunocytochemical identification of certain cell antigens, including cytokeratin,[17, 40, 80, 143] vimentin,[17, 35, 83, 118] carcinoembryonic antigen (CEA),[36, 106, 126, 129, 132, 166, 168] human milk fat globule–derived antigen,[13, 36, 61, 75, 110, 129, 161] TAG-72,[97, 126, 129, 156, 170] Leu-M1,[126, 129, 146, 147, 170] some specific pregnancy proteins,[62, 126, 132] surfactant apoprotein,[123] some blood-group antigens,[123, 126] secretory component (SC),[58, 96, 105, 126] and some incompletely defined or "unspecified" mesothelioma antigens.[52–54, 149, 152] Considerable controversy nevertheless persists regarding the specificity, frequency of expression, and diagnostic value of many of these markers. Discrepancies in the results obtained by different groups can be attributed to several factors, including the selection of cases (the inclusion of equivocal cases) and the type and size of the specimen on which the immunocytochemical procedures are performed. False-negative results can occur in small biopsy specimens where the marker is detectable only in focal areas. The type and source of the antibodies used in the studies, and technical factors such as type and length of fixation or the indiscriminate use of proteolytic enzymes to enhance immunostaining, can be sources of conflicting results. Differing interpretations of the immunocytochemical reactions among observers also lead to conflicting conclusions.[126]

Of all the immunocytochemical markers used to differentiate between mesothelioma and pulmonary adenocarcinoma, CEA is the most widely accepted. Wang and associates[168] were the first to indicate that mesotheliomas do not stain for CEA while adenocarcinomas do. Although this observation was confirmed in a number of studies,[21, 62, 110, 126] other investigators[13, 40, 80, 101, 143] reported positivity in 15% to 35% of the mesotheliomas examined. Since the original description of CEA by Gold and Freedman[63, 64] in 1965, it has become apparent that this molecule is heterogeneous and that its complexity relates to the tumor and tissue specificities of the antibodies that are reactive with CEA.[12, 60, 87] Using monoclonal antibodies and two-dimensional gel electrophoresis, Grunert and colleagues[67] demonstrated differences between the CEA found in bronchogenic carcinomas and that present in breast carcinomas. Similar results were obtained by Jothy and associates,[87] who were able to demonstrate a variable pattern of tissue recognition using a battery of monoclonal antibodies to CEA, indicating a heterogeneous distribution of CEA epitopes. The reported variations in CEA immunoreactivity can probably be attributed to differences in the sensitivity and specificity of the antibodies used.

Leu-M1 is another marker reported to be useful in distinguishing mesothelioma from adenocarcinoma. It is a sugar moiety, lacto-N-fucopentaose III, linked to membranes or intracellular proteins and lipids.[81] This antigen is expressed in a variety of myeloproliferative disorders, in Reed-Sternberg cells in Hodgkin's disease, and in various carcinomas.[146] In a series of 179 adenocarcinomas from various sites, Sheibani and associates[147] found reactivity for Leu-M1 in 105 (59%). In another study, the same group of investigators reported Leu-M1 positivity in 47 of 50 lung adenocarcinomas (94%) but in none of 28 mesotheliomas.[146] In our experience, however, the incidence of Leu-M1 positivity in adenocarcinomas is significantly lower than was reported in those studies. In a group of 23 lung adenocarcinomas, we found reactivity in 14 cases (60.9%) but in none of 19 epithelial mesotheliomas. The results are comparable to those of Warnock and coworkers,[170] who found reactivity for Leu-M1 in 25 of 44 adenocarcinomas (57%) and in 2 (one epithelial and one biphasic) of 33 mesotheliomas, although the reactivity in the latter tumors occurred in only 5% of the tumor cells.

Many conventional and monoclonal antibodies have been raised using as antigen the macromolecules obtained from milk fat globules, which are surrounded by a detached portion of the cell membrane and a thin rim of the subjacent cytoplasm. Most of these antibodies have shown a broad specificity, reacting with both normal lactating breast tissue and breast carcinomas, and also with a variety of nonmammary epithelial tumors, including pulmonary adenocarcinomas. It has been claimed that some of these antibodies can be used to differentiate malignant mesothelioma from pulmonary adenocarcinoma.[158] HMFG-2 monoclonal antibody (Fig. 12–30) has stimulated the most interest and the greatest controversy.

In 1985, Battifora and Kopinski[13] reported reactivity for HMFG-2 in 64 of 100 adenocarcinomas (primary and metastatic to the lung) but in none of 12 mesotheliomas. Because they also found reactivity for CEA in a similar percentage of the adenocarcinomas and in two of the mesotheliomas, they concluded that HMFG-2 was, because of its greater sensitivity and specificity, superior to CEA in the differential diagnosis. In contrast, another study published almost simultaneously by Marshall and colleagues[110] reported reactivity for HMFG-2 in all 27 pulmonary adenocarcinomas and in 12 of 16 mesotheliomas. After these conflicting results had appeared, other studies confirmed[129, 146, 161] or refuted[36, 61, 126] the value of HMFG-2 immunostaining to discriminate between malignant mesothelioma and adenocarcinoma. The reasons for the discrepancy among the reports is not clear, but it may be noted that in the early studies, both Battifora and Kopinski[13] and Marshall and colleagues[110] found membrane staining for HMFG-2 in mesotheliomas but interpreted the reaction differently. Our experience has been that while fewer mesotheliomas react for HMFG-2, this marker does not possess sufficient specificity to discriminate between lung adenocarcinoma and mesothelioma. We have obtained similar results with E29, a monoclonal antibody raised against defatted human milk that recognizes an epithelial membrane antigen (EMA) (Fig. 12–31).[39, 74] In a recent study, we were able to demonstrate immunoreactivity for this marker in 17 of 19 mesotheliomas (89.5%) and in all adenocarcinomas studied.[126]

B72.3 is a murine monoclonal antibody raised against membrane-enriched fractions of a human metastatic adenocarcinoma of breast that recognizes a high-molecular-weight tumor–associated glycoprotein identified as TAG-72.[37, 84] Immunocytochemical studies have demonstrated reactivity with B72.3 in primary adenocarcinomas of various sites including lung.[84, 85, 124, 159] In 1985, Lafebvre and co-workers[97] reported reactivity with this antibody in 17 of 20 adenocarcinomas of the lung but only focal staining in 2 of 10 mesotheliomas and indicated the potential diagnostic use of this antibody for the differentiation of these two types of tumors. Since then, similar results have been reported by others.[126, 129, 155, 170]

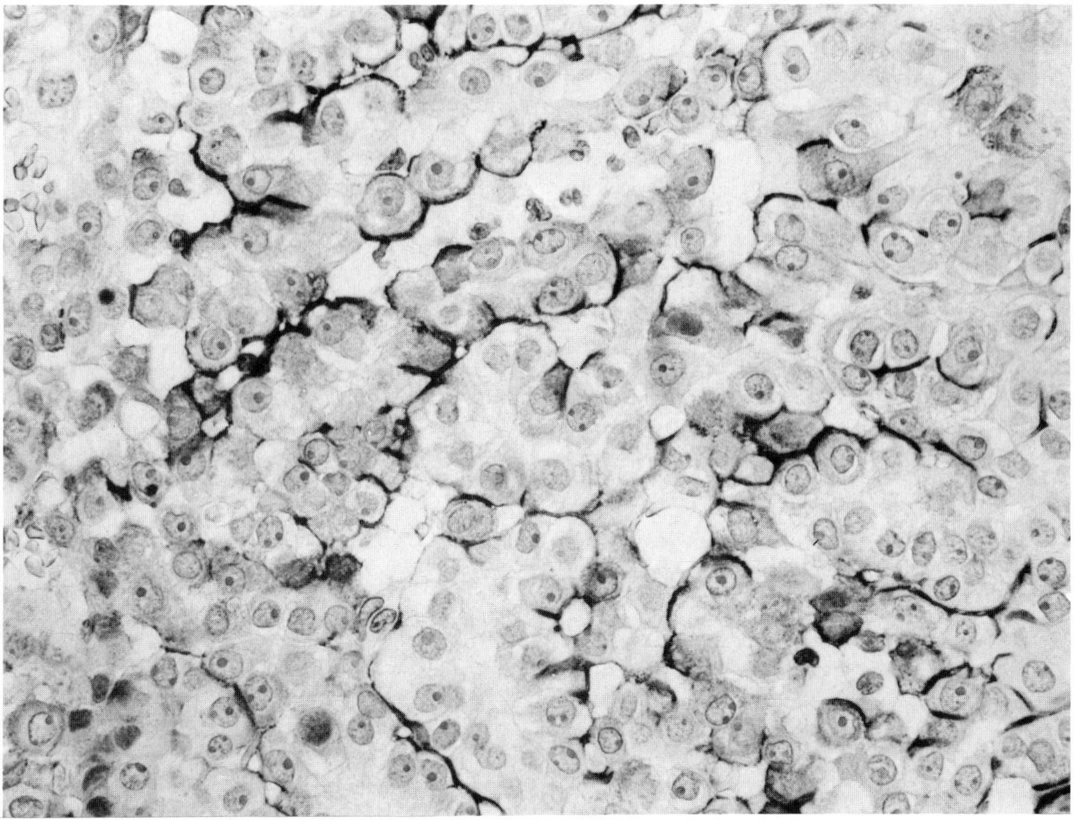

Figure 12–30. Immunoreactivity for HMFG-2 in a pleural mesothelioma.

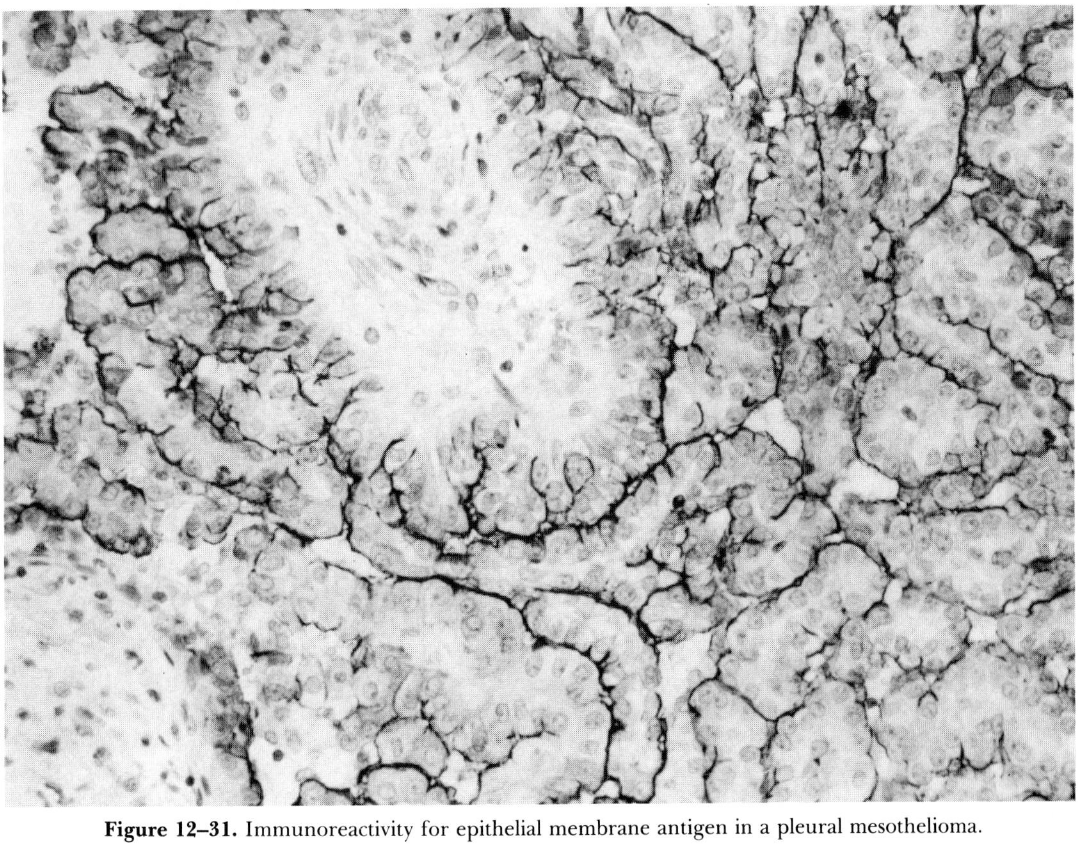

Figure 12–31. Immunoreactivity for epithelial membrane antigen in a pleural mesothelioma.

Blood-group antigens have been reported frequently in gastrointestinal and pulmonary adenocarcinomas.[65, 78, 79] The presence of A-like antigens, regardless of the patient's blood group, has also been reported. In particular, the Tn antigen, which is one of the incompatible A antigens and the precursor of the Thomsen-Friedenreich antigen, was detected in the majority (88%) of the pulmonary adenocarcinomas studied by Hirohashi and colleagues.[77] More recently, Noguchi and coworkers[123] reported reactivity for Tn antigen in 13 of 21 (62%) lung adenocarcinomas but in none of nine mesotheliomas.

The suggestion that most mesotheliomas do not express Lewis blood group antigens, particularly Le^a, received support in a study that demonstrated reactivity for Le^a in 16 of 21 (76%) non-mucin-forming peripheral adenocarcinomas but in only 1 of 11 mesotheliomas.[123]

CA19-9, a sialylated lacto-N-fucopentaose II related to the Le^a blood group,[107] is commonly expressed in ovarian,[127] pancreatic,[108, 109] and gastrointestinal carcinomas.[68, 108] We found reactivity for CA19-9 in 40% of pulmonary adenocarcinomas but in none of 19 epithelial mesotheliomas.[126] CA19-9 may therefore have limited potential for separating pulmonary adenocarcinoma from mesothelioma, but more studies would be needed for confirmation.

Since many peripheral lung adenocarcinomas are positive for surfactant apoprotein, some investigators have suggested that this cell marker can be helpful in the diagnosis of mesothelioma.[117] Noguchi and associates[123] found reactivity for surfactant apoprotein in 13 of 21 (62%) peripheral, non-mucin-producing adenocarcinomas but in none of nine mesotheliomas.

Secretory component (SC) is an antigenically distinct portion of secretory immunoglobulin A found in external secretions and in a variety of normal epithelial cells and their neoplasms.[71, 133] Several studies have shown SC in lung adenocarcinomas, but there have been conflicting accounts of its presence in mesotheliomas. In 1981, Ernst and Brooks[58] found SC in 10 of 16 mesotheliomas. Reactivity for the glycoprotein was found in both pleural and peritoneal mesotheliomas and in all histologic types, including five of nine epithelial mesotheliomas. Loosli and Hurlimann[105] reported the presence of SC in 8 of 15 mesotheliomas. This result contrasts with the observations of Kondi-Paphitis and Addis,[96] who were unable to demonstrate reactivity for SC in any of 11 mesotheliomas, including all histologic types, using an antibody different from that used in the two previous studies. On the other hand, they found reactivity in 25 (62.5%) of 40 lung adenocarcinomas. We found that 14 of 23 (60.9%) adenocarcinomas and no mesotheliomas reacted for SC.[126]

There has been much confusion regarding the expression of intermediate filaments in mesotheliomas and the value of cytokeratin immunostaining in the differentiation of mesothelial tumors from lung adenocarcinomas. According to some authors,[40, 143] strong keratin staining supports mesothelioma whereas negative or weak staining favors adenocarcinoma. Other investigators[80] have failed to confirm these observations. The reason for the conflicting results may be the use in these studies of incompletely defined antibodies against human stratum corneum cytokeratins, antibodies that are known to be of limited usefulness when applied to normal epithelia and neoplasms of internal organs.[17, 88, 153] Using immunofluorescence and two-dimensional gel electrophoresis, LaRocca and Rheinwald[98] found that mesotheliomas have the same cytokeratin polypeptide pattern (Nos. 7, 8, 18, and 19) as many adenocarcinomas, including those arising in the lung.[21] In a similar study, Blobel and co-workers[17] not only confirmed the expression of this keratin pattern in all types of mesotheliomas but also found cytokeratin No. 5 (58 kd) in all epithelial and some biphasic mesotheliomas. Cytokeratins Nos. 4, 6, 14, and 17 were also found, but they varied greatly in frequency and pattern. The authors suggested that the identification of cytokeratin polypeptide No. 5 and, to a lesser degree, Nos. 4, 6, 14, and 17 may help distinguish epithelial and biphasic mesotheliomas from fibrous mesotheliomas, as well as from pulmonary adenocarcinomas. Using immunohistochemistry with different cytokeratin antisera, Walts and co-workers[165] identified the presence of a 63-kd cytokeratin in exfoliated cells of a number of mesotheliomas but of only a few adenocarcinomas. At the present time, none of the antibodies to cytokeratin that is commercially available will differentiate between malignant mesothelioma and pulmonary adenocarcinoma. However, immunostaining for cytokeratin (Figs. 12–32 through 12–34) can serve to distinguish mesothelial cells from macrophages, and this can be useful in cytology specimens.

Although it is generally accepted that vi-

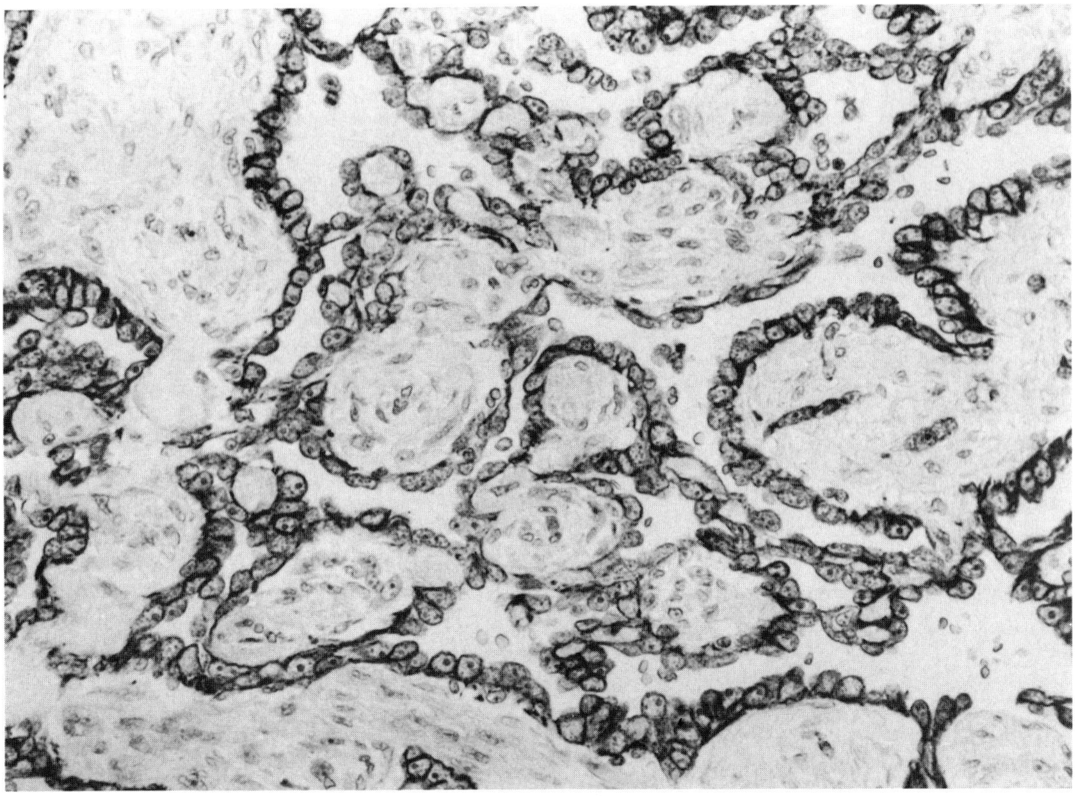

Figure 12–32. Mesothelioma cells showing strongly positive immunostaining for cytokeratin.

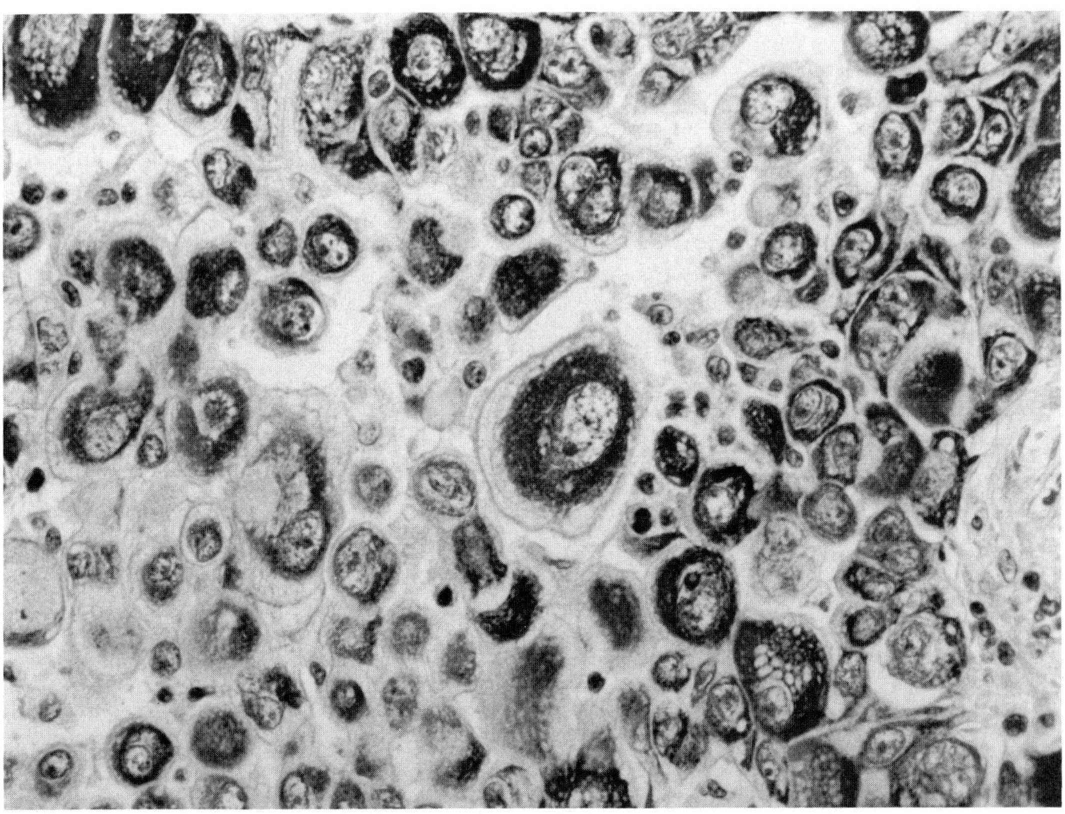

Figure 12–33. At higher magnification than in Figure 12–32, it can be seen that the cytokeratin immunostaining is predominantly perinuclear.

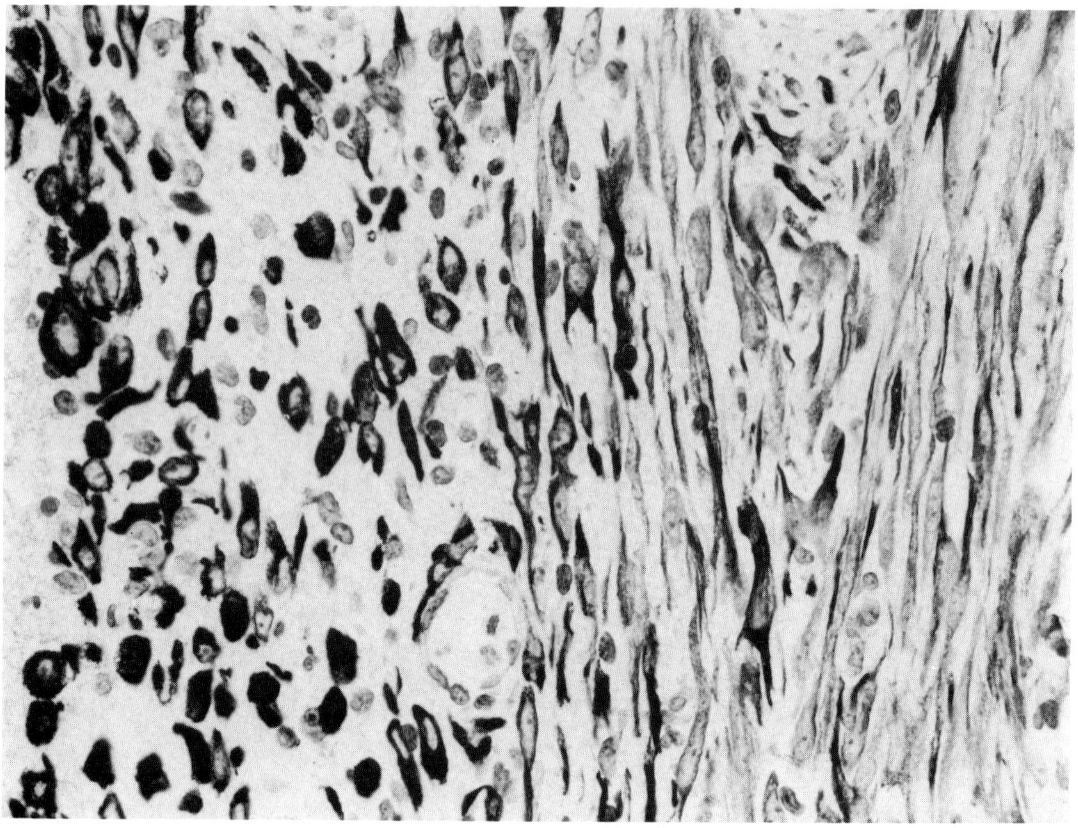

Figure 12–34. Both the epithelial and the spindle cells of this biphasic mesothelioma stain for cytokeratin.

mentin is present in mesotheliomas (Fig. 12–35), the frequency of expression of this marker, particularly in epithelial mesotheliomas, has been a source of controversy. In 1985, Churg[34] reported vimentin in epithelial cells of five of eight mesotheliomas (three epithelial and two biphasic), but in none of three adenocarcinomas. The finding was confirmed by Mullink and colleagues.[118] It might seem, therefore, that coexpression of vimentin and keratin would be helpful in distinguishing mesothelioma from carcinoma of the lung, but we have found that vimentin is expressed in both tumors.

The β_1 pregnancy-specific glycoprotein is one of the so-called specific pregnancy proteins (SPs). Gibbs and associates[62] reported positive reactivity for SP_1 in 85% of 27 adenocarcinomas of the lung but in none of 29 mesotheliomas. On the other hand, Pfaltz and co-workers[132] found reactivity in 13 (59%) of 22 lung adenocarcinomas and three (6%) of 47 mesotheliomas. We found reactivity for SP_1 in 8 of 23 adenocarcinomas (34.5%) but not in any mesotheliomas.

Some investigators have reported that placental lactogen is expressed in some pulmonary adenocarcinomas. Gibbs and associates[62] found this protein in 2 of 27 adenocarcinomas and not in any of 29 mesotheliomas. Our finding of placental lactogen in only 5 of 23 adenocarcinomas and one mesothelioma indicates that the marker has little diagnostic value.

In 1985, Ramussen and Larsen[135] reported positive staining for S-100 protein in three epithelial and two biphasic mesotheliomas, and they suggested that this marker might be useful for the diagnosis of mesothelioma. However, we found reactivity for S-100 in only a small number of lung adenocarcinomas and in none of the mesotheliomas.

None of the markers that have been discussed is specific for mesothelioma, but we believe that CEA immunoreactivity is the single most helpful marker for differentiating epithelial mesothelioma from adenocarcinoma. Other markers, especially TAG-72 (recognized by the B72.3 monoclonal antibody), Leu-M1, SC, and some blood-group antigens, such as Le^a and CA19-9, have some value but they are less sensitive than CEA.

ELECTRON MICROSCOPY

It is widely accepted that electron microscopy is useful to establish the diagnosis of the better-differentiated epithelial mesotheliomas.[18, 21, 27, 38, 47, 48, 50, 70, 169] The profusion of microvilli, often protruding from every free surface of the cells (Fig. 12–36) or filling a lumen (Fig. 12–37), is a distinctive appearance readily recognized and duplicated by few other tumors. The large number of microvilli on neoplastic mesothelial cells coupled with their size and shape is, in the proper clinical context, diagnostic of mesothelioma. The microvilli are long and slender, and they do not have an obvious core of microfilaments (Fig. 12–38). They curve and branch (Fig. 12–39) and tend to clothe many of the free surfaces of the tumor cells. In glandlike structures, the microvilli may be confined to the apical surfaces (Figs. 12–37 and 12–38). They may also line large cytoplasmic vacuoles (Fig. 12–40).

Mature desmosomes between mesothelioma cells are a common finding. Burns and co-workers[27, 28] conducted a morphometric study to compare the desmosomes of adenocarcinomas and malignant mesotheliomas and found that the mean desmosome length was not significantly different between the two tumors but that large (greater than 1 μm) desmosomes were more common in mesotheliomas. Tight junctions (Fig. 12–41) are also found between mesothelioma cells forming glandular structures and therefore they do not serve to distinguish between mesothelioma and adenocarcinoma.

This common problem in differential diagnosis is not always resolved by electron microscopy. When the microvilli are shorter and straighter than typical and present only on the surfaces of cells abutting on lumens (see Fig. 12–36), it may not be possible to exclude adenocarcinoma. Dardick and coworkers[48] appropriately observe that the presence of a few short microvilli does not rule out the diagnosis of epithelial mesothelioma and even complete absence of surface microvilli may be compatible. Clefts between the lateral cell membranes in sheets of cells

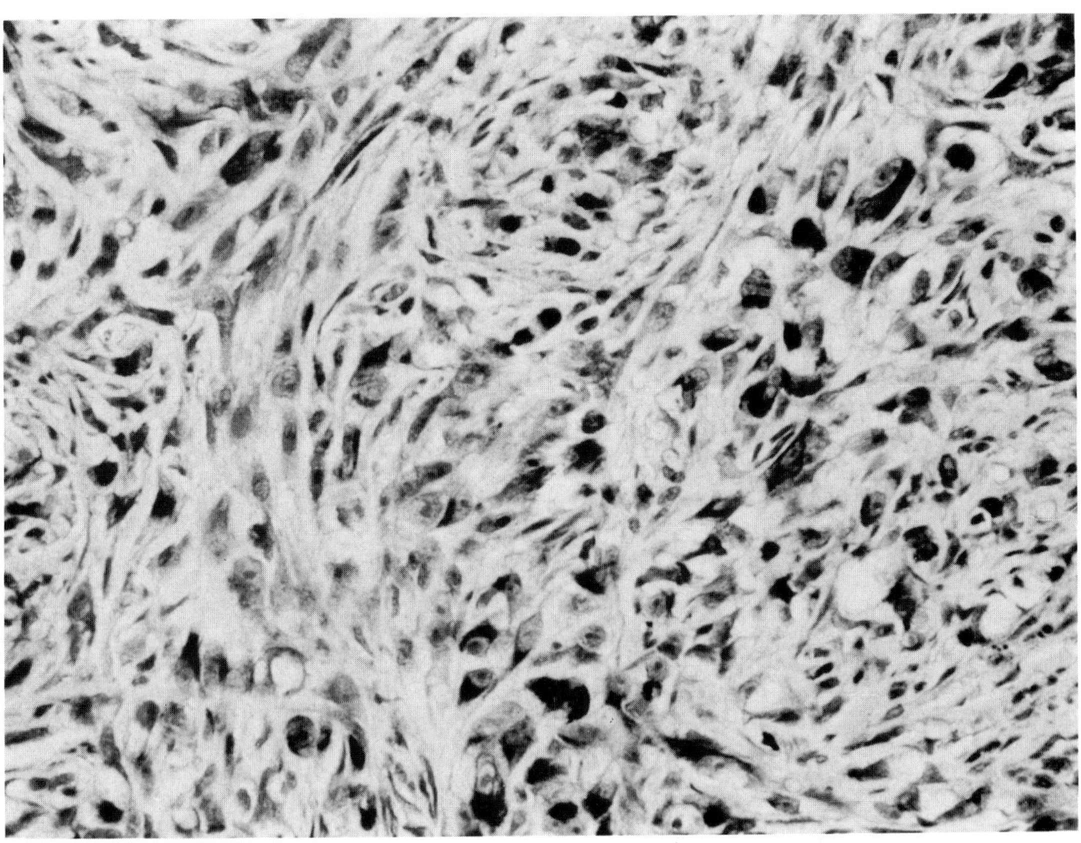

Figure 12–35. Positive immunostaining for vimentin in a pleural mesothelioma.

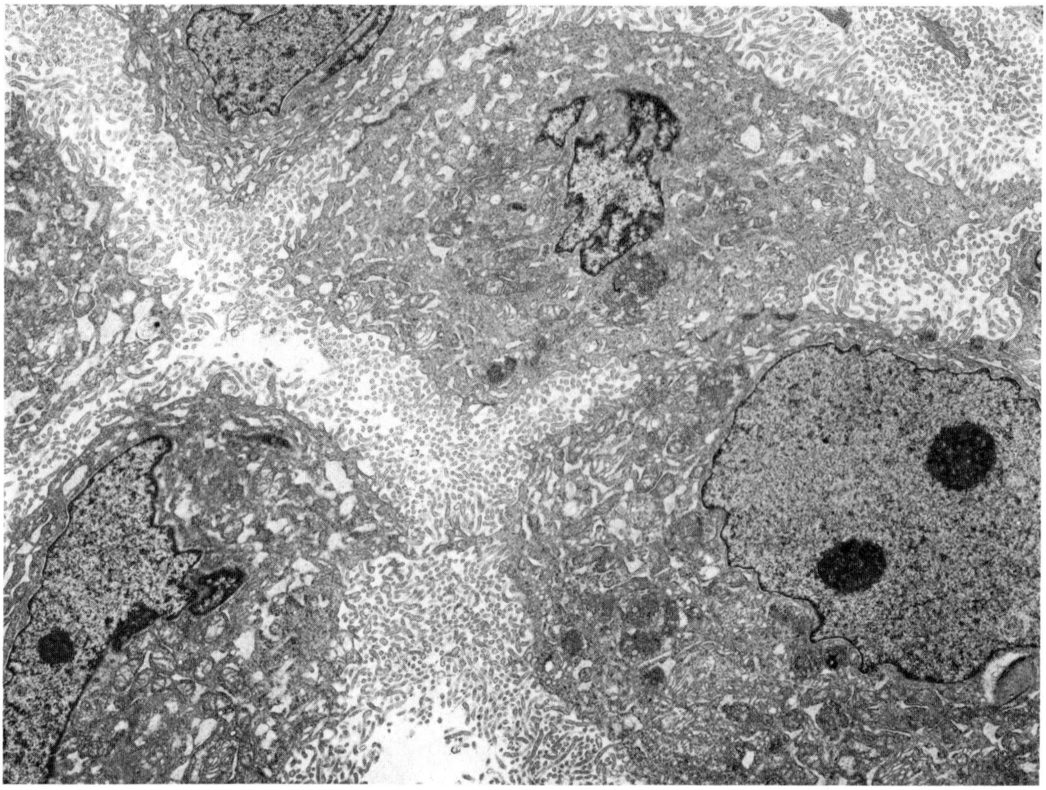

Figure 12–36. The electron micrograph demonstrates the profusion of microvilli occupying the gaps between mesothelioma cells. (×4,300)

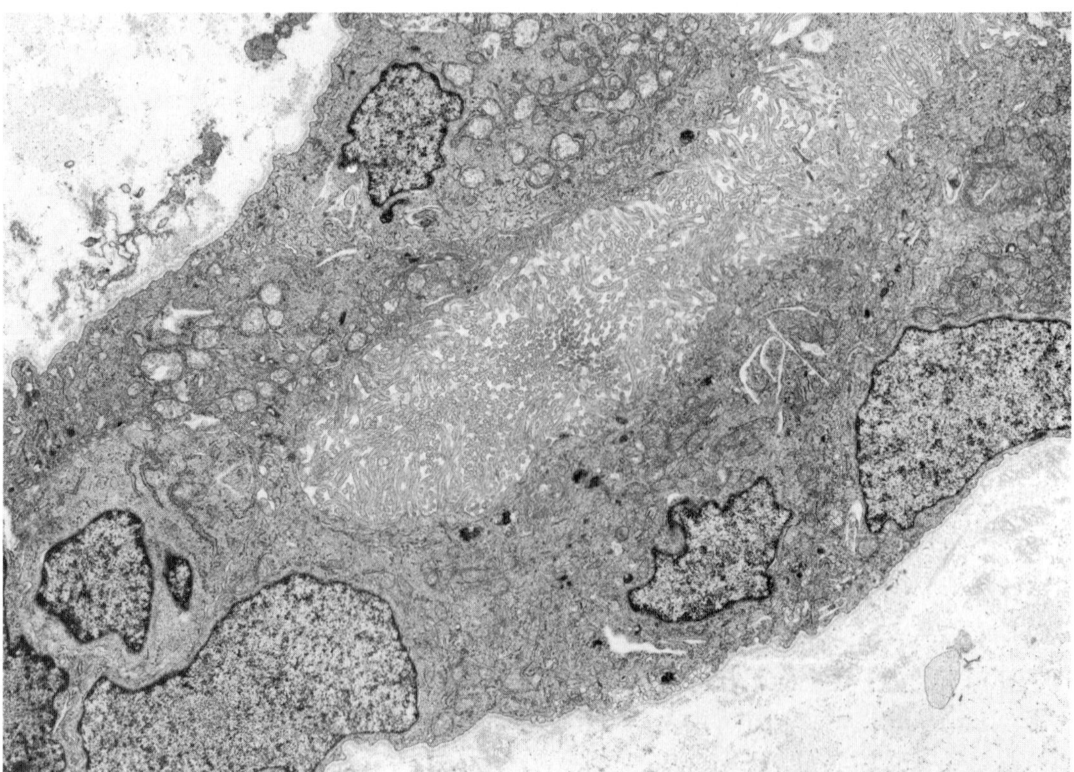

Figure 12–37. The mesothelioma cells are in a glandular configuration bordered at its periphery by a basal lamina. The lumen is filled with microvilli. (×4,100)

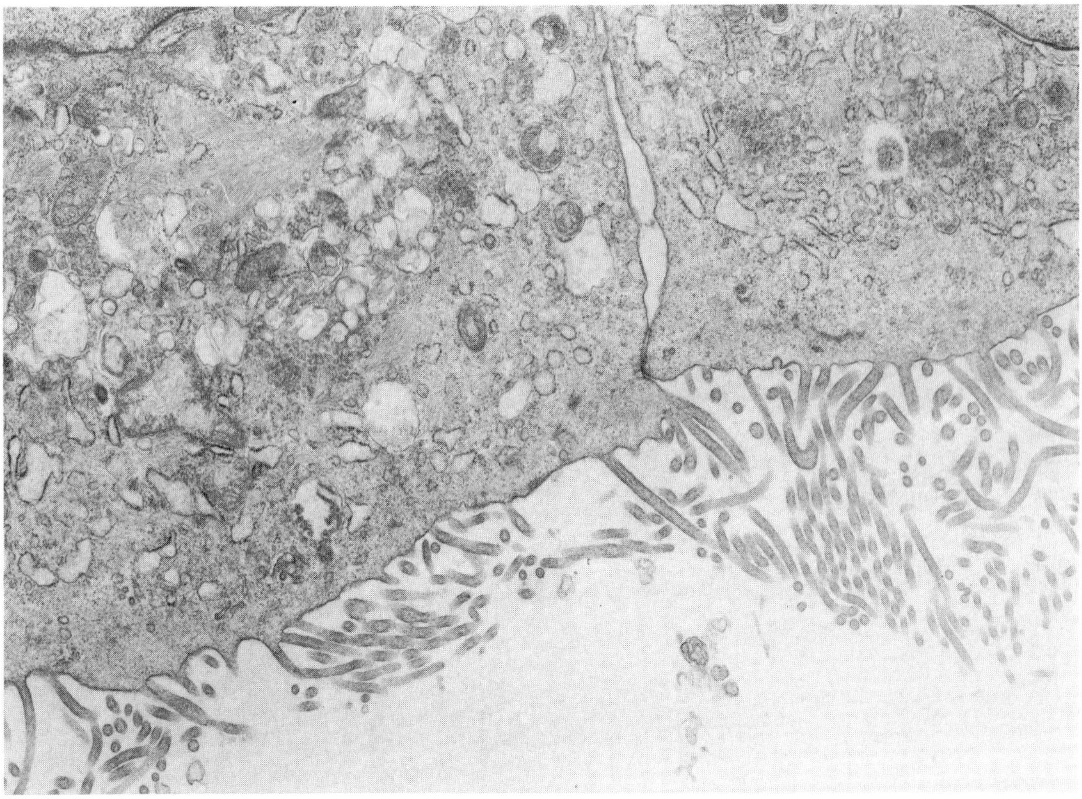

Figure 12–38. Two mesothelioma cells are connected at the luminal margin by a tight junction. (×10,500)

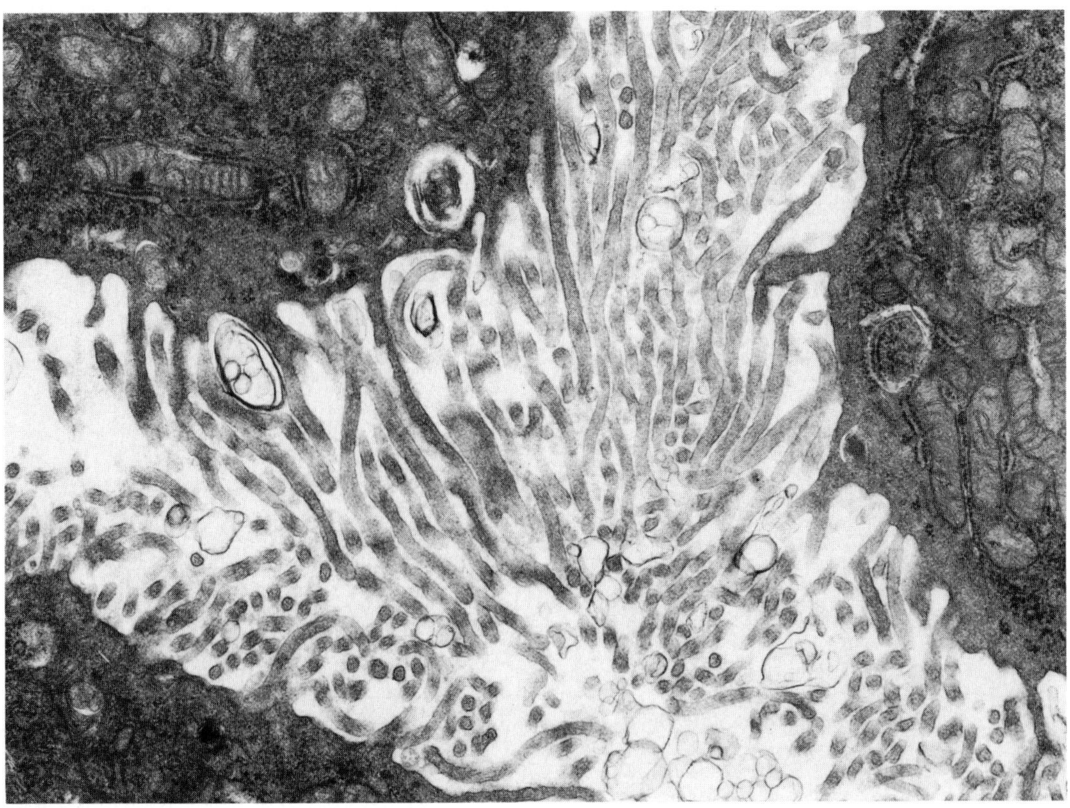

Figure 12–39. The character of the microvilli on mesothelioma cells is illustrated. They are long and slender, and some branch. (×20,000)

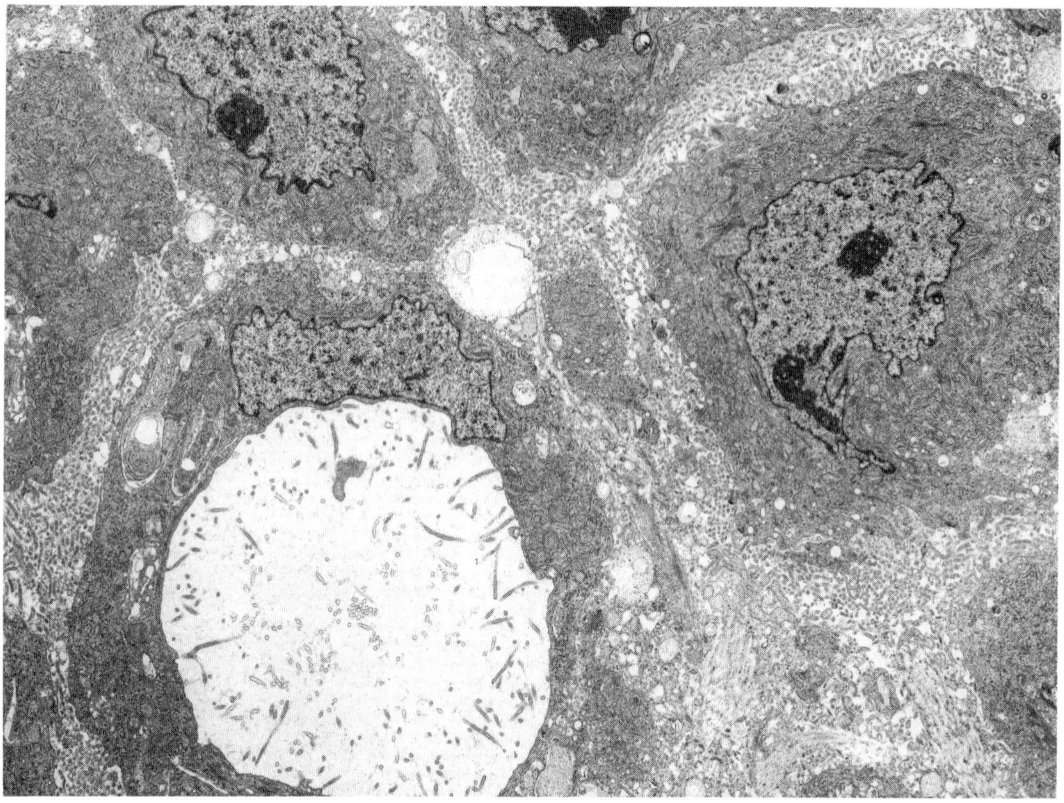

Figure 12–40. In addition to the many microvilli in spaces between the cells, one cell has a cytoplasmic vacuole lined by similar microvilli. (×4,300)

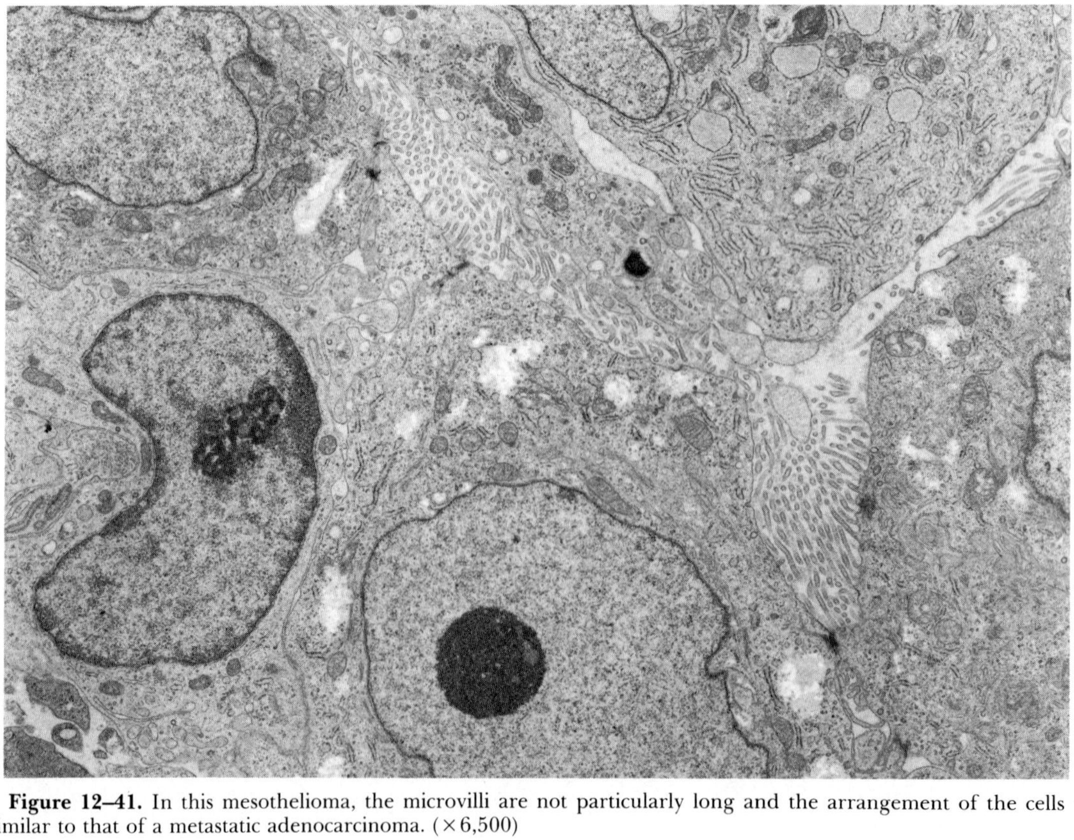

Figure 12–41. In this mesothelioma, the microvilli are not particularly long and the arrangement of the cells is similar to that of a metastatic adenocarcinoma. (×6,500)

are a mesothelial characteristic, but they are seen only in well-differentiated tumors that can be identified by routine light microscopy. Most adenocarcinoma cells contain more organelles than those of mesotheliomas (Fig. 12–42), and the intermediate filaments that are present in many mesotheliomas are in wispy bundles (Fig. 12–43) that tend to encircle the nucleus. The electron microscopic findings may consequently favor one or other diagnosis, but it is the microvilli that constitute the significant criterion: the other fine-structural features can be suggestive but they are not absolute. With loss of differentiation and the assumption of anaplastic morphology, it becomes increasingly unlikely that the diagnosis of mesothelioma will be established by electron microscopy. Dardick and coworkers[46] described five diffuse epithelial mesotheliomas in which most or all of the tumor cells were poorly differentiated with reduced prominence or absence of intermediate filaments, desmosomes, and microvilli.

Electron microscopy has contributed significantly to our understanding of the morphology of sarcomatoid mesotheliomas. Klima and Bossart[95] reported a study of 13 sarcomatous malignant mesotheliomas, including ultrastructural findings on 10 of the tumors. They found that most were composed of primitive cells but some contained foci of rudimentary epithelial differentiation. Our observations have been similar. The tumor cells possess mesenchymal characteristics to varying degrees, but scattered hints of epithelial differentiation are sometimes seen. A small space may contain a number of microvilli (Figs. 12–44 and 12–45). The cells may be intimately apposed in a manner suggestive of epithelial cells but have few or no cell junctions, and the cytoplasm can contain considerable numbers of cisternae (Fig. 12–46). Figure 12–47 shows similar cells, some of them elongated, haphazardly distributed in a collagenous stroma.

At the ultrastructural level, in malignant pleural tumors composed largely or entirely of spindle cells, the cells may appear fibro-

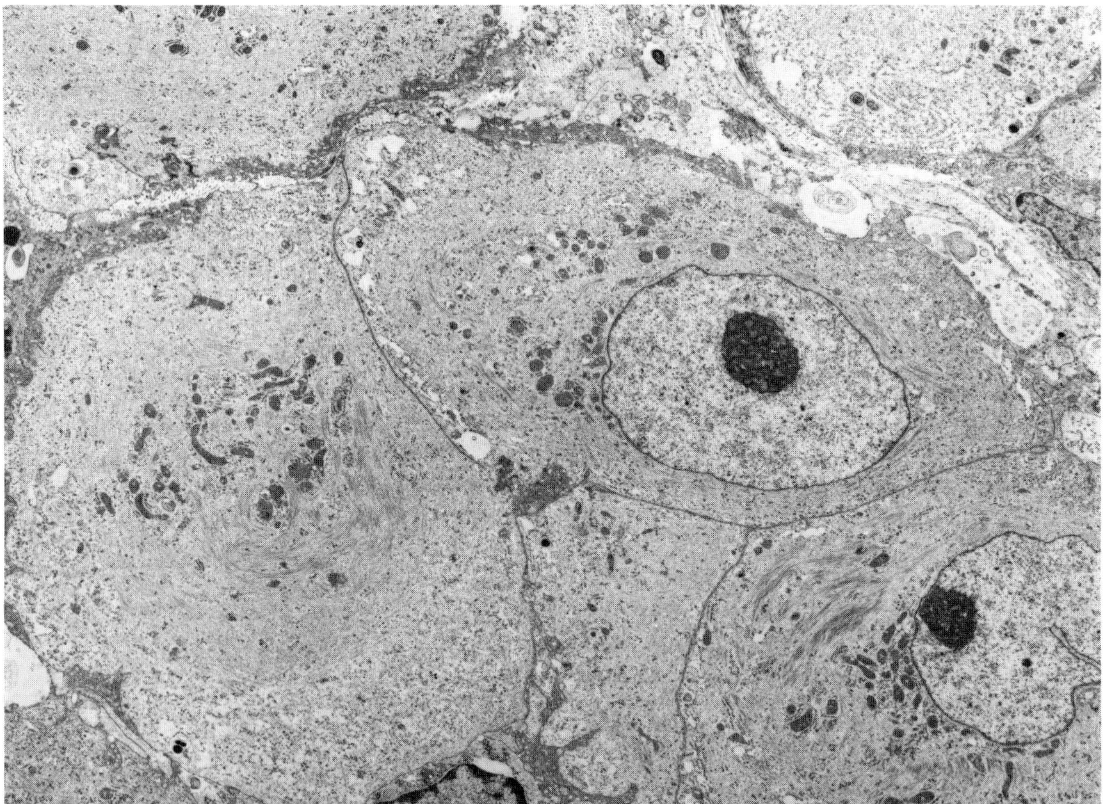

Figure 12–42. The mesothelioma cells do not contain many organelles, but wispy bundles of filaments are visible. (×5,200)

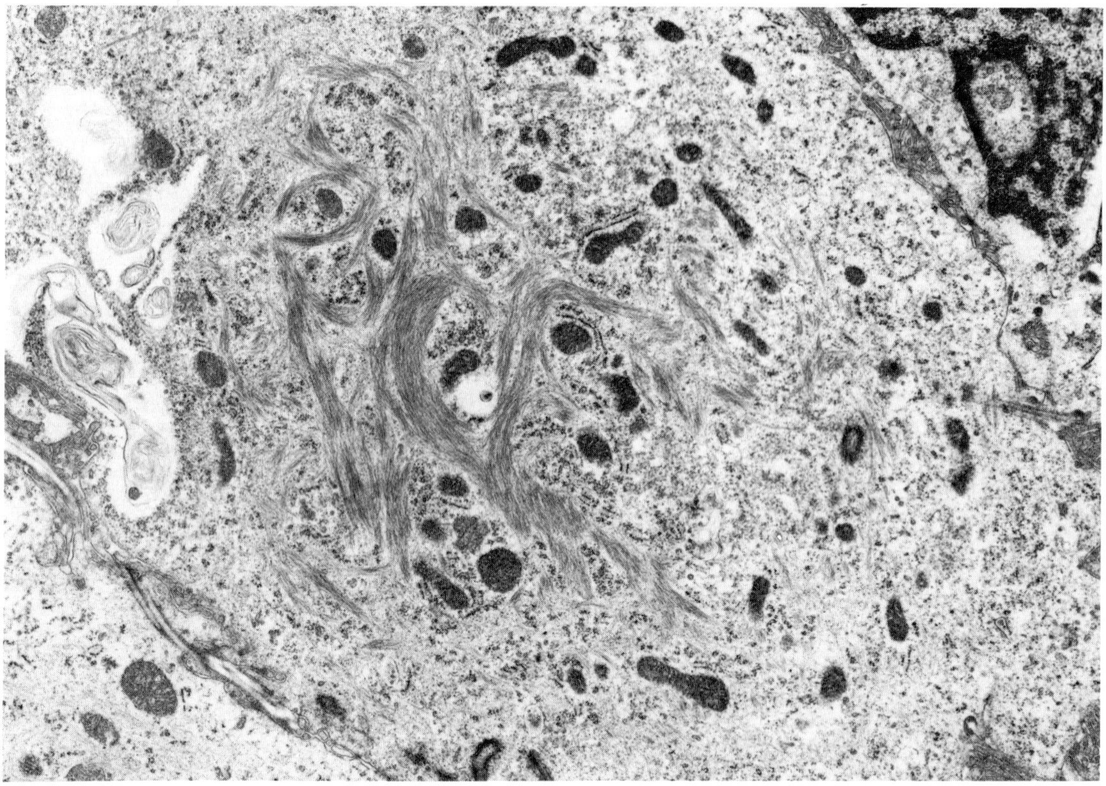

Figure 12–43. Same tumor as in Figure 12–42. The bundles of filaments are shown in more detail. (×7,400)

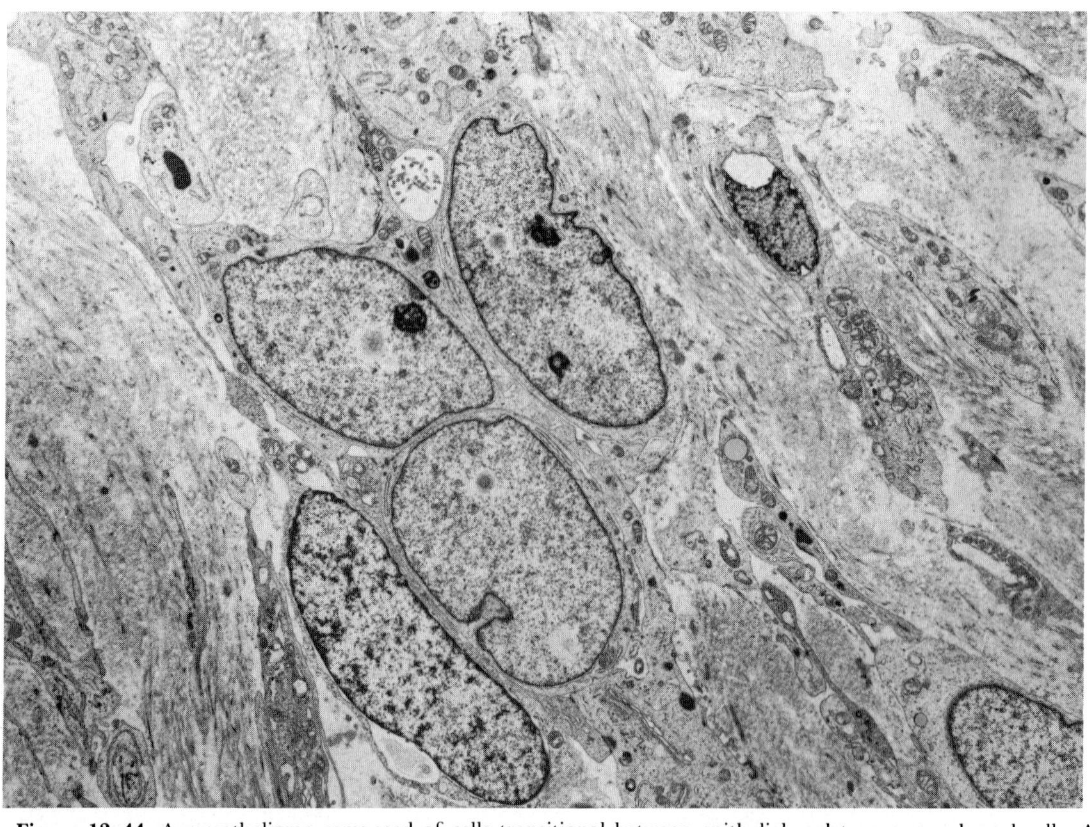

Figure 12–44. A mesothelioma composed of cells transitional between epithelial and true mesenchymal cells. A small space containing microvilli is present. (×3,900)

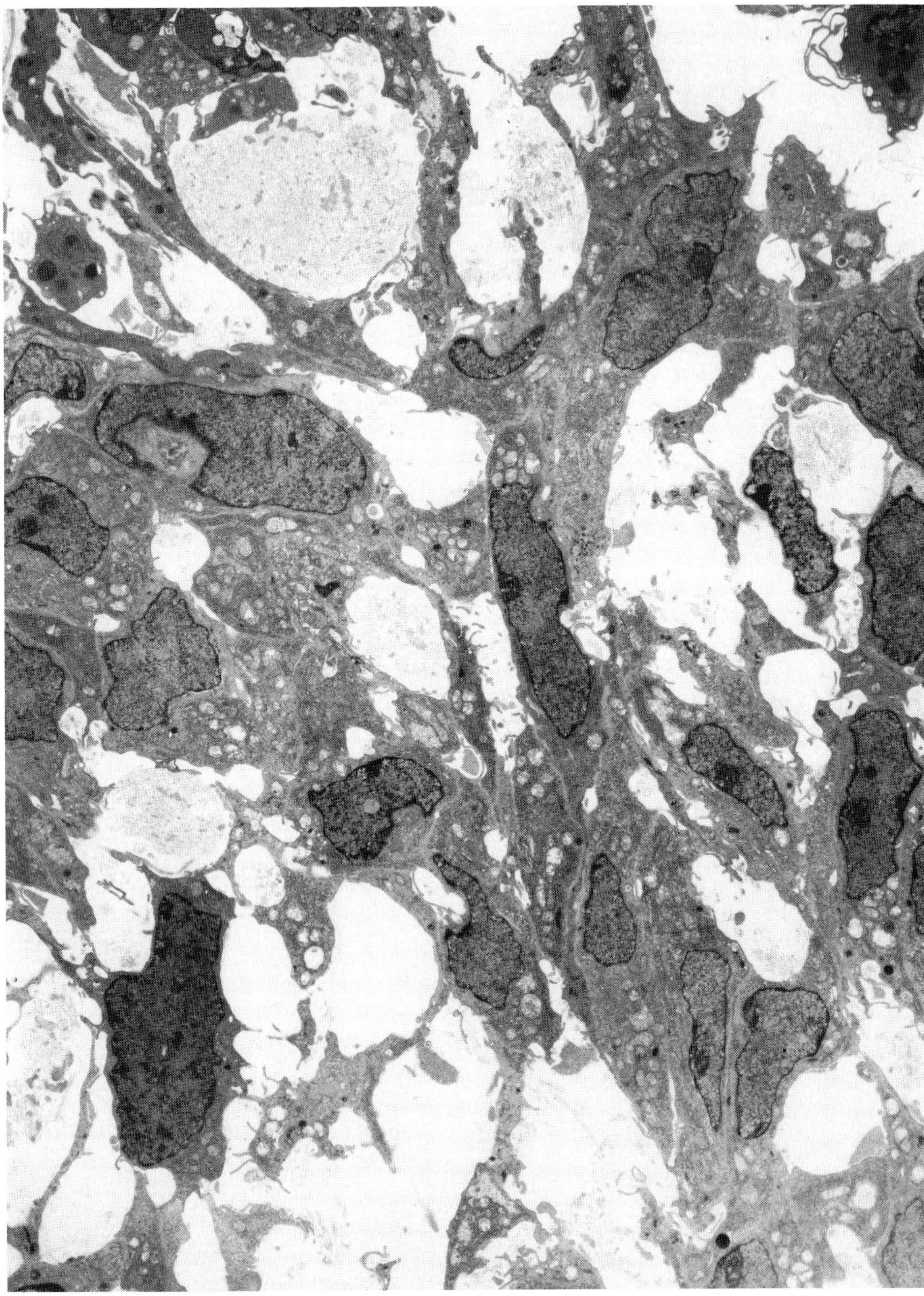

Figure 12–45. Slight epithelial differentiation in a predominantly sarcomatous mesothelioma is shown by the small spaces containing sparse microvilli. (×8,500)

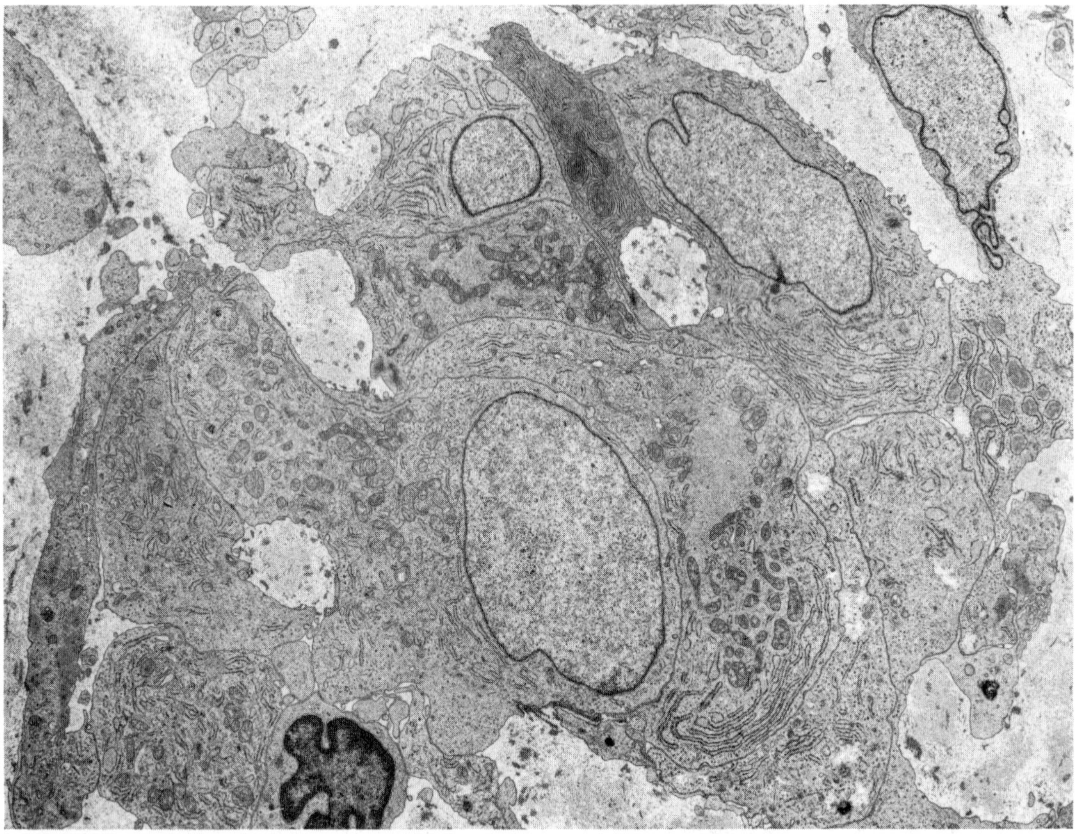

Figure 12–46. Sarcomatous mesothelioma. The cells contain many cisternae. This appearance is indistinguishable from a malignant fibrous histiocytoma. (×4,300)

blastic (Fig. 12–48) or even be myofibroblasts[43] (Fig. 12–49). It can be difficult in these preparations to distinguish between the neoplastic cells and reactive stromal mesenchymal cells, and the importance of identifying entrapped epithelial cells from mesothelium or lung has been stressed. The spindle cells of an authentic mixed mesothelioma may appear primitive or vaguely resemble fibroblasts (Figs. 12–50 and 12–51). The epithelial cells of this tumor were typical, and Burrig[29] reports a localized benign biphasic mesothelioma in which electron microscopy showed true mesothelial differentiation.

TUMORS OF THE CHEST WALL

Primary tumors arising in the chest wall[136, 140] are not common, and in adults most are sarcomas. Tumors of the underlying lung may extend into the soft tissues and bones of the thoracic wall, and it is a relatively frequent location for metastases, so these tumors enter into the differential diagnosis of a mesothelioma.

Two reports from the Mayo Clinic give some indication of the relative frequencies of primary and metastatic tumors in the chest wall. Pairolero and Arnold[130] evaluated 100 consecutive patients accessioned over an 8-year period. There were 55 female and 45 male patients whose ages spanned 12 to 84 years, with a median of 54.5. Fifty patients had primary malignant neoplasms, 32 had metastases, and 18 had benign tumors. King and co-workers[94] studied a series of 90 patients with primary chest wall tumors who underwent surgical resection. The tumor was malignant in 71 (78.9%) and benign in 19. Sarcomas were the most common malignant tumors: 62% of the 90 cases were malignant fibrous histiocytomas, chondrosarcomas, or rhabdomyosarcomas.

A sarcoma may arise in an irradiated chest wall. Souba and associates[150] reported 16 patients who developed sarcomas of the chest wall at a site where a previous malignant neoplasm had been irradiated (ten breast

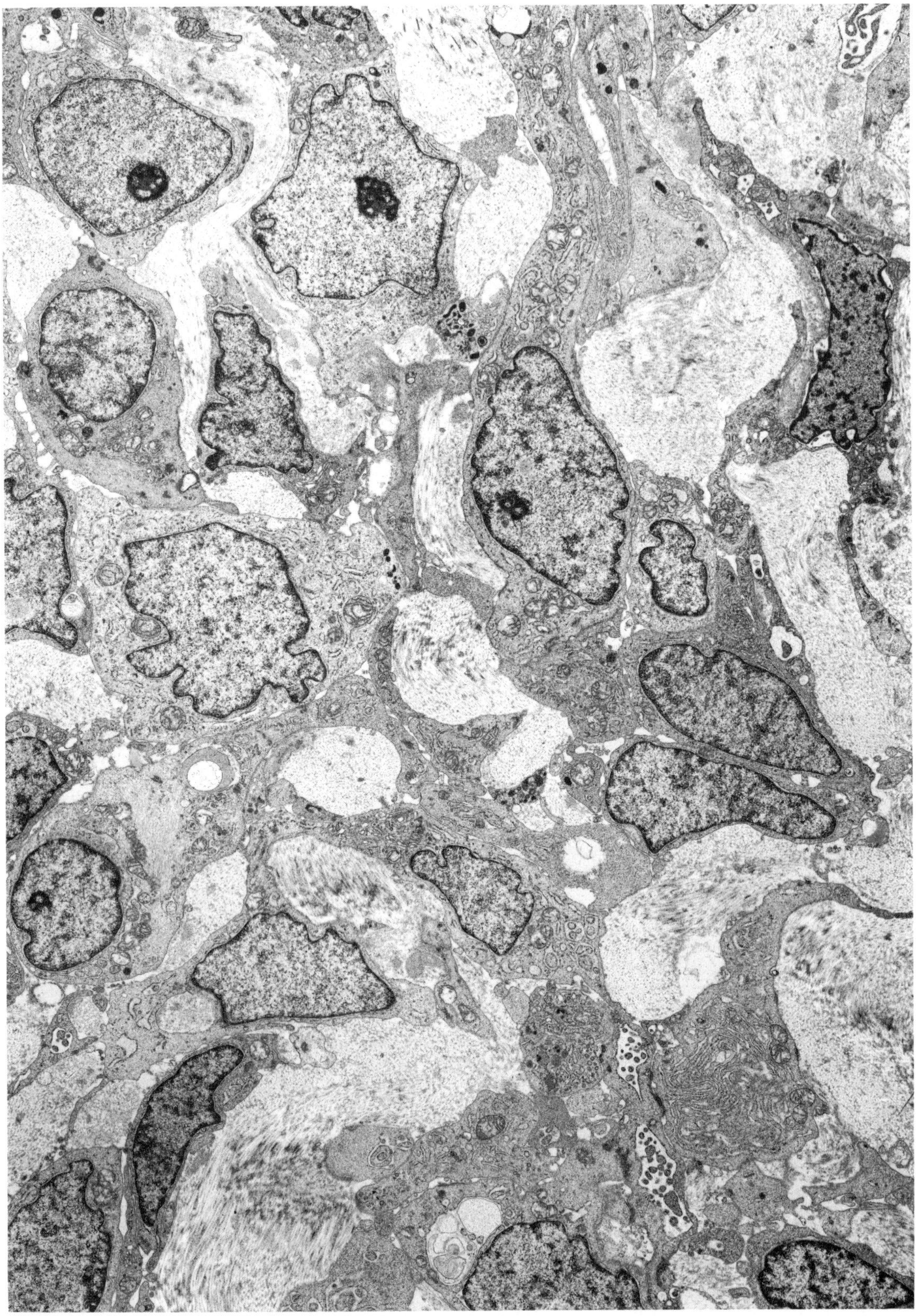

Figure 12–47. Sarcomatous mesothelioma. Some of the cells resemble fibroblasts. (×6,400)

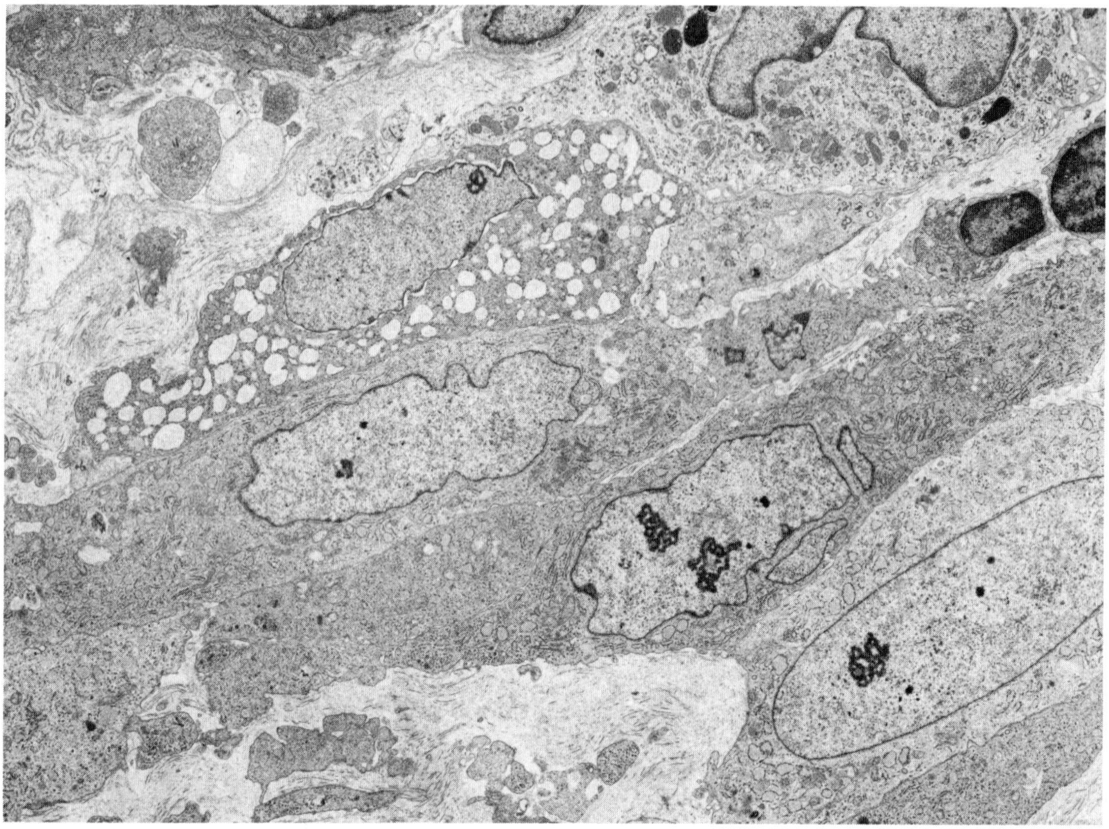

Figure 12–48. A predominantly fibroblastic appearance in a sarcomatous mesothelioma. (×4,000)

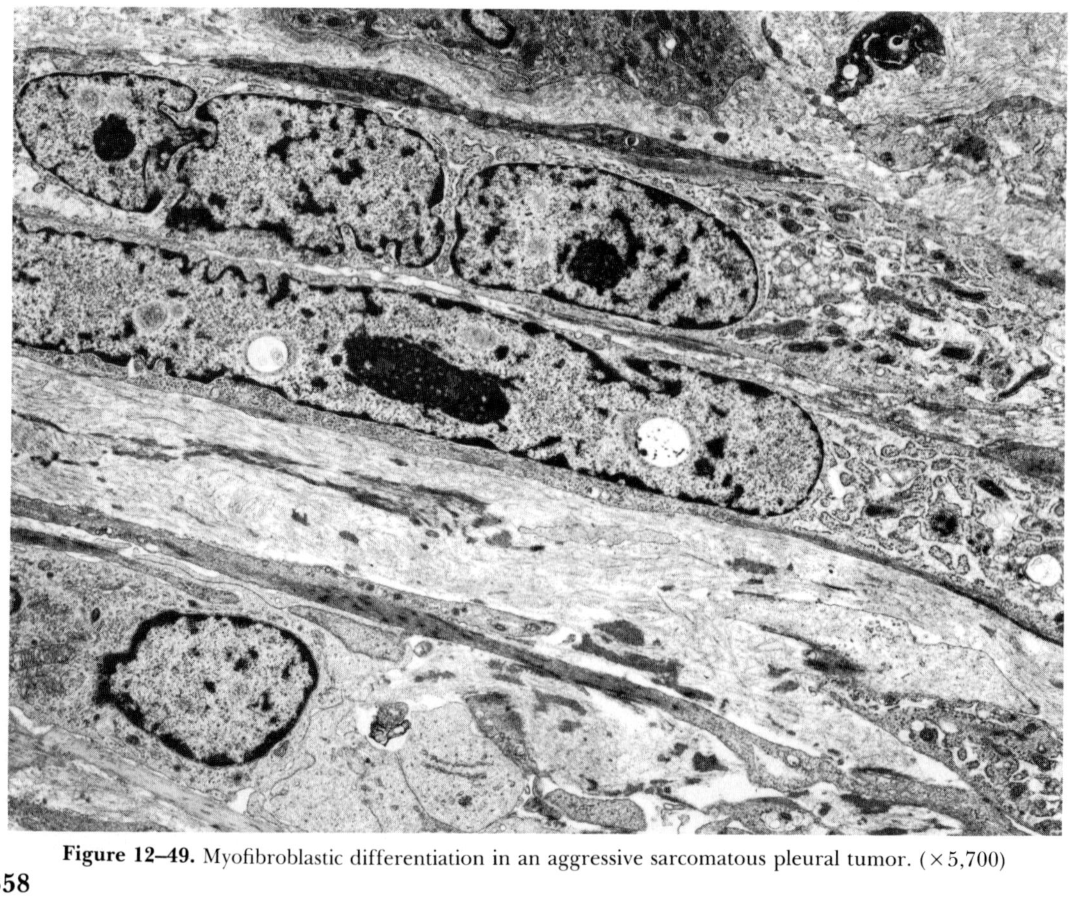

Figure 12–49. Myofibroblastic differentiation in an aggressive sarcomatous pleural tumor. (×5,700)

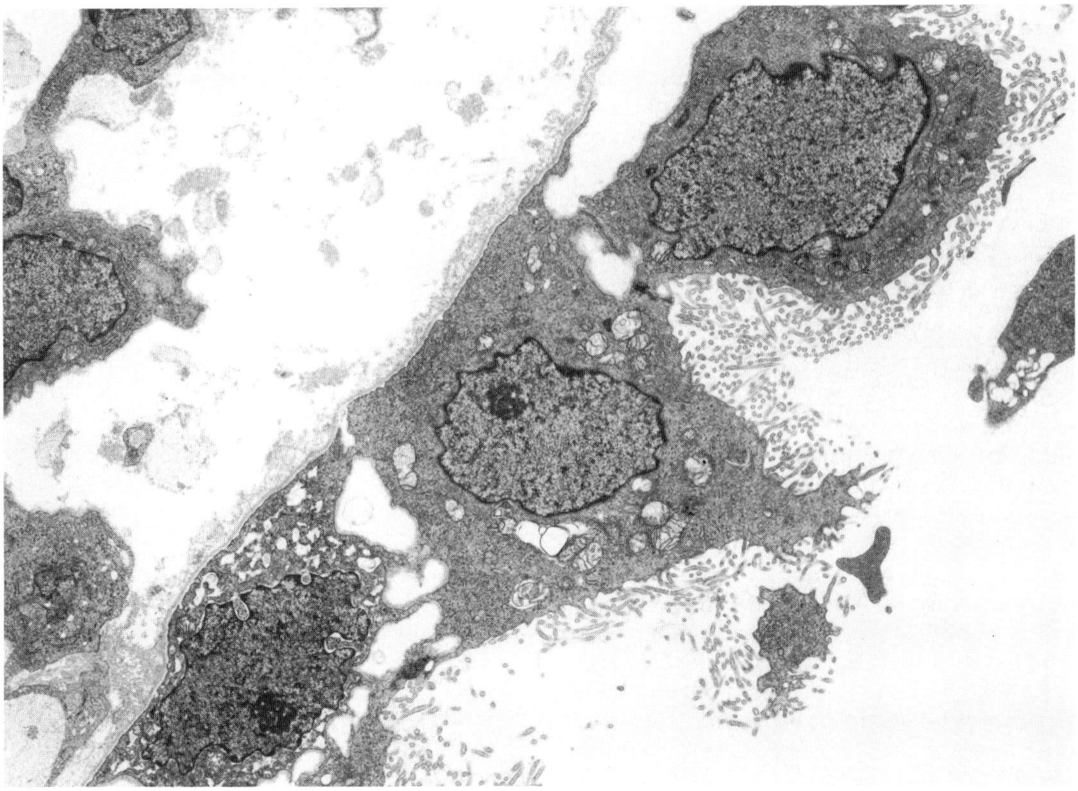

Figure 12–50. Cells of the epithelial component of a biphasic mesothelioma (shown in Figure 12–23) have characteristic microvilli, and clefts between the lateral cell membranes are visible. (×5,100)

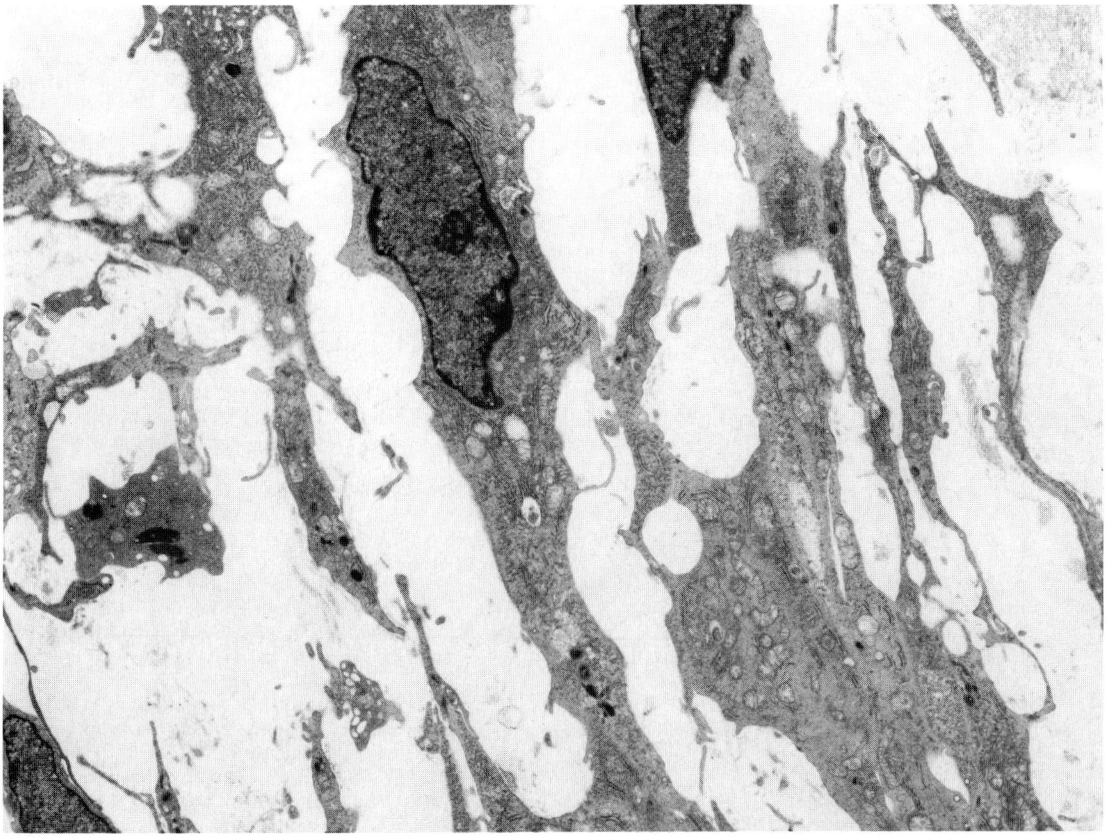

Figure 12–51. Spindle cells in the stroma of the biphasic tumor shown in Figures 12–23 and 12–50 resemble fibroblasts. (×5,700)

carcinomas, four cases of Hodgkin's disease, one primary pulmonary chondrosarcoma, one posterior mediastinal neuroblastoma). The histologic types of the sarcomas were nine malignant fibrous histiocytomas, six osteosarcomas, and a malignant mesenchymoma. Davies and co-workers[49] reported an angiosarcoma arising in irradiated chest wall after mastectomy. The sixth reported liposarcoma of the chest wall, a 3200-g tumor, recurred with features of malignant fibrous histiocytoma.[113] Chondrosarcoma arising in the chest wall has been discussed by McAfee and co-workers.[111] Small cell tumors of the chest wall occur in childhood[66, 145] but are rare after adolescence.

It can be seen that the problem in differential diagnosis between a mesothelioma and primary tumor of the chest wall is likely to involve separation of a pleomorphic mesothelioma from a true sarcoma. Since some mesotheliomas are sarcomatoid and some sarcomas are keratin positive, the distinction is not always possible. Immunocytochemistry and electron microscopy should be attempted, but correlation of the radiologic findings with light microscopy may lead to the correct diagnosis.

REFERENCES

1. Abratt RP, Willcox PA, Casserley RD et al: Mesothelioma—short latent period after industrial asbestos exposure and prolonged survivial. Eur J Surg Oncol 11: 279, 1985.
2. Adams VI, Unni KK: Diffuse malignant mesothelioma of pleura: Diagnostic criteria based on an autopsy study. Am J Clin Pathol 82:15, 1984.
3. Adams VI, Unni KK, Muhm JR et al: Diffuse malignant mesothelioma of pleura. Diagnosis and survival in 92 cases. Cancer 58:1540, 1986.
4. Adamson IYR, Bowden DH: Response of mouse lung to crocidolite asbestos: I. Minimal fibrotic reaction to short fibres. J Pathol 152:99, 1987.
5. Adamson IYR, Bowden DH: Response of mouse lung to crocidolite asbestos: II. pulmonary fibrosis after long fibres. J Pathol 152:109, 1987.
6. Andrews PM, Porter KR: The ultrastructural morphology and possible functional significance of mesothelial microvilli. Anat Rec 177:409, 1973.
7. Antman KH: Current concepts: Malignant mesothelioma. N Engl J Med 303:200, 1980.
8. Antman KH: Clinical presentation and natural history of benign and malignant mesothelioma. Semin Oncol 8:313, 1981.
9. Antman KH, Corson JM: Benign and malignant pleural mesotheliomas. Clin Chest Med 6:127, 1985.
10. Arai H, Kang KY, Sato H et al: Significance of the quantification and demonstration of hyaluronic acid in tissue specimens for the diagnosis of pleural mesothelioma. Am Rev Respir Dis 120:529, 1979.
11. Ayres JG, Crocker JG, Skilbeck NQ: Differentiation of malignant from normal and reactive mesothelial cells by the argyrophil technique for nucleolar organizer region associated proteins. Thorax 43:366, 1988.
12. Banjo C, Shuster J, Gold P: Intermolecular heterogeneity of the carcinoembryonic antigen. Cancer Res 34:2114, 1974.
13. Battifora H, Kopinski MI: Distinction of mesothelioma from adenocarcinoma: An immunohistochemical approach. Cancer 55:1679, 1985.
14. Bernaudin JF, Fleury J: Anatomy of the blood and lymphatic circulation of the pleural serosa. In Chretien J, Bignon J, Hirsch A (eds): The Pleura in Health and Disease, p 101. New York, Marcel Dekker, 1985.
15. Berry PJ, Favara BE, Odom LF: Malignant peritoneal mesothelioma in a child. Pediatr Pathol 5 397 1986.
16. Bilbey JH, Muller NL, Miller RR et al: Localized fibrous mesothelioma of pleura following external ionizing radiation therapy. Chest 94:1291, 1988.
17. Blobel GA, Moll R, Franke WW et al: The intermediate filament cytoskeleton of malignant mesotheliomas and its diagnostic significance. Am J Pathol 121:235, 1985.
18. Bolen JW: Tumors of serosal tissue origin. Clin Lab Med 7:31, 1987.
19. Bolen JW, Hammar SP, McNutt MA: Reactive and neoplastic serosal tissue: A light microscopic, ultrastructural and immunocytochemical study. Am J Surg Pathol 10:34, 1986.
20. Bolen JW, Hammar SP, McNutt MA: Serosal tissue: Reactive tissue as a model for understanding mesotheliomas. Ultrastruct Pathol 11:251, 1987.
21. Bolen JW, Thorning D: Mesotheliomas: A light- and electron-microscopical study concerning histogenetic relationships between the epithelial and the mesenchymal variants. Am J Surg Pathol 4:451, 1980.
22. Boutin C: Thoracoscopy in the early diagnosis of malignant pleural effusions. Endoscopy 12:155, 1980.
23. Brenner J et al: Malignant mesothelioma in children: Report of seven cases and review of the literature. Med Pediatr Oncol 9:367, 1981.
24. Briselli M, Mark EJ, Dickersin GR: Solitary fibrous tumors of the pleura: Eight new cases and review of 360 cases in the literature. Cancer 47:2678, 1981.
25. Bunton RW et al: Pleural fibromas: A clinical review and report of six patients. Ann Thorac Surg 33:609, 1982.
26. Burmer GC, Rabinovitch PS, Kulander BG et al: Flow cytometric analysis of malignant pleural mesotheliomas. Hum Pathol 20:777, 1989.
27. Burns TR, Greenberg SD, Mace M: Ultrastructural diagnosis of epithelial malignant mesotheliomas. Lab Invest 50:5A, 1984.
28. Burns TR, Johnson EH, Cartwright J Jr et al: Desmosomes of epithelial malignant mesothelioma. Ultrastruct Pathol 12:385, 1988.
29. Burrig KF: Localized benign biphasic mesothelioma of the pleura. Histopathology 11:983, 1987.
30. Burrig KF, Kastendieck H: Ultrastructural observations on the histogenesis of localized fibrous

tumours of the pleura (benign mesothelioma). Virchows Arch [A] 403:413, 1984.

31. Butchart EG, Ashcroft T, Barnsley WC et al: Pleuropneumonectomy in the management of diffuse malignant mesothelioma of the pleura: Experience with 29 patients. Thorax 31:15, 1976.
32. Carter D, Otis CN: Three types of spindle cell tumors of the pleura. Fibroma, sarcoma and sarcomatoid meosthelioma. Am J Surg Pathol 12:747, 1988.
33. Chen W-J, Mottet NK: Malignant mesothelioma with minimal asbestos exposure. Hum Pathol 9:253, 1978.
34. Churg A: Immunohistochemical staining for vimentin and keratin in malignant mesothelioma. Am J Surg Pathol 9:360, 1985.
35. Churg A: Malignant mesothelioma in British Columbia in 1982. Cancer 55:672, 1985.
36. Cibas ES, Corson JM, Pinkus GS: The distinction of adenocarcinoma from malignant mesothelioma in cell blocks of effusions: The role of routine mucin histochemistry and immunohistochemical assessment of carcinoembryonic antigen, keratin proteins, epithelial membrane antigen, and milk fat globule-derived antigen. Hum Pathol 18:67, 1987.
37. Colcher D, Hand PH, Nuti M et al: A spectrum of monoclonal antibodies reactive with mammary tumor cells. Proc Natl Acad Sci USA 78:3199, 1981.
38. Coleman M, Henderson DW, Mukherjee TM: The ultrastructural pathology of malignant pleural mesothelioma. Pathol Annu 24(part 1):303, 1989.
39. Cordell J, Richardson TC, Pulford KAF et al: Production of monoclonal antibodies against human epithelial antigen for use in diagnostic immunocytochemistry. Br J Cancer 52:347, 1985.
40. Corson JM, Pinkus GS: Mesothelioma: Profile of keratin proteins and carcinoembryonic antigen: An immunoperoxidase study of 20 cases and comparison with pulmonary adenocarcinomas. Am J Pathol 108:80, 1982.
41. Cotran RS, Karnovsky MJ: Ultrastructural studies on the permeability of the mesothelium to horseradish peroxidase. J Cell Biol 37:123, 1968.
42. Craighead JE: Current pathogenetic concepts of diffuse malignant mesothelioma. Hum Pathol 18:544, 1987.
43. D'Andiran G, Gabbiani G: A metastasizing sarcoma of the pleura composed of myofibroblasts. In Fenoglio CM, Wolff M (eds): Progress in Surgical Pathology, vol 2, p 31. New York, Masson, 1980.
44. Dahl IMS, Laurent TC: Concentration of hyaluronan in the serum of untreated cancer patients with special reference to patients with mesothelioma. Cancer 62:326, 1988.
45. Dahl IMS, Solheim OP, Erikstein B et al: A longitudinal study of the hyaluronan level in the serum of patients with malignant mesothelioma under treatment: Hyaluronan as an indicator of progressive disease. Cancer 64:68, 1989.
46. Dardick I, Al-Jabi M, McCaughey WTE et al: Ultrastructure of poorly differentiated diffuse epithelial mesotheliomas. Ultrastruct Pathol 7:151, 1984.
47. Dardick I, Butler EB, Dardick AM: Quantitative ultrastructural study of nuclei from exfoliated benign and malignant mesothelial cells and metastatic adenocarcinoma cells. Acta Cytol (Baltimore) 30:379, 1986.
48. Dardick I, Jabi M, McCaughey WTE et al: Diffuse epithelial mesothelioma: A review of the ultrastructural spectrum. Ultrastruct Pathol 11:503, 1987.
49. Davies JD, Rees GJ, Mera SL: Angiosarcoma in irradiated post-mastectomy chest wall. Histopathology 7:947, 1983.
50. Dewar A, Valente M, Ring NP et al: Pleural mesothelioma of epithelial type and pulmonary adenocarcinoma: An ultrastructural and cytochemical comparison. J Pathol 152:309, 1987.
51. Donna A, Betta PG: Differentiation toward cartilage and bone in a primary tumour of pleura: Further evidence in support of the concept of mesodermoma. Histopathology 10:101, 1986.
52. Donna A, Betta PG, Bellingeri D et al: New marker for mesothelioma: an immunoperoxidase study. J Clin Pathol 39:961, 1986.
53. Donna A, Betta PG, Jones JSP: Verification of the histologic diagnosis of malignant mesothelioma in relation to the binding of an antimesothelial cell antibody. Cancer 63:1331, 1989.
54. Donna A, Betta PG, Marchesini A: Isolation and characterization of a possible new protein marker for differential diagnosis between metastatic carcinoma and mesothelioma cells in serous effusions: Preliminary findings. Cancer Detect Prev 8:255 1985.
55. Ehya H: The cytologic diagnosis of mesothelioma. Semin Diagn Pathol 3:196, 1986.
56. Ellis K, Wolff M: Mesotheliomas and secondary tumors of the pleura. Semin Roentgenol 12:303, 1977.
57. Ernst CS, Atkinson BF: Mucicarmine positivity in malignant mesothelioma. Lab Invest 42:113, 1980.
58. Ernst CS, Brooks JJ: Immunoperoxidase localization of secretory component in reactive mesothelium and mesotheliomas. J Histochem Cytochem 29:1102, 1981.
59. Frierson HF, Mills SE, Legier JF: Flow cytometric analysis of ploidy in immunohistochemically confirmed examples of malignant epithelial mesothelioma. Am J Clin Pathol 90:240, 1988.
60. Fuks A, Banjo C, Shuster J et al: Carcinoembryonic antigen (CEA): Molecular biology and clinical significance. Biochim Biophys Acta 417:123, 1974.
61. Ghosh AK, Butler EB: Immunocytological staining reactions of anti-carcinoembryonic antigen, Ca, and anti-human milk fat globule monoclonal antibodies on benign and malignant exfoliated mesothelial cells. J Clin Pathol 40:1424, 1987.
62. Gibbs AR, Harach R, Wagner JC: Comparison of tumour markers in malignant mesothelioma and pulmonary adenocarcinoma. Thorax 40:91, 1985.
63. Gold P, Freedman SO: Demonstration of tumor-specific antigens in human colonic carcinomata by immunological tolerance and absorption techniques. J Exp Med 121:439, 1965.
64. Gold P, Freedman SO: Specific carcinoembryonic antigens of the human digestive system. J Exp Med 122:467, 1965.
65. Gong E, Hirohashi S, Shimosato Y: Expression of carbohydrate antigen 19-9 and stage-specific em-

bryonic antigen 1 in nontumorous and tumorous epithelia of the human colon and rectum. JNCI 75:447, 1985.
66. Gonzalez-Crussi F, Wolfson SL, Misugi K et al: Peripheral neuroectodermal tumors of the chest wall in childhood. Cancer 54:2519, 1984.
67. Grunert F, Wank K, Luckenbach GA et al: Monoclonal antibodies against CEA: Comparison of the immunoprecipitates by fingerprint analysis. Oncodev Biol Med 3:191, 1982.
68. Gupta MK, Arciaga R, Bocci L et al: Measurement of a monoclonal-antibody-defined antigen (CA19-9) in the sera of patients with malignant and nonmalignant diseases: Comparison with carcinoembryonic antigen. Cancer 56:277, 1985.
69. Hammar SP, Bockus D, Remington F et al: Familial mesothelioma: A report of two families. Hum Pathol 20:107, 1989.
70. Hammar SP, Bolen JW: Pleural tumors. In Dail DH, Hammar SP (eds): Pulmonary Pathology. New York, Springer-Verlag, 1988.
71. Harris JP, South MA: Secretory component: A glandular epithelial cell marker. Am J Pathol 105:47, 1981.
72. Herbert A: The diagnosis of malignant mesothelioma. J Pathol 143:145, 1984.
73. Hernandez FJ, Fernandez BB: Localized fibrous tumors of pleura: A light and electron microscopic study. Cancer 34:1667, 1974.
74. Heyderman E, Strudley I, Powell G et al: A new monoclonal antibody to epithelial membrane antigen (EMA)—E29: A comparison of its immunocytochemical reactivity with another monoclonal antibody, HMFG-2. Br J Cancer 52:355, 1986.
75. Hilborne LH, Cheng L, Nieberg RK et al: Evaluation of antibody of human milk fat globule antigen in the detection of metastatic carcinoma in pleural, pericardial and peritoneal fluids. Acta Cytol 30:245, 1986.
76. Hillerdal G, Berg J: Malignant mesothelioma secondary to chronic inflammation and old scars: Two new cases and review of the literature. Cancer 55:1968, 1985.
77. Hirohashi S, Clausen H, Yamada T: Blood group A cross-reacting epitope defined by monoclonal antibodies NCC-Lu-35 and -81 expressed in cancer of blood group O or B individuals: Its identification as Tn antigen. Proc Natl Acad Sci USA 82:7039, 1985.
78. Hirohashi S, Ino Y, Kodama T: Distribution of blood group antigens A, B, H and I(Ma) in mucus-producing adenocarcinomas of human lung. JNCI 72:1299, 1984.
79. Hirohashi S, Shimosato Y, Ino Y: Distribution of blood group antigens and CA 19-9 in gastric cancers and nonneoplastic gastric mucosa. Jpn J Cancer Res (Gann) 75:540, 1984.
80. Holden J, Churg A: Immunohistochemical staining for keratin and carcinoembryonic antigen in the diagnosis of malignant mesothelioma. Am J Surg Pathol 8:277, 1984.
81. Hsu SM, Ho Y-S, Li PJ et al: L & H variants of Reed-Sternberg cells express sialylated Leu-M1 antigen. Am J Pathol 122:199, 1986.
82. Janssen JP, Wagenaar SS, van den Bosch JM et al: Benign localized mesothelioma of the pleura. Histopathology 9:309, 1985.
83. Jasani B, Edwards RE, Thomas ND et al: The use of vimentin antibodies in the diagnosis of malignant mesothelioma. Virchows Arch [A] 406:441, 1985.
84. Johnson VG, Schlom J, Paterson AJ et al: Analysis of human tumor-associated glycoprotein (TAG-72) identified by monoclonal antibody B72.3. Cancer Res 46:850, 1986.
85. Johnston WW, Szpak CA, Lottich SC et al: Use of monoclonal antibody (B72.3) as an immuncytochemical adjunct to diagnosis of adenocarcinoma in human effusions. Cancer Res 45:1894, 1985.
86. Jones RD, Smith DM, Thomas PG: Mesothelioma in Great Britain in 1968–1983. Scand J Work Environ Health 14:145, 1988.
87. Jothy S, Brazinsky SA, Chin-A-Loy M et al: Characterization of monoclonal antibodies to carcinoembryonic antigen with increased tumor specificity. Lab Invest 54:108, 1986.
88. Kahn HJ, Huang SN, Hanna WM et al: Immunohistochemical localization of epidermal and Mallory body cytokeratin in undifferentiated epithelial tumors: Comparison with ultrastructural features. Am J Clin Pathol 81:184, 1984.
89. Kannerstein M, Churg J, McCaughey WTE: Asbestos and mesothelioma: A review. Pathol Annu 13:81, 1978.
90. Kannerstein M, McCaughey WTE, Churg J et al: A critique of the criteria for the diagnosis of diffuse malignant mesothelioma. Mt Sinai J Med 44:485, 1977.
91. Katsube Y, Mukai K, Silverberg SG: Cystic mesothelioma of the peritoneum. Cancer 50:1615, 1982.
92. Kawai T, Suzuki M, Shinmei M et al: Glycosaminoglycans in malignant diffuse mesothelioma. Cancer 56:567, 1985.
93. Keating S, Simon GT, Alexopoulou I et al: Solitary fibrous tumour of the pleura: An ultrastructural and immunohistochemical study. Thorax 42:976, 1987.
94. King RM, Pairolero PC, Trastek VF et al: Primary chest wall tumors: Factors affecting survival. Ann Thorac Surg 41:597, 1986.
95. Klima M, Bossart MI: Sarcomatous type of malignant mesothelioma. Ultrastruct Pathol 4:349, 1983.
96. Kondi-Paphitis A, Addis BJ: Secretory component in pulmonary adeoncarcinoma and mesothelioma. Histopathology 10:1279, 1986.
97. Lafebvre MP, Rodriguez F, Schlom J et al: The application of a monoclonal antibody to the differentiation of benign and malignant mesothelial proliferations from adenocarcinomas. Lab Invest 52:38A, 1985.
98. LaRocca PJ, Rheinwald JG: Coexpression of simple epithelial keratins and vimentin by human mesothelium and mesothelioma *in vivo* and culture. Cancer Res 44:2991, 1988.
99. Law MR, Gregor A, Hodson ME et al: Malignant mesothelioma of the pleura: A study of 52 treated and 64 untreated patients. Thorax 39:255, 1984.
100. Law MR, Hodson ME, Turner-Warwick M: Malignant mesothelioma of the pleura: Clinical aspects and symptomatic treatment. Eur J Respir Dis 65:162, 1984.
101. Lee I, Radosevich JA, Chejfec G et al: Malignant meosthliomas: Improved differential diagnosis from lung adenocarcinomas using monoclonal antibodies 44-3A6 and 624A12. Am J Pathol 123:497, 1986.

102. Legha SS, Muggia FM: Pleural mesothelioma: Clinical features and therapeutic implications. Ann Intern Med 87:613, 1977.
103. Levine RJ (ed): Asbestos: an Information Resource. Prevention Branch, Division of Cancer Control and Rehabilitation, US Department of Health, Education and Welfare. Washington, DC, US Government Printing Office, 1978.
104. Lewis MI, Horak DA, Yellin A et al: The case of the moving intrathoracic mass: Pedunculated benign localized pleural mesothelioma. Chest 88:897, 1985.
105. Loosli H, Hurlimann J: Immunohistological study of malignant diffuse mesotheliomas of the pleura. Histopathology 8:793, 1984.
106. Lucas JG, Tuttle SE: Diagnostic histochemical and immunohistochemical studies in malignant mesothelioma. J Surg Oncol 35:30, 1987.
107. Magnani JL, Nilsson B, Brockhaus M et al: A monoclonal antibody-defined antigen associated with gastrointestinal cancer is a ganglioside containing sialylated lacto-N-fucopentaose II. J Biol Chem 257:14365, 1982.
108. Magnani JL, Steplewski Z, Koprowski H et al: Identification of the gastrointestinal and pancreatic cancer-associated antigen detected by monoclonal antibody 19-9 in the sera of patients as a mucin. Cancer Res 43:5489, 1983.
109. Makovitzky J: The distribution and localization of the monoclonal antibody-defined antigen 19-9 (CA19-9) in chronic pancreatitis and pancreatic carcinoma: An immunohistochemical study. Virchows Arch [B] 51:535, 1986.
110. Marshall RJ, Herbert A, Braye SG et al: Use of antibodies to carcinoembryonic antigen and human milk fat globule to distinguish carcinoma, mesothelioma, and reactive mesothelium. J Clin Pathol 37:1215, 1984.
111. McAfee MK, Pairolero PC, Bergstralh EJ et al: Chondrosarcoma of the chest wall: Factors affecting survival. Ann Thorac Surg 40 535 1985.
112. McCaughey WT, Al-Jabi M: Differentiation of serosal hyperplasia and neoplasia in biopsies. Pathol Annu 21 (part 1): 271, 1986.
113. McGregor DH, Dixon AY, Moral L et al: Liposarcoma of pleural cavity with recurrence as malignant fibrous histiocytoma. Ann Clin Lab Sci 17:83, 1987.
114. McNicholas KW et al: Resection of giant benign fibrous mesothelioma of pleura. NY State J Med 80:626, 1980.
115. Mengeot PM, Gailly C: Spontaneous detachment of benign mesothelioma into the pleural space and removal during pleuroscopy. Eur J Respir Dis 68 141 1986.
116. Miles JM, Hart WR, McMahon JT: Cystic mesothelioma of the peritoneum: Report of a case with multiple recurrences and review of the literature. Cleve Clin Q 53:109, 1986.
117. Mizutani Y, Nakajima T, Morinaga S: Immunohistochemical localization of pulmonary surfactant apoproteins in various lung tumors, with special reference to nonmucus producing lung adenocarcinomas. Cancer 61:532, 1988.
118. Mullink H, Henzen-Logmans CS, Alons-van Kordelaar JJM: Simultaneous immunoenzyme staining of vimentin and cytokeratins with monoclonal antibodies as an aid in the differential diagnosis of malignant mesothelioma from pulmonary adenocarcinoma. Virchows Arch [B] 52:55, 1986.
119. Nakano T, Fujii J, Tamura S et al: Thrombocytosis in patients with malignant pleural mesothelioma. Cancer 58:1699, 1986.
120. Nakano T, Fujii J, Tamura S et al: Glycosaminoglycan in malignant pleural mesothelioma. Cancer 57:106, 1986.
121. Nguyen H, Briere J, Clavier J et al: Five new cases of solitary fibrous mesothelioma of the pleura. Poumon Coeur 39:167, 1983.
122. Nichols DM, Johnson MA: Calcification in a pleural mesothelioma. J Can Assoc Radiol 34:311, 1983.
123. Noguchi M, Nakajima T, Hirohashi S et al: Immunohistochemical distinction of malignant mesothelioma from pulmonary adenocarcinoma with anti-surfactant apoprotein, anti-Lewis, and anti-Tn antibodies. Hum Pathol 20:53, 1989.
124. Nuti M, Teramoto YA, Mariani-Costantini R et al: A monoclonal antibody (B72.3) defines patterns of distribution of a novel tumor-associated antigen in human mammary carcinoma cell populations. Int J Cancer 29:539, 1982.
125. Olesen LL, Thorshaughe H: Thrombocytosis in patients with malignant pleural mesothelioma. Cancer 62:1194, 1988.
126. Ordonez NG: The immunohistochemical diagnosis of mesothelioma: Differentiation of mesothelioma and lung adenocarcinoma. Am J Surg Pathol 13:276, 1989.
127. Ordonez NG, Freedman RS, Herlyn M et al: Lewis and related tumor associated determinants in ovarian carcinoma. Gynecol Oncol 26:1, 1987.
128. Osamura RY: Ultrastructure of localized fibrous mesothelioma of the pleura: Report of a case with histogenetic considerations. Cancer 39:139, 1977.
129. Otis CN, Carter D, Cole S et al: Immunohistochemical evaluation of pleural mesothelioma and pulmonary adenocarcinoma: a bi-institutional study of 47 cases. Am J Surg Pathol 11:445, 1987.
130. Pairolero PC, Arnold PG: Chest wall tumors: Experience with 100 consecutive patients. J Thorac Cardiovasc Surg 90:367, 1985.
131. Pepper JR: Thoracoscopy in the diagnosis of pleural effusions and tumours. Br J Dis Chest 72:74, 1978.
132. Pfaltz M, Odermatt B, Christen B et al: Immunohistochemistry in the diagnosis of malignant mesothelioma. Virchows Arch [A] 411:387, 1987.
133. Poger ME, Hirsch BR, Lamm ME: Synthesis of secretory component by colonic neoplasms. Am J Pathol 82:327, 1976.
134. Prakash UB, Reiman HM: Comparison of needle biopsy with cytologic analysis for the evaluation of pleural effusion: Analysis of 414 cases. Mayo Clin Proc 60:158, 1985.
135. Ramussen OO, Larsen KE: S-100 protein in malignant mesotheliomas. Acat Pathol Microbiol Immunol Scand [A] 93:199, 1985.
136. Reck T, Bartsch M, Kockerling F et al: Primary and secondary chest wall tumors—diagnosis, therapy and results. Langenbecks Arch Chir 372:791, 1987.
137. Roboz J et al: Hyaluronic acid content of effusions as a diagnostic aid for malignant mesothelioma. Cancer Res 45:1850, 1985.
138. Rosai J, Dehner LP: Nodular mesothelial hyper-

plasia in hernia sacs: A benign condition simulating a neoplastic process. Cancer 35:165, 1975.
139. Ruttner JR et al: Squamous cell carcinoma of the pleura. Thorax 32:497, 1977.
140. Sabanathan S, Salama FD, Morgan WE et al: Primary chest wall tumors. Ann Thorac Surg 39:4, 1985.
141. Sahn SA: State of the art: The pleura. Am Rev Respir Dis 138:184, 1988.
142. Said JW, Nash G, Banks-Schlegel S et al: Localized fibrous mesothelioma: An immunohistochemical and electron microscopic study. Hum Pathol 15:440, 1984.
143. Said JW, Nash G, Tepper G et al: Keratin proteins and carcinoembryonic antigen in lung carcinoma: An immunoperoxidase study of fifty-four cases, with ultrastructural correlations. Hum Pathol 14:70, 1983.
144. Seggewiss H, Menami K, Khorfer R: Localized benign mesothelioma of the pleura: Case report and review of the literature. Thorac Cardiovasc Surg 34:330, 1987.
145. Shamberger RC, Grier HE, Weinstein HJ et al: Chest wall tumors in infancy and childhood. Cancer 63:774, 1989.
146. Sheibani K, Battifora H, Burke J et al: Leu-M1 antigen in human neoplasms: An immunohistologic study of 400 cases. Am J Surg Pathol 10:227, 1986.
147. Sheibani K, Battifora H, Burke JS: Antigenic phenotype of malignant mesotheliomas and pulmonary adencoarcinomas: An immunohistologic analysis demonstrating the value of Leu-M1 antigen. Am J Pathol 123:212, 1986.
148. Sienkowski IK, Russell AJ, Dilly SA et al: Peritoneal cystic mesothelioma: An electron microscopic and immunohistochemical study of two male patients. J Clin Pathol 39:440, 1986.
149. Singh G, Whiteside TL, Dekker A: Immunodiagnosis of meosthelioma: Use of antimesothelial cell serum in an indirect immunofluorescence assay. Cancer 43:2288, 1979.
150. Souba WW, McKenna RJ, Meis J et al: Radiation-induced sarcomas of the chest wall. Cancer 57 610 1986.
151. Spirtas R, Beebe GW, Connelly RR et al: Recent trends in mesothelioma incidence in the United States. Am J Ind Med 9:397. 1986.
152. Stahel RA, O'Hara CJ, Waibel R et al: Monoclonal antibodies against mesothelial membrane antigen discriminate between malignant mesothelioma and lung adenocarcinoma. Int J Cancer 41:218, 1988.
153. Sun TT, Shih C, Green H: Keratin cytoskeletons in epithelial cells and internal organs. Proc Natl Aca Sci USA 76:2813, 1979.
154. Sweetman WR: Pleural fibromas masquerading as coin lesions in lung. Am Surg 43:719, 1977.
155. Szpak CA et al: Antigenic expression among malignant mesotheliomas of the pleura and adenocarcinomas of the lung as defined by monoclonal antibodies B72.3, B1.1, and pooled AE1, AE3. Lab Invest 54:62A, 1986.
156. Szpak CA, Johnston WW, Roggli V et al: The diagnostic distinction between malignant mesothelioma of the pleura and adenocarcinoma of the lung as defined by a monoclonal antibody. Am J Pathol 122:252, 1986.
157. Talerman A et al: Diffuse malignant peritoneal mesothelioma in a 13-year-old girl: Report of a case and review of the literature. Am J Surg Pathol 9:73, 1985.
158. Taylor-Papadimitrious J, Peterson JA, Arklie J et al: Monoclonal antibodies to epithelium-specific components of the human milk fat globule membrane: Production and reaction with cells in culture. Int J Cancer 28:17, 1981.
159. Thor A, Gorstein F, Ohuchi N et al: Tumor-associated glycoprotein (TAG-72) in ovarian carcinomas defined by monoclonal antibody B72.3. JNCI 76:995, 1986.
160. Triol JH, Conston AS, Chandler SVD: Distinguishing adenocarcinoma from mesothelioma in effusions. Hum Pathol 18:969, 1987.
161. Tron V, Wright JL, Churg A: Carcinoembryonic antigen and milk-fat globule protein staining of malignant mesothelioma and adenocarcinoma of the lung. Arch Pathol Lab Med 111:291, 1987.
162. Utley JR, Parker JC Jr, Hahn RS et al: Recurrent benign fibrous mesothelioma of the pleura. J Thorac Cardiovasc Surg 65:830, 1973.
163. Wagner JC, Sleggs CA, Marchand P: Diffuse pleural mesothelioma and asbestos exposure in the Northern Western Cape Province. Br J Ind Med 17:260, 1960.
164. Walker AM, Loughlin JE, Friedlander ER et al: Projections of asbestos-related disease 1980–2009. J Occup Med 25:409, 1983.
165. Walts AE, Said JW, Banks-Schlegel S: Keratin and carcinoembryonic antigen in exfoliated mesothelial and malignant cells: An immunoperoxidase study. Am J Clin Pathol 80:671, 1983.
166. Walts AE, Said JW, Shintaku IP et al: Keratins of different molecular weight in exfoliated mesothelial and adenocarcinoma cells: An aid to cell identification. Am J Clin Pathol 81:442, 1984.
167. Wang NS: The preformed stomas connecting the pleural cavity and the lymphatics in the parietal pleura. Am Rev Respir Dis 111:12, 1975.
168. Wang NS, Huang SN, Gold P: Absence of carcinoembryonic antigen–like material in mesothelioma: An immunohistochemical differentiation from other lung cancers. Cancer 44:937, 1979.
169. Warhol MJ, Corson JM: An ultrastructural comparison of mesotheliomas with adenocarcinomas of the lung and breast. Hum Pathol 16:50, 1985.
170. Warnock ML, Stoloff A, Thor A: Differentiation of adenocarcinoma of the lung from mesothelioma: Periodic acid–Schiff, monoclonal antibodies B72.3, and Leu M1. Am J Pathol 133:30, 1988.
171. Weilbaecher TG, Sarma DP: Localized fibrous mesothelioma of the pleura. J Surg Oncol 25:67, 1984.
172. Weiss NS, Suarez L, Honchar PA et al: Review of mesothelioma incidence and mortality in Texas. Tex Med 84:44, 1988.
173. Xu Z, Armstrong BK, Blundson BJ et al: Trends in mortality from malignant mesothelioma of the pleura, and production and use of asbestos in Australia. Med J Aust 143:185, 1985.
174. Yousem SA, Hochholzer L: Malignant mesotheliomas with osseous and cartilaginous differentiation. Arch Pathol Lab Med 111:62 1987.
175. Yousem SA, Flynn SD: Intrapulmonary localized fibrous tumor: Intraparenchymal so-called localized fibrous mesothelioma. Am J Clin Pathol 89:365, 1988.

Chapter

13

TUMORS OF THE MEDIASTINUM

In the evaluation of a mediastinal mass, metastatic lung carcinoma must be distinguished from primary lesions and neoplasms of the mediastinum. Some of these tumors are uncommon, a number occur mainly in childhood, and others are so different in their histology from lung carcinomas that confusion is unlikely when suitable material is available for study. This chapter provides a brief review of the pathology of the more common mediastinal tumors, other than soft tissue tumors, as it pertains to the differential diagnosis of metastatic lung carcinoma.

ANATOMY OF THE MEDIASTINUM

Subdivision of the part of the thorax that lies between the pleurae into four compartments is convenient for descriptive purposes since many lesions occur predominantly within one region. The middle mediastinum is clearly defined by the pericardium. The superior compartment may be combined with the anterior and posterior compartments to form the anterosuperior and posterosuperior mediastinal compartments.

DIAGNOSTIC TECHNIQUES

The relatively inaccessible location of some lesions and the presence of the great vessels and other vital structures complicate the invasive procedures that are used to obtain tissue from mediastinal masses, but newer diagnostic techniques including radioisotopic scanning, computed tomographic scans, and magnetic resonance imaging have greatly enhanced the accuracy of the preoperative diagnosis of mediastinal lesions.[16] The findings from these studies may provide a strong indication of the nature of a lesion and facilitate a decision on how tissue for pathologic evaluation should be obtained. Percutaneous needle aspiration biopsy is particularly useful for detecting metastatic carcinoma,[2] but it can also aid in the diagnosis of primary mediastinal lesions.[75] Linder and coworkers[38] reviewed 32 fine-needle aspiration biopsy specimens from 29 patients: 18 aspirates contained malignant cells, and in 13 of these a definite cell type was identified, usually metastatic lung carcinoma. In 16 of the 29 patients (55%), thoracotomy was avoided because of the findings from the aspiration biopsy.

Paratracheal lesions may be inspected and biopsied by mediastinoscopy, but the tissue specimens are small and they tend to be fragmented and are prone to distortion from crushing. Larger and better specimens can be obtained by anterior mediastinotomy,[20] and this approach may be used to establish a diagnosis in patients in whom thoracotomy is contraindicated. Best and colleagues[9] reported their experience with 62 consecutive patients who underwent anterior mediastinotomy. The overall diagnostic specificity was 64.5%, and the diagnostic sensitivity was 98%.

Since it is often difficult to identify the nature of a mediastinal tumor by conventional light microscopy, it should be routine practice to procure smears or sections for immunocytochemistry and a small quantity of tissue for electron microscopy whenever one is biopsied. The immunostaining procedures that are used in the differential diagnosis of a mediastinal mass can usually be performed on formalin-fixed, paraffin-embedded material, but if lymphoma is suspected, frozen tissue sections should be prepared and held for possible marker studies.

CLASSIFICATION OF MEDIASTINAL MASSES

In spite of the difficulty that may be entailed in obtaining acceptable biopsy material, the nature of a mediastinal mass should be determined by histologic or cytologic examination before any therapy is instituted. Some lesions that are suspected clinically or radiologically to be tumors turn out to be benign or nonneoplastic, and the mediastinum is a common location for metastatic tumors.

In Davis and co-workers' series of 400 consecutive patients with primary mediastinal lesions, 17% were thymic tumors, 16% were lymphomas, 14% were neurogenic tumors, and 11% were germ cell tumors.[16] Forty-two percent of the neoplasms were malignant. Fifty-four percent of the lesions involved the anterosuperior mediastinum, 26% the posterior mediastinum, and 20% the middle mediastinum. Eighty-three percent of the lesions detected on routine chest radiographs were benign, whereas 57% of the lesions in symptomatic patients were malignant.

Cysts[69] and neoplasms of the mediastinum and their common locations are listed in Table 13–1. Cysts of the thymus may occur anywhere along the path of embryonic migration of the thymic primordia from the branchial region to the anterior mediastinum. The cyst lining is formed by columnar or squamous cells, and thymic parenchyma is present in the tissues forming the cyst wall.

Thyroid and parathyroid neoplasms rarely cause confusion with metastatic lung cancer. Zapatero and associates[83] reported two ectopic goiters in the anterior mediastinum, which comprised 5.1% of intrathoracic goiters and 1.3% of mediastinal tumors in their series. Of the mediastinal parathyroid tumors studied by Clark,[15] 52 were situated in the anterior mediastinum and 12 were in the posterior mediastinum. A benign mixed tumor of salivary type is rare in the mediastinum: Feigin and colleagues[18] reported one that formed a large middle mediastinal mass and noted that they had seen salivary inclusions in hilar lymph nodes in a lobe resected for lung adenocarcinoma.

Soft tissue tumors may present at any site in the mediastinum, and Schwann cell neoplasms are the most common type. If an adequate biopsy specimen is procured, a mesenchymal tumor can usually be distinguished from metastatic lung carcinoma, although immunostaining for cytokeratins may be needed to identify the occasional sarcomatoid carcinoma. Posterior mediastinal tumors may require thoracotomy to secure sufficient representative material.[26] Approximately 20% of neuroblastomas occur in the mediastinum,[28] but almost all are tumors of childhood. Ganglioneuroblastomas may however be encountered in adult patients: Talerman and co-workers[70] reported a primary ganglioneuroblastoma in the anterior mediastinum, an incidental finding at autopsy in a 61-year-old woman.

In the brief review of the more common mediastinal tumors (thymoma, carcinoid, lymphomas, germ cell tumors) that follows, the emphasis is on distinguishing between them and metastatic tumors from the lung.

Table 13–1. Mediastinal Tumors and Cysts

Anterosuperior	Middle	Posterosuperior
Thymoma	Cardiac tumors	Neurogenic tumors
Thymic carcinoma	Pericardial cyst	Neuroblastoma
Thymic carcinoid	Bronchogenic cyst	Ganglioneuroma
Germ cell tumor		Bronchogenic cyst
Lymphoma		Enteric cyst
Hodgkin's disease		Fibromatosis
Parathyroid neoplasms		
Thyroid neoplasms		
Lipoma		
Lymphangioma		

THYMOMA

Most thymomas are confined to the anterior mediastinum, but occasionally one presents in another mediastinal compartment or even within the neck, and infiltrating tumors can extend into the pleural cavity. Thymomas are rare in children. Among 283 patients with thymoma from the Mayo Clinic, Lewis and co-workers[37] found an age range of 16 to 90 years with a mean of 52 years; 136 patients were male and 147 were female. Associated syndromes, when present, provide a clue to the diagnosis: more than half of patients with myasthenia gravis have a thymoma, and many others have lymphoid hyperplasia of the thymus, characterized by the presence of lymphoid follicles that are rare or absent in the normal thymus. Forty-six percent of Lewis and co-workers' patients had myasthenia, and 10% had other paraneoplastic syndromes.[37] Hypogammaglobulinemia is reported in approximately 10% of patients with thymoma, and erythroid hypoplasia occurs in 5%.

Thymomas vary greatly in size, and some are large. Radiology shows a lobulated shadow, occasionally with foci of calcification. About 90% of thymomas have a well-defined capsule that may be thick and contain calcified areas.[47] Careful inspection of the capsule of a resected thymoma is important since infiltration of the capsule may be the only evidence that the tumor is behaving aggressively. Lewis and co-workers[37] found that 32% were locally invasive, with metastases to lung or pleura in 6%; and 15% of the totally resected tumors recurred, 3% with distant metastases. Maggi and colleagues[41] reviewed 165 surgically treated thymomas with a 28-year follow-up, and the survival figures at 3, 5, and 10 years were 84%, 79%, and 65%, respectively. Patients with macroscopic findings indicating invasive behavior had a 5-year survival of 67% versus 85% for noninvasive tumors.

A thymoma is composed of epithelial cells and lymphocytes in greatly varying proportions, ranging from apparently pure epithelial neoplasms to lymphocytic lesions with barely discernible foci of epithelial cells. A marked predominance of epithelial cells or lymphocytes may lead to a thymoma being subtyped as epithelial or lymphocytic, but every tumor contains both cell types. Even in an apparently pure epithelial tumor, small numbers of lymphocytes can be detected. Subtyping is pertinent, however, since largely epithelial thymomas tend to behave more aggressively.[37]

Variations in the histologic pattern of a thymoma are produced by the number and arrangement of the epithelial cells. They may form diffuse sheets, cords, clusters, or rosettes, or only isolated epithelial cells may be detected amid a sea of lymphocytes. Usually these apparently solitary epithelial cells are parts of small clusters, and scrutiny of a predominantly lymphocytic thymoma will often reveal tiny groups and facilitate the diagnosis. In the majority of thymomas, the epithelial cells are more or less round in paraffin sections, and they have a central round nucleus with a smooth profile, finely dispersed chromatin, and a rather small nucleolus (Fig. 13–1). The bland nuclear appearance coupled with the plentiful, rather pale cytoplasm helps to distinguish the cells from those of metastatic carcinoma. Nomori and co-workers[54] measured the nuclear areas of the epithelial cells in 42 thymomas, 14 thymic hyperplasias, and 10 normal thymuses and found that the nuclei of the epithelial cells were significantly larger than in the hyperplasias and normal thymuses and that those of invasive thymomas were significantly larger than in noninvasive tumors. The epithelial cells may assume a spindle shape in part or all of a thymoma, and they occasionally form intersecting fascicles, although the pattern is rarely well developed.

A secondary component may be present in a thymoma. Skeletal muscle differentiation is sometimes found, and focal neuroblastomatous differentiation has been reported in a thymic carcinoma.[3] The term *thymic carcinoma* connotes an epithelial neoplasm of the thymus with cytologic features that indicate aggressive behavior, and the histology may be similar to that of carcinomas from other sites including lung (squamous, small cell), or the tumor may be undifferentiated. Distinction from a metastatic tumor of the lung may be difficult or impossible from the histopathology and will then depend on the clinical findings.

When the material furnished for pathologic examination is adequate in quantity and quality, most thymomas can be identified with confidence. When there is difficulty, recourse to immunostaining and/or electron microscopy should resolve the problem.

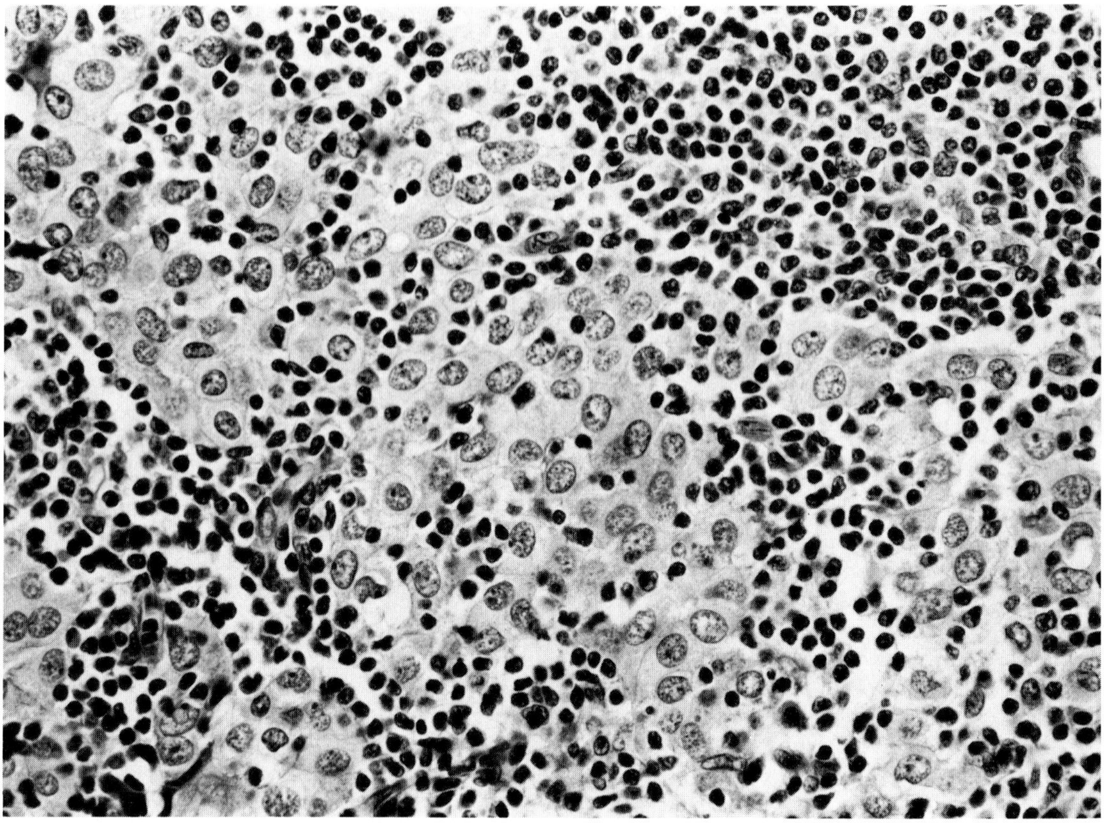

Figure 13–1. Thymoma. Irregular groups of epithelial cells are present among the small lymphocytes.

Immunocytochemistry

Since the epithelial cells of thymomas react for cytokeratin, immunostaining with broad-spectrum antibodies for this intermediate filament can assist in establishing the diagnosis (Fig. 13–2). In most thymomas, cytokeratin immunostaining reveals a greater number of epithelial cells than are detected in the hematoxylin-eosin–stained sections. The diagnosis of thymoma is consequently facilitated in cases in which only a small amount of tissue is available for examination,[7, 49] and immunocytochemical studies using antibodies to cytokeratin and leukocyte common antigen can be very helpful in differentiating thymoma from lymphoma or seminoma. A positive reaction for carcinoembryonic antigen (CEA) in the epithelial cells of thymomas may help differentiate this tumor from mesotheliomas, which are almost always CEA negative.[63] Kodama and co-workers[31] reported Leu-7 reactivity in 17 thymomas but in none of five squamous cell carcinomas, suggesting that Leu-7 may be of some value in differentiating thymomas from thymic or bronchogenic squamous cell carcinomas.

Several investigators[14, 35, 46, 62] have demonstrated that predominately lymphocytic and mixed-type thymomas contain a distinct subset of T lymphocytes showing the OKT6 epitope and containing terminal deoxynucleotidyl transferase (TdT). These T cells, which are also found in the thymic cortex, are regarded as immature lymphocytes. Some studies[19] have indicated that recognition of the TdT^+ $OKT6^+$ phenotype can help to differentiate thymomas arising in unusual sites, (*e.g.*, lung and pleura) from other neoplasms with which they can be confused, including small cell carcinoma and some mesotheliomas. This is particularly liable to be a problem when the tissue available for examination is limited or heavily infiltrated by inflammatory cells. Recognition of a thymic-derived T-cell phenotype can help to separate thymomas and immunoblastic lymphomas from other lymphomas and inflammatory pseudotumors.

Electron Microscopy

The admixture of epithelial cells and lymphocytes is obvious at the ultrastructural level

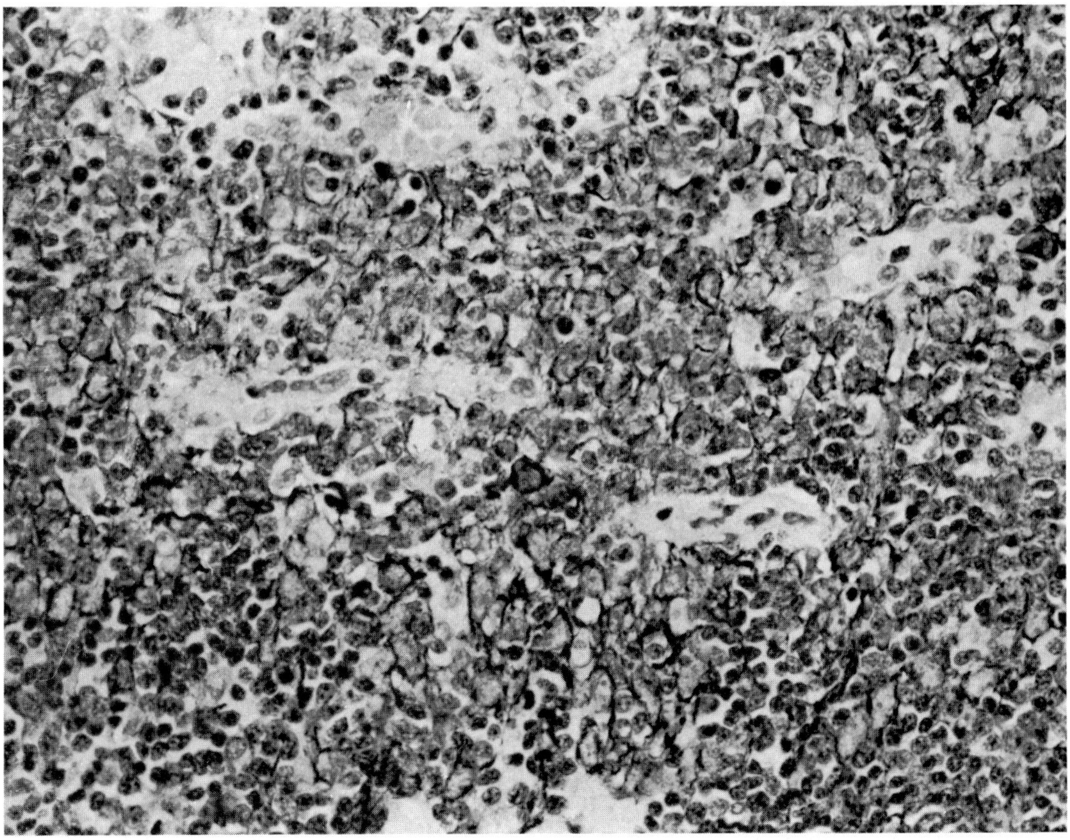

Figure 13–2. Thymoma. Immunostaining for cytokeratin is positive in the cytoplasm of the epithelial cells.

(Fig. 13–3), and the former are found to be more plentiful than was suspected from the paraffin sections. The lymphocytes are small with dense nuclei and scanty cytoplasm and organelles, but a few larger lymphocytes with more cytoplasm are a common finding. Lymphocytes are often intimately apposed to epithelial cells and may even be within their cytoplasm (emperipolesis).[55] A word of caution is appropriate: the electron microscopist should avoid mistaking epithelial cells from the thymic remnant for tumor cells, just as cytokeratin immunoreactivity in these residual cells within a lymphoma must not be misinterpreted as evidence for a thymoma.

The epithelial cells of thymomas vary in size, but they are invariably larger than the small lymphocytes, with bigger nuclei and more cytoplasm. They have smooth cell and nuclear profiles, and the nuclear chromatin is typically fine and evenly dispersed.[55] Clustering of the epithelial cells may be detected, and a group of cells is often bordered by a basal lamina (Fig. 13–4). Cytoplasmic extensions link neighboring cells, and at low magnification a cell may appear stellate because of the radiating arms of cytoplasm. The cell junctions are particularly distinctive. They are mature desmosomes with prominent intermediate lines and are often long: they are more conspicuous when several form a chain (Fig. 13–5). Tonofilaments are visible at the desmosomes, but it is difficult to trace them as they leave the subplasmalemmal region. At low magnification, the desmosomes are usually noticeable as linear densities. In an occasional thymoma, cell junctions are sparse and difficult to find.

Organelles are not plentiful in the epithelial cells of a thymoma. Some cells contain moderate numbers of mitochondria, but endoplasmic reticulum is confined to a few slender cisternae. A few dense bodies and some lipid droplets may be seen. Filaments within the cytoplasm are quite variable in number and appearance. They are commonly present as diffuse aggregates, but in a few tumors, condensed bundles are found.

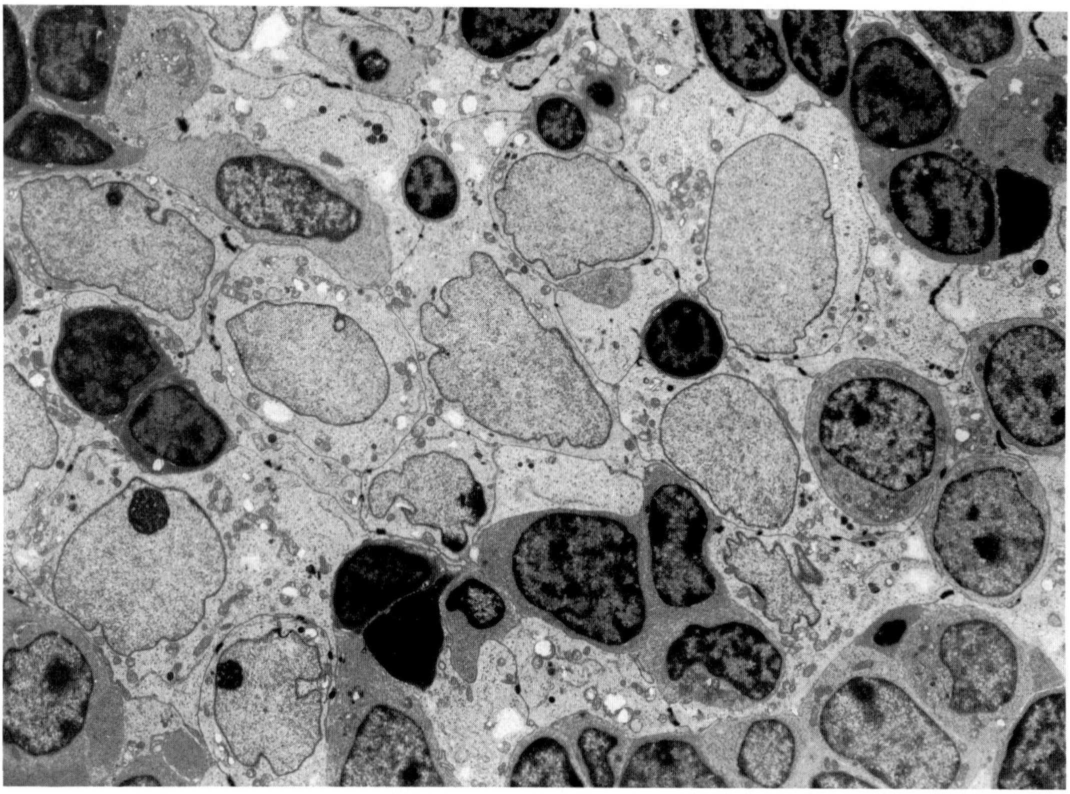

Figure 13–3. Thymoma. The electron micrograph shows the contrast between the pale epithelial cells and the smaller lymphocytes with their scanty cytoplasm and dense nuclei. Even at this low magnification, desmosomes between the epithelial cells can be distinguished. (×2,800)

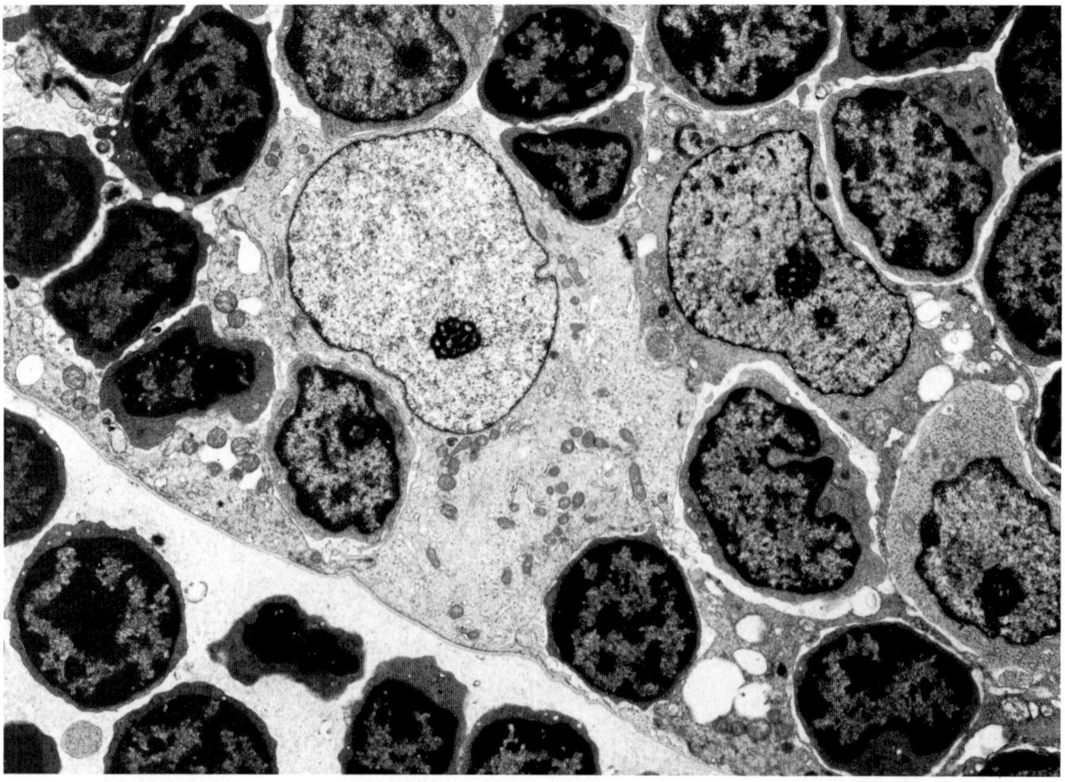

Figure 13–4. Thymoma. The periphery of a nest of tumor cells is bordered by a basal lamina. The epithelial cells contain a few mitochondria and diffuse intermediate filaments. (×4,800)

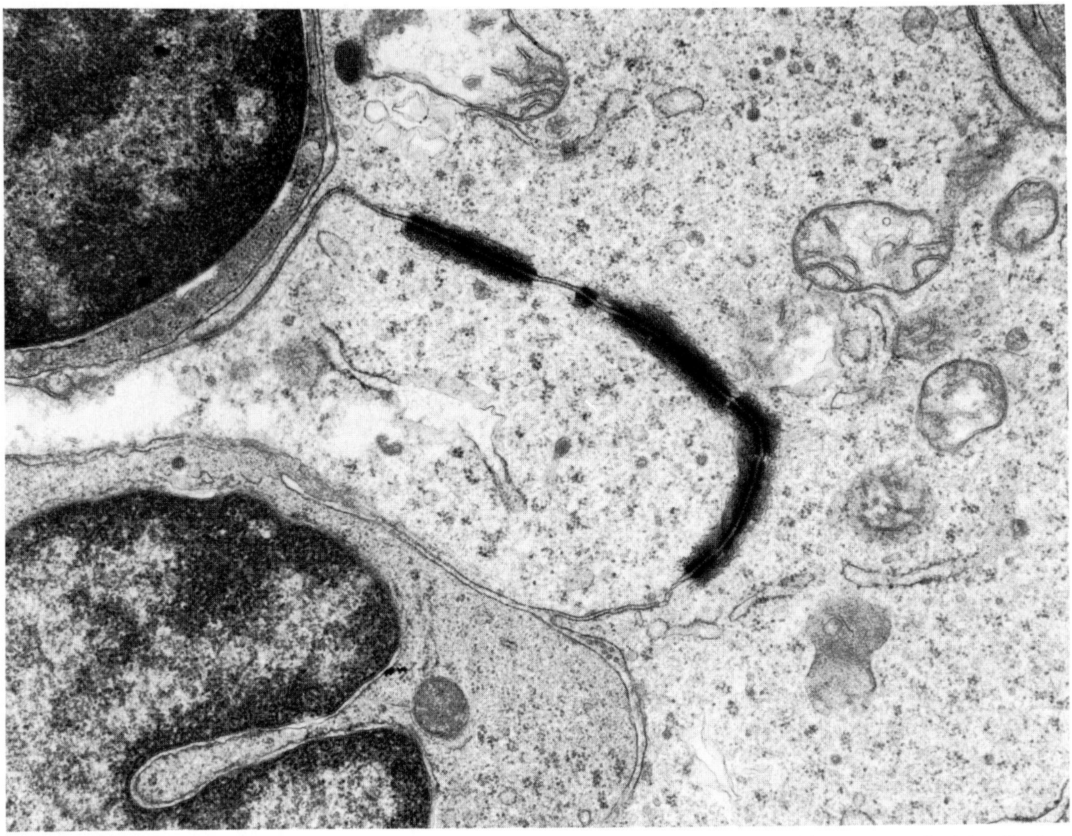

Figure 13–5. Thymoma. A chain of desmosomes connects two epithelial cells. Tonofilaments can be identified only immediately adjacent to the desmosomes. (×21,000)

The filaments can often be followed into the arms of cytoplasm that connect the cells. In a few tumors, the cytoplasmic processes are as numerous as in many Schwann cell neoplasms and they then tend to form parallel bundles (Fig. 13–6).

This description pertains to the typical thymoma and encompasses the great majority of the tumors. A few variants are encountered with unusual features at the ultrastructural level (Figs. 13–7 and 13–8).[55]

MEDIASTINAL CARCINOID TUMOR

Because of the occurrence of a rosette pattern in some thymomas, a carcinoid tumor in the anterior mediastinum is readily confused with thymoma by conventional light microscopy. The histology of mediastinal carcinoids is similar to that of carcinoid tumors arising in lung or gastrointestinal tract, and the immunocytochemical findings and ultrastructural features are comparable.[10, 22, 27, 43] Occasionally the carcinoid tumor is responsible for endocrine symptoms, or a syndrome of multiple endocrine neoplasia may be present. Wick and co-workers[76, 80] reported six patients with ectopic ACTH secretion, and five of them had Cushing's syndrome. Metastases were present in 11 patients (73%), appearing as long as 8 years after diagnosis. Lagrange and co-workers[33] found melanocytic differentiation in a neuroendocrine carcinoma from a patient with the ectopic ACTH syndrome. Warren and Yum[74] recorded the unusual situation of a carcinoid tumor arising in a treated primary mediastinal germ cell tumor.

A mediastinal paraganglioma[17] will contain dense-core granules and may be indistinguishable from a carcinoid tumor by light microscopy or at the ultrastructural level.

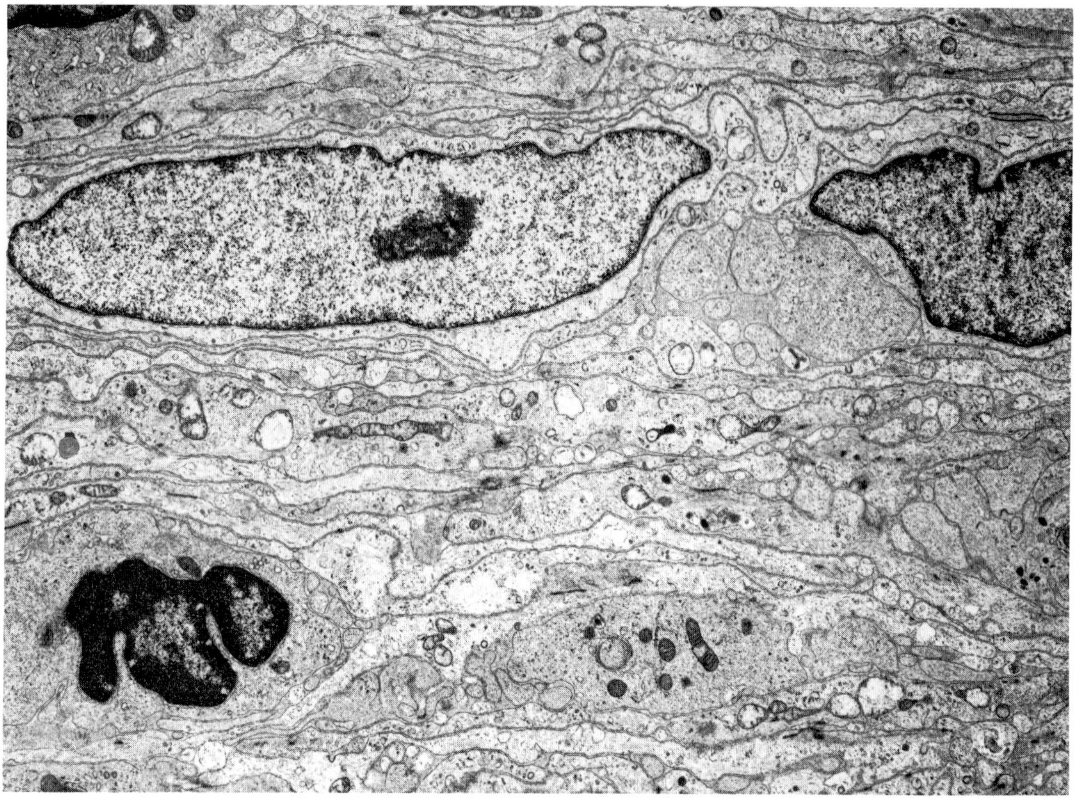

Figure 13–6. Thymoma. In this tumor, the processes of the cell cytoplasm were unusually well developed. (×6,500)

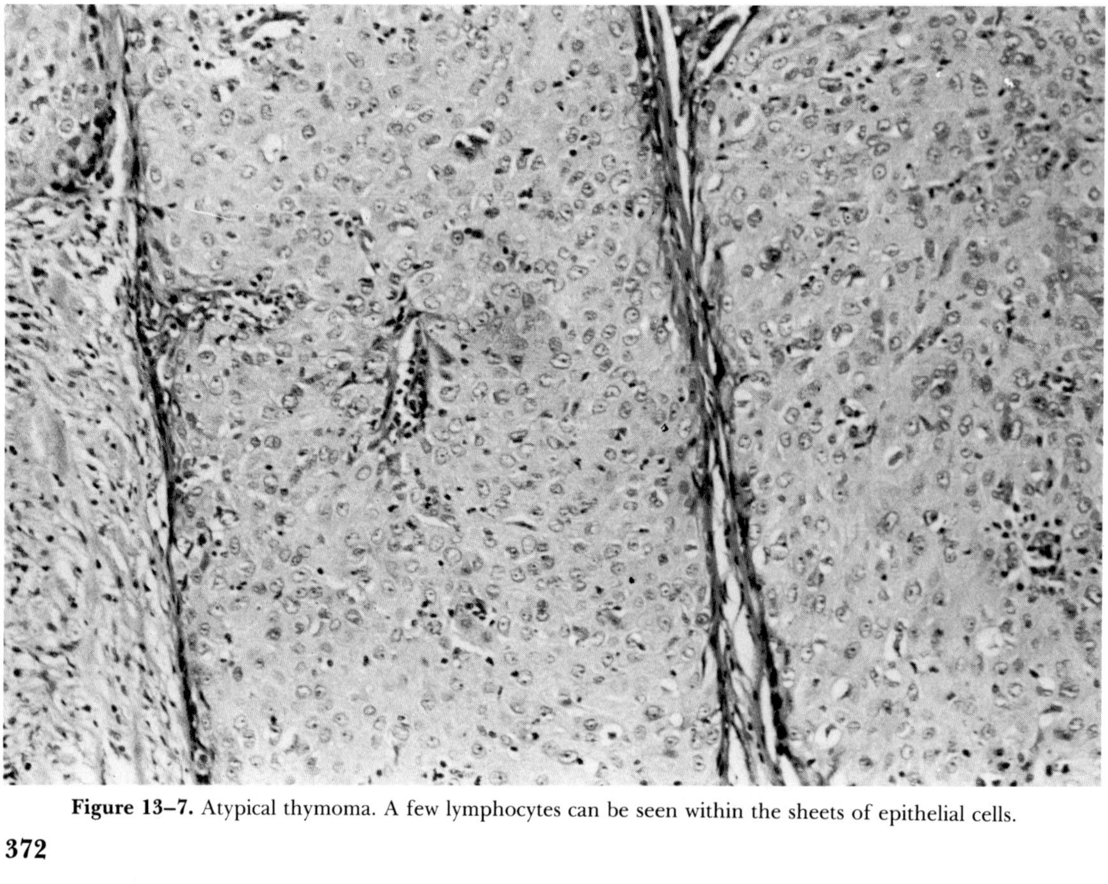

Figure 13–7. Atypical thymoma. A few lymphocytes can be seen within the sheets of epithelial cells.

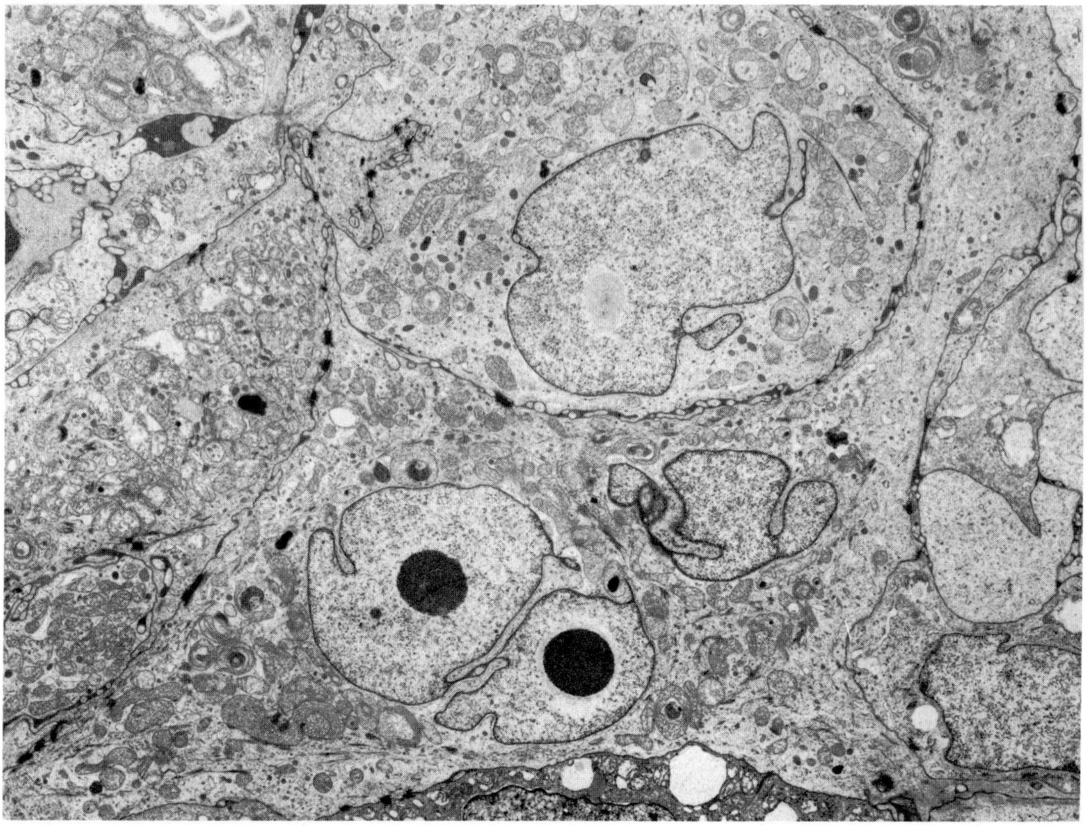

Figure 13–8. Atypical thymoma. The same tumor as Figure 13–7. The electron micrograph shows epithelial cells with irregular nuclear profiles, prominent nucleoli, considerable numbers of mitochondria, and dense bodies presumed to be lysosomes. (×5,000)

Pheochromocytomas may occur in the middle mediastinum,[65] and they also contain granules, often with eccentric cores.

Immunocytochemistry

The diagnosis and cell characterization of endocrine tumors can be facilitated by the use of general immunocytochemical markers. Those most commonly used are the gamma-gamma dimer of 2-phospho-D-glycerate hydrolase (neuron-specific enolase), Leu-7, chromogranin, and synaptophysin.[77] Because of their high specificity and sensitivity for endocrine differentiation, chromogranin and synaptophysin are the two most useful markers for the immunocytochemical diagnosis of thymic and other endocrine tumors. In view of their limited specificity for endocrine differentiation, we believe that neuron-specific enolase and Leu-7 have little value in the diagnosis of mediastinal carcinoids. Neuron-specific enolase is often expressed in a variety of nonendocrine tumors, including some bronchogenic carcinomas,[57] large cell lymphomas,[51] and seminomas,[32] all of which can be confused with thymomas when they occur in the mediastinum.

The thymic carcinoids associated with Cushing's syndrome reported by Wick and co-workers[79] were shown to express ACTH by immunocytochemical procedures. Production of other neuropeptides including somatostatin, β-endorphin, and Leu- and Met-enkephalins has also been documented.[5, 58, 77, 79] Serotonin, not associated with carcinoid syndrome, has been demonstrated in both carcinoid and small cell carcinoma of the thymus.[78, 79]

GERM CELL TUMORS

Origin from ectopic germ cells is the favored explanation for the occurrence of germ cell tumors in the mediastinum. In the anterior mediastinum, they can be intimately related to the thymus. Some indication of their frequency relative to other mediastinal neoplasms is provided by the study of Davis and co-workers,[16] who analyzed 400 patients with mediastinal masses and reported that 42 (11%) had germ cell tumors and that they made up 10% of 2,399 primary mediastinal tumors in 13 published series. The same subtypes that occur in the testis are seen in the mediastinum. From a review of 56 patients with primary malignant mediastinal germ cell tumors, Knapp and colleagues[30] reported that the mean age was 29 years and that 86% were male and 14% were female. A single germ cell element was found in two thirds, and varying combinations were present in the remaining one third. Martini and associates[44] found 20 embryonal cell carcinomas and 10 seminomas among 30 cases. Wirtanen and co-workers[82] reviewed 1,064 exploratory thoracotomies performed at the Mayo Clinic between 1929 and 1968 for mediastinal masses: 99 (9.3%) resulted in a diagnosis of teratoma, of which 16 (1.7%) were malignant.

The findings of Luna and Valenzuela-Tamariz[40] on mediastinal germ cell tumors point out the importance of evaluating retroperitoneal lymph nodes. In an autopsy study of 20 anterior mediastinal germ cell tumors, all from male patients aged 14 to 45 years, the testes were carefully examined. Occult tumor was found in one case of embryonal cell carcinoma, and a well-defined scar with calcification was present in the testis of a patient with choriocarcinoma. These two patients were the only ones in the series who had lower retroperitoneal lymph node metastases, and only in 4 patients were the retroperitoneal nodes above the level of the renal arteries involved.

Most patients with mediastinal seminomas are young men. The 21 examples reviewed by Schantz and associates[64] were from male patients with a mean age of 29.8 years, and the tumors were from 2 to 13 cm in size. The histology is usually closely similar to that seen in the testis, and the cells contain abundant glycogen (Fig. 13–9). However, Burns and McCaughey[13] reported three cystic examples

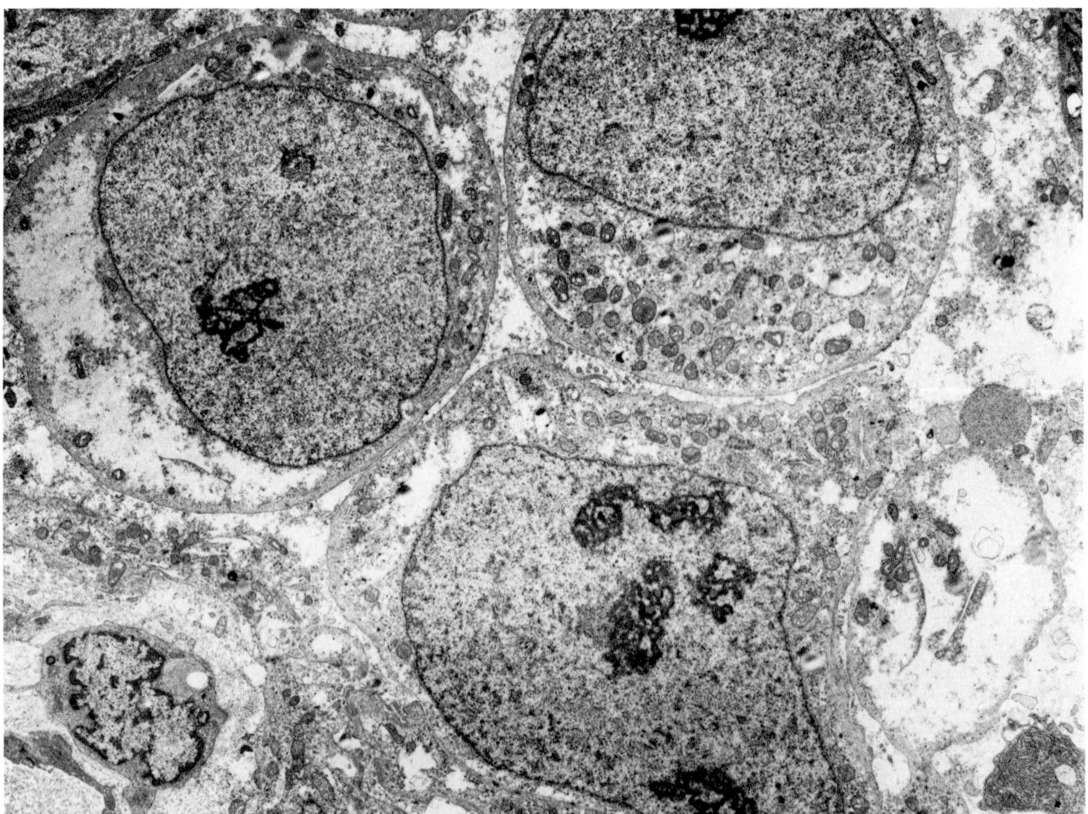

Figure 13–9. Mediastinal seminoma. Three detached tumor cells. The clear areas represent lakes of cytoplasmic glycogen. The nucleoli have a loose, skeinlike pattern. (×3,800)

in which a combination of epithelioid granulomas and fibrosis coupled with reactive follicular hyperplasia obscured the seminoma component.

Embryonal cell carcinoma arising in the mediastinum is more aggressive than seminoma. The histology is again similar to that of a testicular primary lesion, and α-fetoprotein levels can be elevated. A yolk sac component with its distinctive glomeruloid bodies may be present. Truong and co-workers[72] state that only 49 primary mediastinal endodermal sinus tumors had been reported prior to their presentation of seven new cases, in which they emphasized the occurrence of periodic acid–Schiff (PAS)-positive material within and outside the cells.

Mature teratoma is the most common type of mediastinal germ cell tumor. It is usually detected in early adult life. Some of these tumors are large and cause damage to adjacent organs by pressure. Radiologic examination may reveal cystic areas and calcification. In microscopic sections, various tissue elements can be seen.[61] Rarely an endocrine component of a mediastinal teratoma is functional. Malignant teratomas are relatively uncommon in the mediastinum, and almost all occur in men. While the cut surface will show hemorrhage and necrosis, it may not be possible to distinguish a malignant from a mature teratoma by inspection alone, and histologic verification is mandatory. Landanyi and Ray[34] reviewed 19 published cases of hematologic malignancies associated with mediastinal germ cell tumors and report two immature teratomas with focal yolk sac differentiation associated with histiocytosis, one clearly malignant and the other cytologically benign.

A primary choriocarcinoma is rare in the mediastinum.[29, 60] Most of the reported cases have been in young men, and they have been aggressive tumors with a poor prognosis.

Immunocytochemistry

Several studies have indicated that primitive germ cell tumors do not contain cytokeratins, yet cytokeratins are expressed in early embryos and extraembryonic tissues.[36] Seminoma, a neoplasm made up of primitive, nondifferentiated germ cells, does not express cytokeratins, while all other germ cell tumors, being characterized by embryonal or extraembryonal differentiation, show reactivity for this marker.[6, 45, 59] Cytokeratin can also be expressed in the trophoblastic-like cells seen in some classic seminomas.[6]

Placental alkaline phosphatase (PLAP) is a marker often reported to be expressed in seminomas and other germ cell tumors, especially in embryonal carcinoma.[42, 52] Staining for this marker is most commonly confined to the plasma membranes of seminoma cells (Fig. 13–10) and could help in differentiating seminomas from lymphomas and melanomas. However, since it can also be expressed in a wide variety of carcinomas including those originating in the lung,[81] the diagnostic value of PLAP is somewhat limited.

Recently, Bailey and colleagues[4] developed a monoclonal antibody (M2A) against a human ovarian epithelial cell line. The antibody has been reported to react with seminomas and dysgerminomas but not to stain other gonadal or extragonadal tumors. In our experience, it is specific for seminoma, but a drawback exists in that it reacts only on frozen tissue and not on routinely fixed and processed specimens.

Endodermal sinus tumor can readily be confused with poorly differentiated adenocarcinomas secondarily involving the mediastinum, and the immunocytochemical demonstration of α-fetoprotein can then help to resolve the differential diagnosis.[72] We have found that most endodermal sinus tumors express this marker and that carcinomas, with the exception of liver cell carcinomas, do not. Other markers, including α_1-antitrypsin, ferritin, PLAP, and CEA,[24, 52, 72] can be expressed in endodermal sinus tumors, but because of low specificity for this tumor, their diagnostic value does not compare well with that of α-fetoprotein. About one third of embryonal carcinomas also express α-fetoprotein.

Immunostaining for the β-unit of human chorionic gonadotropin (β-hCG) can help in the identification of choriocarcinomas arising in the mediastinum and lung, but other tumors, including lung carcinomas, can also express this marker.

LYMPHOMA

The common lymphomas arising in the mediastinum are the nodular sclerosing form of Hodgkin's disease, and among the non-Hodgkin's lymphomas, diffuse large cell lymphoma and lymphoblastic lymphoma.[73]

Hodgkin's disease involving mediastinal

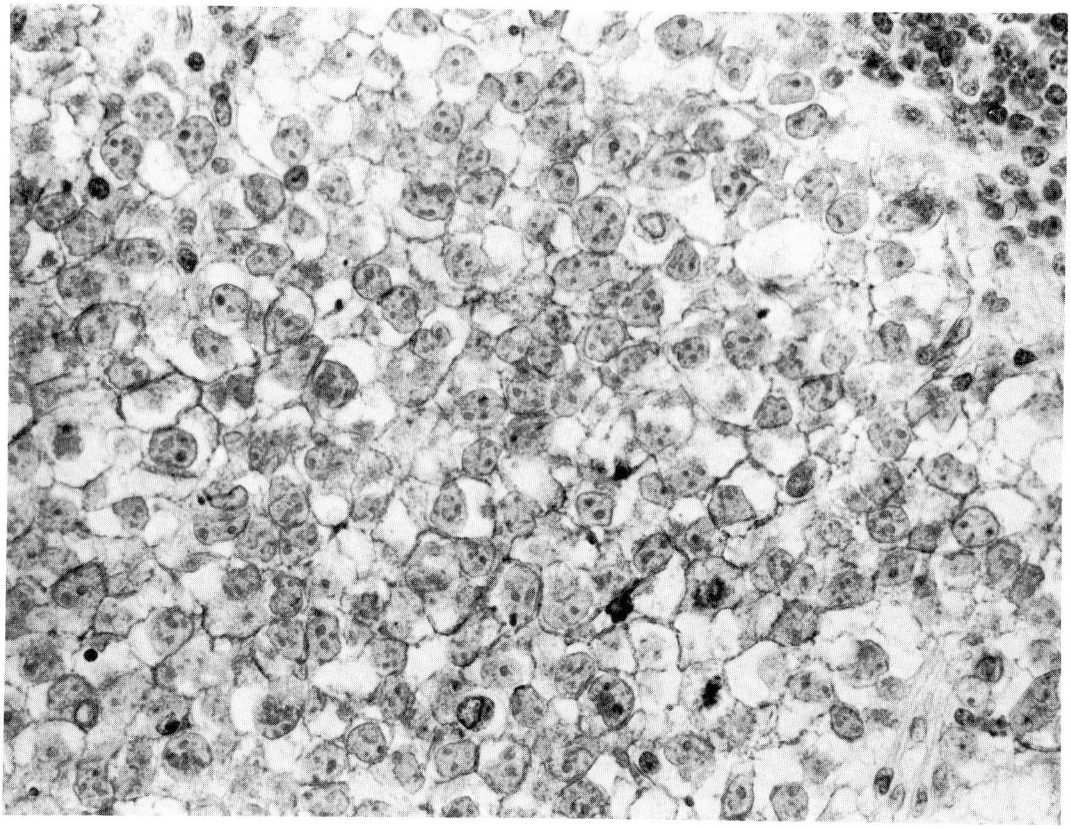

Figure 13–10. Mediastinal seminoma. Immunoreactivity for placental alkaline phosphatase is confined to the plasma membranes of the tumor cells.

lymph nodes can encroach on or appear within the thymus. Mediastinal Hodgkin's disease is commonly of the nodular sclerosing type, and the lacunar cell predominant form may simulate a thymoma or carcinoma. Recognition of the bizarre nuclear profiles may indicate the diagnosis, and marker studies will confirm it.

Lymphoblastic lymphoma can form a large mass in the upper mediastinum of children or adolescents, and it may be accompanied by leukemic manifestations. Confusion with a thymoma containing a large content of lymphocytes is possible, but convoluted nuclei are present in at least half of the cases and immunostaining or electron microscopy should provide the diagnosis.

Large cell lymphoma[1] (Fig. 13–11) may involve mediastinal lymph nodes or the thymus or quite frequently both, and, particularly in a small biopsy specimen, distinction from an epithelial thymoma or metastatic carcinoma by routine light microscopy is sometimes difficult. Surface marker studies will help, and electron microscopy should be diagnostic. Jacobson and co-workers[25] studied 30 adults with large cell lymphoma predominantly located in the mediastinum. Median age of the 20 women and 10 men was 34 years. The mass was larger than 10 cm in 65%, and its size was a significant prognostic factor. A superior vena cava syndrome and large pleural and pericardial effusions were common. Eighty percent of patients achieved complete remission, and 59% had failure-free survival at 5 years.

Histiocytosis X may involve the mediastinum and affect the thymus,[12] but it mostly occurs in young patients. Hamoudi and co-workers[21] examined the thymuses from 32 pediatric patients with histiocytosis X and found abnormalities in 27 (84%). Siegal and colleagues[67] reported four cases in patients aged from 2 months to 8 years, and in two the disease was restricted to the thymus. Plasma cell tumors rarely present in the mediastinum,[48, 53] and granulocytic sarcoma is also uncommon.[71]

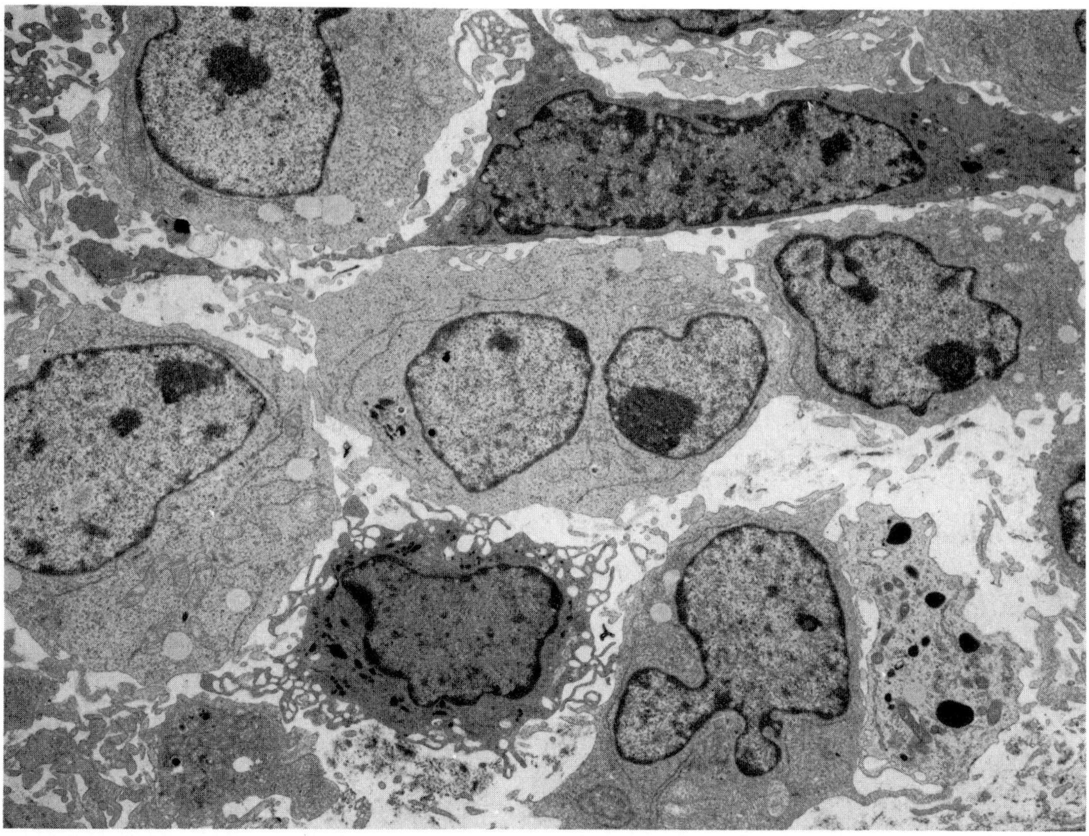

Figure 13–11. Mediastinal large cell lymphoma. Several cells with the ultrastructural features of transformed lymphocytes are present together with macrophages. (×4,500)

Immunocytochemistry

The differentiation of lymphomas from other small cell and poorly differentiated tumors involving the mediastinum can be aided by the application of immunohistochemical procedures. In addition to the antibodies to cytoskeletal proteins and other tissue and cell markers that help differentiate lymphomas from carcinomas, sarcomas, and melanomas on routinely processed specimens, a variety of antibodies that mark lymphocytes in formalin-fixed, paraffin-embedded tissues have been developed. They include various murine monoclonal antibodies (MAbs) that react broadly like leukocyte common antigen (LCA) and some that are more restricted to B or T lymphocytes.[39, 56]

LCA constitutes a group of four related glycoproteins (185, 200, 215, and 230 kd) that are present on the cell membrane of a variety of hematopoietic cells, including granulocytes, lymphocytes, macrophages/monocytes, and immature erythroid cells. Since the molecular weights of the glycoproteins that define LCA closely average 200 kd, the generic term anti-T200 is frequently used to refer to these antibodies.[56] Many MAbs to T200 that differ in their capacity to recognize lymphoid cells have recently been developed. For example, the MAbs PD7/26 and 2B11 react strongly with B cells and T cells, respectively. It has been our experience that the use of a mixture of these two antibodies can distinguish most lymphomas from other poorly differentiated neoplasms of the mediastinum. This mixture also has the advantage over other commonly used anti-T200 antibodies, such as T29/33, in that it can be used on paraffin-embedded tissues.

The diagnosis and classification of B-cell lymphomas using paraffin-embedded tissues have long been based on the demonstration of monotypic intracytoplasmic reactivity for immunoglobulin. This is relatively easy when the tumor cells secrete large amounts of immunoglobulins, but the staining is usually negative if they contain a lower content of these proteins. In addition, surface immunoglobulins, as well as a variety of other surface markers, are undetectable in paraffin-embedded tissues since they are usually inactivated during tissue processing. Recently, a variety of MAbs exhibiting varying sensitivity and specificity for B lymphocytes on paraffin-embedded tissue sections have been developed. Among them, the most widely used are L26, MB1, and LN2, which have attributes of pan-B cell antibodies.[23, 39] Staining with these antibodies is seen in both germinal center and follicular mantle zones, as well as in most B-cell lymphomas. Different MAbs that react selectively to T lymphocytes in routinely processed tissues have also been generated.[39, 68] The most widely used are UCHL1, MT1, Leu-22, and T2/48. Although the sensitivity and specificity of these antibodies vary, they can nevertheless be of diagnostic value.

Because histologic similarities exist between Hodgkin's disease and some T-cell lymphomas, certain MAbs that detect Leu-M1 antigen have been used to distinguish between these two conditions.[39, 66] It was emphasized that Reed-Sternberg cells react positively for this marker and not for LCA,[39] but the specificity of this immunostaining pattern has been questioned since Leu-M1 has been reported in certain non-Hodgkin's lymphomas, and LCA reactivity in Reed-Sternberg cells has also been observed.

Antibodies to lysozyme, α_1-antitrypsin, and α_1-antichymotrypsin have been used to identify true histiocytic neoplasms in paraffin-embedded tissues and might appear to have potential to distinguish between true histiocytic lymphoma and malignant histiocytosis. Unfortunately, lysozyme, while specific, lacks sensitivity, and α_1-antitrypsin and α_1-antichymotrypsin are highly sensitive but have limited specificity.

Histiocytosis X can be distinguished from other "histiocytic" disorders by its strong reactivity with the monoclonal antibody OKT6 in frozen sections, as well as with anti-HLA-Dr (Ia) reagents. The OKT6 reactivity has been the justification for claims that histiocytosis X is a proliferative disorder of Langerhans' cells or a close relative thereof.[8, 11] Histiocytosis X cells, like cutaneous Langerhans' cells, also react for S-100 protein in formalin-fixed, paraffin-embedded tissue specimens.[8, 50] Staining for lysozyme, α_1-antitrypsin, and α_1-antichymotrypsin is negative.[8]

REFERENCES

1. Addis BJ, Isaacson PG: Large cell lymphoma of the mediastinum: A B-cell tumor of probable thymic origin. Histopathology 10:379, 1986.
2. Adler OB, Rosenberger A, Peleg H: Fine-needle aspiration biopsy of mediastinal masses: Evaluation of 136 experiences. AJR 140:893, 1983.
3. Alguacil-Garcia A, Halliday WC: Thymic carcinoma with focal neuroblastoma differentiation. Am J Surg Pathol 11:474, 1987.
4. Bailey D, Baumal R, Law J et al: Production of a monoclonal antibody specific for seminomas and dysgerminomas. Proc Natl Acad Sci USA 83:5291, 1986.
5. Baker J, Holdaway IM, Jagusch M et al: Ectopic secretion of ACTH and met-enkephalin from a thymic carcinoid. J Endocrinol Invest 5:33, 1982.
6. Battifora H, Sheibani K, Tubbs RR et al: Antikeratin antibodies in tumor diagnosis: Distinction between seminoma and embryonal carcinoma. Cancer 54:843, 1984.
7. Battifora H, Sun TT, Bahu RM et al: The use of antikeratin antiserum as a diagnostic tool: Thymoma versus lymphoma. Hum Pathol 11:635, 1980.
8. Beckstead JH, Wood GS, Turner RR: Histiocytosis-X and Langerhans cells: Enzyme histochemical and immunologic similarities. Hum Pathol 2:11, 1984.
9. Best LA, Munichor M, Ben-Schakhar M et al: The contribution of anterior mediastinotomy in the diagnosis and evaluation of diseases of the mediastinum and lung. Ann Thorac Surg 43:78, 1987.
10. Blom P, Johannessen JV: Mediastinal mass in a young male. Ultrastruct Pathol 4:391, 1983.
11. Bos JD, Sillevis SJH, Krieg SR et al: Acute disseminated histiocytosis X: *In situ* immunophenotyping with monoclonal antibodies. J Cutan Pathol 11:59, 1984.
12. Bramwell NH, Burns BF: Histiocytosis X of the thymus in association with myasthenia gravis. Am J Clin Pathol 86:224, 1986.
13. Burns BF, McCaughey WT: Unusual thymic seminomas. Arch Pathol Lab Med 110:539, 1986.
14. Chan W, Zaatari GS, Tabei S et al: Thymoma: An immunohistochemical study. Am J Clin Pathol 82:160, 1984.
15. Clark OH: Mediastinal parathyroid tumors. Arch Surg 123:1096, 1988.
16. Davis RD Jr, Oldham HN Jr, Sabiston DC Jr et al: Primary cysts and neoplasms of the mediastinum: Recent changes in clinical presentation, methods of diagnosis, management, and results. Ann Thorac Surg 44:229, 1987.
17. Evora PR, Bongiovani HL, Sgarbieri RN et al: Nonfunctioning paraganglioma of the posterior mediastinum: Case report. Scand J Thorac Cardiovasc Surg 22:294, 1988.
18. Feigin GA, Robinson B, Marchevsky A: Mixed tumor of the mediastinum. Arch Pathol Lab Med 110:80, 1986.
19. Fukuyama M, Maeda Y, Funata N et al: Pulmonary and pleural thymoma: Diagnostic application of lymphocyte markers to the thymoma of unusual site. Am J Clin Pathol 89:617, 1988.
20. Goldstraw P: Mediastinal exploration by mediasti-

noscopy and mediastinotomy. Br J Dis Chest 82:111, 1988.
21. Hamoudi AB, Newton WA, Mancer K et al: Thymic changes in histiocytosis. Am J Clin Pathol 77:169, 1982.
22. Huntrakoon M, Lin F, Heitz PU et al: Thymic carcinoid tumor with Cushing's syndrome. Arch Pathol Lab Med 108:551, 1984.
23. Ishii Y, Takami T, Yuasa H et al: Two distinct antigen systems in human B lymphocytes: Identification of cell surface and intracellular antigen using monoclonal antibodies. Clin Exp Immunol 58:183, 1984.
24. Jacobsen GK, Jacobsen M, Clausen PP: Distribution of tumor associated antigen in the various histologic components of germ cell tumors of the testis. Am J Surg Pathol 5:257, 1981.
25. Jacobson JO, Aisenberg AC, Lamarre L et al: Mediastinal large cell lymphoma: An uncommon subset of adult lymphoma curable with combined modality therapy. Cancer 62:1893, 1988.
26. Joseph SG, Tellis CJ: Posterior mediastinal mass with intraspinous extension. Chest 93:1101, 1988.
27. Judge DM, Changaris DG, Harvey HR et al: Malignant APUDoma (carcinoid) of the anterior mediastinum: Simplified methods of demonstrating biogenic amines in endocrine neoplasms. Arch Pathol Lab Med 110:491, 1976.
28. Kajanti M: Neuroblastoma in 88 children: Clinical features, prognostic factors, results and late effects of therapy. Ann Clin Res 15(suppl 39):1, 1983.
29. Kathuria S, Jablokow BR: Primary choriocarcinoma of medinastinum with immunohistochemical study and review of the literature. J Surg Oncol 34:39, 1987.
30. Knapp RH, Hurt RD, Payne WS et al: Malignant germ cell tumors of the mediastinum. J Thorac Cardiovasc Surg 89:82, 1985.
31. Kodama T, Watanabe S, Sato Y et al: An immunohistochemical study of thymic epithelial tumors: I. Epithelial component. Am J Surg Pathol 10:26, 1986.
32. Kuzmitz R, Schernthaner G, Krisch K: Serum neuron-specific enolase: A marker for response to therapy in seminoma. Cancer 60:1017, 1987.
33. Lagrange W, Dahm HH, Karstens J et al: Melanocytic neuroendocrine carcinoma of the thymus. Cancer 59:484, 1987.
34. Landanyi M, Roy I: Mediastinal germ cell tumors and histiocytosis. Hum Pathol 19:586, 1988.
35. Lauriola L, Maggiano N, Marino M et al: Human thymoma: Immunologic characteristics of the lymphocytic component. Cancer 48:1992, 1981.
36. Lehtonen E, Lehto VP, Vartio T et al: Expression of cytokeratin polypeptides in mouse oocytes and preimplantation embryos. Dev Biol 100:158, 1983.
37. Lewis JE, Wick MR, Scheithauer BW et al: Thymoma: A clinicopathologic review. Cancer 60:2727, 1987.
38. Linder J, Olsen GA, Johnston WW: Fine-needle aspiration biopsy of the mediastinum. Am J Med 81:1005, 1986.
39. Linder J, Ye Y, Armitage JO et al: Monoclonal antibodies marking B-cell non-Hodgkin's lymphoma in paraffin-embedded tissue. Mod Pathol 1:29, 1988.
40. Luna MA, Valenzuela-Tamariz J: Germ-cell tumors of the mediastinum: Postmortem findings. Am J Clin Pathol 65:450, 1976.
41. Maggi G, Giacconi G, Donadio M et al: Thymomas: A review of 169 cases, with particular reference to results of surgical treatment. Cancer 58:765, 1986.
42. Manivel JC, Jessurun J, Wick MR et al: Placental alkaline phosphatase immunoreactivity in testicular germ cell neoplasms. Am J Surg Pathol 11:21, 1987.
43. Marchevsky AM, Dikman SH: Mediastinal carcinoid with an incomplete Sipple's syndrome. Cancer 43:2497, 1979.
44. Martini N, Golbey RB, Hajdu SI et al: Primary mediastinal germ cell tumors. Cancer 33:763, 1974.
45. Miettinen M, Virtanen I, Talerman A: Intermediate filament proteins in human testis and testicular germ-cell tumors. Am J Pathol 120:402, 1985.
46. Mokhtar N, Hsu SM, Lad RP et al: Thymoma: Lymphoid and epithelial components mirror the phenotype of normal thymus. Hum Pathol 15:378, 1984.
47. Mori K, Eguchi K, Moriyama H et al: Computed tomography of anterior mediastinal tumors: Differentiation between thymoma and germ cell tumor. Acta Radiol 28:395, 1987.
48. Muller C, Chantelot JM, Kemeny JL et al: Plasmacytoma of the mediastinum: A new case. Rev Pneumol Clin 44:39, 1988.
49. Muller-Hermelink HK, Marno M, Palestro G: Pathology of thymic epithelial tumors. Curr Top Pathol 75:207, 1986.
50. Nakajima T, Watanabe S, Sato Y et al: An immunoperoxidase study of S-100 protein distribution in normal and neoplastic tissues. Am J Surg Pathol 6:715, 1982.
51. Nemeth J, Galian A, Mikol J et al: Neuron-specific enolase and malignant lymphomas (23 cases). Virchows Arch [A] 412:89, 1987.
52. Niehans GA, Manivel JC, Copland GT et al: Immunohistochemistry of germ cell and trophoblastic neoplasms. Cancer 62:1113, 1988.
53. Niwa K, Tanaka T, Mori H et al: Extramedullary plasmacytoma of the mediastinum. Jpn J Clin Oncol 17:95, 1987.
54. Nomori H, Horinouchi H, Kaseda S et al: Evaluation of the malignant grade of thymoma by morphometric analysis. Cancer 61:982, 1988.
55. Osborne BM, Mackay B, Battifora H: Thymoma: A clinicopathologic study of 23 cases. Pathol Annu 20 (part 2):289, 1985.
56. Pinkus GS: Leukocyte common antigen. In DeLellis RA (ed): Advances in Immunohistochemistry. New York, Raven Press, 1988.
57. Premi T, Battifora H, Menderino GL et al: A monoclonal antibody against neuron-specific enolase: Immunohistochemical comparison with a polyclonal antiserum. Am J Clin Pathol 88:146, 1987.
58. Pullan PT, Clement-Jones V, Corder R et al: Ectopic production of methionine-enkephalin and beta-endorphin. Br Med J 280:758, 1980.
59. Ramaekers F, Feitz W, Moesker O et al: Antibodies to cytokeratin and vimentin in testicular tumour diagnosis. Virchows Arch [A] 408:127, 1985.
60. Rusch VW, Logothetis C, Samuels M: Endodermal

sinus tumor of the mediastinum: Report of apparent cure in two patients with extensive disease. Chest 86:745, 1984.

61. Saabye J, Elbirk A, Andersen K: Teratomas of the mediastinum. Scand J Thorac Cardiovasc Surg 21:271, 1987.
62. Sato Y, Watanabe S, Mukai K et al: An immunohistochemical study of thymic epithelial tumors: II. Lymphoid component. Am J Surg Pathol 10:862, 1986.
63. Savino W, Durand D, Dardenne M: Immunohistochemical evidence for the expression of the carcinoembryonic antigen by human thymic epithelial cells *in vitro* and in neoplastic conditions. Am J Pathol 121:418, 1985.
64. Schantz A, Sewall W, Castleman B: Mediastinal germinoma: A study of 21 cases with an excellent prognosis. Cancer 30:1189, 1972.
65. Shapiro B, Sisson J, Kalff V et al: The location of middle mediastinal pheochromocytomas. J Thorac Cardiovasc Surg 87:814, 1984.
66. Sheibani K, Battifora H, Burke JS et al: Leu-M1 antigen in human neoplasms: An immunohistochemical study of 400 cases. Am J Surg Pathol 10:227, 1986.
67. Siegal GP, Dehner LP, Rosai J: Histiocytosis X (Langerhans' cell granulomatosis) of the thymus: A clinicopathologic study of four childhood cases. Am J Surg Pathol 9:117, 1985.
68. Smith SH, Brown MH, Rowe D et al: Functional subsets of human helper-induced cells defined by new monoclonal antibody UCHL1. Immunology 58:63, 1986.
69. Snyder ME, Luck SR, Hernandez R et al: Diagnostic dilemmas of mediastinal cysts. J Pediatr Surg 20:810, 1985.
70. Talerman A, Gratama S: Primary ganglioneuroblastoma of the anterior mediastinum in a 61-year-old woman. Histopathology 7:967, 1983.
71. Toback A, Hasbrouck DJ, Blaustein J et al: Granulocytic sarcoma of the anterior mediastinum. Am J Med Sci 290:206, 1985.
72. Truong LD, Harris L, Mattioli C et al: Endodermal sinus tumor of the mediastinum: A report of seven cases and review of the literature. Cancer 58:730, 1986.
73. Waldron JA, Dohring EJ, Farber LR: Primary large cell lymphomas of the mediastinum: An analysis of 20 cases. Semin Diagn Pathol 2:281, 1985.
74. Warren JS, Yum MN: Carcinoid tumor arising in a treated primary germ cell tumor of the mediastinum. South Med J 80:259, 1987.
75. Weisbrod GL: Percutaneous fine-needle aspiration biopsy of the mediastinum. Clin Chest Med 8:27, 1987.
76. Wick MR, Carney JA, Bernatz PE et al: Primary mediastinal carcinoid tumors. Am J Surg Pathol 6:195, 1982.
77. Wick MR, Rosai J: Neuroendocrine neoplasms of the thymus. Pathol Res Pract 183:188, 1988.
78. Wick MR, Scheithauer BW: Oat cell carcinoma of the thymus. Cancer 49:1652, 1982.
79. Wick MR, Scheithauer BW: Thymic carcinoid: A histologic, immunohistochemical and ultrastructural study of 12 cases. Cancer 53:475, 1984.
80. Wick MR, Scott RE, Li CY et al: Carcinoid tumors of the thymus: A clinicopathologic report of seven cases and review of the literature. Mayo Clin Proc 55:246, 1980.
81. Wick MR, Swanson PE, Manivel JC: Placental-like alkaline phosphatase reactivity in human tumors: An immunohistochemical study of 520 cases. Hum Pathol 18:946, 1987.
82. Wirtanen GW, Stephenson JA, Wiley AL: Primary anterior mediastinal malignant teratoma: A case report with long-term survival. Cancer 63:1823, 1989.
83. Zapatero J, Baamonde C, González-Aragonesses F et al: Ectopic goiters of the mediastinum. Jpn J Surg 18:105, 1988.

Chapter

14

TECHNICAL PROCEDURES FOR LUNG TUMOR SPECIMENS

At many points in this book the importance to the pathologist and cytopathologist of material adequate in quantity and quality has been stressed. Imprecise or incorrect diagnoses, or failure to reach a diagnosis, are more often due to inadequate specimens than to their not being representative. Care in the procurement, handling, and processing of specimens yields preparations that can make the pathologist's task a great deal easier and may save the clinician and the patient considerable time and expense by avoiding the need to repeat a diagnostic procedure.

In this chapter, technical methods applicable to the various types of specimens that are obtained from patients with lung cancer are briefly reviewed, with comments on how the specimens should be submitted to the laboratory and some suggestions for processing that can improve the worth of the final product.

BRONCHOSCOPY

When a lesion is beyond the subsegmental bronchial division, brush or biopsy instruments used with the fiberoptic bronchoscope can be directed under fluoroscopic control into the abnormal area, so direct visualization of a tumor is not essential.[10, 21, 27] The advantage of the rigid bronchoscope is that it is wider and can provide a larger biopsy specimen and also better control of bleeding, but the procedure may require a general anesthetic and the rigid instrument does not penetrate as deeply in the bronchial tree.

The overall accuracy of a bronchoscopic biopsy is between 55% and 80%, but it is of course higher for central lesions and low for small peripheral lesions. In one series, 87% of tumors more than 2 cm in diameter located in the inner third of the lung were accurately diagnosed by bronchoscopy, but when the tumor was less than 2 cm in size and was in the outer third, accuracy fell to 23%.[38] Two areas that are difficult to reach with the fiberoptic bronchoscope are the superior segments of the lower lobes and the most medial portions of the apical segments of the upper lobes.

Transbronchial needle aspiration has extended the value of bronchoscopy for lesions that do not reach the lumen, and it can be used for subcarinal node involvement and for aspirating peripheral nodules under fluoroscopic control.[8, 19, 23, 39, 44, 47, 48]

Biopsy specimens obtained with the bronchoscope are small, often compressed or fragmented, and prone to drying artifact, so they should be placed in fixative as soon as possible. Generally, a single biopsy fragment cannot be subdivided and is submitted in its entirety for light microscopy. If it can be anticipated that electron microscopy will be needed as well, a second biopsy specimen should be requested.

MEDIASTINOSCOPY

Mediastinoscopy[13, 28, 54] is essentially a paratracheal exploration and is used mainly as a staging procedure, but it often provides adequate material for diagnosis. The tissue specimens are commonly submitted for intraoperative evaluation by frozen section. The diagnostic yield is high if there is radiologic evidence of mediastinal involvement and correspondingly low when the radiograph of the mediastinum appears normal.

LUNG RESECTION SPECIMENS

Segmental and Wedge Resection

Since bronchopulmonary segments are distinct anatomic units, it is possible to perform segmental resections on many smaller lesions that are confined to these anatomic units.[40] A segmental or wedge resection allows the optimum preservation of healthy lung parenchyma. It may be used for a small primary cancer or for multiple peripheral metastatic foci.

The following points should be kept in mind when processing a segmental or wedge resection.

1. Indicate from which lobe the wedge or segment was removed.
2. Orient the specimen with relation to the hilum and pleura and inspect and palpate the margin of resection.
3. Record the distance of the lesion from the pleura and from the margins of resection, and note the appearance of the overlying pleura.
4. Measure the tumor in millimeters, preferably in three dimensions.
5. Take specimens as required for frozen section, permanent sections, and electron microscopy. Frozen section evaluation will include determining whether the resection margin is free of tumor.
6. If the tumor is believed to be metastatic and the primary site is not known, cut additional slides from the frozen section block for immunohistochemistry.

Lobectomy

The resected lobe should be identified, measured, and weighed and the pleural surface examined for exudate, hemorrhage, adhesions, puckering, scarring, and lymphatic involvement. The lobe is palpated gently to determine the location of the tumor (*i.e.*, central, mid lung, or peripheral). Major segmental bronchi are opened, their mucosa is examined, and the relation of the tumor to any involved bronchus is recorded. The distance of the tumor from the bronchial margin of resection and from the pleura should be documented. Major blood vessels are opened to look for vascular invasion, thrombi, or emboli. All hilar, bronchopulmonary, and segmental lymph nodes should be identified and their precise location recorded to facilitate accurate surgical staging. Areas of the lobe that show pathologic changes such as infarction, emphysema, pneumonia, or granuloma should be identified. The dimensions of the tumor in millimeters and the gross appearance of the cut surface should be recorded, and the presence and extent of cavitation, hemorrhagic areas, and necrosis should be noted.

Some or all of the following tissue sections may be submitted from a lobectomy specimen:

1. The bronchial margin of resection
2. Normal peripheral lung including pleura
3. Tumor tissue for frozen section
4. Tumor for light microscopy
5. Sections representing pathologic processes other than tumor, such as pneumonia, granuloma, emphysema, and infarction
6. All lymph nodes for complete surgical staging
7. For immunocytochemistry, additional unstained slides prepared from frozen section blocks (ten slides), and a small piece of tumor placed in 95% ethanol, methacarn, or Carnoy's solution
8. Representative tissues for biochemical analysis, flow cytometry, and genetic and research studies
9. A thin slice in 2% glutaraldehyde for electron microscopy if the need is anticipated.

Pneumonectomy

Pneumonectomy, often referred to as total pneumonectomy, is the surgical excision of an entire lung. In the early 1930s, pneumonectomy was considered proper treatment for carcinoma of the lung. In the decade from 1930 to 1940, 75% of lung cancer patients were treated by total pneumonectomy, but with improvements in surgical techniques over the past 30 years, lobectomy and lesser resections are now preferred.[59]

Radical pneumonectomy, which requires more extensive dissection of mediastinal and hilar lymph nodes, offers no special advantage over simple pneumonectomy and increases both morbidity and mortality without an accompanying increase in survival.[59] When possible, the entire lung and lymph nodes are removed *en bloc* to prevent spillage of cancer cells into the chest.[57] Total pneumonectomy and radical pneumonectomy are performed sparingly, the main reason being the presence of a metastasis or a second primary lesion in another lobe on the ipsilateral side.

When a pneumonectomy specimen is received in the laboratory, it should be weighed and measured and the pleural surface on each lobe and in the interlobar fissures examined for pathologic changes. The lobes are palpated for tumor, and all lymph nodes in the hilar, bronchopulmonary, lobar, segmental, and subsegmental areas are recorded and submitted for paraffin embedding. The tumor should be sampled for light microscopy at intervals of 1 cm or less. The bronchial resection margin and a portion of the tumor will often be evaluated by frozen section, but this should be performed with as little disturbance of the architecture of the specimen as possible. In an academic institution, there are frequently requests for tissue for research purposes, and some may even be required sterile; it can be difficult to honor these requests without mutilating the specimen, and care must be exercised to retain sufficient viable tumor for the pathologic studies.

Extrapleural pneumonectomy has been used to totally eradicate extensive unilateral infectious disease, predominantly tuberculous empyema with or without bronchopleural fistula. It has also been used in the treatment of main bronchial stump fistulas, for bronchogenic carcinoma with localized malignant pleural effusion, and for the treatment of diffuse malignant mesothelioma. It is an attempt to remove by *en bloc* dissection a whole lung with its investing envelope, in order to prevent and control the spread of the infectious process. The extrapleural plane is entered beneath the periosteum of the resected rib, and by blunt dissection the parietal pleura is removed from the chest wall, diaphragm, pericardium, and hilar area. The pleural contents ideally can be removed without contamination of the chest cavity. Since malignant mesothelioma is currently incurable by all forms of therapy, extrapleural pneumonectomy for mesothelioma is only palliative, but it extends the lives of some patients.[18]

The specimen received in the laboratory is an entire lung completely surrounded by both visceral and parietal pleura. It is weighed, measured, and palpated to detect any fluid that may be present in an area where the pleural space is not obliterated. If fluid is present, it is aspirated and processed as an effusion. The tumor can then be exposed, and the specimen can be dissected and the lymph nodes recovered.

CYTOLOGY

The clinical information accompanying a cytology specimen is often meager. It would appear that many clinicians regard a cytology specimen as being in the same category as a blood specimen sent to the laboratory for mechanical analysis.

In Sweden, air-dried smears stained with the May-Grunwald-Giemsa stain are currently in vogue. In the United States, rapid smearing and quick fixing in 95% ethanol or with spray fixatives is common, and the ethanol fixation is the procedure we follow. It eliminates air-drying artifact (cell enlargement, cytoplasmic swelling, and nuclear smudginess), and the preparations compare favorably with the appearance of the same lesion in the subsequently resected lung. For lymphomas and leukemias, Diff-Quik or similar Romanovsky preparations are added.

An accurate interpretation of the specimen requires not only a properly processed specimen but also explicit clinical information. The cytologist must have a brief history with information on the precise location of the lesion and whatever therapy the patient has already received. Short cuts in processing and inadequate information can lead to faulty interpretation and meaningless reports.

The Papanicolaou staining technique is used for cytologic smears of all nonlymphoma cases. In order to give the results in a few minutes, a modified quick-staining technique is used in our superficial aspiration clinic. Since most of the aspiration specimens are usually bloody, the slides are fixed in Carnoy's solution for 3 to 5 minutes prior to staining. Details of the staining procedure are given in the Appendix.

The Diff-Quik stain is a rapid-staining method used (in conjunction with the modified Papanicolaou stain) in the initial evaluation of material taken during fine-needle aspiration biopsies. The staining procedure yields results similar to the staining pattern obtained with the Wright or Wright-Giemsa stains. This three-step staining procedure, detailed in the Appendix, produces stained slides in less than 30 seconds.

We have found that Liu's stain is excellent and more quickly performed than Wright's stain, and in our laboratory Liu's stain is performed on all specimens from patients with a history of lymphoma, leukemia, histiocytosis, or myeloma. Specimens to be stained with Liu's stain should be processed on frosted tip slides and allowed to air dry. The staining technique is given in the Appendix.

Sputum

The initial diagnosis of lung carcinoma is frequently made from cytologic evaluation of sputum preparations,[6, 36] but the preparatory techniques are of considerable importance. The specimen submitted to the cytopathologist is always physically altered. Secretions continue while the patient is sleeping, and sputum samples collected in the morning have frequently been lying in the patient's bronchial tree throughout much of the night. When such a specimen is compared with a specimen obtained by bronchial washing, the degenerative changes can be obvious. Sputa should therefore be submitted in a fixative solution in order to retard degeneration.

Sputum from a hospital patient can be expectorated directly into a Petri dish and "hand-picked," but this practice has its drawbacks because clumping of the cells and the presence of blood, mucus, or inflammatory cells may interfere with the staining procedure and will occasionally disguise tumor cells and prevent their detection.

Most cytopathology laboratories require that sputum specimens be submitted in a fixative so that processing by homogenization may be performed. Either the Waring blender or the Biosonic IV, an ultrasound instrument, may be used for this purpose. Boluses of mucus are dispersed, and the smears prepared from the homogenate show a uniform distribution of cells and stain evenly. This type of processing also has some disadvantages. It alters the architectural pattern of small tissue fragments, and when the cells are fragile, as in small cell carcinomas, processing by the blender may totally denude the nucleus of cytoplasm. For details of the procedures, see the Appendix.

Sputum Processing by "Pick and Smear" Method

Deep cough specimens contain cells from the lower respiratory tract. If there is a cell-shedding tumor in this area, it is possible to detect it cytologically by careful selection of material, preparation of thin smears, adequate fixation, good staining techniques, and careful screening by cytotechnologists.

This technique is used for specimens obtained from patients with a history of undifferentiated small cell carcinoma. These specimens are not sonified since it is desirable to retain the characteristic cohesive clusters of tumor cells.

Bronchial Washings and Brushings

The quality of the cytologic preparations obtainable from washing and brushing specimens is clearly superior to that of typical sputum smears, and identification and subclassification of a primary lung tumor is often possible with representative material.[7, 30, 33, 42] The instrumentation usually dislodges clusters of cells and may cause brisk bleeding. It is distinctly more difficult to perform immunocytochemical or even routine histochemical stains on smears that contain excessive blood and are air dried. This type of background reduces the sensitivity of the staining procedures and may render the preparations technically unsatisfactory.

Bronchial washing specimens are brought to the cytology laboratory unfixed and are processed immediately, following the procedure detailed in the Appendix.

Processing Alveolar Lavage Specimens for *Pneumocystis carinii*

The policy for handling contaminated specimens should be strictly followed when processing specimens from patients suspected of having *Pneumocystis carinii* infection. The usual specimen is alveolar lavage fluid. More detail on the procedure is given in the Appendix.

Fine-Needle Aspiration Biopsies

Two different slide procedures are used for examining aspiration biopsy specimens. Direct smears of the aspirate are prepared on totally frosted slides for staining by the quick Papanicolaou technique, and in addition a Diff-Quik stain is performed on frosted-tip slides on which the sediment is air dried. The Diff-Quik–stained smears enable the cytopathologist to quickly assess the adequacy of the aspirate and to determine whether additional lung punctures will be required for the preparation of smears for immunocytochemical studies.

As a further step, the syringe is rinsed in a conical tube containing 15 ml of a 1:1 mixture of Ringer's solution and 50% ethanol. The rinse is centrifuged for 10 minutes at 1800 rpm (600 *g*) and two cytospin preparations are made from the sediment and fixed in modified Carnoy's solution. These fixed smears are stained with the standard Papanicolaou stain. If sufficient material is available, a cell block may be prepared from which paraffin sections can subsequently be cut for histologic study. Many immunostaining procedures can be effectively performed on these sections.

Effusions

When a pleural fluid aspiration is contemplated, heparin (Liquaemin 1:10,000) should be added to the container in which the fluid is to be collected. The amount of heparin adequate to prevent clotting is 1 ml/330 ml of fluid. If processing is delayed overnight or longer, the container should be refrigerated until it can be processed. In the processing laboratory the container is agitated to resuspend the cells, or if sedimentation has occurred, the supernatant may be decanted and saved until specimen processing is completed and reported. Usually the cells are resuspended and aliquots of fluid are poured into 50-ml centrifuge tubes and centrifuged. It may be necessary to combine the sediment from two or more tubes to obtain an adequate specimen. A drop of the sediment is removed by pipette, placed immediately on completely frosted slides, and smeared evenly. The smears are then immersed in Carnoy's solution for 15 to 30 minutes. Carnoy's solution lyses red blood cells, penetrates both cytoplasm and nucleus, and preserves cell detail with minimum distortion. Maximum cell preservation coupled with optimal staining results in preparations of superior quality and aids in greater diagnostic accuracy. Conversely, poor technique often results in failure to classify neoplastic cells and may actually prevent their detection. If after concentration the sediment is found to be scanty, the sediment from all centrifuge tubes may be combined, placed on filter paper, and inserted into a cassette, which is submitted to the histology laboratory in 10% buffered neutral formalin for processing as a cell block.

IMMUNOCYTOCHEMISTRY

Immunofluorescence is the earliest method developed for immunocytochemical study. Frozen sections are cut in a cryostat and stained by the direct method of immunofluorescence, which is simpler and satisfactory for routine purposes, or by the indirect method when extra sensitivity is needed. In the direct method, a fluorochrome (fluorescein or rhodamine) conjugated to a primary antibody is applied directly to the tissue or cytology specimen. The indirect method is a two-step staining procedure: first, a primary unconjugated antibody is applied, then a secondary fluorochrome-labeled antibody derived from a second species is directed against the globulin fraction of the first antibody. The site of the antigen–antibody reaction is visualized under ultraviolet light using a darkfield microscope. Because of the high contrast characteristic of the immunofluorescent reaction, we found this method to be particularly useful in the cellular localization of small amounts of antigen, such as those present in cell junctions (*i.e.*, desmoplakins). In addition, it is a simple method that can be used for "double labeling" through the simultaneous use of different fluorochrome labels to identify different antigens in the same preparation.

Immunoenzymatic Techniques

Because these techniques do not require a special fluorescent microscope and have the advantage of localizing antigens in relation to preserved tissue section morphology, immunoenzymatic methods have largely supplanted immunofluorescent techniques in diagnostic pathology. They also are applied on routinely processed, paraffin-embedded tissues; in addition, the immunohistochemical preparation can be stored indefinitely without significant fading, depending on the choice of enzyme and substrate used.

The immunoenzyme methods that are more commonly used are the unconjugated immunoenzyme techniques, particularly the peroxidase–antiperoxidase (PAP),[50] and the avidin–biotin–immunoperoxidase complex (ABC)[24, 25] methods, which not only have proved to be more sensitive than the immunofluorescence technique but also have circumvented some of the disadvantages inherent in conjugation procedures, such as denaturation of the antibody, inactivation of the enzyme, and residual free antibody. Free antibody, or antibody conjugated to inactivated enzyme, binds competitively with active conjugated antibody, reducing the sensitivity of the reaction, while the denaturated antibody and free enzyme increase nonspecific staining.

The PAP and the ABC immunoperoxidase methods are illustrated in Figures 14–1 and 14–2, respectively. The PAP method is a sequential application of a primary antibody, an antibody (bridge) with specificity directed toward the globulin fraction of the primary antibody, and a soluble peroxidase–antiperoxidase complex generated in the same species as that of the primary antibody. The

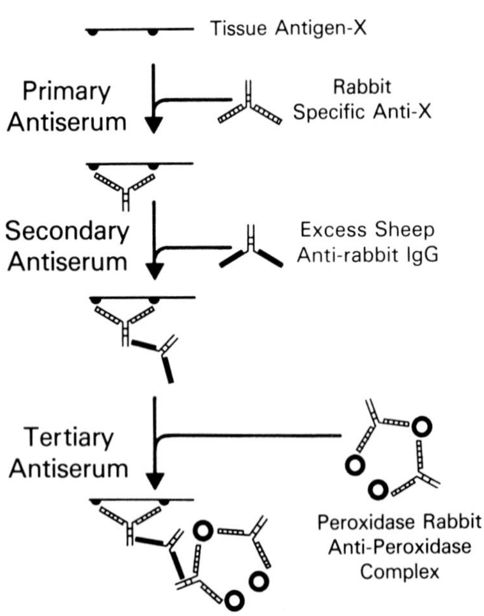

Figure 14–1. Diagrammatic representation of the peroxidase–antiperoxidase (PAP) method.

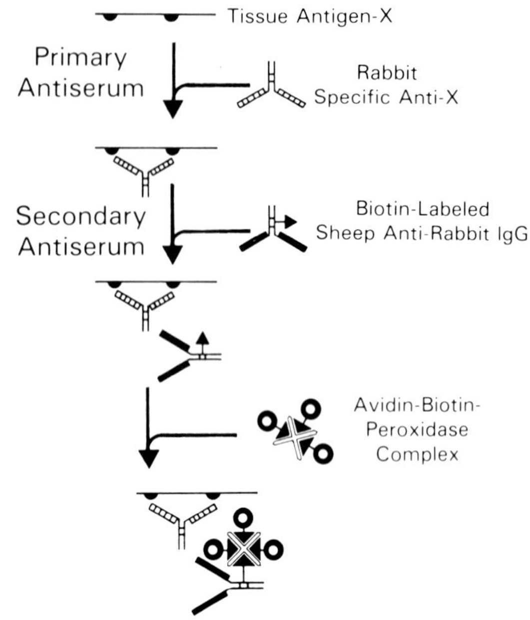

Figure 14–2. Diagrammatic representation of the avidin–biotin–peroxidase complex (ABC) method.

ABC method is the immunocytochemical method most commonly used in most diagnostic immunocytochemistry laboratories. Reagents are relatively inexpensive and readily available as complete "kits," including primary antibodies and buffers. The principle of this method is the stoichiometric affinity of avidin to bind four molecules of biotin. In the first step, the primary antibody reacts with the specimen. This is followed by a biotin-labeled secondary antibody capable of binding to the primary antibody. The third step involves the use of a complex of peroxidase-conjugated biotin and avidin: the free sites on the avidin molecule allow binding of the biotin to the secondary antibody. Then the peroxidase (and consequently the original antigen) is visualized with the use of the appropriate chromogen (3,3′-diaminobenzidine, 3-amino-9-ethylcarbazole, or tetramethyl benzidine).[17, 32]

Specimen Procurement

The success of the immunostaining greatly depends on the adequacy of the specimen on which the procedure is performed. Insufficient attention to the handling of the specimen not only may result in complete failure of the immunostaining but also may cause a misinterpretation of the results and a misdiagnosis of the pathologic condition. Before

Appendix: Techniques and Procedures

PAPANICOLAOU QUICK-STAINING TECHNIQUE

SOLUTION	TIME
1. Water	10 dips
2. Harris hematoxylin	3 to 5 seconds
3. Water	10 dips
4. 95% ethanol	10 dips
5. OG-6	1 minute
6. 95% ethanol	10 dips
7. EA—modified	2 minutes
8. 95% ethanol	10 dips
9. 100% ethanol	10 dips
10. Xylene	10 dips or until cleared

The slides are then covered with coverslips and are ready to be examined. The regressive method Papanicolaou staining procedure is used for cytologic smears of all nongynecologic specimens. (For instructions on how to prepare Harris hematoxylin, OG-6, and EA—modified, refer to Keebler C, Reagan JW: A Manual of Cytotechnology, 6th edition, Am Soc Pathol Press, Chicago, 1983.)

Destaining and Restaining Slides with the Papanicolaou Technique

Occasionally, as a result of improper timing or faulty solutions, it is necessary to destain and restain slides. This is accomplished by the following steps:

1. The slide is placed in xylene until the coverslip is removed. (Time is variable in this step and may take as long as several hours or overnight.)
2. The rack is carried in reverse order through the solutions except in the staining solutions.
3. When the hydrochloric acid is reached, the rack is left in a dish containing 70% ethanol with 1% HCl until all visible color is removed. (This may require minutes to an hour.)
4. The hematoxylin is skipped, and the rack is placed in the water preceding the stain.
5. Restaining is begun at this point. Proceed with the usual staining technique starting with the hematoxylin, adjusting the time accordingly.

Lysing Red Blood Cells and Restaining Previously Stained Cytologic Smears

Occasionally, as a result of poor processing technique, including failure to lyse red blood cells, it becomes necessary to decolorize and restain previously stained slides. The steps below should be followed.

SOLUTION	TIMING	PURPOSE
1. Xylene	Variable (approx. 1 day)	Remove coverslip and permount
2. 100% ethyl alcohol	20 dips	Remove xylene
3. 100% ethyl alcohol stain (OG and EA)	30 minutes	Remove color
4. 95% alcohol	30 minutes	
5. Modified Carnoy's solution	15 minutes	Remove blood
6. Equal parts Carnoy's solution and glacial acetic acid	30 minutes	Remove excess blood
7. Glacial acetic acid	30 minutes	Remove blood

At this point the slides should be free of blood. If they are still bloody, leave slides longer in acetic acid.

SOLUTION	TIMING	PURPOSE
8. Modified Carnoy's solution	20 dips	Rinse off acid
9. 95% ethyl alcohol	10 minutes	Rinse off acid
10. 1% HCl in 70% alcohol	Variable	Destain the nucleus 6 hours or overnight, until all color is removed
11. 95% ethyl alcohol	20 dips	
12. Running water	1 hour	
13. Hematoxylin	1 minute	Stain the nucleus
14. 1% HCl in distilled water	1 slow dip	Remove excess hematoxylin
15. Running water	10 minutes	Rinse off HCl

Check the stain at this point. Check for nucleus stain.

SOLUTION	TIMING	PURPOSE
16. 95% ethyl alcohol	10 dips	Dehydrate the cells
17. OG-6	1 slow dip	Stain keratin
18. 95% ethyl alcohol	10 dips	
19. 95% ethyl alcohol	10 dips	
20. EA—modified	5 minutes (variable)	Counterstain for cytoplasm
21. 95% alcohol		Rinse and dehydrate
22. 95% alcohol		Rinse and dehydrate
23. 100% alcohol	20 dips	Dehydrate

If the slides look grossly red at this point, follow steps 24 through 28; otherwise, proceed to step 29.

SOLUTION	TIMING	PURPOSE
24. Equal parts of solution and acetic acid	10 dips	
25. Glacial acetic acid	5–10 minutes until the slide turns green	Remove excess red coloring
26. Equal parts of solution and acetic acid	10 dips	
27. 95% alcohol	5 minutes	Remove acid
28. 100% alcohol	5 minutes	Dehydrate and clear
29. 100% alcohol	5 minutes	Dehydrate and clear
30. Xylene	20 dips	Clearing
31. Xylene	20 dips	Clearing

Modified Carnoy's Solution

FIXATIVE FOR BLOODY FLUIDS

1200 ml 70% ethanol
200 ml Glacial acetic acid

FORMALIN 10% SOLUTION
(used for cell blocks)

1000 ml	2000 ml
100 ml formaldehyde	200 ml formaldehyde
900 ml water	1800 ml water

1% HCl SOLUTION IN 70% ALCOHOL
(used for destaining slides)

1980 ml of 70% alcohol
20 ml concentrated HCl

1% HCl SOLUTION IN WATER
(used for removing excess hematoxylin)

1980 ml of water
20 ml of concentrated HCl

SOLUTION	TIMING	PURPOSE
1. 95% alcohol	5 minutes	Remove acid
2. 100% alcohol	5 minutes	Dehydrate and clear
3. 100% alcohol	5 minutes	Dehydrate and clear
4. Xylene	20 dips	Clearing
5. Xylene	20 dips	Clearing

DIFF-QUIK STAINING PROCEDURE

The Diff-Quik stain set* is composed of three different solutions:

*Available from Harleco, Division of American Hospital Supply Corporation, 480 Democrat Road, Gibbstown, NJ 09027.

Also available as Hemacolor Stain Set from American Scientific Products, Cat. #65044/93.

STAINING	TIME
Fixative solution I	5 seconds (1 dip per second)
Solution II	5 seconds (1 dip per second)
Solution III	5 seconds (1 dip per second)

1. Rinse slide with distilled or deionized water.
2. Allow to dry.
3. Coverslip.

LIU'S STAINING PROCEDURE

1. Cover the slides with solution A and allow to stand for 15 to 30 seconds.
2. Add solution B† drop by drop to solution A on the slide and mix by blowing slowly. Allow to stand for 1½ to 2 minutes (greenish metallic layer should be seen during this time).
3. Rinse with water.
4. Air dry and coverslip.

Liu's Stain

SOLUTION A

Eosin Y	0.17–0.18 g
Methylene blue	0.05 g
Methanol (absolute)	100 ml

Dissolve eosin Y in methanol. Add methylene blue to the solution and shake solution well. Allow the solution to stand for 24 hours. Filter and store in brown bottle. *Always filter before use.*

SOLUTION B

Methylene blue	0.7 g
Azure A	0.6–0.7 g
Na_2HPO_2	12.6 g
KH_2PO_4 Monobasic	6.25 g
Distilled water	500 ml

Dissolve Na_2HPO_4 and KH_2PO_4 in distilled water. Put azure A in beaker or flask and add the solution (Na_2HPO_4 + KH_2PO_4) gradually. Add methylene blue to the solution. Shake solution vigorously. Filter after 24 hours in brown bottle. *Always filter before use.* It can be preserved for a long time. The effect increases by aging.

SPUTUM PROCESSING BY SONIFICATION

The sonification of sputa is accomplished through the use of a 2% Carbowax/50% ethanol solution and the Biosonic IV ultrasound unit to produce a homogeneous sputum specimen devoid of mucus. Sputum is collected in the 2% Carbowax/50% ethanol solution.

Equipment needed:

- Biosonic IV ultrasound unit
- Cold drink cup for rinsing off probe
- Medi-wipes
- Extra Carbowax solution for increasing volume
- Conical centrifuge tubes (50 ml)
- Tube rack
- Wash bottle containing 95% ethanol
- Wax glassware marker for identifying centrifuge tubes
- Completely frosted slides (2–4)
- Castell pen or lead pencil for identifying slides
- Disposable Pasteur pipets
- Rubber bulbs
- Paper towels

Procedure Using Biosonic IV Ultrasound Unit

1. Add Carbowax solution to sputum container to reach a volume of 40 ml.
2. Rinse Biosonic probe with 95% ethanol and wipe dry with a tissue.
3. Place the sputum container below the probe of the Biosonic.
4. Raise the container until the probe is into the specimen about 1/16 an inch below the level of the specimen. Do not allow the probe to touch the sides or bottom of the specimen container.
5. Turn on power control to 400 W.
6. Set timer and homogenizer for 3 to 8 seconds (variable).
7. Shut off time control knob.
8. Rinse probe with 95% ethanol and wipe clean with medi-wipes (facial tissue).
9. Pour specimen into conical tubes and centrifuge for 10 minutes.
10. Pour off supernatant and pipette sediment onto four frosted slides. Distribute specimen thinly and evenly.
11. Allow to air dry completely.
12. Occasionally the centrifugate may appear to be sparse and watery. These specimens may be processed using the Shandon Cytospin.
13. Rack slides and place in a dish of 95% ethanol for at least 5 minutes prior to staining.
14. If smear appears grossly to be bloody, place it into a Coplin jar of modified Carnoy's solution for 15 minutes prior to staining.

Sonification Chart

GROSS APPEARANCE OF SPUTA	APPROXIMATE TIME	INTENSITY
Slightly mucoid	3–4 seconds	400 watts
Mucoid with fragments	4–5 seconds	400 watts
Thick and viscous	5–8 seconds	400 watts

SPUTUM PROCESSING BY PICK AND SMEAR METHOD

1. A paper towel is placed on the counter for each specimen. On this towel place the specimen, four frosted slides, two wooden sticks, and a bottle of 95% ethanol.
2. Transfer the accession number on the container to the slides.
3. If the specimen is mucoid, add 3 or 4 ml of 95% ethanol and allow the material to harden for about 15 minutes. With the wooden sticks, carefully select a small amount of material, picking out any gray particles or discolored areas. *Note:* Yellow areas will generally contain pus; hemorrhagic areas contain red blood cells in excessive quantities. Place the selected material on slide A (first slide).
4. Grasp the number end of slide A between fingers of the left hand with the frosted side upward. With the right hand, grasp the numbered end of slide B with the frosted side downward. Press and rotate the material until a fine monolayer of cells is evenly distributed on the slides (see note).
5. If flecks of tissue are not visually evident, add a small amount of 95% ethanol to the specimen container and agitate. Smear any material that precipitates.
6. Prepared slides are spray-fixed and stained using Papanicolaou stain.

Note: If the material selected is hard, fragile, or difficult to process, the addition of a few drops of water will help dissolve the specimen and make it easier to smear.

Instruments:
Shandon Cytospin II (Shandon Inc.,
171 Industry Drive,
Pittsburgh, PA 15275)
Biosonic IV (Braun Sonik 2000,
Curtin-Matheson Scientific, Inc.,
9999 Veterans Memorial Drive,
Houston, TX 77038)

PROCESSING BRONCHIAL WASHINGS AND BRUSHINGS

1. The specimen is centrifuged for 10 minutes at 1800 rpm.
2. The supernatant is decanted, and the sediment is placed on four prenumbered frosted slides.
3. The slides are gently rotated together, spreading the specimen evenly over each slide.
4. The slides are immersed in a Coplin jar containing modified Carnoy's solution.
5. If the centrifugate appears to be watery and of scanty volume, Cytospin preparations may be prepared and placed into a Coplin jar of modified Carnoy's solution for 10 to 15 minutes prior to staining.
6. Slides are stained by a modified Papanicolaou technique.

Bronchial brushing specimens are submitted in either of two separate methods: If smears are to be made at the time of bronchoscopy, the brushed material is quickly placed on frosted slides and immediately immersed in a container of 95% ethanol. Otherwise the brushing specimen may be collected in 1:1 solution of 50% ethyl alcohol and Ringer's solution and sent to the laboratory for processing as follows:

1. The solution containing the brush is placed in a 50-ml conical tube and vortexed for 20 to 30 seconds to allow cells to dislodge from the brush.
2. The vortexed solution is centrifuged for 10 minutes at 1800 rpm.
3. The centrifuge is discarded, and the sediment is pipetted onto two to four totally frosted slides and smears prepared.
4. The slides are placed in a Coplin jar of modified Carnoy's solution and allowed to fix for 10 to 15 minutes.
5. Slides are stained by the modified Papanicolaou technique.

PROCESSING ALVEOLAR LAVAGE SPECIMENS FOR *PNEUMOCYSTIS CARINII*

1. The specimen is centrifuged at 1800 rpm for 10 minutes.
2. If the centrifugate is mucoid and sufficient material is available, four direct smears are made using fully frosted slides. Two smears are alcohol-fixed and stained with Papanicolaou stain; the other two are submitted to the histology section for staining with Gomori's methenamine silver.
3. If the centrifugate is sparse (thin/watery), four Cytospin preparations are made. The smears are fixed in Carnoy's solution apportioned in the same manner as explained in step 2 of this procedure.

With specimens obtained from patients with known or suspected hematologic disorders, air-dried smears are prepared using frosted tip slides and stained with Wright's, Wright-Giemsa, or Liu's stain.

PREPARATION OF ELECTRON MICROSCOPY FIXATIVE

1. Prepare buffer and fixative solution under fume hood.
   a. 0.2M cacodylate buffer (sodium dimethylarsinic acid): dissolve 42.8 g sodium cacodylate trihydrate of 32.0 g anhydrous sodium cacodylate in sufficient distilled water to make 1000 ml.

b. 2% glutaraldehyde in cacodylate buffer: 50% glutaraldehyde can be purchased in 5- or 10-ml vials.

2. Add 40 ml of 50% glutaraldehyde to 960 ml 0.2M sodium cacodylate buffer.

Preparation of Fine-Needle Aspirate for Electron Microscopy

1. The aspirate is promptly expressed into a vial containing 10 ml of 2% buffered glutaraldehyde, and the container is gently agitated to prevent clotting and maintain dispersion of the cells. After 1 hour, any floating material is withdrawn using a plastic Pasteur pipette and is transferred to buffer and processed as specimen A.
2. The remainder of the specimen is filtered through a 20-μm woven filter screen.[29]
3. Semi-thin sections of the embedded filtrate are examined by light microscopy to select suitable areas for ultrastructural study.

Preparation of Effusion Fluid for Electron Microscopy

An effusion that is not frankly bloody can be centrifuged to provide a pellet that is then fixed in 2% buffered glutaraldehyde. If the effusion contains many red blood cells, they can be removed by brief lysis, filtration, or Ficoll-gradient separation.

Index

Note: Page numbers in *italics* refer to illustrations; page numbers followed by (t) refer to tables.